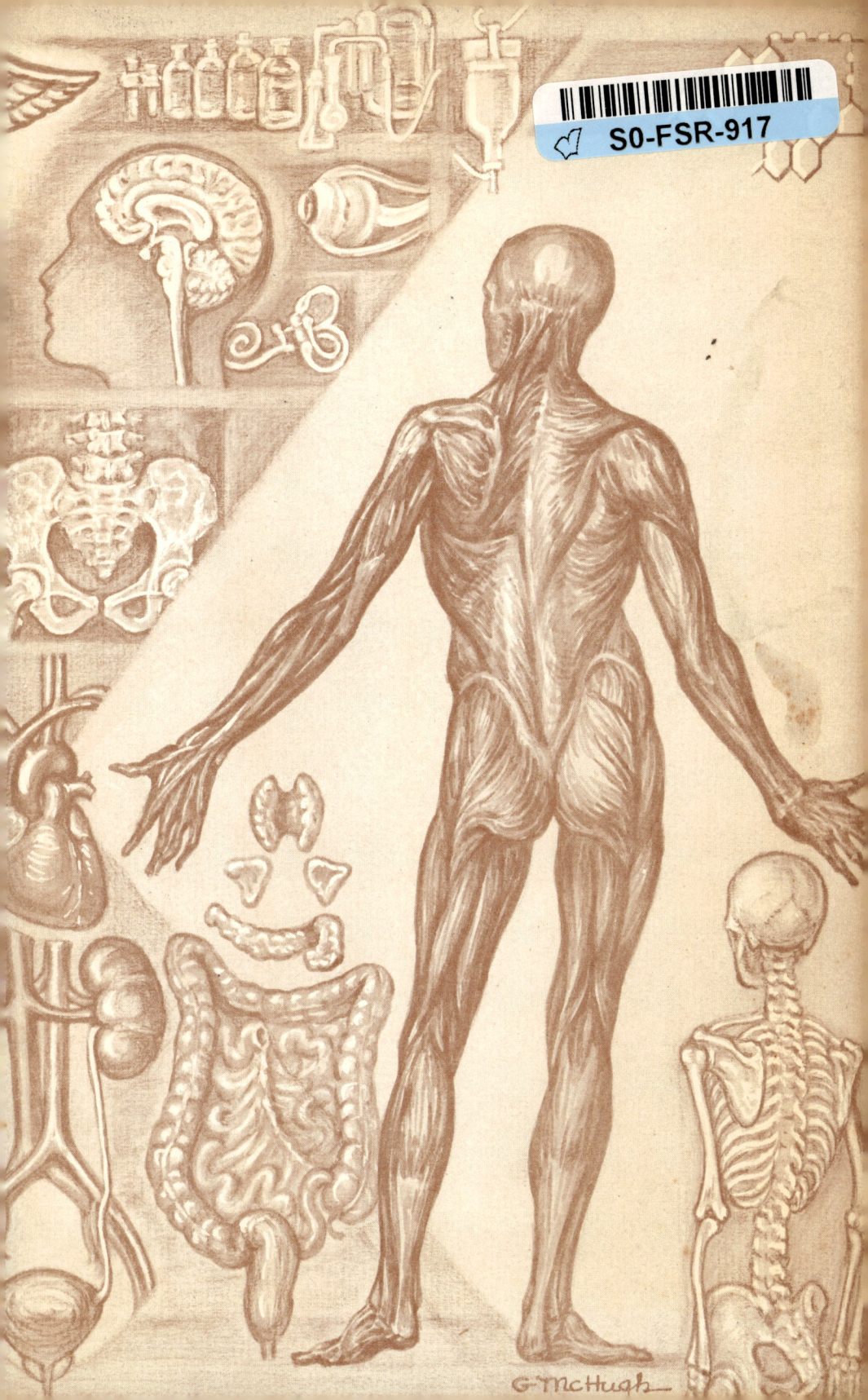

ILLUSTRATED

MEDICAL
AND
HEALTH
ENCYCLOPEDIA

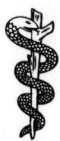

VOLUME 7
PREGNANCY (continued) — SKIN

A Modern Medical and Health Library for the Family
. . . Includes all the Articles From "THE MODERN
HOME MEDICAL ADVISOR" and "THE POPULAR
MEDICAL ENCYCLOPEDIA" Plus Additional
Articles, Photographs and Charts.

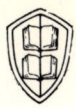

ILLUSTRATED
MEDICAL
AND
HEALTH
ENCYCLOPEDIA

EDITED BY

MORRIS FISHBEIN, M.D.

EDITOR, MEDICAL PROGRESS; EDITOR, MODERN HOME MEDICAL
ADVISER; MEDICAL EDITOR, BRITANNICA BOOK OF THE YEAR;
CONTRIBUTING-EDITOR, POST GRADUATE MEDICINE; AND
FOR 25 YEARS EDITOR OF THE JOURNAL OF
THE AMERICAN MEDICAL ASSOCIATION

WITH THE COLLABORATION OF LEADING
SPECIALISTS IN MEDICINE AND SURGERY

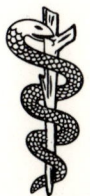

H. S. STUTTMAN CO., *Publishers*
NEW YORK, N. Y.

Copyright © 1957, 1959, 1963, 1966 by Doubleday & Company, Inc.
All Rights Reserved

ILLUSTRATED MEDICAL AND HEALTH ENCYCLOPEDIA contains new entries and illustrations plus material from THE MODERN HOME MEDICAL ADVISOR. (Copyright © 1935, 1939, 1940, 1941, 1942, 1948, 1951, 1953, 1956, by Doubleday and Company, Inc.) and THE POPULAR MEDICAL ENCYCLOPEDIA, revised and enlarged edition, (Copyright © 1946, 1950, 1953, 1956) by Doubleday and Company, Inc.

PRINTED IN THE UNITED STATES OF AMERICA
BY ROTARY GRAPHIC PRESS INC., NEW YORK 16, N. Y.
33P—11-67—15R

Some people think that the sex of the baby is indicated by the shape of the mother. There is no basis for this belief. Some people think that a baby will always be lucky or will have second sight if he is born with a caul or a veil. That is just a condition of birth and has not the slightest significance. Anybody who believes in second sight will believe anything.

Not long ago a man listed the superstitions in Adams County, Illinois, relative to pregnancy. Here are some samples:

1. A woman who lays her coat and hat on a strange baby's bed will get a baby.
2. If outgrown baby clothes are given away, the mother will soon need them again.
3. If a couple get married and go to a picture show within the first three days, they will have twins.
4. A poor man is certain to have many children.
5. When a boy is born, it means that the husband has more strength than his wife.
6. Boys are born more frequently to youthful than to elderly parents.
7. A baby born on a stormy night will be cross and nervous.
8. A child born at four o'clock in the afternoon will be moderately rich.
9. A baby born with an open hand will be openhanded and of a generous disposition.
10. There are still people in Adams

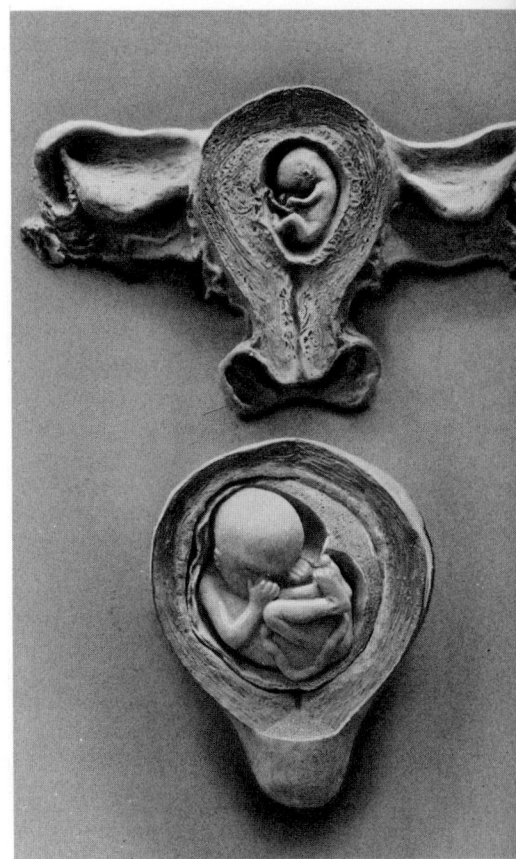

Uterus open with 2½- and 3½-month-old embryo. The placenta and cord are visible.
Cleveland Health Museum

County who think that the stork brings babies, that the doctor brings the children in his satchel, and there are some who say that babies are found in hollow tree stumps. This is not peculiar to Adams County. There are still people all over the world who do not know even a fraction of the simplest facts about life and living.

DIET OF THE PROSPECTIVE MOTHER —A woman who is going to have a child must remember that her food supplies the child with the essential materials for his growth. The food supply of the child comes to the baby through the blood vessels which connect him to the mother. If the food of the mother lacks these necessary substances, they are likely to be extracted from her tissues and organs for the growth of the child.

There used to be an idea that a mother had to lose a tooth for every baby. Now we know that proper attention to the teeth of the mother and to her diet makes unnecessary any loss of teeth during pregnancy. This does not mean that the prospective mother ought to overeat. Overeating will throw an excess burden on her digestive organs and make her carry around extra weight, which will mean increased fatigue and disability. A slight increase of weight in the prospective mother is normal. Any abnormal increase in weight will have a bad effect.

The prospective mother should not think that she can keep down the weight of the baby by starving herself. The baby's weight is not dependent entirely on the amount of food that his mother eats. A good general rule for the prospective mother is to eat the foods that she usually eats but to make certain that she gets plenty of milk and more fresh fruits and vegetables than she would take ordinarily. She should watch particularly her supply of vitamins and such mineral salts as calcium, phosphorus, iron, and iodine. She ought to have eight to ten glasses of water each day unless her doctor tells her that she should restrict her fluid for some reason. The necessary proteins are supplied by meat, eggs, milk, and such vegetables as peas and beans. Fats are important—particularly butter, cream, and cheese because they provide vitamin A. The sugars and starches, including bread, potatoes, and cereals, are needed to provide the materials for energy.

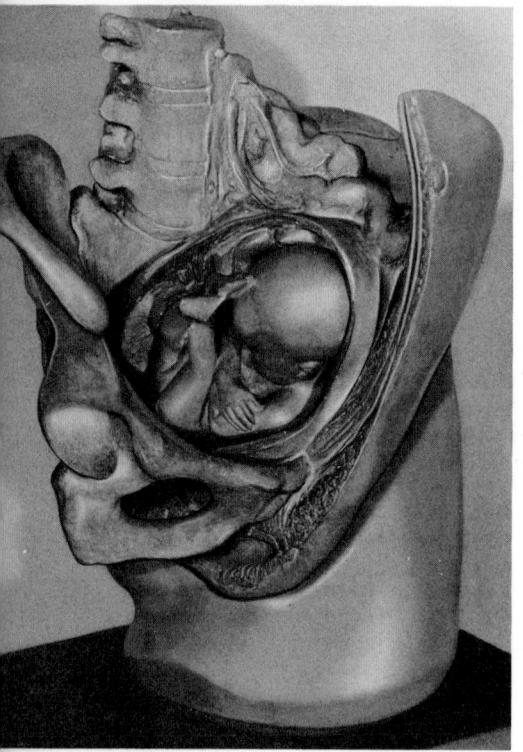

Uterus with fetus at 4½ months. The pelvic organs and skeletal structure in standing posture are shown.
Cleveland Health Museum

PREGNANCY

Besides getting a rich supply of vitamins A, B, and C from fresh fruits and vegetables, particularly citrus fruits and tomatoes, the prospective mother may require extra cod-liver oil or halibut-liver oil, as prescribed by her doctor, so that she will get adequate amounts of vitamins A and D.

Alcohol should be avoided altogether, and cigarettes should be smoked in moderation. Moderation means around five or six cigarettes daily as a maximum for the prospective mother.

The nausea and vomiting that occur during the early months of pregnancy are sometimes helped by replacing the regular three meals daily with small amounts of food taken every two and one half hours.

HYGIENE—The amount and kind of exercise that the expectant mother takes depends largely on her previous habits. She should never exercise to the point of fatigue but should stop as soon as she begins to feel tired.

Walking is the best exercise. It may be taken outdoors except during extremely bad weather. When walking, the pregnant woman should wear shoes with low heels and wide toes because high-heeled shoes may cause her to slip more easily, with the possibility of accident.

Women who are accustomed to strenuous sports, such as tennis, can stand more exercise than those who have usually led an indoor life.

In summer the expectant mother should be cautious about walking in the hot sun. She should walk slowly and avoid crowds. Two miles daily is an average distance.

Among the strenuous sports particularly to be avoided are running, tennis, swimming, skating, and horseback riding. A little dancing may be enjoyed in the early months. The prospective mother should never dance in a crowd where she is likely to be bumped or pushed about.

If the woman is used to driving her own car, she may continue to do so during the early months but should certainly give up driving later. Rough roads and bouncing should always be avoided.

The prospective mother must remember to rest frequently. If she has not been taking a nap in the afternoon, she should develop the habit and lie down for half an hour daily if circumstances permit. If she is not able to sleep, the reclining position will rest the heart and relax the body generally.

A pernicious notion is the belief that bathing during pregnancy is harmful. Cleanliness at all times is necessary for the health of the human body. There are many kinds of baths, including shower, sponge, or tub. Hot baths cause fatigue

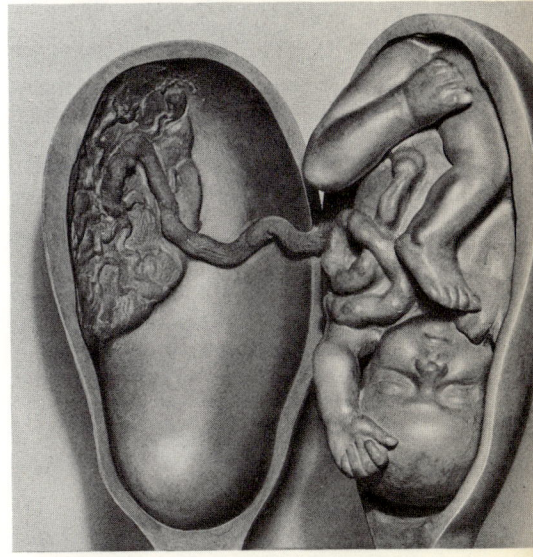

Opened uterus with 7-month fetus. Babies born at this time are likely to survive.
Cleveland Health Museum

but produce some relaxation. The best temperature of water for ordinary baths is between 85 and 90 degrees Fahrenheit. Even those who are accustomed to cold baths in the morning will find it best to increase the temperature of the bath while carrying a prospective child. Extraordinary kinds of baths like cold showers, ocean baths, Turkish and Russian sweat baths should never be taken during pregnancy except with the advice of the doctor.

BIRTH OF THE BABY—Before the baby comes, the mother should assemble the materials that will be required at childbirth. If she is going to a hospital, and the vast majority of women now have their babies in the hospital, she will need at least two nightgowns, a bathrobe, two pairs of stockings, a pair of slippers, a few handkerchiefs, a toothbrush, some toothpaste or tooth powder, and a comb and brush.

In most hospitals the baby's clothes are provided until the baby is ready to leave. The day before the mother expects to leave the hospital with the baby she should be provided with a shirt, a band, a petticoat, a pair of stockings, some safety pins, a few diapers, a sweater, a cap, and two blankets, all of which may be necessary for the baby en route to his home. The more experienced mother will have available a good many other clothes for the baby because babies grow fast and need many changes before they become one year old.

In most cases the time required for childbirth for a first baby will be between sixteen and eighteen hours and for later babies between eight and ten hours. There is no reason to be panicky when the first symptoms appear. A wise mother will have consulted her physician about having a baby even before pregnancy begins and will be in touch with her doctor throughout the pregnancy and after the baby is born.

There is a common belief that more babies are born at night than in the daytime. Actual investigations show, however, that births vary little from hour to hour in the course of a day. A slightly larger number occur between three and four o'clock in the morning than between nine and ten o'clock at night, but the number from hour to hour varies little indeed.

The body of the woman returns in most instances to normal six to eight weeks after childbirth. During this period rest and quiet are important. About the fourth day after childbirth the mother may begin light exercise, sitting up in bed and increasing her activity. The

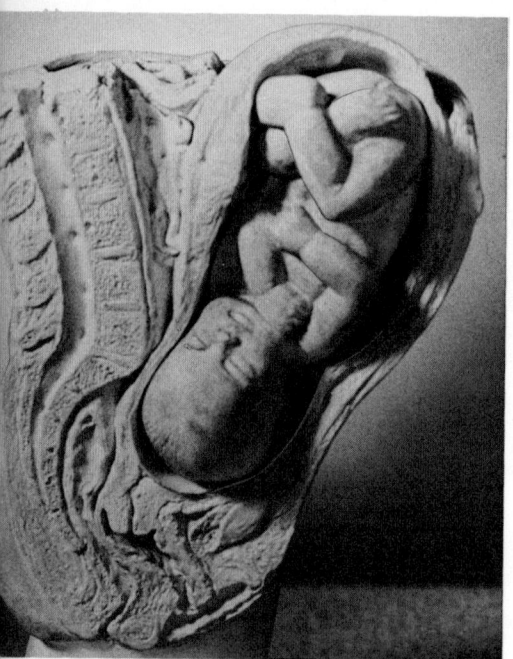

Model of abdomen of standing woman with full-term pregnancy.
Cleveland Health Museum

PREGNANCY

tendency nowadays is to get the mother up much earlier than used to be the case. Nevertheless, it is still not advisable for the mother who leaves the hospital on the tenth or twelfth day following childbirth to go up three flights of steps to an apartment, if she lives in an apartment building. If possible, someone should carry her. If she must walk, she should walk slowly and rest frequently. It is usually best for the mother to leave the hospital in the afternoon so that she can go home and get right to bed.

Women of different races and different spheres of life have different habits in regard to how much they undertake after childbirth. Many women incline to overdo the social side of pregnancy. Too many visits and visits that last too long cannot do any good. Long telephone calls are frequently more boring and weakening than actual conversation with visitors. People with colds or infections should never visit a woman who has just had a baby and certainly should be kept out of any contact with the baby or baby's room.

CHILDBIRTH—care of mother before and after: See BIRTH, article CARE OF MOTHERS BEFORE AND AFTER CHILDBIRTH.

CHILDBIRTH—fever: See HEART, article DISEASES OF THE HEART AND CIRCULATION.

CHILDBIRTH—misconceptions: See BIRTH, article CARE OF MOTHERS BEFORE AND AFTER CHILDBIRTH.

CHILDBIRTH—pituitary extract to cause contraction: See article ENDOCRINOLOGY.

CHILDBIRTH—reason for difficulty: See article SEX HYGIENE.

CHILDBIRTH—superstitions: See BIRTH, article CARE OF MOTHERS BEFORE AND AFTER CHILDBIRTH.

PREGNANCY—abortion during early months: See BIRTH, article CARE OF MOTHERS BEFORE AND AFTER CHILDBIRTH.

PREGNANCY—afterpains: See BIRTH, article CARE OF MOTHERS BEFORE AND AFTER CHILDBIRTH.

PREGNANCY—antepartum care, importance of: See BIRTH, article CARE OF MOTHERS BEFORE AND AFTER CHILDBIRTH.

PREGNANCY—appetite, perversion of: See BIRTH, article CARE OF MOTHERS BEFORE AND AFTER CHILDBIRTH.

PREGNANCY—asthma: See article ALLEGRY.

PREGNANCY—bathing: See BIRTH, article CARE OF MOTHERS BEFORE AND AFTER CHILDBIRTH.

PREGNANCY—belching: See BIRTH, article CARE OF MOTHERS BEFORE AND AFTER CHILDBIRTH.

PREGNANCY—beriberi: See article DEFICIENCY DISEASES.

PREGNANCY—bowels, care of: See BIRTH, article CARE OF MOTHERS BEFORE AND AFTER CHILDBIRTH.

PREGNANCY—breasts, care of: See BIRTH, article CARE OF MOTHERS BEFORE AND AFTER CHILDBIRTH.

PREGNANCY—cathartics: See BIRTH, article CARE OF MOTHERS BEFORE AND AFTER CHILDBIRTH.

PREGNANCY—clothing: See BIRTH, article CARE OF MOTHERS BEFORE AND AFTER CHILDBIRTH.

PREGNANCY—constipation: See BIRTH, article CARE OF MOTHERS BEFORE AND AFTER CHILDBIRTH.

PREGNANCY—corsets: See BIRTH, article CARE OF MOTHERS BEFORE AND AFTER CHILDBIRTH.

PREGNANCY—cramps, leg: See BIRTH, article CARE OF MOTHERS BEFORE AND AFTER CHILDBIRTH.

PREGNANCY—delivery at home: See BIRTH, article CARE OF MOTHERS BEFORE AND AFTER CHILDBIRTH.

PREGNANCY—dental care: See TEETH, article THE CARE OF THE TEETH.

PREGNANCY—diabetes: See BIRTH, article CARE OF MOTHERS BEFORE AND AFTER CHILDBIRTH; article DIABETES.

PREGNANCY—diet: See BIRTH, article CARE OF MOTHERS BEFORE AND AFTER CHILDBIRTH.
PREGNANCY—disappearance of menstruation: See WOMEN, article HYGIENE OF WOMEN.
PREGNANCY—dizziness: See BIRTH, article CARE OF MOTHERS BEFORE AND AFTER CHILDBIRTH.
PREGNANCY—douches: See BIRTH, article CARE OF MOTHERS BEFORE AND AFTER CHILDBIRTH.
PREGNANCY—estimating date of birth: See BIRTH, article CARE OF MOTHERS BEFORE AND AFTER CHILDBIRTH.
PREGNANCY—exercise: See BIRTH, article CARE OF MOTHERS BEFORE AND AFTER CHILDBIRTH.
PREGNANCY—fainting: See BIRTH, article CARE OF MOTHERS BEFORE AND AFTER CHILDBIRTH.
PREGNANCY—fruits: See BIRTH, article CARE OF MOTHERS BEFORE AND AFTER CHILDBIRTH.
PREGNANCY—gall-bladder disease: See article DIGESTION AND DIGESTIVE DISEASES.
PREGNANCY—gastroposis: See article DIGESTION AND DIGESTIVE DISEASES.
PREGNANCY—genitals, care of: See BIRTH, article CARE OF MOTHERS BEFORE AND AFTER CHILDBIRTH.
PREGNANCY—German measles serious: See CHILDHOOD DISEASES, article INFECTIOUS DISEASES OF CHILDHOOD.
PREGNANCY—goiter, prevention of: See BIRTH, article CARE OF MOTHERS BEFORE AND AFTER CHILDBIRTH.
PREGNANCY—hair, care of: See BIRTH, article CARE OF MOTHERS BEFORE AND AFTER CHILDBIRTH.
PREGNANCY—hair affected by: See SKIN, article THE SKIN.
PREGNANCY—hair lost: See HAIR, article THE HAIR.
PREGNANCY—heartburn: See BIRTH, article CARE OF MOTHERS BEFORE AND AFTER CHILDBIRTH.
PREGNANCY—hemorrhoids: See BIRTH, article CARE OF MOTHERS BEFORE AND AFTER CHILDBIRTH.
PREGNANCY—housework: See BIRTH, article CARE OF MOTHERS BEFORE AND AFTER CHILDBIRTH.
PREGNANCY—hypertension: See article BLOOD PRESSURE.
PREGNANCY—indicated by temperature record: See WOMEN, article HYGIENE OF WOMEN.
PREGNANCY—iodine requirement increased: See article ENDOCRINOLOGY.
PREGNANCY—iron deficiency anemia: See BLOOD, article THE BLOOD AND ITS DISEASES.
PREGNANCY—kidney disease: See KIDNEY, article THE KIDNEY: ITS DISEASES AND DISTURBANCES.
PREGNANCY—kidney disturbances: See KIDNEY, article THE KIDNEY: ITS DISEASES AND DISTURBANCES.
PREGNANCY—kidney poisoning: See KIDNEY, article THE KIDNEY: ITS DISEASES AND DISTURBANCES.
PREGNANCY—kidneys, care of: See BIRTH, article CARE OF MOTHERS BEFORE AND AFTER CHILDBIRTH.
PREGNANCY—labor, signs of beginning: See BIRTH, article CARE OF MOTHERS BEFORE AND AFTER CHILDBIRTH.
PREGNANCY—laxatives: See BIRTH, article CARE OF MOTHERS BEFORE AND AFTER CHILDBIRTH.
PREGNANCY—massage: See BIRTH, article CARE OF MOTHERS BEFORE AND AFTER CHILDBIRTH.
PREGNANCY—miscarriage during early months: See BIRTH, article CARE OF MOTHERS BEFORE AND AFTER CHILDBIRTH.
PREGNANCY—modesty: See BIRTH, article CARE OF MOTHERS BEFORE AND AFTER CHILDBIRTH.
PREGNANCY—nephritis: See BIRTH, article CARE OF MOTHERS BEFORE AND AFTER CHILDBIRTH.
PREGNANCY—neuritis: See BIRTH, article CARE OF MOTHERS BEFORE AND AFTER CHILDBIRTH.

PREGNANCY—physician to be consulted: See article SEX HYGIENE.

PREGNANCY—piles: See BIRTH, article CARE OF MOTHERS BEFORE AND AFTER CHILDBIRTH.

PREGNANCY—possible even in absence of menstruation: See BIRTH, article CARE OF MOTHERS BEFORE AND AFTER CHILDBIRTH.

PREGNANCY—prenatal care, importance of: See BIRTH, article CARE OF MOTHERS BEFORE AND AFTER CHILDBIRTH.

PREGNANCY—prepared for by progesterone: See article ENDOCRINOLOGY.

PREGNANCY—puerperium: See BIRTH, article CARE OF MOTHERS BEFORE AND AFTER CHILDBIRTH.

PREGNANCY—pyelitis: See BIRTH, article CARE OF MOTHERS BEFORE AND AFTER CHILDBIRTH; KIDNEY, article THE KIDNEY: ITS DISEASES AND DISTURBANCES.

PREGNANCY—recreation: See BIRTH, article CARE OF MOTHERS BEFORE AND AFTER CHILDBIRTH.

PREGNANCY—rest: See BIRTH, article CARE OF MOTHERS BEFORE AND AFTER CHILDBIRTH.

PREGNANCY—serious symptoms: See BIRTH, article CARE OF MOTHERS BEFORE AND AFTER CHILDBIRTH.

PREGNANCY—sexual intercourse: See article SEX HYGIENE; BIRTH, article CARE OF MOTHERS BEFORE AND AFTER CHILDBIRTH.

PREGNANCY—signs: See BIRTH, article CARE OF MOTHERS BEFORE AND AFTER CHILDBIRTH.

PREGNANCY—skin stretched: See SKIN, article THE SKIN.

PREGNANCY—teeth, care of: See BIRTH, article CARE OF MOTHERS BEFORE AND AFTER CHILDBIRTH.

PREGNANCY—travel: See BIRTH, article CARE OF MOTHERS BEFORE AND AFTER CHILDBIRTH.

PREGNANCY—trouble, sign of: See BIRTH, article CARE OF MOTHERS BEFORE AND AFTER CHILDBIRTH.

PREGNANCY—urine tests: See BIRTH, article CARE OF MOTHERS BEFORE AND AFTER CHILDBIRTH.

PREGNANCY—varicose veins: See BIRTH, article CARE OF MOTHERS BEFORE AND AFTER CHILDBIRTH.

PREGNANCY—vegetables: See BIRTH, article CARE OF MOTHERS BEFORE AND AFTER CHILDBIRTH.

PREGNANCY—visits to physician: See BIRTH, article CARE OF MOTHERS BEFORE AND AFTER CHILDBIRTH.

PREGNANCY—vitamin K to prevent hemorrhages: See article DEFICIENCY DISEASES.

PREMATURE BABIES The chances for survival of babies born prematurely depend somewhat on the weight of the babies at birth. Babies who weigh five pounds or over have a 93 per cent chance of living; those who weigh four pounds have a 70 per cent chance; and those who weigh just over two and a half pounds have a 50 per cent chance. In France a survey made to determine the subsequent survival of prematurely born babies showed that the outlook for survival is favorable provided there have been no serious complications at the time of birth and provided the baby has a good home. Premature birth is not in itself a cause of either physical or mental retardation. Among the famous people who were born prematurely are Newton, Darwin, Voltaire, Renoir, Victor Hugo, and Churchill.

PRENATAL CARE In accordance with the dictates of modern medical science, a woman should consult her physician even before she becomes a prospective mother. He is able from a study of the heredity of the husband and wife, from a study of the incidence of disease in the family, and from an examination of the physical condition of the woman, to give advice as to whether or not it is desirable for the parents concerned to have a child.

Certainly just as soon as a woman believes she is to become a mother she should consult her physician. He will then make the necessary scientific examinations to determine with certainty that she is in the expectant state. These examinations include laboratory studies which are now well-nigh positive as to whether the answer is yes or no. They include also physical examinations, tests of the excretions of the body, and a record of symptoms.

Then the physician makes a complete physical examination, which includes a study of the blood, the blood pressure, and the kidneys, to determine the presence or absence of inflammations and of diabetes. He makes accurate measurements of the organs concerned in childbirth and thus is able to anticipate any difficulties which are likely to arise.

Examinations continue at first at intervals of one month, unless extraordinary symptoms arise, later at more frequent intervals of perhaps two weeks, or indeed every week if that seems necessary. On each occasion the doctor will question the prospective mother carefully as to fatigue, vision, and the presence of any unusual swellings or headaches. Should the answers be suggestive, he will then make the necessary examinations to determine the exact significance of any such symptoms. By those examinations he is able again to anticipate difficulties and in most instances to prevent serious complications.

Diet—A prospective mother usually gains about 14 per cent in weight during the nine months previous to the birth of the child. Most experts are convinced that a gain of anything more than twenty pounds is far too much.

The authorities are agreed, however, that the prospective mother requires in addition to her normal well-balanced diet, more protein, calcium, phosphorus, iron, and the established vitamins. We know that some proteins have higher biologic values—that is, more value for the building and conserving of human tissues—than others. The proteins especially important are the so-called animal proteins, including milk and meat. The proteins of cereals and vegetables and fruits are less important.

The prospective mother must have enough vitamins A and D, calcium, and phosphorus, to provide for the calcium needs of her baby and also those of the growing baby. Milk and milk products provide most of the necessary calcium, but the doctor may choose to recommend additional calcium in the diet if he thinks it necessary.

Our diets are ordinarily low in iron, and iron is absolutely necessary for the building of red blood cells. Obviously the prospective mother needs extra iron. The fact that many a baby is born slightly anemic is now demonstrated by careful scientific studies. Therefore the mother should be sure to eat plenty of the iron-containing foods and, if necessary, should have extra iron prescribed by the physician.

Finally, among the mineral salts iodine is of great importance. Much of our modern salt is enriched by the addition of extra iodine or indeed by the restoration of iodine that has been removed in the refining process. We know that a lack of sufficient iodine in the

---

To insure the well-being of the developing infant, the mother's diet should be well-balanced. For some pregnant patients the curtailment of certain foods may be necessary. The advice of the physician should be strictly followed.

Relation Of Pregnant Mother's Diet To Infant's Health At Birth
(ACCORDING TO A HARVARD–BOSTON LYING-IN HOSPITAL STUDY)

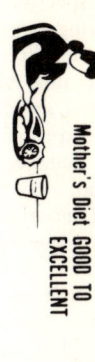

Mother's Diet GOOD TO EXCELLENT

← INFANT'S CONDITION ←

42% 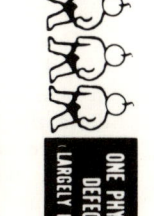 SUPERIOR 2.5%

45% 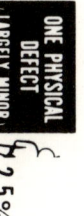 ONE PHYSICAL DEFECT (LARGELY MINOR) 2.5%

10% 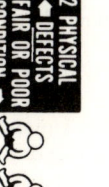 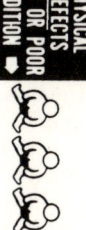 2 PHYSICAL DEFECTS ← FAIR OR POOR CONDITION ↓ 28%

3% 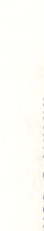 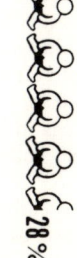 CONGENITAL DEFECTS, STILLBORN, ETC.

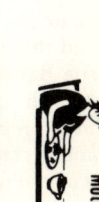

Mother's Diet POOR TO VERY POOR

← INFANT'S CONDITION ←

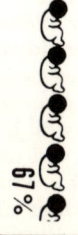 67%

Charts by Graphics Institute, N.Y.C.

diet of the mother may influence not only her own thyroid gland but that of the prospective child.

HEALTH OF THE PROSPECTIVE MOTHER—When a prospective mother finds that her wedding ring is getting too tight or that her shoes feel too tight or that her vision is becoming blurred, she must realize that these are danger signals. She should never disregard persistent vomiting, bleeding, nausea, or any difficulty with her vision.

During the months before the child is born the prospective mother should wear comfortable clothing. She should avoid any constrictions around the waist. She should be careful about wearing elastic garters that constrict the blood vessels because this helps to cause varicose veins.

The prospective mother should try to be contented and avoid undue emotional reactions or excitement. She need not fear that her mental condition will affect the physical body of the prospective child. However, nervous irritation, undue fatigue, or exhaustion associated with excess emotional reactions may harm both her and the developing child.

EQUIPMENT FOR BABY—After the end of the third month the prospective mother can begin to prepare for the baby by providing some necessary equipment. This includes as a minimum the following:

Three abdominal bands, about 6 inches by 20 inches, torn from fine, firm flannel and not hemmed. A half yard of 22-inch flannel may have the selvage torn off, then may be torn in three equal strips. Bands are not necessary after the navel heals, unless the physician particularly orders them.

Three shirts, size 2, silk and wool, or cotton and wool mixed, for the winter baby; cotton for the summer baby. These shirts should be large enough to slip on easily and not be outgrown too rapidly. Those that open down the front and are tied in place are most convenient.

Three dozen or more diapers, size 20 by 40 inches, preferably of bird's-eye or good quality outing flannel; the new gauze type is quite popular with some mothers. A more expensive type is the paper or cotton-filled diaper that may be used once and destroyed. These are especially nice for traveling or for people who can afford such luxuries. Knitted soakers are also used and are preferred to rubber diapers or pants, but neither is advisable for constant wear because they cause irritation of the skin.

Three nightgowns, made of soft outing flannel, 27 inches long, with drawstring in hem and wrists. These should open down the back.

Three or four kimonos of medium weight, flannelette, with little or no trimming, opening down the back and fastening with ties. Simple dresses with "gertrudes" are preferred by some mothers but kimonos are more practical.

Sleeping bag or baby bunting, a sleeveless square slip with hood attached, with zipper or tie front, will be useful for out of doors for a cold-weather baby.

Three pairs of soft stockings, socks, or booties. For small infants many prefer to wrap feet and legs in extra diaper.

Blankets, three cotton and two wool, 1 yard square.

Two flannel or cashmere sacks or crocheted jackets are useful.

Two quilted pads for lap protectors or square of rubber sheeting.

It is also desirable to have suitable preparation in the home, including a bed or a bassinette. A new clothes-basket will make an ideal bed for the first six months. If the husband can do a little plain carpentering, he can make a platform with legs which will hold the basket securely and which will raise it above the floor level. In this basket is put a plain mattress which is also made of quilting or padding material. A rubber sheet is placed over the mattress.

The mother will need a tub in which to bathe the baby and a tray to hold sterile water, a jar of sterile cotton, nipples and bottle caps, nursing bottles for holding water and artificial feedings if they are to be used.

CAESAREAN SECTION—See entry CAESAREAN OPERATION.

CHILDBIRTH—care of mother before and after: See BIRTH, article CARE OF MOTHERS BEFORE AND AFTER CHILDBIRTH.

CHILDBIRTH—delivery at home: See BIRTH, article CARE OF MOTHERS BEFORE AND AFTER CHILDBIRTH.

CHILDBIRTH—estimating date: See BIRTH, article CARE OF MOTHERS BEFORE AND AFTER CHILDBIRTH.

CHILDBIRTH—fever: See HEART, article DISEASES OF THE HEART AND CIRCULATION.

CHILDBIRTH—misconceptions: See BIRTH, article CARE OF MOTHERS BEFORE AND AFTER CHILDBIRTH.

CHILDBIRTH—out of wedlock: See article SEX HYGIENE.

CHILDBIRTH—pituitary extract to cause contraction: See article ENDOCRINOLOGY.

CHILDBIRTH—reason for difficulty: See article SEX HYGIENE.

CHILDBIRTH—superstitions: See BIRTH, article CARE OF MOTHERS BEFORE AND AFTER CHILDBIRTH.

CONFINEMENT—See BIRTH, article CARE OF MOTHERS BEFORE AND AFTER CHILDBIRTH.

PREGNANCY—See entry PREGNANCY.

PRESBYOPIA When people get old, their eyes change. The word "presbyopia" merely means "sight of an old man." The ability to see normally slightly changes after the age of forty, increasingly toward the age of 70. There is a gradual decline of the power of the eye to accommodate due to a loss of elasticity of the lens of the eye, which becomes more rigid and flatter. As a result the near point of distinct vision moves and reading becomes increasingly difficult at the usual distance. At this time it is difficult for anyone who has the condition to read fine print or to do any kind of near work without the aid of convex glasses.

This change in the eye is not a disease but a natural change which occurs in the human being with age. The lens of the eye in youth is an elastic tissue. By action of one of the muscles of the eye the elastic capsule of the lens becomes relaxed, which allows it to become more globular. However, as age goes on, the lens becomes hardened and cannot easily become more globular.

People with presbyópia see well at a distance. This is likely to give them a great deal of encouragement, particularly on a golf course when they can see the flight of a golf ball for hundreds of yards. When, however, they try to read the telephone book, they find that that is an entirely different matter. As the condition becomes worse, the person with farsightedness pushes the book away and holds the head back. However, even with this help it is still difficult to see the book well. Reading at night becomes especially troublesome because the pupil of the eye dilates, owing to poor illumination.

One of the chief symptoms of presbyopia is a feeling of tiredness on reading, culminating in many people with headaches toward the end of the day. Women find it especially difficult to thread needles or to work on fine patterns because the patterns fade away and become almost obliterated and the eyes become tired if they persist in the work.

There is just one thing for a person with such a change in the eyes to do and that is to consult a specialist in conditions affecting the eyes, who will measure the amount of change that has taken place and will prescribe suitable convex lenses to meet the situation. The specialist in conditions affecting the eye is likely to take into account the occupation of the person concerned because the distance at which the work is usually done is important. In reading, writing, and sewing, 13 inches is usually a comfortable working distance but a piano player may require 20 to 25 inches, so that the glasses that he will need would be weaker than those required by a printer. Some people require two sets of glasses, one for reading and the other for their work.

Every few years it is desirable to consult a specialist again because the eyes continue to change up to a certain point.

PRESCRIPTIONS Many a patient has puzzled inordinately over the prescription handed to him by the doctor. Once prescriptions were written almost altogether in Latin. This was not done to mystify the patient. Latin was the classical language used by all learned men in the Middle Ages; at that time medicine was studied in Latin. True, there is some advantage in having the confidence of the patient in the prescription. He is more likely to respect a long technical term that he does not understand. However, modern times tend to remove the mystery and secrecy from science. People are being educated in medical matters. Furthermore, the writing of prescriptions in English tends to oppose charlatanism and quackery.

The official books used by doctors and druggists as guides to the drugs that are prescribed by the doctor and put into prescriptions in the drugstore will, during the coming years, use the English titles as the main titles, with the Latin supplementary.

Many people wonder why there is an R with a cross on the top of the doctor's prescription. Some have suggested that this sign represents an invocation to Jupiter and that it is a carry-over from the days when people believed in mythical gods and goddesses. More recent studies indicate that the cross at the end of the R is not a symbol but a substitute for a period to indicate that this R is an abbreviation. The letter R is the first letter of the Latin word *recipe,* which means take. Thus the doctor instructs the druggist to take the amount specified of each of the substances mentioned in the prescription and to mix them according to the directions, which are usually given in Latin at the bottom of the prescription. The most common direction in any prescription is the word *misce,* which is another Latin word, meaning mix. Quite often the doctor abbreviates this with a capital letter M.

Once prescriptions were noted for the large number of ingredients that they contained. A doctor of an earlier day would inquire as to the various symptoms about which the patient complained and would put something in the prescription to cover every symptom. Nowadays, however, scientific medicine limits itself to a smaller number of drugs of higher power and of more specific effect on the human body. The modern doctor is likely to include only a few ingredients in any prescription. He is more concerned with controlling the cause of the disease and healing and somewhat less with relieving all of the individual symptoms. Control of the cause and healing of the disease remove the symptoms.

PRESCRIPTIONS—not to be kept for the future: See MEDICINE CHEST, article THE FAMILY MEDICINE CHEST.

PRESCRIPTIONS—See entry MEDICINE CHEST.

PRESSURE (See also *Blood Pressure, High; Blood Pressure, Low*) Your blood pressure is a measure of the activity of your heart in pumping, and of the resistance created by the size and the hardness of the walls of the blood vessels. When the doctor measures your blood pressure he puts an inflatable cuff around your arm, then stops the blood flow by pumping air into the cuff; then he listens with a stethoscope to get the pressure at the time when the heart has contracted—systolic pressure—and when it has dilated or relaxed—diastolic pressure. The pressure is taken by a column of mercury measured in millimeters or by a spring device calibrated to the mercury column.

Normal or average blood pressure may range from 95 to 160 systolic and 65 to 90 diastolic. There may be a range in the systolic pressure from 85 to 300 and in the diastolic pressure from 40 to 160. The pressure may vary with sleeping or waking, sitting or standing, with exercise, lack of oxygen or anemia; with chilling, anger, anxiety, frustration or the height of pleasure.

People with blood pressure somewhat below the average used to be said to suffer from low blood pressure. The condition was called hypotension. Now records are available of great numbers of people with somewhat lower blood pressures who nevertheless feel quite well, and who seem to be likely to live long. Hypotension is recognized as a condition in which the systolic pressure is under 80 mm. of mercury or 20 mm. below the usual average of the person concerned. The blood pressure may be quite low after prolonged rest in bed or with malnutrition. The blood pressure may also be lowered by conditions affecting the spinal cord or by the operation which cuts off the sympathetic nervous system.

A feeling of faintness or weakness may be the only indication that the blood pressure is lower than it should be.

HIGH BLOOD PRESSURE—HYPERTENSION—High blood pressure or hypertension is diagnosed by the doctor when, after repeated examination, the pressure is found to be above the average for healthy young people in the area in which the person lives. In the United States levels are around 120 to 140 systolic and 80 to 90 diastolic. The pressure may reach 180 systolic and 100 diastolic without the appearance of any symptoms.

If the person suffers with acute hypertension, such symptoms as convulsions, loss of vision, severe headaches and kidney inflammations may be indications. In chronic high blood pressure dizziness, headaches, hemorrhages in the eye or the brain, heart failure and uremia may be present. Still cases are known in which people with definitely high blood pressures on measurement have failed to manifest any of these symptoms.

Associated with high blood pressure the doctor may find disturbances of the function of the kidneys; disturbances of function of the adrenal glands; or in some instances apparently no immediate cause except some psychologic problem. When a cause cannot be found the case is called "essential hypertension." Often the first indication of the condition may be changes in the blood vessels at the back of the eye which the doctor sees with an ophthalmoscope. Definite relationships have been established between the blood-flow through the kidneys and the pressure of high blood pressure. A high salt or sodium chloride intake may set up high blood pressure. The kidney condition is believed to indicate some substances are elaborated by the kidney which may establish high blood pressure. The pressure with high salt intake is associated with functioning of the adrenal glands.

In an examination of the patient with high blood pressure study of the urine which indicates the condition of the kidneys is important. A low specific gravity—under 1020—and the presence of albumin or pus may show that the kidney condition is responsible. If the kidney function as determined by a variety of tests is normal, the doctor then sees if the adrenal activity is proper. A number of laboratory and functional tests are available which the doctor can use.

Wise physicians recommend that patients be reassured and do not disturb themselves about the pressure in the absence of severe symptoms and in failure to find anything wrong about the blood vessels of the retina of the eye, the heart size and action and the kidney function. If the patient has vague symptoms and sound organs, suggests Dr. William Dock, search should be made for sources of anxiety and frustration. The facts determined by the doctor in his study determine the nature of the treatment that may be prescribed.

The suggestion has been made that the first steps are reassurance of the patient, sedation with the appropriate drugs and restricted use of salt. Rigid elimination of salt from the diet is recommended when there is headache, dizziness, and heart failure. Several drugs are known which will lower blood pressure but all are difficult to use and may have unfavorable effects. The operation called sympathectomy is tried when the condition cannot be controlled but always with a recognition that it may have after effects with annoying symptoms and disability. The rice diet is a form of salt restriction which also reduces weight.

Weight reduction, adequate rest, suitable mental hygiene, are among the best measures that can be recommended in a majority of cases of high blood pressure.

PRICKLY HEAT Frequently the skin becomes irritated due to excessive perspiration after exposure to heat. Wearing excessive clothing in hot weather is a contributing cause. The Inflammation occurs most often in the folds of the skin about the neck, under the breasts, but occasionally also on the chest and back and between the thighs.

The reddened skin develops little tiny, transparent blisters filled with a clear fluid. The itching and burning may be severe. Prevention of contact of the surfaces of the skin will give the inflamed area a chance to heal.

As recovery from the irritation occurs the dead skin may peel away. The greatest danger arises, however, from too much treatment which increases the inflammation and gives opportunity for pus germs to invade.

The utmost cleanliness is important in all irritations of the skin, because damaged tissue gives opening to dangerous germs. The inflamed area may be washed with warm water and a bland soap, then dried carefully by patting without rubbing and powdered with a suitable powder. The physician will often prescribe a soothing lotion, like calamine lotion.

PROSTATE In the male human being just at the neck of the urinary bladder is an organ known as the prostate. The prostate surrounds the urethra, the tube which carries the urine from the bladder, like the insulation around a pipe. The muscle fibers of the prostate act as a sort of valve mechanism which shut off the urinary bladder so that urine does not come into contact with the male sperm cells.

When the prostate becomes infected, as it usually does in severe cases of gonorrhea, there are all the usual signs of infection including a rise in temperature, pain at the area of infection, and frequently a discharge. Sometimes an infection in the prostate persists to the point of abscess, which either breaks into the urethra or the surrounding tissues or else is evacuated by a surgical procedure.

The most common condition affecting the prostate gland is the simple enlargement that comes on with advancing years. The exact cause of this enlargement of the prostate is not known. Sometimes it enlarges slowly for many years without symptoms, the chief sign being a falling off of the power to urinate. Another sign, however, is a more frequent desire to urinate, so that the man who is affected gets up frequently at night. Associated with this there may be some retention of fluid in the bladder, so that it is not completely emptied at the time of urination.

Among the greatest advances made by medicine in recent years is the improvement of treatment in this condition. Modern treatments include the use of glandular substances which help to bring about control of the hypertrophy of the gland. In an earlier day the operative procedure for enlargement of the prostate included a two-stage operation which was a major operation in every sense of the word. Nowadays a new technic permits removal of the enlarged material through a tube which is passed up from the outside and through which the gland is removed by electrical dissection. Formerly the death rate in surgical operations on the prostate was very high; nowadays it is minimal.

PROSTATE GLAND—See article SEX HYGIENE.

PROSTATE GLAND—cancer: See articles SEX HYGIENE; CANCER; OLD AGE.

PROSTATE GLAND—examination: See article CANCER.

PROSTATE GLAND—growth affected by testosterone: See article ENDOCRINOLOGY.

PROSTATE GLAND—hypertrophy: See article CANCER.

PROSTATE GLAND—kidney disease: See KIDNEY, article THE KIDNEY: ITS DISEASES AND DISTURBANCES.

PROTEINS Proteins are one of the principle building materials of the body. They are the important foodstuff found in meat. Cheese, beans, and egg white are other important sources of dietary protein. The minimum daily requirement of protein can be had in about 3½ to 4 ounces of lean meat. Of course, if one is engaged in strenuous work or play, more is needed.

Chemically, proteins are huge molecules made of smaller molecules. These smaller molecules, called amino acids, have both acid and anti-acid (basic) properties. There are about twenty different kinds of these amino acids in animal protein, and hundreds of them are combined to make up one protein molecule. When protein is digested it is broken down in the stomach and small intestine into individual amino acids. These are absorbed into the blood and are carried to the liver and other organs to be synthesized into human protein. The composition or protein in each species of animal differs in the type, number and arrangement of its constituent amino acids. The protein-forming organs select the proper combination from the amino acids circulating in the blood. It is evident, therefore, that some kinds of protein are more valuable than others, the most valuable being those which most resemble human protein.

The body is constantly "wearing out" its proteins and these must be replaced. Those amino acids which are not used for replacement are burned for energy. Besides carbon, hydrogen and oxygen, nitrogen is the most important element in the amino acid molecules. (Sulfur, phosphorus, and other elements may also be present.) When the amino acids are burned, nitrogenous waste products

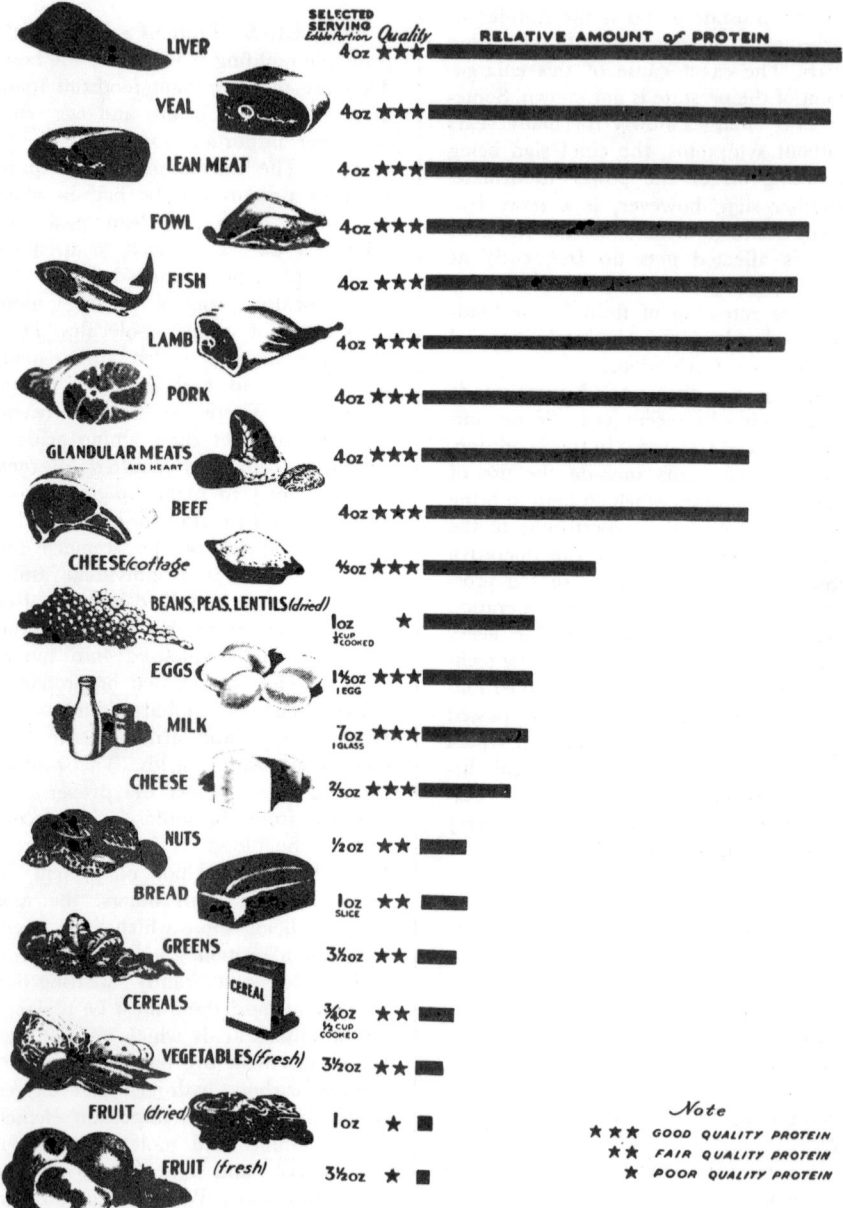

are formed. It is the duty of the kidney to dispose of these waste products.

Proteins have a large number of other functions in the body. One of these functions is the holding of water within the circulatory system. In cases of starvation water leaks out of the vessels and accumulates in the tissues and body cavities. Because of this collection of fluid, starved persons have protruding abdomens and puffy feet and legs. Blood, enzymes, some hormones, body fluids, connective tissue and all cells contain protein.

PRURITUS See *Itching*.

PSITTACOSIS The popular name for psittacosis is parrot's disease. However, the disease is transmitted not only by parrots but also by all kinds of birds, including parakeets, lovebirds, and canaries, and also by infected human beings.

Just as human beings who are apparently well can transmit infectious disease, so also may a bird that is apparently well transmit psittacosis. In most cases, however, the parrot will seem to be ill. Because of the illness of the bird the owner is likely to fondle it and give it much more personal attention, with the result that the owner gets the psittacosis. As might be expected, a disease that can pass from a parrot to a man may also infect chickens, rabbits, mice, and guinea pigs. Strangely the disease affects chiefly the intestinal tract of birds but in almost every instance specifically the lungs of human beings. Cases are recorded in which the infection has reached a human being because he fed the parrot by the mouth-to-mouth method. Most often it occurs merely from handling the sick birds. Not infrequently a person who becomes sick will pass the disease on his infected hands to other members of the same family.

In the United States during the past few years there have been several serious outbreaks of psittacosis in California, Pennsylvania, and in Boston, Massachusetts. The United States has forbidden the importation of birds, particularly during the war period, because of the danger of bringing psittacosis into the country.

The cause of psittacosis is another one of those filtrable viruses—the toxic agents which are so small that they can pass through the pores of a clay filter.

Usually from eight to fourteen days after a person has been exposed to the infection he will feel sick, have a headache, backache, pains in the eyes, and chills. Soon he begins to cough, and in at least one fourth of the cases serious nosebleeds occur. There is an inflammation of the lungs which has the symptoms of pneumonia but does not have the congestion of the lungs and other signs that are typical of pneumonia. The disease is likely to be confused with all forms of pneumonia caused by other germs and viruses. The disease may be exceedingly serious, causing death, but many cases probably recover and, because they are exceedingly mild, are never diagnosed as psittacosis.

Regardless of the love or attachment of the owner to the bird, any bird that is shown to be infected with psittacosis should be sacrificed. Not only the bird but the cage and any other materials which have come in contact with the bird should be destroyed by fire.

California investigators have examined 125 parakeets in a pet shop, 100 parakeets from breeders in the San Francisco Bay area, and a considerable number of squab from a squab farm. Records showed that adult parakeets carry psittacosis, a condition like pneumonia caused by a virus. By injections of tetracycline two or three times a day for a period of two to three weeks the birds were freed of the disease and of the danger of infecting their owners. This drug has been successful in getting the human death rate from psittacosis, which used to be 20-40%, down to 0.5 to 5%. The birds most frequently infected are the green Panama parrots and many Australian birds which are brought into the United States.

PSITTACOSIS—See article TRANSMISSIBLE DISEASES.

PSORIASIS Psoriasis is one of the ten most frequent of all skin diseases, actually making up about 6 per cent of all of the cases of skin diseases for which people consult specialists.

Cases have been reported in babies six days old, but usually psoriasis does not appear until after fifteen years of age. This skin eruption affects women and men alike. It is non-infectious, but there seems to be a tendency to psoriasis in certain families.

Psoriasis is the most puzzling of all skin diseases because exact information as to its source is not available. Many dermatologists believe that psoriasis is related to difficulty in digesting fat. Some believe that it is related to a disturbance of the nervous system. There are from time to time papers published which seem to indicate that certain germs or viruses may be responsible, but thus far the evidence in behalf of any of these causes is not considered well established by the medical profession.

Usually psoriasis begins by a little pinhead-size, bright red eruption. These little spots group to form larger ones, finally resulting in great patches of reddened skin. The healing occurs from the center, leaving a red or reddish-brown stain. Characteristic of psoriasis also are the scales, which are thick and silvery white. When the scales are pulled off, small bleeding points remain.

Eruption is seen most frequently on the elbows, knees, and backs of the arms and legs; less frequently the chest and abdomen are involved. Occasionally the lesions become infected, and this results in the usual formation of pus. Also in chronic psoriasis the fingernails and toenails may be affected.

When the cause of the disease is unknown, treatment is likely to be widely varied. Psoriasis has been treated by diets, most of which seem to have been ineffective, except low fat diets. Vitamins are usually prescribed because people who are on special diets may miss important vitamins. Arsenic is frequently prescribed by specialists. Because it is a

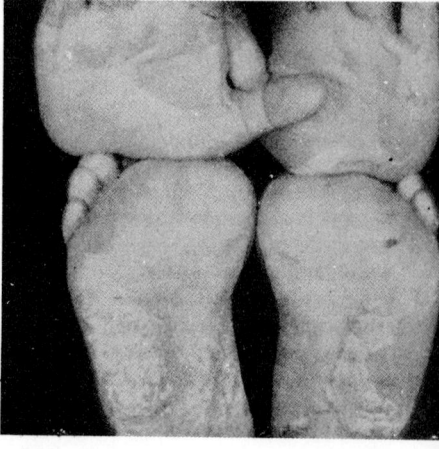

Psoriasis on palms of the hands and soles of the feet. Psoriasis is a skin disease characterized by red patches and scaly eruptions. It is commonly found on the scalp, nails, lower back and the extremities, particularly the knees and elbows. Most often the condition is recurrent and resistant to treatment. The cause is unknown.
Postgraduate Medicine

poisonous drug, it should never be taken except in doses prescribed by the dermatologist. As might have been expected, all of the sulfonamide drugs and the antibiotic drugs have been tried in psoriasis but without any special effect.

Many patients with psoriasis improve with sunlight or with artificial sunlight such as comes from ultraviolet rays. Here again the dosage must be carefully selected by a specialist in diseases of the skin, since overexposure may make the condition worse.

Several special drugs have been developed for the treatment of psoriasis, including particularly one called chrysarobin, which has been found by dermatologists to bring about improvement in many cases.

With the point of view that psoriasis might be due to glandular deficiencies, some cases have been treated recently with male and female sex hormones. In a few instances, but certainly not in all, these hormones occasionally bring about improvement.

A few cases have made great improvement when treated with Cortisone and later relapsed.

A study based on information on 464 consecutive patients with psoriasis showed more men than women affected. There was no relationship between the sex of the patient and that of any other member of the family who happened to be affected. Neither was there established any particular relationship of psoriasis to the order of birth. The data assembled indicated the presence of some sort of hereditary component in the causation of psoriasis but the exact mechanism of the hereditary has certainly not yet been established.

During the last 25 years a dozen new treatments have been tried including the use of glandular products and new drugs. None of these has proved specifically curative. Special diets, including meatless and low fat diets, have been tried. While they are sometimes helpful they are not specifically curative. A recent suggestion made to the American College of Allergists involves the use of histamine which is itself responsible for many symptoms associated with allergic skin reactions. Histamine causes dilation of the blood vessels in the skin. Texas dermatologists who tried histamine on 8 cases of psoriasis say the method gave better results than any other treatment they had tried previously. Because psoriasis is a chronic condition with phases during which it seems spontaneously to get better or worse, the passage of time and tests of many more cases will be needed before the exact merit of histamine for psoriasis can be evaluated accurately.

A substance called animopterin was tried in psoriasis. Investigators reported that 72 out of 171 patients who were treated had complete clearing of the skin lesions from two to three weeks. Seventy-one were greatly improved but 28 did not have any benefit. This drug has dangerous as well as good possibilities and the margin between the beneficial and toxic doses is exceedingly narrow. Use of this drug must always be under the direction of a physician.

PSORIASIS—See SKIN, article THE SKIN.

PSORIASIS—vitamin B2 helpful in treatment: See SKIN, article THE SKIN.

PSYCHOLOGY OF WEIGHT REDUCTION (See also, *Weight, Over* and *Diets.*)

When an underlying psychological reason for overeating is absent, and the patient's overweight is merely the result of a long-continued habit of excess nibbling, reduction of weight is easy. When overeating is mixed with emotional satisfactions, removal of the overeating may be associated with disturbing mental reactions. The doctor has to find the mental conflicts that are the real basis of the overweight. Dr. George Thorn has called attention to the difference in care of the fat girl led into the doctor's office by an anxious and yet domineering mother from that of the girl who wants to increase her personal attractiveness in order to achieve certain social relationships. For that reason control of overeating is much easier with a sixteen-year-old girl than with one approaching thirteen.

With older people, fear of such conditions as diabetes, high blood pressure or arthritis or heart failure may be the reason for weight reduction. Nevertheless, older people have established habits of life including regular meetings of luncheon clubs, banquets, parties and what not which make dieting difficult. For such people a trip away from their accustomed surroundings to a health resort is advantageous because the environment is more conducive to restricted eating.

An eminent authority on dieting suggested recently the organization of a group which he wanted to call "Calories Anonymous" because people can, in this way, have their own will power reinforced by that of the group. Weight reduction classes are successful because of the factor of competition, exchange of ideas, joint participation in exercises, group walking, dancing, and similar activities.

At the appearance of any sign of distress associated with a weight reduction program, the patient should consult his doctor. If the program needs to be modified, the earlier it is done the better.

PSYCHOSIS This term is used to describe any disturbance of the mind, varying from exaggerated emotional outbreaks to serious disturbances such as used to be called insanity.

Psychosis—See entry MENTAL DISEASE.

PSYCHOSOMATIC MEDICINE

Psychosomatic medicine is concerned with the relationship between emotional conflicts and bodily symptoms. In recent years psychosomatic medicine has proved beyond any question of doubt that many symptoms and even changes in the organs and tissues of the body may result from unconscious emotional conflicts.

Many patients consult physicians without any demonstrable bodily disease to account for their symptoms. These patients complain of a large variety of symptoms, often changing from day to day or week to week. Careful physical and laboratory examinations prove entirely negative. The physician is at a complete loss to account for their complaints. These are classified as the hypochondriacs. They enjoy ill health; they get pleasure from medical attention. There is a second group whose symptoms are partially traceable to emotional factors. These people actually have disturbed functioning of some of their organs, but the organic change itself may be the result of psychic disturbances. Peptic ulcer, ulcerative colitis, and some forms of heart disease belong to this group. A third group, which was formerly classified as purely physical, would include asthma, high blood pressure in the young, migraine, possibly some of the allergic manifestations, and some cases of anorexia (loss of appetite), including anorexia nervosa (a condition in which the person's inability to retain food may result in actual self-starvation).

The manner in which a psychic conflict may eventually result in organic changes is well illustrated in some cases of peptic ulcer. The ulcer patient indicates that his illness began with symptoms in the stomach or duodenum which were purely emotional. In time actual physical change takes place in the organ itself as a result of the constant tension and interference with the secretions of the stomach. Probably the same may be said of high blood pressure, which begins as what is termed essential hypertension, meaning that the cause is not demonstrable and is in the beginning a state of tension in the arteries resulting ultimately in a loss of muscular elasticity in the walls of the blood vessels.

We also know from experience that many people who suffer from asthma, urticaria (hives), neurodermatitis, eczema, acne, hay fever, arthritis, diabetes, obesity, and varying degrees of malnutrition have been greatly improved by intensive psychotherapy. Probably we have barely touched the surface of the many diseases that will eventually be proven to have been precipitated by the emotional environment to which patient has been subjected.

PSYCHOSOMATIC SKIN DISEASE (See also discussion under *Acne, Itching, Skin*) At least two forms of skin disturbances are now considered to have a psychosomatic basis: disturbances in people who think the skin is diseased when it is not and skin disturbances definitely related to mental outlook. In addition, there are the conditions called neurodermatitis which definitely have a basis through stimulation coming from the nervous system. Psychosomatically scratching has been found to be an aggressive act that removes something unpleasant whether real, imagined or something else. Itching around the genital organs and the rectum is significant; specialists find that although extreme itching in these areas may be caused by infection or by infestation with germs or fungi, it may also be associated with a feeling of guilt over some illicit action. Sometimes skin eruptions occur in emotionally insecure people who need more affection and attention. Also, the pimples and blackheads that appear on the adolescent's skin are related to the glandular function and sometimes become worse under emotional stress.

PTOMAINE POISONING See *Food Poisoning.*

PULMONIC STENOSIS, SURGERY IN (See also *Heart,* Surgery of the) Pulmonic stenosis is an obstruction in the valve between the heart and the artery which carries blood into the lungs. Until recently, the only treatment attempted was the construction of an artificial bypass to detour the blood around the obstruction. This operation is of limited value, adding a man-made malformation to the already imperfect heart. While this operation was done entirely outside the heart, the new technique involves corrective surgery within the heart itself. The surgeon inserts a miniature knife through a tiny slit in the heart wall, and working by touch, eliminates the obstruction in or near the valve. Forty-one such cases were reported without any operative mortality.

PULSE When blood passes through an artery, the impulse of the pumping by the heart is carried down so that a finger applied to the artery anywhere near the surface permits a counting of the pulse rate. The number of pulsations in a minute varies with adults from 67 to 72. Infants may have a normal pulse rate anywhere between 100 and 120. The most rapid pulse rate ever recorded was something over 300 beats per minute. This condition is called tachycardia. A slow pulse is known as bradycardia. Many long-distance runners have exceedingly slow pulses—indeed as low as 40 to 65.

PURPURA HEMORRHAGICA

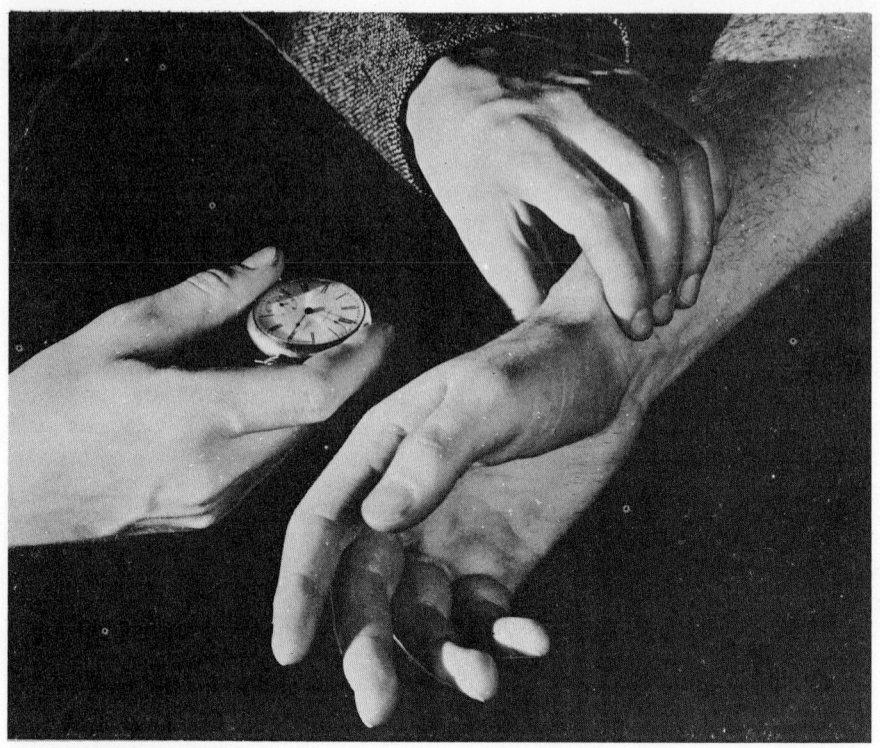

Proper technic for taking the pulse. With the index finger, not the thumb, the pulse beat is found on the thumb side of the wrist and the beats are counted for a full minute.

PULSE—See article BLOOD PRESSURE.

PULSE—irregularities: See HEART, article DISEASES OF THE HEART AND CIRCULATION.

PULSE—rapid, in exophthalmic goiter: See HEART, article DISEASES OF THE HEART AND CIRCULATION.

PULSE—test for danger of death from failure of respiration: See article FIRST AID.

PURPURA HEMORRHAGICA

Whenever there is a shortage of platelets—certain formed elements—in the blood, bleeding will occur almost spontaneously, particularly from the mucous membranes in the nose and in the mouth. Bleeding underneath the skin is frequent, giving the appearance of bruising. Sometimes this condition is associated with poisoning by drugs of the benzol type or with the poisoning that occurs from the action of certain types of germs, such as those of diphtheria, tuberculosis, and the streptococcus. Cases occasionally follow poisoning with the drugs that are used in the treatment of syphilis. The number of platelets may be lessened as a result of some action on the bone marrow, in which the cells giving rise to the platelets are formed. A lessened number of platelets may result from a lessened formation of the cells or from a toxic action which destroys these cells more rapidly than they are formed. In many women a lessening of the platelets occurs with each menstruation.

By a safety mechanism of the body the number of platelets tends to increase whenever a slight hemorrhage starts in the body of a normal person. Also the platelets that are left develop increased ability to form clots. If there has been an extensive attack on the blood-forming organs, the lessening of the number of platelets is associated with the lessening of the number of red blood cells and of the white blood cells as well. In some instances the lessening of the number of platelets occurs only at irregular intervals, between which the bleeding does not occur.

Purpura hemorrhagica occurs most commonly in people between the ages of twelve to twenty-five years, although it may occur at any age. The condition may come on gradually so that it is not possible for the person concerned to say just when the condition started. Some cases are so severe that the person bleeds to death in a few days or weeks. In others the condition goes on with varying severity throughout a long life.

Many different methods have been discovered for treating patients with this condition with a view to bringing about benefit, if not cure. One of the simplest methods is the injection of blood directly into the body, sometimes into the veins, sometimes into the muscles or under the skin. Transfusion of blood is today one of the most useful methods in the treatment of disease. The use of the venom of the moccasin snake has been found to be of value, and tests have been discovered for determining whether or not the case is of the type which will be benefited by the use of the venom.

In severe cases the removal of the spleen by surgical operation has been shown to be of value. This operation has been used now in many hundreds of cases, apparently with advantage in most instances. Still other treatments involve the taking of large amounts of vitamin C, the feeding of a high vitamin diet, and the use of a new chemical called vitamin P.

Most of the methods of treatment are considered to be experimental for the individual case. In every case a study should be made to see if the person is sensitive to some protein and if the platelet disturbance is associated with such sensitivity.

Purpura—due to absence of platelets: See Blood, article The Blood and Its Diseases.

Purpura—nosebleed: See Ear, article The Ear, Tongue, Nose, and Throat.

PYELITIS (See also *Kidneys*) Inflammation of the kidney is called pyelitis. Infection is usually associated with pain and tenderness, irritability of the bladder, fever, sometimes blood or pus in the urine. Pyelitis is described as hemorrhagic or suppurative, depending on whether or not the blood or the pus is the most prominent feature. A pyelogram is an X-ray picture of the kidney. Pyelonephritis is another term for infection of the kidney and its pelvis. The treatment of pyelitis nowadays involves, first, a scientific diagnosis as to the nature of the condition and, second, the use of such drugs as the sulfonamides, penicillin, streptomycin, and mandelic acid, which are known to be efficient in removing the infection. When, however, control by drugs becomes impossible, surgical procedures are used.

Pyelitis—See Kidney, article The Kidney: Its Diseases and Disturbances.

Pyelitis—albuminuria may arise in:

See Kidney, article The Kidney: Its Diseases and Disturbances.

Pyelitis—infants: See Infancy, article Care and Feeding of the Child.

Pyelitis—pregnancy: See Birth, article Care of Mothers Before and After Childbirth; Kidney, article The Kidney: Its Diseases and Disturbances.

Pyelitis—prostate gland enlarged: See Kidney, article The Kidney: Its Diseases and Disturbances.

PYEMIA Any infection with germs that produces pus which gets into the blood is known as pyemia.

Pyemia—endocarditis may occur: See Heart, article Diseases of the Heart and Circulation.

PYLORUS The pylorus is the valve which releases food from the stomach into the intestines. Ulcers may occur in this area with subsequent scarring and constriction. Sometimes a spasm of the pylorus occurs, particularly in babies. Serious conditions affecting the pylorus are usually treated by surgery.

Pylorus—See Infancy, article Care and Feeding of the Child; article Digestion and Digestive Diseases.

PYORRHEA Pyorrhea alveolaris refers to a purulent inflammation of the gums and the outer covering of the roots of the teeth. As a result the teeth become loose and there is a flow of pus from the roots of the teeth. Pyorrhea can be prevented by suitable dental attention to the teeth at regular intervals. Treatment involves not only a high quality of dental care, including the use of specific remedies against infection, but also a study of the general health of the person concerned.

Pyorrhea—See Teeth, article The Care of the Teeth.

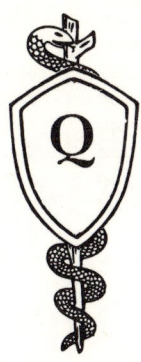

Q FEVER Q fever is a disease something like influenza or atypical pneumonia. It is caused by a rickettsial organism similar to the type of organism that causes typhus. The condition was first definitely established in Australia but now cases have been reported in Texas, Illinois, Montana, Arizona, and California. In Los Angeles doctors have seen more than 300 cases and three deaths have been reported. Apparently the condition can be carried by raw milk that has not been properly pasteurized. Cases of Q fever have been found also in Italy, in the Balkans, in Panama, and in Switzerland.

Q fever usually begins suddenly with symptoms like those of any common infectious disease, including fever with slowness of the heartbeat, headache, occasionally chills and drenching sweat. When the doctor examines the patient he finds that there is some inflammation of the lungs accompanied by a mild cough but with little expectoration and accompanied also by pains in the chest but examination by stethoscope or X ray does not reveal changes such as those typical of pneumonia or tuberculosis. In many ways the appearance of Q fever under the X ray is more like atypical virus pneumonia. Q fever has been treated with the sulfonamide drugs and with penicillin but without definitely affecting the course of the disease. Streptomycin has been more beneficial than either of these drugs, and aureomycin is even more beneficial than streptomycin. All of these drugs must be prescribed by the physician in the amounts suited to the individual case. In exceedingly severe cases transfusions of blood and inhalation of oxygen have been helpful. Such diseases as Q fever indicate how important is proper pasteurization and control of milk as a means of preventing the spread of infectious disease.

QUACKS In times of great stress, in pain or in sorrow, human beings frequently forget everything they have learned about science and truth and resort to incantation, prayer, and magic. The human being in fear of an incurable disease will grasp at any suggestion that may be offered to him, never stopping to inquire as to the motives of those who sell the cures and never inquiring as to the basis on which the claims of cures may rest.

All over the world there are still people who explain all disease as a seizure of the body by some evil influence. To them the cure of disease rests on conjuring that evil influence out of the body. Out of that belief have come all of the magical cures, which include charms, amulets, suggestion, and a good many medicines that are without any virtue except such as resides in the faith that the patient has in the medicine and in the doctor.

Human beings crave miracles. Modern science gives them miracles like penicillin and the sulfa drugs, like modern surgery and blood plasma. But familiarity with these miracles soon takes away their magic.

The quack in medicine today does not have the opportunity he had in a previous generation to victimize millions of people. Once quacks had unlimited use of the radio, the mails, and newspaper advertising. Today the new Food, Drug and Cosmetic Act, the regulations of the Federal Trade Commission, the ethical standards adopted by newspapers, radio stations, and similar mediums of public education limit the most gross varieties of quacks from any use of their mediums for securing public attention. A few quacks still prevail, but they are largely limited to local areas and to small groups of susceptible people who are always willing to try something weird or mystical before they try science in the healing of disease.

The quacks are marked by certain definite characteristics. They claim knowledge that they do not possess. They put after their names long appendages of degrees, most of which were never conferred on them by any university. They make exaggerated claims as to their ability to cure disease. They do not even hesitate to guarantee a cure if that seems necessary to secure a patient. They are likely to charge far more than the traffic will bear or else to build up a tremendous group of followers by charging just a trifle to thousands of people. Finally, they always claim to be able to perform functions in the field of healing which are far beyond the ability claimed by others in the community.

The public can tell a good doctor by the fact that he is just the opposite of the list of attributes that has just been mentioned. A good doctor will have graduated from a good medical school, he will have had an internship in an approved hospital, he will be a member of leading medical organizations, and he will be a member of the staff of a reputable hospital. If he is a specialist, he will have the certificate of one of the certifying boards in the various specialties. He will not be an advertiser. He will not pass out handbills. He will not have a big electric sign in front of his office. He will never guarantee a cure or promise to cure a serious disease in one or two treatments. He will be a reputable citizen of his community.

QUACKS—cancer treatment: See article CANCER.

QUACKS—distinguishing from ethical physicians: See PHYSICIAN, article THE CHOICE OF A PHYSICIAN.

QUACKS—gonorrhea: See VENEREAL

Diseases, article The Venereal Diseases.

Quacks—kidney disease: See Kidney, article The Kidney: Its Diseases and Disturbances.

Quacks—syphilis: See Venereal Diseases, article The Venereal Diseases.

QUARANTINE The word "quarantine" comes from an Italian word meaning forty. The Italians of the Middle Ages would prevent people who arrived on ships from entering port until forty days had passed if there was a case of plague aboard the ship. Nowadays the word "quarantine" is applied to any instance in which a human being or an animal is detained for the purpose of preventing infection. For instance it is impossible to take a dog into England or Hawaii without a quarantine period, which is used to make certain that the animal does not have rabies, or hydrophobia.

A sick person who is kept to himself is not quarantined but isolated. It is customary to isolate sick people with infectious conditions until they are well and free from germs of contagious disease. For every infectious disease there is a period of quarantine and a period of isolation. For example, if a child has scarlet fever, other members of the family are likely to be quarantined for a certain period of time to make sure that they will not spread the disease. The patient himself is isolated until he is free from the infection, including discharges from the nose and throat.

The isolation and quarantine periods vary for different diseases. For meningitis the period of quarantine is two weeks. For measles and for German measles the minimum time is one week from the appearance of the rash or the first symptoms of the disease.

A child who has had diphtheria is not released to play with other children while there are still germs of diphtheria in his throat. In most cases of diphtheria germs can still be found in the throat a week or two after all other signs of the disease have disappeared. It is customary, therefore, not to release the child until at least two cultures from the throat have been negative—that is, free from germs of diphtheria.

Whooping cough is one of the diseases in which the practice of quarantine and isolation is most difficult. Cases are known in which the germs that are associated with whooping cough may still be found in the throat for months after all the other symptoms have disappeared. Therefore, if the weather is pleasant, children who have had whooping cough are permitted to be outdoors in the sunshine, but they are not permitted to make close contacts with other children as long as the whoop and the germs persist.

Mumps is most contagious during the early days. Once the patient begins to convalesce, the danger of catching mumps is not so great.

It is a safe rule, whenever a child has an infectious disease, to make certain that he is entirely free from secondary complications like running nose, cough, infection in the ear, and similar disturbances before the child is permitted to go back to school or to mingle otherwise with other children.

Isolation—pneumonia: See Respiratory Diseases, article The Respiratory Diseases.

Isolation—smallpox: See Infectious Disease, article The Prevention and Treatment of Infectious Disease.

Quarantine—mumps: See Childhood Diseases, article Infectious Diseases of Childhood.

Quarantine—whooping cough: See Childhood Diseases, article Infectious Diseases of Childhood.

QUICKENING When a pregnant woman feels motion inside the uterus, commonly called "feeling life," this is called quickening. The first recognizable movements appear usually from the sixteenth to the twentieth week of pregnancy.

QUINIDINE (See also discussion under *Fibrillation, Heart, Leukocytes, Thrombocytopenia, Quinine*) A remarkable observation was made relative to the manner in which people react to certain drugs by great diminution in some of the blood factors. Certain types of anemia and certain disorders in which bleeding occurs constantly were found to be associated with the taking of the drug quinidine. The usual pattern was as follows: The patient was given quinidine for an illness, usually for irregularity or arrhythmia of the heart. The drug was taken at irregular intervals without any reaction. Then shortly after the drug was given purple spots developed all over the body together with blood blisters in the mouth and with bleeding from the gums and the nose. Investigation of these cases showed there was a severe reduction in the blood platelets. A substance had formed in the blood which had the power to clump the platelets. However, this acted only in the presence of the drug quinidine. An antibody had formed against the platelets. This observation suggests that similar mechanisms may be a part of other reactions to drugs and chemicals.

As a result of this observation, scientists now theorize that the reactions to certain antiepileptic drugs, to antibiotics,, to other drugs used against arthritis and high blood pressure may be a part of a similar phenomenon. Fortunately, withdrawal of the offending drug results in most instances in recovery. However, a great shortage of white cells might lead to lack of the body's defense against infections. Customarily therefore an adequate dose of a strong antibiotic is prescribed to prevent such infections.

QUININE Quinine is a drug used specifically in the treatment of malaria. Because of the shortage which occurred during World War II, a substitute called atabrine was developed which is also used as a specific against malaria. This product is called quinacrine hydrochloride in the United States Pharmacopoeia. Quinine was long used as a tonic and as bitters. It has also been used for certain forms of muscle weakness. The great shortage of quinine during World War II has limited its use almost exclusively to the treatment of malaria. One of the substances derived from quinine called quinidine is used in the treatment of fibrillation of the heart muscle. It acts to slow the heart and lengthen the time of conduction of the heartbeat.

All of these drugs are toxic when taken in wrong dosage and should never be used except when prescribed by the physician.

ATABRINE—See article TRANSMISSIBLE DISEASES.

QUININE—hives caused by: See SKIN, article THE SKIN.

QUININE—malaria: See article TRANSMISSIBLE DISEASES.

QUININE—occupational hazard: See article OCCUPATION AND HEALTH.

QUININE—poisoning: See article FIRST AID.

QUINSY (See also discussion under *Tonsils*) Quinsy is a term applied to abscess in the area around the tonsils. Such abscesses must be treated by a specialist in conditions affecting the throat; he will open the abscess and supply treatment against the infection, such as the use of the sulfa drugs.

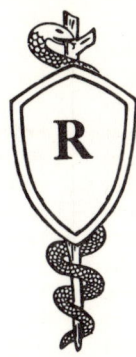

RABBIT FEVER See *Tularemia.*

RABIES Summer is the time of the year when pet and domestic animals run free and, therefore, the time when rabies is most frequent.

The dog is the animal most frequently attacked by rabies, although any animal may be infected. Most people think that a dog with rabies, or hydrophobia, will run wildly through the street, snapping at every human being who crosses its path. Not every animal with rabies has reached this stage of the disease when it bites a human being. In many animals the first signs of rabies are merely irritableness and restlessness. Ultimately, however, the animal develops difficulty in swallowing, paralysis which makes the mouth hang open, and the drooling of saliva, which are the marks of the animal with hydrophobia.

In the final stages of rabies an infected dog will howl, snap at people and other animals, will run and bite. Eventually the infected animal becomes paralyzed, has convulsions, and dies. Under modern conditions, however, such an animal will probably be picked up if it is in the city or killed if it happens to be in the country before it reaches the final stages of rabies.

Human beings get rabies from the bite of an animal infected with the disease. Rabies is caused by a virus which appears in the saliva of the animal several days before it has serious symptoms. When this virus gets into the body of a human being, either by the bite of an animal or in any other way, the virus affects the nervous system and eventually reaches the central nervous system, including the spinal cord and brain. The closer the entrance of the virus to the brain, the quicker come the serious symptoms. Bites on the face, lips, and hands are more serious than on the feet and legs because the point of inoculation of the virus is nearer to the brain.

Considerable epidemics of rabies have appeared in the United States in recent years. During 1944 the disease was especially prevalent in Maryland, Indiana, and in the Bronx in New York.

People can do a great deal to prevent the spread of rabies by taking proper care of dogs. Dogs should wear muzzles when out of doors. The dog that is kept in a good home is usually watched carefully, kept from contact with savage dogs, and therefore is not likely to be involved as is the dog that runs free. Homeless animals should be picked up and disposed of by the methods that prevail in the particular area.

Because of the terrible possibilities of rabies, just one course should be followed after every dog bite. The animal should be captured alive, if possible, and kept secured for at least ten days, during which time it will either die or develop the symptoms of hydrophobia if it has that disease. If the dog dies (or, in fact, if the dog does not die, it may be desirable to destroy the animal), the brain should be examined in order to make certain whether or not it has the signs in the brain that are characteristic of rabies.

If a person is bitten on the face or on the hands, the Pasteur treatment should be begun immediately because of the short time that may elapse between the time the bite occurs and the time the virus reaches the brain and nervous system.

The onset of rabies usually follows the bite of an infected animal in from twenty to ninety days. During this period the symptoms may include restlessness, apprehension, with irritation and tingling at the site of the bite. When the disease begins, the horrible symptoms which give hydrophobia its name appear. A slight huskiness of the voice is followed by a sense of choking because the muscles of swallowing and breathing go into spasms. The infected person may refuse to take water because of the pain associated with swallowing. The physician who is called to see such a patient will wish to treat the bite by cauterizing it with a strong acid, sometimes by laying the wound open with a knife in order that the treatment may reach all parts of the wound. Then the Pasteur treatment is given, during which the patient may usually go about his business.

The old term "dog days" refers to the period when dogs were thought to be most likely to run about mad. It is a misnomer. Dogs may run loose and bite people in any season of the year.

RABIES — See articles FIRST AID; TRANSMISSIBLE DISEASES.

RABIES—control: See article TRANSMISSIBLE DISEASES.

RABIES—deaths: See article TRANSMISSIBLE DISEASES.

RABIES—incubation period: See article TRANSMISSIBLE DISEASES.

RABIES—meaning of words: See article TRANSMISSIBLE DISEASES.

RABIES—nervous system: See INFECTIOUS DISEASE, article THE PREVENTION AND TREATMENT OF INFECTIOUS DISEASE.

RABIES—Pasteur treatment: See article TRANSMISSIBLE DISEASES.

RABIES—superstition concerning "dog days": See article TRANSMISSIBLE DISEASES.

RABIES—symptoms: See article TRANSMISSIBLE DISEASES.

RABIES—transmissible disease: See article TRANSMISSIBLE DISEASES.

RABIES—vaccine: See articles TRANSMISSIBLE DISEASES; ALLERGY.

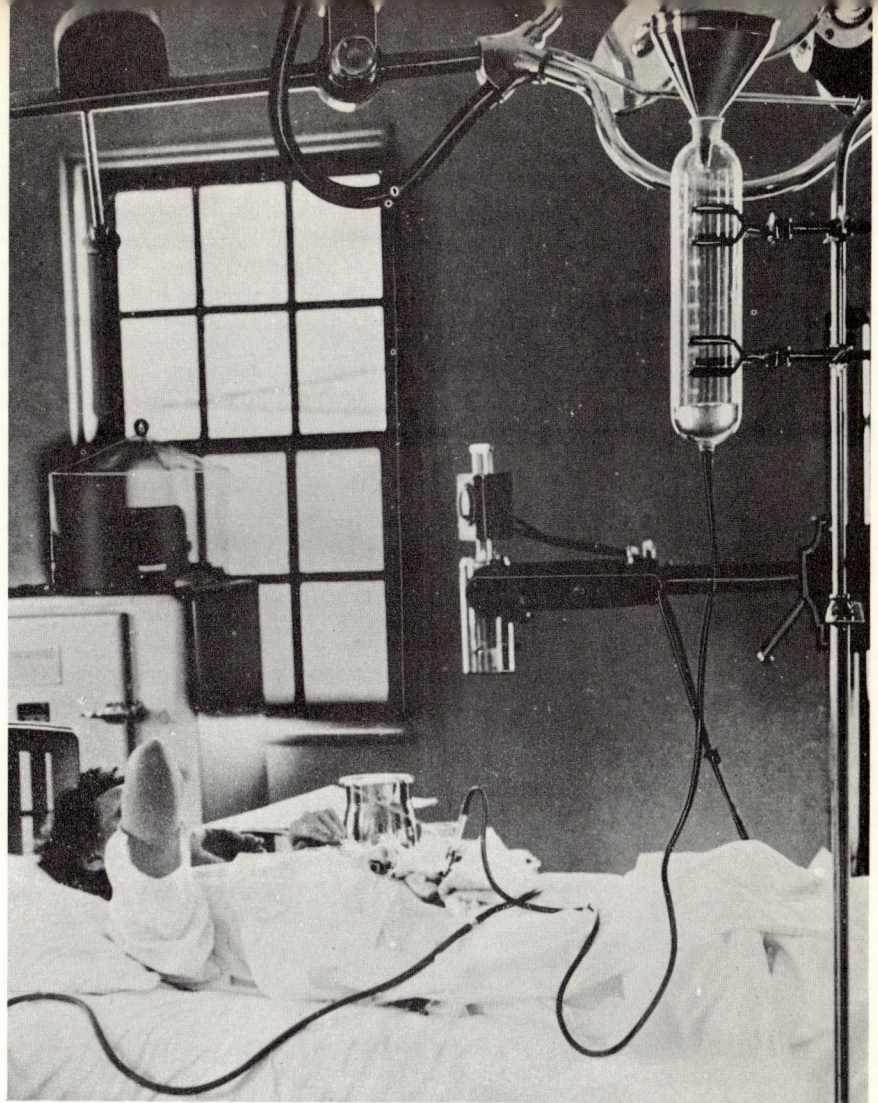

Solution containing radioactive chlorine 38 is funneled into the glass container (right above) for administration to a patient suffering from cancer. The use of chlorine 38, one of the short-lived radioisotopes, is being explored in medicine. Chlorine 38 loses half of its radioactivity every 38 minutes, so speed, precision and care are necessary in getting these isotopes from the nuclear reactor to the hospital. On the average, a total of only 15 minutes elapses from the time the isotope is removed from the reactor until it has been transported to the hospital, dissolved in a sterile solution, and administered to the patient. In 350 minutes only insignificant traces of radioactivity will remain.

Brookhaven National Laboratory

RADIATION Radiation is used in medicine to describe the action of rays of various types and also the divergence from a common center of sensations and stimuli. The term "radiography" is used to describe the use of the X ray as well as roentgenography, which comes from Roentgen, the inventor of the X ray.

RADIATION RESEARCH (See also discussion under *Atomic Energy, Cancer, Detection of Brain Tumors, Leukemia, Lung Cancer, Medical Reactor, First, Research in Cancer, Radioactivity*) Nowadays we hear much about betatrons, cyclotrons and synchrotrons. In addition there are cobalt bombs and

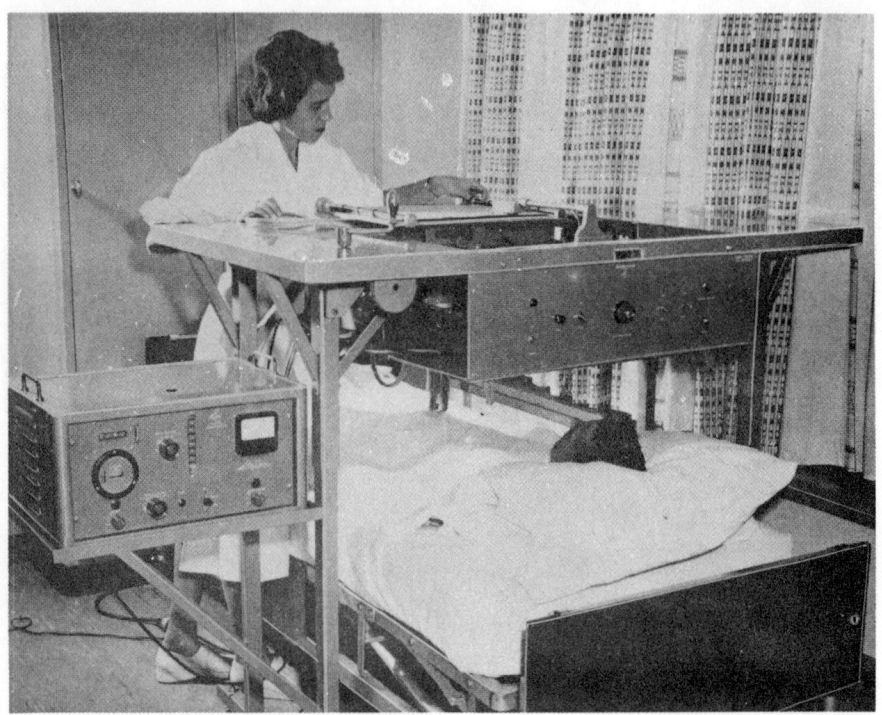

A sensitive machine used to measure the distribution of radioisotopes in organs or body cavities. The patient either drinks or is injected with radioactive substance. The machine is able to pick up the radiation emitted by the radioisotopes. Radioactive isotopes have been a great contribution of our atomic age to medicine. They can be formed from many elements, such as gold, iodine, cobalt and phosphorus. Production of isotopes and equipment for their use are expensive, but the number of well-equipped centers are steadily growing to meet the demands of research, diagnosis and treatment.

Postgraduate Medicine

high voltage x-ray machines as well as radium in many different forms used to attack the growth of cancer cells. Tremendous amounts of research are necessary to establish the effects of the different types of radiation on the chemical reactions and on the hereditary structure of cells of various types and forms. Much needs to be learned about the way in which radiation affects living matter. This gives rise to a new science called radiobiology.

There are studies that indicate the great hazards of radiant energy not only in relationship to such conditions as leukemia but also for its effects on the growing cells of the body. For long it has been known that persons exposed to radioactivity might produce malformed children. Among the hazards of various occupations, now must be included exposure of specialists in x-ray to such dangerous rays. The evidence from Hiroshima showed that radioactivity could damage the germ cell and cause the birth of deformed babies. Questionnaires were sent to 3,800 radiologists and 3,800 other medical specialists to find out the percentage of children in such families who were formed with congenital defects. Radiologists as a result of their exposure to frequent doses of ionizing radiation were found to have a higher incidence of congenital defects in their children than did other doctors.

RADIATION SICKNESS People are continually exposed to minute amounts of radiation that comes not only from the various forces in the atmosphere surrounding the world but also from naturally radioactive materials that occur in soil and water and in other materials in our environment. Fortunately this radiation is so small in amount that it does not seem to have any significant effect on the body. Also a certain amount of radiation may come from X-ray tubes or from radium or from the taking of various radioactive isotopes. There is no way in which an untrained person can find out whether or not he is being subjected to radiation. For that reason various means have been developed for determining the presence of radiation in our atmosphere.

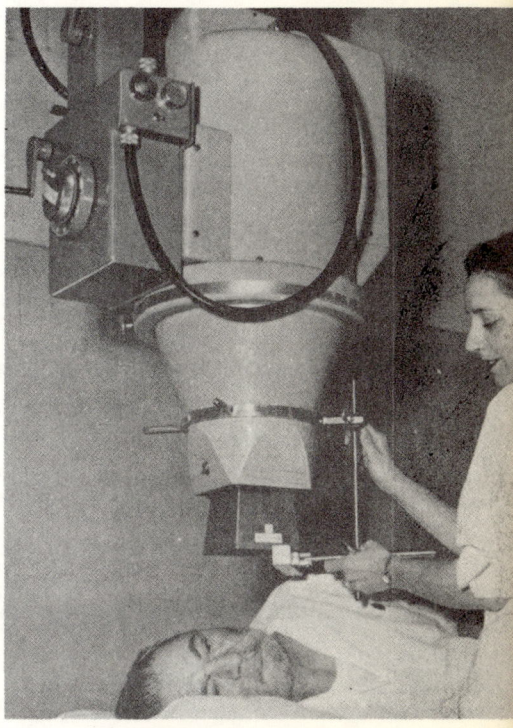

Patient being treated with radiocobalt for cancer of the tonsil. The assistant is adjusting the machine so the rays will strike the diseased area. Proper doses of radiocobalt will interfere with the growth of cancerous tissue but will not affect healthy tissue.
Postgraduate Medicine

These include the exposure of photographic film and devices like the Geiger counter.

The physicists have classified the radiation into various types of waves and particles which vary greatly in their effects on the living tissue of the body. Some rays penetrate more than do others. The irradiation affects the protoplasm of the tissues and brings about certain chemical and physical effects. Some cells of the body are more sensitive to radiation than are others. When radiation is used against tumors, the physician knows the sensitivity of the cells to the radiation and the extent to which it can be counted on to stop cellular growth.

Radiation sickness results from absorption of the products of disintegration of the protein of the body. The chief symptom of radiation sickness is mild to severe nausea and, in some instances, there may be diarrhea due to the response of the intestinal tissues to the irritation.

Another type of radiation sickness results from irradiation of the entire body over a short period of time. This begins suddenly with severe illness that may go to the point of prostration. There may be thereafter a phase of relative well-being followed by severe illness and ultimately by death.

The most sensitive cells of the body are the white blood cells of the blood.

RADIOACTIVE GOLD – Au 198
FOR INTRACAVITARY USE IN METASTASIZED CANCER

COLLOIDAL GOLD IN SHIELD
TO PERITONEAL OR PLEURAL CAVITY
SALINE SOLUTION

ADVANTAGES:
1 - INHIBITS FORMATION OF CAVITARY FLUID
2 - REDUCES PAIN
3 - HELPS RETURN PATIENT TO NORMAL ACTIVITY

USAEC-ID 18A

RADIATION SICKNESS

Radiation can damage the blood-forming organs so that the cells fall below normal with subsequent hemorrhage due to destruction of the thrombocytes in the blood and increased permeability of the capillaries from damage to the cells. Obviously with loss of blood comes severe anemia. The effects of radiation can be such as to produce sterility, but permanent sterility is not expected from irradiation because the dose necessary to sterilize the male sex gland is close to what is a fatal dose. In the woman also the radiation may produce transient sterility; permanent sterility is rare.

At present the best method of treatment for irradiation is the transfusion of whole blood, the use of antibiotic drugs to control infection and forced nutrition to enable the body to overcome the damage that has occurred.

RADIOACTIVE IODINE

RADIOACTIVE GOLD (See also discussion under *Detection of Brain Tumor and Radioactivity*) Radium emanation from seeds of radium encased in glass tubes and implanted in tumors has been used to treat the growths. Now radioactive gold is being used in a similar way. Fifty-one patients were treated by implantation in a tumor of a thread of radioactive gold sealed in a thin, inactive tube. Most of the patients for whom this was done were reported to have benefited from the treatment.

RADIOACTIVE IODINE (See also discussion under *Angina Pectoris, Cancer, Goiter, Heart, Thyroid and the Heart, Radioactivity*) Physicians in the Cedars of Lebanon Hospital in Los Angeles gave radioactive iodine for

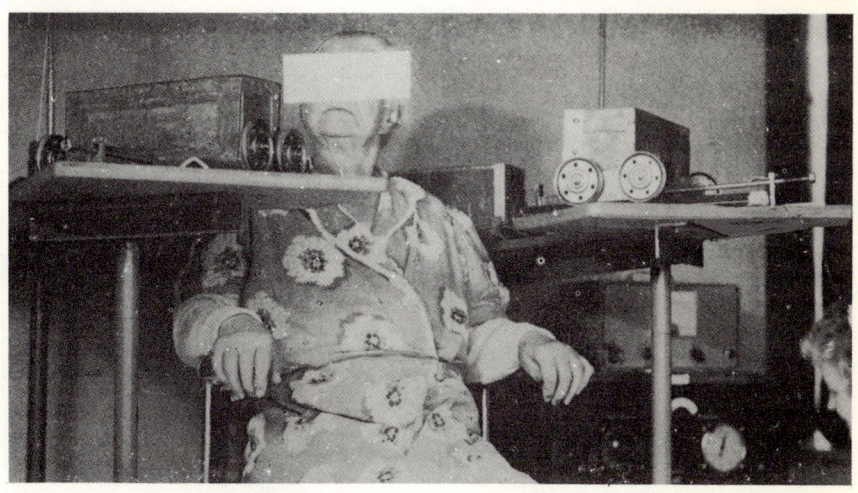

Patient being treated for cancer of the thyroid gland. A dose of radioactive iodine is given to the patient and the thyroid gland absorbs the radioiodine. The boxes shown are Geiger counters used to detect the amount of radioiodine absorbed and the areas of the gland in which it is localized. Radioactive iodine enables the doctor to make an accurate diagnosis of the activity of the thyroid gland.

Postgraduate Medicine

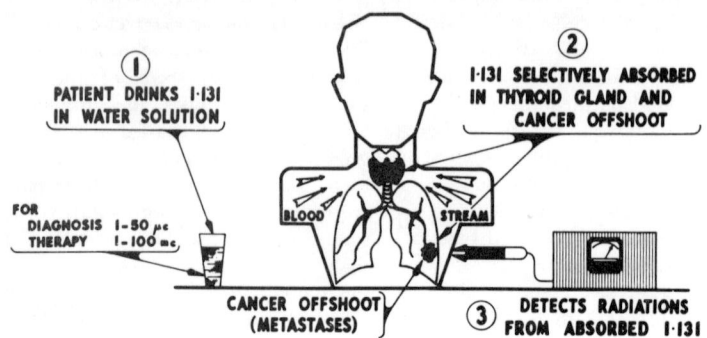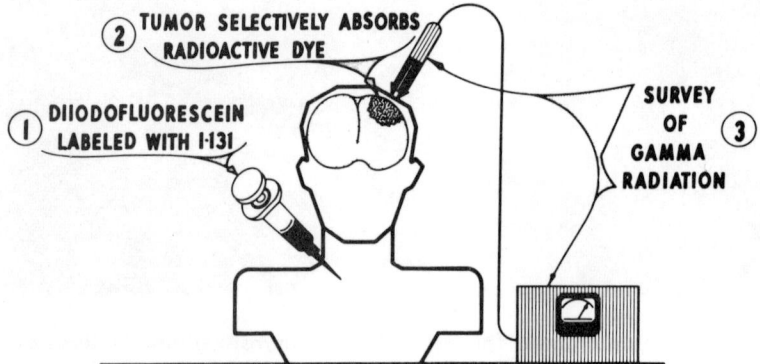

periods of six months to four years to patients with advanced stages of heart disease. These people had angina pectoris or congestive heart failure and some of them a combination of the two conditions which are painful and which make it difficult for the heart to maintain the circulation. The effect of the radioactive iodine was to reduce the output of the hormone from the thyroid gland. As a result, the heart beats more slowly and its work is lessened. Fifty-three per cent of 231 patients were classed as having made excellent progress and an additional 33 per cent made good progress. Only 14 per cent were found not to have improved.

RADIOACTIVE ISOTOPES—cancer research: See article CANCER.

RADIOACTIVE ISOTOPES—cancer treatment: See article CANCER.

RADIOACTIVE ISOTOPES—leukemia: See article CANCER.

RADIOACTIVE ISOTOPES — occupational diseases in handling: See article OCCUPATION AND HEALTH.

RADIOACTIVITY—discovery: See article OCCUPATION AND HEALTH.

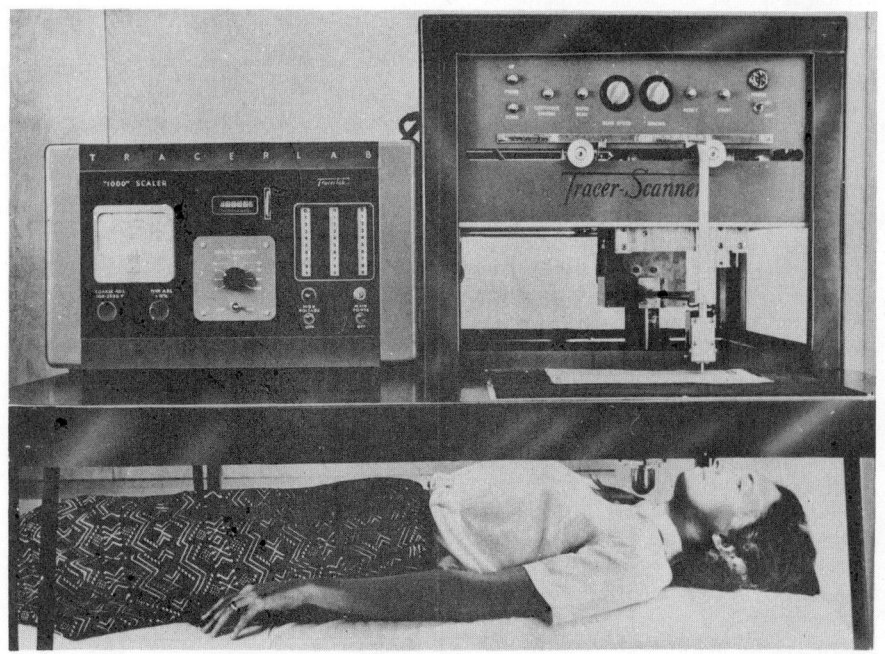

A clinical device used for determining the location of radioactive iodine in the thyroid. This tracer scanner automatically draws a diagram, indicating distribution of the radioactive iodine in the thyroid area. At the same time it records the level of activity in various parts of the thyroid. This is used extensively in thyroid diagnosis.

Tracerlab, Inc.

ROENTGEN, WILLIAM—See article OCCUPATION AND HEALTH.

RADIOACTIVITY (See also discussion under *Arteriosclerosis, Atomic Energy, Bladder Condition, Detection of Brain Tumor, Goiter, Keloid, Medical Reactor, First, Radiation, Radiation Research, Radioactive Gold, Radioactive Iodine, Radium, Thyroid and the Heart, X Ray*) Medicine long ago began to study the potentialities of radioactive substances for research and in the treatment of disease. According to an educational bulletin of the Metropolitan Life Insurance Company the X-ray apparatus is one of the first standard implements of medicine to undergo change in keeping with radiological advances. In 1954, a portable X-ray unit was developed which employs radioactive thulium, a rare earth metal, as its source of radiation. A small amount of this substance encased in lead, which affords full protection to personnel, produces radiographs without the use of electricity, water, or darkroom facilities. The unit, which weighs only 40 pounds, is simple to operate and produces a finished radiograph ready for inspection in five to ten minutes.

The radioisotopes, 150 of which are now in use, are perhaps the most notable by-products of the current atomic energy program. One isotope, artificially radioactivated iodine, has provided a most sensitive indicator of thyroid gland activity. The activity has heretofore been largely determined by the basal metabolic test. A much more accurate determination of thyroid activity can now be achieved by measuring the gland's uptake of radioactive iodine.

Many isotopes have been used to apply radiation for treatment both externally and internally. A notable example is cobalt-60 for deep therapy of cancer. The great energy of the radiations emitted by this substance is evidenced by the fact that their penetration of body tissues is approximately the same as that of the radiation from a 2-million-volt X-ray machine. It has been estimated that $47 million worth of radium would be required to do the work of a large cobalt-60 source.

The first "cobalt bomb" was manufactured in the Chalk River Plant of the Canadian Atomic Commission. This agency also supplied hospitals in the United States and Europe with "cobalt bombs."

A unique beam has been developed which provides energy capable of obliterating completely the pituitary gland of rats. Thus, it may someday be possible to perform "surgery" by radiation.

Valuable as the isotopes are in retarding the growth of some forms of cancer and arresting a few diseases, they are essentially investigative tools rather than therapeutic agents.

The isotopes, which carry their radioactivity wherever they go in the body, are revealing new facts about vital processes. Iron can be "tagged" and its integral part in the production of red blood cells elucidated by following the activated mineral. The average length of life of a red corpuscle has been established by labeling the iron in the cell's hemoglobin. An average lifetime of about 44 days was found.

Studies with isotopes are being conducted on what happens to the chemical elements in food when they are transformed into tissue or energy—the process called metabolism. The role of cholesterol, the fatty molecule believed to be partly responsible for arteriosclerosis, is likewise becoming better understood with the aid of isotopes. More is being learned about how the body uses sugar. When sugar is not metabolized properly, diabetes usually results. The course of sugar through the body is fol-

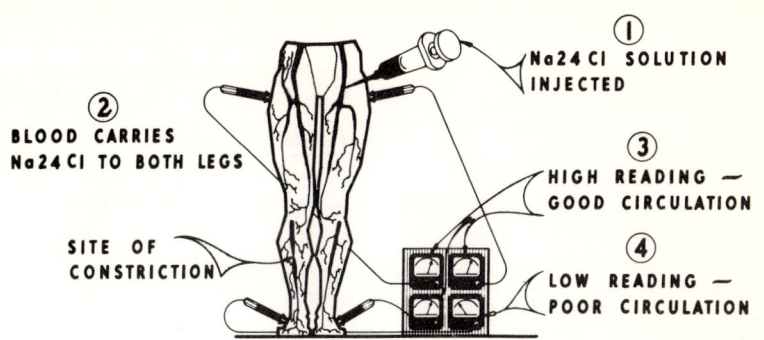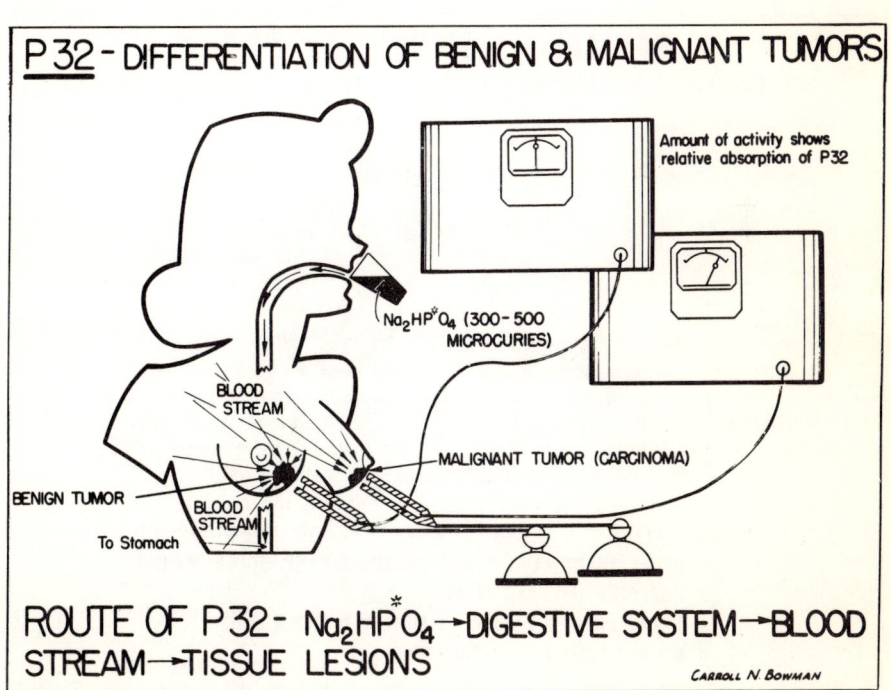

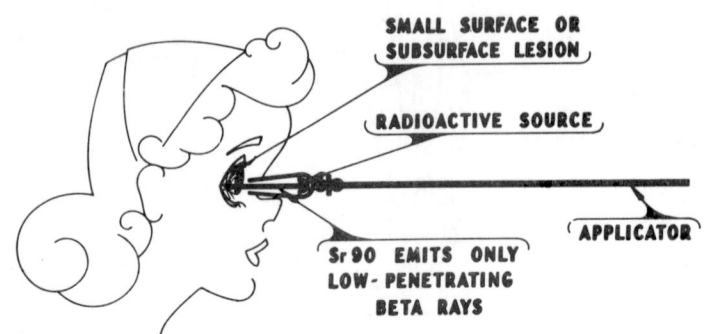
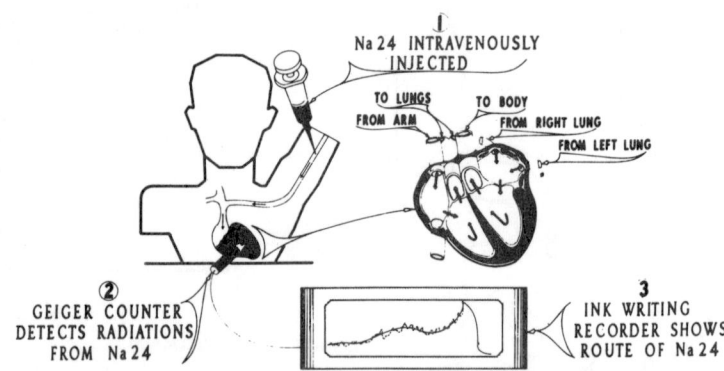

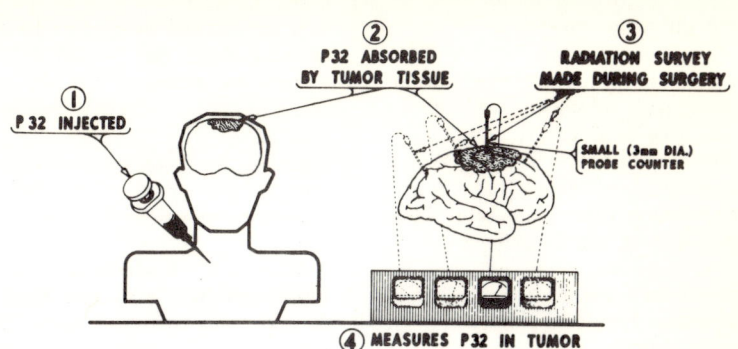

RADIOACTIVE PHOSPHORUS – P 32
FOR LOCATING EXTENT OF BRAIN TUMORS

ADVANTAGES:
1 - ABSORPTION GREATER (5-100 TIMES) IN TUMOR THAN NORMAL BRAIN TISSUE
2 - LIMITS OF TUMOR MASS ACCURATELY DETERMINED
3 - METHOD CAN BE USED DURING SURGERY

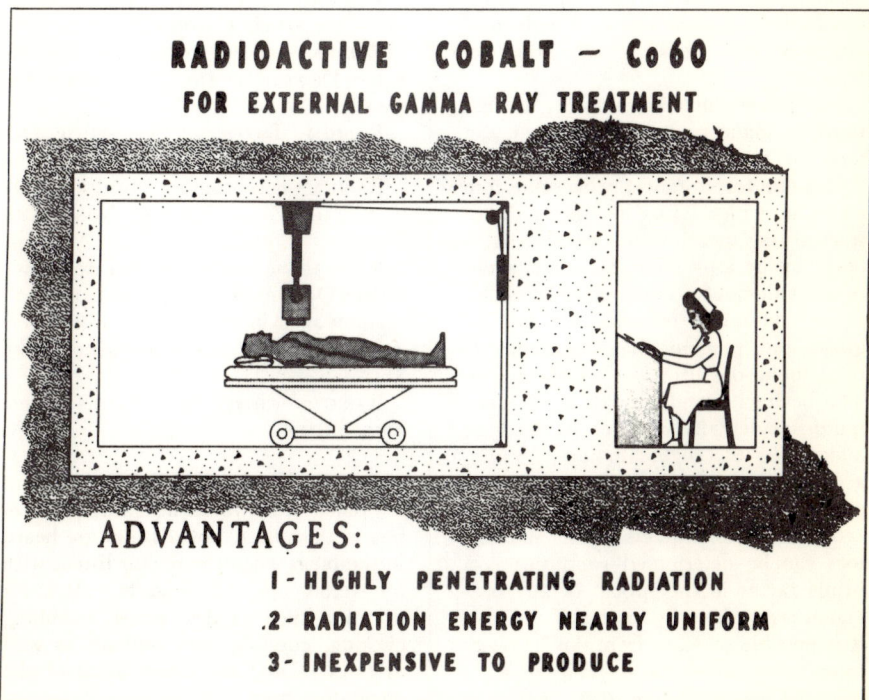

RADIOACTIVE COBALT – Co 60
FOR EXTERNAL GAMMA RAY TREATMENT

ADVANTAGES:
1 - HIGHLY PENETRATING RADIATION
2 - RADIATION ENERGY NEARLY UNIFORM
3 - INEXPENSIVE TO PRODUCE

lowed by incorporating radioactive carbon into the sugar molecule.

In drug therapy, the isotopes have been put to many uses. Knowledge of how medicinal substances act in the body has been fragmentary and inexact. How does the body use a drug? Where does it accumulate? What "breakdown" or end products does it liberate? How long does a drug remain active?

These questions could not be answered precisely before the advent of the isotopes because biological and chemical methods available were not sufficiently sensitive. With the isotopes, the course of a drug can be followed through all the body's organs and tissues, and through the urine and feces. The sensitivity of this new technique is revealed by experiments in which 1 milligram of digitalis was traced, over a period of 35 days, in a human subject to whom this "heart drug" was administered. This delicate method will provide new facts about the way drugs behave in the body.

Mosquitoes, including those types that transmit malaria and yellow fever, can now be tagged with isotopes. Radiostrontium, for instance, when put into water in which larvae of the malaria-transmitting mosquito are developnig, is taken up by a peculiar gland, analagous to the kidney of a mammal. The radioactive substance concentrates in this gland and remains there permanently throughout the life cycle of the insect. The bevhavior and growth of the mosquito, incidentally, are not in the least affected by the slight amount of radioactivity which the insect harbors in its anatomy.

The migratory habits of the mosquitoes can be determined—and this is a prime factor in the spread of any contagion transmitted by insects. Then, too, it is possible to learn from the "tagged" mosquitoes more about their span of life, the places where they prefer to breed, how far they may fly, or whether they are carried by natural forces, such as winds, from one locality to another. Data thus obtained can be used in planning more effective programs for controlling diseases borne by insects, especially in those regions of the world that are still ravaged by the winged vectors of infection.

RADIUM Radium is a rare metal discovered by Pierre and Marie Curie in 1899 and is known particularly because it emits rays which have the power to control the growth of human tissue. Radium rays have been used in the treatment of all sorts of skin diseases, cancers and other new growths of the skin, hemorrhage, and infections.

RADIUM—birthmarks: See SKIN, article THE SKIN.

RADIUM—cancer caused by overexposure: See article CANCER.

RADIUM—cancer treatment: See articles DIGESTION AND DIGESTIVE DISEASES; CANCER.

RADIUM—discovery: See article OCCUPATION AND HEALTH.

RADIUM—nose tumors: See EAR, article THE EAR, TONGUE, NOSE, AND THROAT.

RADIUM—occupational diseases: See article OCCUPATION AND HEALTH.

RADIUM—skin unprotected from overexposure to rays: See SKIN, article THE SKIN.

RADIUM—warts: See SKIN, article THE SKIN.

RÂLE The word "râle" comes from a French word meaning rattle and refers to the various sounds that are heard in the lungs when the doctor listens with his stethoscope. He describes all kinds of râles, such as dry, moist, bubbling, clicking, gurgling, and sibilant, as well as râles related to certain areas of the respiratory tract.

RATBITE FEVER The bite of a rat, or less commonly of other animals like the ferret, the cat, the dog, the weasel, the squirrel, and the pig, sometimes injects into the body of human beings organisms which are capable of setting up infection with fever, nervous symptoms, and serious disability. The infection is called ratbite fever.

Another condition like ratbite fever is called Haverhill fever. It also is caused by the bite of a rat, and sometimes by taking food and drink which have been contaminated with an organism similar to that conveyed by ratbite.

Japanese investigators were first to discover that the bite of the rat injects into the body of the person bitten a spiral organism which is responsible for the symptoms.

Haverhill fever is so named because the first epidemic which was studied occurred in Haverhill, Massachusetts. Since that time other cases have been found in other portions of the United States.

It is apparent that the germs responsible live in the noses and throats of rats without disturbing them, but cause a variety of diseases with fever when conveyed to human beings.

Ratbite fever has been found in practically every part of the world. It is seen most often in infants and children, the youngest child on record being an infant who was bitten on the eleventh day of his life and died from the infection.

Not every rat has the infection. In the United States the largest and most vicious species are the Norway or sewer rats which are found mostly in underground places and the sleeping quarters of poorly constructed houses. This is the type of rat responsible in most cases of ratbite fever.

There is an incubation period for infection from ratbite fever ranging from one to four weeks. Then when the disease begins, there is fever which goes up and down and which disappears briefly from time to time. Occasionally there is a skin rash.

Haverhill fever is distinguished from ratbite fever by the fact that its incubation period is much shorter and the fever does not come and go as in ratbite fever. If there is any skin eruption, it is small. Usually in Haverhill fever the joints are involved as part of the condition.

Most patients recover, particularly if the condition is diagnosed early and if treatment is given promptly. Anyone bitten by a rat should, of course, have the wound cauterized at once by a physician, who will use a solution of carbolic acid; then strong antiseptic solutions are applied to destroy such germs as may remain in the wound.

The spiral germs of ratbite fever are controlled by the giving of preparations of arsphenamine. The treatment of Haverhill fever is still under investigation. It has been found, however, that the sulfonamide drugs and salicylic acid do not control this infection.

RATBITE FEVER—See article TRANSMISSIBLE DISEASES.

RATS—encephalitis: See article TRANSMISSIBLE DISEASES.

RATS—thallium used in poisons: See article OCCUPATION AND HEALTH.

RATS—typhus carried by: See SKIN, article THE SKIN.

RAT CONTROL Scientists estimate that rats cause an annual loss of property in the United States of almost a billion dollars.

A new rat killer called ANTU can destroy rats as DDT destroys insects. The letters ANTU stand for a chemical substance known as alpha-naphthyl-thiourea.

A similar product was first used to test taste because of a special bitter quality. Tests were carried out first on rats because rodents have the special ability of being able to select nourishing foods and to avoid poisonous substances.

The day after the first test made with this chemical on the rats all of them were dead. Human beings had tasted the substance without harm. The investigators found that laboratory rats would eat enough of this chemical, which was called phenylthiourea, to poison them; but that wild rats, which had been trapped in city dumps, objected to the bitter taste and would not eat bait that had been treated with it. The chemists then selected twenty-four different substances like phenylthiourea for tests and finally chose ANTU.

ANTU affects dogs, cats, and other pets but it is so much less poisonous for them that it will not injure them. A single dose will kill a half-pound rat quickly but will have little effect on a ten-pound dog.

ANTU kills rats in a peculiar manner. After the rat has taken a small quantity the lungs fill up with body fluid, which suffocates the rat exactly as if it had been drowned. Strangely, ANTU is less effective against the common house mouse than against the brown Norway rat.

As an indication of the effectiveness of ANTU, one pound of the substance is sufficient to kill 200,000 rats. The product is mixed with finely ground corn or wheat or as a spray or dust on cut-up vegetables, tomatoes, or potatoes that are readily eaten by rats.

REACTION TIME OF OLDER PEOPLE (See also discussion under *Accidents, Degenerative Changes, Senescence*) Older people's common fear of falling and their frequent accidents while crossing streets are probably due to the fact that older people need more time to get information from their surroundings. Reaction time measurements were made on 54 men ranging in age from 18 to 83 years. Older men reacted significantly slower than young men even when alerted in advance of the appropriate moment for making a response. The speed of response was measured in a finger movement operation when there was a time interval between a warning signal (a light) and reaction signal (buzzer). The mean reaction time was .31 seconds for the elderly; corresponding values for young men were .21 seconds.

REDUCING SCIENTIFICALLY (See also entries on *Diet*) The ability of the body to retard destruction of its own tissue for fuel during starvation was widely confirmed in the survival of prisoners in concentration camps during the war. There is no evidence that overfeeding produces an opposite effect resulting in an increased basal and total energy expenditure which tends to maintain body weight at a constant level. Therefore obesity can not be attributed to the failure of such a mechanism. The obese individual does not use food more economically than the normal. Under equal conditions his energy requirement exceeds that of the normal individual of the same age, height, and sex.

Obesity is not uniformly associated with glandular disorders. Where they occur together the obesity is frequently present before the onset of the disease. Where it has followed the disease it can be attributed to decreased activity associated with a good appetite.

Weight reduction can be accomplished by limitation of caloric intake to sufficiently low levels. A failure to achieve weight loss can always be attributed to water retention. If the lowered intake is continued the tissues will release the water, with resulting weight loss.

The causes of overeating are varied. The childhood environment may have been one in which the habit of eating rich foods was established. The overfed appearance of many businessmen may be the result of conducting business over the luncheon table. The parent who has experienced economic difficulty in obtaining food may stress its importance too much in training the child. He may consider a large appetite an expression of good health and encourage immoderate eating. The enjoyment of the flavors of food and the comfort of a full stomach may lead to excessive intake. The housewife may eat to break her dull work routine or the one who lives alone may eat to relieve the monotony of his day. Availability of food is a factor. Occupations involving food preparation often result in overweight workers. Appetite may be exaggerated in time of emotional strain. Eating may lessen anxiety caused by failures, family difficulties, or illnesses. In some individuals fatigue may lead to overeating. The onset of obesity may occur when the individual is bedridden and continues his established eating habits. Indulgence in food may serve as compensation for a disabling disease.

Stare has stated that he believes "excessive caloric intake is the single most extensive nutritional problem affecting public health in this country." The continuance of early food habits after the need for food intake has been reduced is one of the most insidious and easily avoided causes of overeating. A regular checking of weight and immediate adjustment of caloric intake can prevent overweight. People should be taught to avoid obesity. Teaching of good nutrition should be a part of the school program. The school lunch offers both teaching and practice material for nutrition education. The school-lunch program should be directed by a nutritionist who meets the same academic standards as other members of the faculty and receives her salary from the same source.

Training in his nutritional needs should be a part of the child's education. The eating of a well-balanced lunch should be a part of his practice of good nutrition. Cost to the child should be for the prepared food. There is no more justification for including cost of equipment used in preparation of the lunch in his meal check than there is for charging him for the desk at which he learns arithmetic.

If we fail to prevent obesity we must find a cure. Growth in stature in obese children is in excess of the average normal but is in harmony with that of children who mature early. Bruch has pointed out that the low-caloric diets used for adults are not suitable for these children. The well-balanced diets used for normal children are prescribed and the child permitted to grow up to his weight. In the meantime effort should be made to gain the confidence of the child and to train him and his parents in good nutrition practice.

Brown and Ohlson have called attention to the fact that the greatly restricted diets used in some reducing programs for adults do not allow for skeletal growth and the deposit of soft tissue in adolescents and young adults. A report of their studies indicates that young obese and formerly obese women must continue low-caloric diets for years in order to maintain weight at normal levels. A more generous allowance seems indicated in view of the length of time low-calorie feeding must be continued.

No attempt will be made to present a program for the grossly overweight individual whose reducing regimen should be started in a hospital under the observation of his physician. There he can adjust to the diet without temptation to supplement it. He will have the guidance of his physician in understanding the reasons for the diet and sympathetic aid in adjusting the causes of overeating. He will learn to weigh his diet and have the opportunity to observe its effectiveness. When he leaves the hospital he will be confident of his ability to carry on the reducing program.

Once the moderately obese adult has the approval of his physician he can follow a reducing plan without disturbing his normal routine to any marked degree. In deciding to embark upon a program of weight reduction certain facts must be acknowledged:

Overweight is the result of overfeeding.
The practice of overfeeding is well established and will be difficult to abandon.
Worth-while weight loss will not be accomplished by half-way measures.
Unless there is a willingness to change established eating habits weight at the normal level will not be maintained.
Obesity will not be cured by waiting until tomorrow to limit caloric intake.

Improved health, more attractive appearance, greater ease in performing work, and preservation or recovery of ability to earn a living are excellent reasons for weight reduction. However, the fat person must believe the reasons outweigh in importance his craving for food if he is to pursue the course to a successful conclusion. Once a goal has been set thought must be directed toward its attainment, not in recalling pleasant memories of food.

For the moderately obese young adult and adult a plan is offered for a reducing program in which diets at different caloric levels are planned to meet the recommended daily dietary allowances advised by the Food and Nutrition Board of the National Research Council. This is not a minimum standard, but one believed to make generous allowance for body needs.

Moderate reducing plans range from 1000–1500 calories for women and 1500–2000 calories for men. These allowances roughly approximate the basal needs for normal adults. The basal metabolic need is the energy requirement of the body while at rest and fasting for twelve to eighteen hours. It may be estimated grossly as ten calories per pound of body weight. Ideal weight for height may be determined from the early chapters of this subject. If the figure for ideal weight is used rather than actual weight a lower figure for caloric allowance will be obtained. If used in selecting a reducing diet, a more rapid rate of weight reduction can be expected than from one based on actual weight.

A diet providing food energy (calories) equal to ten times the ideal weight will provide for the basal needs of the individual. The need for energy to perform work must then be supplied by the oxidation of body tissue. Protein in body tissue is associated with water equal to three times its weight and fat with water equal to one tenth its weight. When protein and fat are burned as fuel the water is released and excreted. Weight loss will equal the sum of protein and fat used plus associated water. Each pound of body fat oxidized will result in a weight loss of 1.1 pounds.

If there is a deficit of 900 calories per day, or 6300 calories per week, in the diet, the body must give up 700 grams of fat for fuel (700 × 9 calories per gram = 6300 calories). The total weight loss will equal 770 grams, or approximately one pound ten ounces. Since the body gives up this water unwillingly, the fat may be consumed without an immediate weight loss. A temporary gain may even occur because the body is withholding additional water as well. This maintenance of body weight in spite of tissue destruction may continue for as long as two weeks. If the diet is continued the tissues will release the water and the total expected loss will occur suddenly.

The obese individual is less likely to lose body protein on a diet of limited intake than the individual of normal weight. It is important that only body fatty tissue be used for energy expenditure in weight reduction. The protein included in this diet plan is adequate in quantity and of high quality. The 1000-calorie diet is somewhat below the recommended iron allowance for women. If liver is used once a week or kidney or heart twice a week as the source of meat the iron content is raised to the recommended level. In the 1000 and 1200-calorie diets the proportion of vitamin A contributed by carotene is greater than the two thirds average value of unrestricted diets on which the recommendation was based. Since carotene is presumed to have less than one half the value of vitamin A, the available vitamin will be low unless there is a wise selection of foods. In planning the menu two leafy green vegetables should be chosen. It is intended that a green lettuce shall be used for salads in these diets. These selections will improve the iron and niacin content of the diet as well.

Since obesity is the result of overeating, these diets have been planned to provide for a loss in weight and to set a dietary pattern that can be followed after weight reduction has been accomplished. The foods included in the pattern supply the ingredients of an adequate diet. Once normal weight has been achieved food to supply energy for body activity can be added.

It is not expected that the individual can resume his former eating habits without an accompanying weight gain. Once the reducing plan has been decided upon it should be pursued until the desired weight has been reached. Foods can then be added to maintain weight at the normal level.

Diets have been planned to supply body nutritional needs with the exception of calories. It is expected that the individual following a diet plan will change his habits. His obesity indicates that he has followed the practice of overeating. He must establish new eating habits that can be continued with certain modifications when weight loss has been achieved. Some adjustments relating to family and associates must be made. The less conspicuously these can be accomplished the better. Everyone is familiar with talk of diet which is either a bid for sympathy or the result of a hope that someone will urge the use of forbidden food. It is wiser to postpone discussion of the diet until an obvious weight loss indicates the use of one worth talking about.

Omission of meals is undesirable, since there is a temptation to overeat if one is very hungry. However, it is usually possible to omit some foods from other meals of the day if one is to be a guest and cannot refuse food inconspicuously. With this in mind it is well to establish the habit of eating slowly, since one is not urged to take a second serving if the plate is still half full.

A common source of energy in many diets is the cream and sugar added to coffee. The addition of only one teaspoon of sugar and two of cream to a cup of coffee will add 40 calories. Multiply this by three or even six, and 120-240 calories have been added to the daily diet. If this intake is in excess of body need it will be stored as fat. In one week three and one half to seven ounces of fat could be stored from this source alone. Black coffee yields no energy. It is preferred by those who have learned to drink it. The taste, once acquired, will eliminate the temptation to return to a practice that contributed to the condition of overweight. The use of saccharin in coffee is not encouraged, since it only serves to continue a taste for sweets that may interfere later in following a maintenance diet.

The individual who must lose weight or guard against a gain in weight may order black coffee without adding to his caloric intake while his friends drink Coca-Cola, or he may add a few calories as orange juice while they consume a soda. The caloric yield of alcoholic beverages bars their use in any reducing program.

Muscle tone in body areas where fat has been withdrawn will probably be improved by moderate exercise. Strenuous exercise interferes with adherence to the diet by stimulation of the appetite. Since one must walk thirty-six miles to destroy one pound of fatty tissue, exercise is not a practical means of weight reduction.

The diets in this plan are based in the use of milk in greater amount than in the average adult diet. Milk provides high quality protein at lower cost than other sources. The caloric value is low. At the same time its contribution to the total allowance of other dietary essentials is high. A taste for it can be acquired easily. Milk lends itself to menu planning.

All foods listed above the double line in the diet pattern are essential if the diet is to supply the recommended nutrients. These foods are to be included in the diet each day. Permitted substitutions are given for foods listed below the double line.

3½ OUNCES VEGETABLE
Asparagus, 9 medium spears—4″ × ¾″
Broccoli, head—3½″ diam. × 5″ long
Brussels sprouts, 7—1¼″ diam.
Carrot strips, 28—³⁄₁₆″ strips, 6″ long
Celery heart, 1½″ diam. × 4½″ long
Green pepper, 1½—2″ diam. × 4¾″ long
Leaf lettuce, 18—5″ × 6″ leaves
Potato, 1—2½″ diam.
Radish, 14—1″ diam.
Tomato, 1—2¼″ diam. × 2″ thick

Cabbage, shredded ⎫
Carrot, shredded ⎪
Celery, diced ⎪
Green pepper, diced ⎬ 1 cup
Green onion, diced ⎪
Head lettuce, diced ⎪
Radish, sliced ⎭
Chicory, chopped 1½ cup
Cucumber, sliced ¾ cup
Green beans, cooked ¾ cup
Beets, diced cooked ½ cup
Beet greens ½ cup
Cabbage, cooked ¾ cup
Carrots, cooked diced ¾ cup
Cauliflower, cooked ⅔ cup
Mustard greens ½ cup
Sauerkraut ⅔ cup
Spinach, cooked ½ cup
Squash, mashed ½ cup
Turnip greens, cooked ½ cup
Tomatoes, stewed ½ cup
Tomato juice ½ cup

3½ OUNCES FRUIT—FRESH
Apple, ⅔—2¾″ diam.
Apple, 1—2″ diam.
Blueberries, ⅔ cup
Cantaloupe, ½ cup pulp
Cantaloupe, ⅓—4½″ melon
Cherries, ⅔ cup
Grapefruit, ½—3¾″ diam.
(80 size)
Grapes, Malaga, 17—1½″ × ¾″ diam.
Grapes, Rebier, 12—1¼″ × 1″ diam.
Orange, 1—3″ (176 size)
Peach, 1—2½″ diam.
Pear, ⅔—3¼″ × 2⅜″
Raspberries, fresh, 1 cup
Strawberries, fresh, ⅔ cup

3½ OUNCES FRUIT—
   CANNED WITHOUT SUGAR
Apricots, 3—1½″ diam.
Cherries, 14—¾″ diam.
Peaches, 2 halves—2½″ diam.
Pears, 2 halves—2½″ × 2¼″ diam.
Pineapple, 2½ slices—3″ slice, ⁷⁄₁₆″ thick

⅔ OUNCE CEREAL
Branflakes ½ cup
Cooked cereals ½ cup

Cornflakes	1 cup
Corn Soya	⅜ cup
Grapenuts	¼ cup
Puffed Rice	1¼ cup
Puffed Wheat	1 cup
Rice Krispies	¾ cup

LEAN MEAT

2 ounces, 2" × 4½" × ½"
3 ounces, 3" × 4½" × ½"
4 ounces, 4" × 4½" × ½"

Measures are given for three-and-one-half-ounce servings of fruits and vegetables in the menu plan.

The caloric value of vinegar dressing is negligible and may be used on salads as desired.

½ cup vinegar
½ teaspoon salt
¼ teaspoon paprika
1 grain saccharin
1 tablespoon of grated onion or clove of garlic

Oil-and-vinegar dressing is permitted only when and in amounts allowed in the diet. One tablespoon of dressing will be equivalent to two squares of butter or two teaspoons of oil.

½ cup salad oil
¼ cup vinegar
2 teaspoons salt
clove of garlic

The diet allowance is divided into three meals with approximately equitable distribution of the protein. This distribution should be maintained. Protein digests more slowly than carbohydrates, and the meals will give greater satisfaction if protein is spread throughout the day. If for greater convenience it is desirable to shift a part of the lunch to the evening meal neither milk nor meat should be changed. The milk may be saved for a midafternoon feeding if the dinner hour is very late.

The foods in the diet supply all the nutrients needed by the body, calories excepted. After ideal weight has been achieved they should continue to form the basis of the diet. A regular check of body weight will serve as a guide to the amount of food that should be eaten to maintain the body in a state of good nutrition.

DIET PLAN FOR REDUCING SCIENTIFICALLY

CALORIES	1000	1200	1400	1600	1800	2000
PROTEIN	69	81	83	86	86	91
All foods listed above double line to be included each day						
Egg	1	1	1	1	1	1
Citrous fruit	3½ oz.	3½ oz.	3½ oz.	3½ oz.	3½ oz.	3½ oz.
Fruit—fresh or unsweetened canned	7 oz.	7 oz.	7 oz.	7 oz.	7 oz.	7 oz.
Leafy green vegetable—raw	3½ oz.	3½ oz.	3½ oz.	3½ oz.	3½ oz.	3½ oz.
Additional leafy green or yellow vegetable	3½ oz.	3½ oz.	3½ oz.	3½ oz.	3½ oz.	3½ oz.
Additional vegetable	3½ oz.	3½ oz.	3½ oz.	3½ oz.	3½ oz.	3½ oz.
Skim milk	1½ pt.	1½ pt.	1½ pt.	1½ pt.	—	—
Whole milk	—	—	—	—	1½ pt.	1½ pt.
Butter (squares cut 72 to lb. or 18 to ¼ lb.)	1 sq.	2 sq.	5 sq.	5 sq.	3 sq.	5 sq.
Bread (commercial thin slice = ⅔ oz.)	⅔ oz. (1 slice)	1⅔ oz. 2½ slices)	1⅔ oz. (2½ slices)	1⅓ oz. (2 slices)	2 oz. (3 slices)	2⅔ oz. (4 slices)
Cereal	—	—	—	⅔ oz.	⅔ oz.	1 oz.
Potato—2½″ diam.	—	—	1	1	1	2
Lean meat, fish, or fowl	5 oz.	7 oz.	7 oz.	7 oz.	7 oz.	7 oz.
Bacon (⅔ oz. = 1 slice, 1½″ × 9″ × ⅛″)	—	—	—	⅔ oz.	—	—
Fat or oil	—	—	—	—	2 tsp.	—
Sugar	—	—	—	—	1 tbs.	1 tbs.

The following substitutes may be made in foods listed below double line:

Omit		1½ slices bread	1½ slices bread	½ slice bread	½ slice bread	1½ slices bread
Add		⅔ oz. cereal	⅔ oz. cereal 3½ oz. vegetable			3½ oz. fruit
Omit		2 squares butter			Oil and ½ square butter	2½ squares butter
Add		1 tbs. oil-vinegar dressing or 2 tsp. mayonnaise or 1 tbs. French dressing			⅔ oz. bacon	⅔ oz. bacon
Omit		Cereal			Cereal	Cereal
Add		Potato			Potato	2 slices bread
Omit					Sugar	Sugar
Add					3½ oz. fruit or ⅔ oz. cereal	
Omit	2 oz. meat	3 oz. meat	3 oz. meat	3 oz. meat	3 oz. meat	3 oz. meat
Add	½ cup cottage cheese, ⅝ cup cottage cheese, or 2 eggs or 8 oz. skim milk plus ½ square butter					
Omit			1 potato	1 potato	1 potato	1 potato
Add			Banana (5″ × 1⅜″) or green lima beans (½ cup) or sweet potato (3″ × 1¾″) or peas (¾ cup) or rice (⅜ cup) or macaroni (⅜ cup)			

MENU PLAN

CALORIES	1000	1200	1400	1600	1800	2000
Breakfast						
Citrous fruit	3½ oz.	3½ oz.	3½ oz.	3½ oz.	3½ oz.	3½ oz.
Egg	1	1	1	1	1	1
Skim Milk	8 oz.	8 oz.	8 oz.	8 oz.	—	—
Whole Milk	—	—	—	—	8 oz.	8 oz.
Bread (1 thin commercial slice = ⅔ oz.)	⅔ oz.	⅔ oz.	⅔ oz.	⅔ oz.	⅔ oz.	⅔ oz.
Butter (squares 72 to lb.)	½ sq.	½ sq.	1 sq.	1 sq.	1 sq.	1 sq.
Cereal	—	—	—	⅔ oz.	⅔ oz.	1 oz.
Bacon	—	—	—	⅔ oz.	—	—
Sugar	—	—	—	—	½ tbs.	½ tbs.
Black coffee (no caloric value)	may be used as desired.					
Lunch						
Lean meat	2 oz.	3 oz.	3 oz.	3 oz.	3 oz.	3 oz.
Vegetable salad—leafy green	3½ oz.	3½ oz.	3½ oz.	3½ oz.	3½ oz.	3½ oz.
Skim milk	8 oz.	8 oz.	8 oz.	8 oz.	—	—
Whole milk	—	—	—	—	8 oz.	8 oz.
Fruit	3½ oz.	3½ oz.	3½ oz.	3½ oz.	3½ oz.	3½ oz.

Bread (1 thin commercial slice = ⅔ oz.)	—	⅔ oz.	⅔ oz.	⅔ oz.	⅔ oz.	1⅓ oz.
Butter	—	½ sq.	1 sq.	1 sq.	1 sq.	2 sq.
Potato	—	—	—	—	—	1
Vinegar dressing (no caloric value)	may be used as desired.					
Black coffee or plain tea (no caloric value)	may be used as desired.					
Dinner						
Lean meat	3 oz.	4 oz.	4 oz.	4 oz.	4 oz.	4 oz.
Skim milk	8 oz.	8 oz.	8 oz.	—	—	—
Whole milk	—	—	—	8 oz.	8 oz.	8 oz.
Vegetable salad—leafy green	3½ oz.	3½ oz.	3½ oz.	3½ oz.	3½ oz.	3½ oz.
Vegetable	3½ oz.	3½ oz.	3½ oz.	3½ oz.	3½ oz.	3½ oz.
Fruit	3½ oz.	3½ oz.	3½ oz.	3½ oz.	3½ oz.	3½ oz.
Bread	—	⅓ oz. (½ slice)	—	—	⅔ oz. (1 slice)	⅔ oz. (1 slice)
Butter	½ sq.	1 sq.	3 sq.	3 sq.	1 sq.	2 sq.
Potato	—	1	1	1	1	1
Oil and vinegar dressing	—	—	—	—	—	1 tbs.
Vinegar dressing (no caloric value)	may be used as desired.					
Black coffee (no caloric value)	may be used as desired.					

REFLEX The word "reflex" is used to describe a reaction or movement which is reflected from some stimulus far away. Essentially a reflex is an involuntary action. Among the reflexes most commonly known are the knee jerk, which is absent in many diseases of the brain and spinal cord, and other similar responses related to tests on other parts of the body. The oculocardiac reflex is a slowing of the rhythm of the heart that follows compression of the eyeball. A slowing of 5 to 13 beats per minute is normal. Anything more or less than that is not normal. Laughter brought on by tickling is also a reflex action, also vomiting when the throat is tickled with a feather. The swallowing reflex takes place when some substance is put on the back of the tongue. If a baby jumps when he hears a loud sound, that is called a startle reflex.

REGRESSION (See also discussion under *Emotions, Mental Depression, Middle-Life Disturbances, Neurosis, Senescence*) The progress of regression in older people, sometimes referred to as "second childhood," can be reversed in many instances, according to Dr. M. E. Linden, Director of the Division of Mental Health in the Philadelphia Department of Public Health. Many of these symptoms of senility result from a state of panic in the aged person when he feels that he has been rejected by society. Whether or not the feeling of neglect and isolation is real or imagined, the person reacts by building up tighter psychological defenses against his environment, or by losing all of his usual defenses. In either case, regression takes place.

The amount of regression varies, and in some cases is extreme. The stage of past psychological development to which the senile person regresses provides a clue to neurotic disturbances which may have lain dormant throughout his life.

Treatment must be designed to deal with specifically diagnosed psychiatric conditions.

RESEARCH IN CANCER (See also discussion under *Cancer*) So vast is the amount of material regularly published on cancer that a complete review is well nigh impossible in a volume much larger than this. Recently Dr. Cornelius Rhoads of the Sloan-Kettering Institute has surveyed the present attack on cancer. He points out that better means for early diagnosis are continually being found, that surgical and radiological treatments of cancer have been improved and much information is being obtained as to various approaches to cancer by the use of ionizing radiation of various energies. This has been made possible through our knowledge of atomic energy. Means have been found for measuring the ability of chemicals to control some forms of cancer and each new technique that is offered is tested by these means. The chemists are putting together new formulas which have the power to control cancer. Some types of human cancer have been grown outside the human body and are thus studied. Scientists have found that certain viruses have the power to attack cancer. Much more information has been obtained relative to the relationship of the glands such as the pituitary and the adrenal glands in the growth of cancer. Study has also been devoted to the function of the thyroid gland and particularly to thyroid cancer.

Much is being done toward the prevention of cancer by educating people as to recognition of the earliest possible symptoms. The steroid hormones such as the hormones formed by the sex glands in the adrenal glands are known to be able to affect cancer as will be discussed later. Certain types of cancer in animals can be prevented by giving these hormones. Evidence is developing as to the effect of various cancer causing agents in the air and in smoke. Information has developed new techniques for preventing cancer of the uterus in women. All of this points to the understanding that cancer is not just a single condition affecting a portion of the tissues of the body but a condition in which all of the body may play a part in development, in maintenance and in control.

In 1915 two Japanese produced malignant tumors by painting rabbits ears with tar. The knowledge that this could be accomplished gave a new method to the scientists for studying cancer. By 1948 scientists demonstrated that substances which contain only carbon and hydrogen could cause tumors. The hydrocarbons as they are called are of many different varieties. The one that has been most definitely proved to be cancerogenic is 3, 4-benzpyrine. This has now been proved to be a constituent of many industrial smokes and wastes and its presence in such materials may be definitely related to the rise of cancer of the lung.

In 1775 cancer of the sex organs in men who were chimney sweeps was definitely related to the accumulation of soot on the skin of the testes. Benzpyrine has been isolated from domestic soot, from carbon blacks, from atmospheric dust in cities, and from oils used in industries.

The accumulation of new knowledge about cancer is largely a triumph of teams including chemists, physicists, biologists and pathologists. Such teams demonstrated that the hormones contain chemical structures which are definitely related to the activity of human cells. This has given rise to the view that cancer may result from an unknown substance that arises in the body from altered use by the body of steroid substances. Experimental observations have proved that proliferation of tissues of the vagina, the uterus and the breast of female mice might be brought about through stimulation by ovarian hormones. Studies on mice have indicated the possibility of causing cancer of the breast by such action and investigators were able to reduce the rate of formation on the breast to zero or almost zero by the removal of the ovaries of the mice at the time of their beginning sexual maturity.

The ovarian secretions are known now to play a definite role in the inducing of cancer of the breast in animals which have a high hereditary susceptibility to cancer. Similarly there has been found a relationship to natural estrogenic hormones and cancer of the breast in men. Huggins of the University of Chicago showed the effects of male and female sex hormones on the prostate gland. Similarly cancer of the breast in women may be inhibited by the male sex hormone. Now it is known that the hormones of the pituitary glands are also related to the growth of tissue in the body. Experiments have been done involving the surgical removal of the entire pituitary gland with a view to stopping the rapid advance of cancer. The proof that hormones are the direct causes of cancer does not exist but the possibility of production within the body of cancer-causing substances as by-products of the body's action on steroids is being continually investigated. The hormones do exert effects on the rates of growth and development of the cells. In the processes of growth enzymes and vitamins are of course intimately involved.

Although repeated studies have not been able to demonstrate the presence of virus in human cancers, evidence definitely exists to the effect that viruses can be associated with growths. Thus viruses can cause the rapid growth of warts. Even if the viruses are not directly related to the production of cancer, they may be involved secondarily in stimulating growth. Viruses grow only in living cells, and often stimulate the growth of such cells followed by cell destruction. The viruses pick out certain kinds of tissue on which they live but viruses change their ways and change the ways of the tissues they attack. Viruses can remain latent in tissues from infancy to late in life. They cause one type of lesions in young people and perhaps others in older people.

Much attention has been given to a virus known as the Bittner virus which is transmitted in milk and which definitely affects the incidence of cancer of the breast in mice. Bittner demonstrated that the factor was commonly transferred in the milk during nursing by the mice. This is a highly specialized phenomenon which cannot be translated directly into any relationship to human cancer.

During World War II extensive studies were made as to the effects of poison gases on the tissues of the body. Evidence was accumulated that they stopped growth by interfering with the ability of cells to divide and reproduce. After all, cancer represents a speeded up process of this kind. Actual experiments in the armed forces proved that certain types of cancer of blood-forming tissue could be halted by nitrogen mustard war gas. A number of chemical substances related to war gases have been developed and have been applied to various forms of cancer in animals before being used on human beings. The beneficial effects they exert are small except for cancer of blood-forming tissues but even in these disorders the effects are limited.

The human cells contain a substance called nucleic acid which conveys inherited properties from parent to daughter cells during the course of their division and growth. The chemical substances that affect cancers act on this chemical process. The development of nucleic acid in the cells of the body requires a vitamin called folic acid. This vitamin is essential to the growth particularly of blood cells and in fact folic acid is now used in cases of pernicious anemia. Substances have been prepared which are antifolic acid substances and have been used in acute leukemia in children. One such new compound which affects nucleic acid is called 6-Mercaptopurine. This chemical is now perhaps the most widely used compound employed in the treatment of leukemia. While it is not curative, it definitely affects the condition and prolongs life.

Also new in the attack on cancer in the Sloan-Kettering Institute for cancer research is the development of anti-cancer viruses. Viruses as has already been explained reproduce only by acting on certain types of cells, sometimes causing the death of the host cells. The virus of the common cold kills the cells lining the nose. The virus of infantile paralysis attacks certain cells in the brain and spinal cord. These examples indicate that viruses can injure some kinds of cells and leave others unharmed. Experiments on animals with some of the new viruses developed in the Institute have shown that a possibility does exist of developing viruses which might attack cancer cells and not disturb ordinary normal cells.

The Respiratory Diseases

BY

MORRIS FISHBEIN, M.D.

Former Editor, *Journal American Medical Association,* Chicago; Editor, *Excerpta Medica, Bulletin World Medical Assn.; Post-graduate Medicine.*

The Common Cold

WHEN WILLIAM OSLER wrote his *Principles and Practice of Medicine,* the most popular textbook of medicine ever published, he began with typhoid fever, probably because typhoid was one of the most serious and incapacitating diseases affecting a vast number of people. Students learned to study diseases according to the way in which William Osler systematized knowledge of typhoid. Today typhoid is definitely under control and really disturbs but few people.

Now one of the most widely used textbooks of medicine begins with the common cold—and rightly. Infections of the nose, throat, and sinuses are responsible for more than one half the time lost by wage earners due to sickness. Everybody knows how to cure a cold, and, even if he does not, will tell *you.* You can put your feet in a mustard bath, drink several glasses of hot lemonade, carry a buckeye in your right rear pocket, wear an iron ring, indulge freely in many of the widely advertised remedies, and even take some of the beverages that once required a doctor's prescription and about which the government expressed considerable doubt as to curative value—and at the end of three days you will probably begin to get well almost regardless of the treatment.

The common cold is essentially a self-limited disease. Unfortunately, however, it does not, like an attack of measles or scarlet fever, induce in the person who has it a resistance or immunity which will prevent him from having a cold soon again. People who have colds seem to have them often. Those who are easily susceptible constitute about 23 per cent; they have colds four or more times a year. Sixty per cent of people have colds two or three times a year and 17 per cent once a year or not at all.

There is a great difference between the common cold and epidemic influenza of the type that devastated the world in 1918. That was a definite infectious disease, highly contagious, affecting vast numbers of people and causing a terrific number of deaths. The history of medicine shows that at least eight great pandemics of influenza had previously swept the world, beginning with one in 1580, the seventh occurring in 1889–1892. The common cold is something quite different.

CAUSES OF COLDS

Changes in the weather have been incriminated as a cause of colds from the time of Hippocrates. Geologists, geographists, physiographers, and biometricians have tried to find certain relationships between changes in the weather and the occurrence of colds; as a result, some definite knowledge is now available. Most colds occur in October; then comes a slight drop in the incidence, with a new peak in January and in February, working up to a rather high point in March; then another gradual drop with a low rate in summer, the rate rising gradually to the October maximum. From October to April, whenever the maximum temperature, the average temperature, or the dry bulb temperature falls below the ordinary figures, there is a slight tendency of the incidence of colds to rise. It has not been found, however, that there is any relationship between the maximum temperature, humidity, rainfall, wind velocity, sunshine, or atmospheric pressure. In the warm period, from April to October, whenever the maximum temperature, the average temperature range, the dry bulb temperature, the vapor pressure, or the pecentage of sunshine falls below the ordinary level, there is likely to be a rise in the number of colds. Apparently there is a great deal in the general effect of atmosphere on the human being, but it is rather difficult to determine just how these effects are brought about.

Some time ago investigators in a large clinic proved that the ability of a person with rheumatism to predict a change in the weather is an actual ability, and that it is based on changes that take place in the body before the change in weather occurs. The opinion of at least twenty centuries that there is a definite relationship between sudden changes in the weather and catching cold tends to be borne out by modern scientific investigations but is not absolutely established. A professor of hygiene in the University of Amsterdam found a definite relationship between changes in temperature and the occurrence of the common cold in seven thousand people who kept a careful record of their colds while he kept a record of the weather. If it can be shown that difficulties with the heat regulation of the human body are fundamental to catching cold, the obvious way to prevent colds will be to develop methods for keeping the heat of the body constant.

The noted British physiologist, A. V. Hill, believes that cold weather brings about a large number of colds because people shut themselves up in warm, stuffy rooms and perspire; then submit themselves to the outdoor air without proper protection. The statistician for our largest insurance company found that a sudden drop of 10 degrees in the temperature brought an increase of eighteen colds per week among 6,700 employees in his office. Moreover, Prof. E. O. Jordan of the University of Chicago discovered that 90 per cent of colds occur at a time when there is less ventilation in both public and private dwellings. Here certainly is well established evidence that changes in the weather are associated with colds.

Everybody has experienced the development of a cold following a night in a sleeping car, a swim in the pool, or a shower bath immediately after being overheated by exercise. Investigators are convinced that the overheated and dehydrated air in the homes and in offices in the United States lowers the resistance of the membranes of the nose; then germs, which are almost constantly present among human beings, begin their work of infection.

There are several ways of emphasizing this fact. Extreme cold does not cause colds. Eskimos seldom have colds. A group of explorers found on visiting one Eskimo settlement that there was not one cold among the Eskimos from the tiniest infant to the most ancient patriarch of the tribe. Seventy-two hours after the expedition, which included several people who had colds, arrived in the settlement, practically every one of the Eskimos developed the characteristic symptoms. That ought to be sufficient proof that there is some transmissible agent which produces the infection. It correlates with the fact that germs do well on new soil.

Obviously, therefore, some search must be made for a specific virus as a cause of the common cold. When the cause is isolated, specific measures of prevention may follow. It is conceivable, indeed, that not one but several different organisms may produce the symptoms.

Granted that the cold is caused by an infectious organism, there must apparently be other factors or all of us would have colds all the time. These factors constitute what are called predisposing causes. Tobacco, dust, gas, the amount of sleep, sitting in a draft, constipation, perspiration, and footwear have all been suggested as possible predisposing elements. A research made by investigators at Cornell University failed to incriminate definitely any one of them. Changes in the weight and quality of underwear that is worn have been suggested. Enough evidence is available to indicate that the wearing of woolen underwear is not a panacea; besides, it itches!

Experts in diseases of the nose and throat feel that obstruction in the nose and enlarged tonsils are important in relationship to the number of colds. Numerous studies recently made failed to prove that either one of them is a certain factor. Obstructions in the nose ought to be taken care of because they interfere with breathing and perhaps bring about congestion. Enlarged and infected tonsils are a menace to health and should be removed. But the person concerned may have just as many colds, if not more, after these factors are attended to than he had previously.

Our modern methods of living may be largely responsible for the increased incidence of colds. We are crowded together in offices, in motion-picture houses, at football and basketball games. We are packed into elevators and subway cars. We breathe constantly, cough frequently, and sneeze unexpectedly in one another's faces. Moreover, our hands are constantly in contact with door knobs, pencils, dishes, and other utensils, also handled by other people. We carry our hands to our mouths and to our noses and thus transmit by what is called hand-to-mouth infection.

SYMPTOMS OF COLDS

Because of its symptoms and its rather poorly understood character in relationship to other diseases, the common cold is variously called by a number of high-sounding scientific titles, in most instances related to the part of the body particularly affected. What is known as a head cold is called coryza. Because of the increase in the temperature and the outpouring of fluid from the nose, the cold has been called acute catarrhal fever. Because the running is principally from the nose, it has been called acute catarrhal rhinitis. If the throat is hoarse, the portion affected may give the title to the disease so that it becomes acute pharyngitis, acute laryngitis, or acute tracheitis.

These anatomical designations nevertheless hardly convey the stuffiness, the chills, the irritability, the loss of appetite, and the other symptoms that are commonly associated with this disorder. The chief changes in the tissues involved are those which affect the mucous membranes of the nose and throat. The lining of the nose is red and swollen, and from it pours continuously the fluid that causes much sniffling and blowing. With the sniffling and blowing comes irritation of the skin around the nose and mouth, and, if the trouble extends down far enough, there is coughing without much discharge from the throat. The mouth is held open during sleep so that the tongue becomes thick and coated.

PREVENTION OF COLDS

What everyone wants to know is how to prevent a cold, how to stop a cold, and how to cure one. In every infection of the human body three factors are concerned: First, contact with the infecting substance; second, sufficient virulence in the infecting germ to overcome the resistance of the body, and third, sufficient resistance in the body to overcome the infecting germ.

The human family, particularly in large cities, is so crowded that it is practically impossible to avoid contact with those who have respiratory infections. Our modern apartment dwellings are simply great barracks into which families are packed, and individual dwellings are like cans into which the individual members of the family are crowded closely together.

If a single organism is responsible for the common cold, it may, of course, vary in virulence from time to time exactly as diphtheria, scarlet fever, and similar infections vary in their potency. However, what is called a variation in virulence may really be the reflection of lessening of resistance or the development of a new generation that has not the resistance of a previous generation. One conception of epidemic influenza emphasizes the fact that it occurs in cycles of some thirty years which permit the development of new generations of human beings not capable of resisting the infection. Since the germs are living organisms, it is conceivable that they may vary in their power from one occasion to another exactly as human beings vary.

Germs may be affected exactly as human beings are affected by the atmosphere in which they live, the soil on which they rest, the diet on which they thrive. The organism of the common cold may die readily on the surface of the skin but grow happily on a mucous membrane. It may die readily on a normal mucous membrane, but multiply exceedingly on a mucous membrane that has been vitiated by the continuous residence of its possessor in a hot, dry, stuffy, dusty room. Here then comes the question of proper ventilation as a factor in the onset and in the prevention of the common cold. Investigators from the United States Public Health Service studied various ventilation systems in their relationship to catching cold by children in seven schools in Connecticut. In three schools ventilation was controlled by windows, in three by fans, and in one by a special ventilating system. About thirty-six hundred pupils attended the schools. Records were kept of their absences, the daily temperature of the rooms, and the occurrence of coughs and colds among the children. The total number of absences on account of coughs and colds among the children in rooms with artificial ventilation was much larger than that among those in rooms ventilated by the open-window method—indeed, almost twice as much. Of course, the children were in school only eight hours of the day. This need not be taken, therefore, as a general condemnation of all mechanical systems of air conditioning. Assembly rooms, theaters, motion-picture houses, and places seating great crowds of people simply cannot be properly ventilated by the open-window method. In general, however, authorities on ventilation are agreed that window ventilation provides the best system for changing the air and keeping it healthful.

The most serious problem is the question of proper heating and the provision of sufficient moisture in the air. Private homes should be heated to 68 or 70 degrees, and large halls to 60 or 65 degrees F. The large halls require less heat because human beings will provide from their own bodies enough extra heat to make up the deficiency. Equally important with heat is moisture. A sufficient amount of humidity prevents chilling. Moisture can be obtained either by special devices built into furnaces which are now widely advertised and which have been proved to be efficient, or by special electric devices which have been developed for moistening the air.

The common impression that chilling, dampness, and fatigue are predisposing factors in catching cold is, as has been shown, supported by much good scientific evidence. The theory is that chilling and dampness induce a cold through disturbing the heat-regulating mechanism of the body by sudden evaporation of moisture from the surface of the body. For example, one who is quite well may sit in front of an electric fan and get up after fifteen minutes with the nose congested and with all of the beginning symptoms of a cold. The draft from the electric fan brings about chilling of the surface of the body and disturbs the circulation of the blood in the mucous membranes of the nose.

Conditioning against colds has behind it the acceptance of many hygienic authorities. The technic of conditioning involves the building of resistance through proper hygiene and a few special measures directed specifically against the predisposing causes. One of these technics is the cold-bath technic. A cold shower is all right for anyone who wants it, provided he rubs himself thoroughly thereafter with towels so as to restore a brisk circulation to the congealed surface. The majority of people probably do better with a lukewarm bath taken primarily for purposes of cleanliness and only secondarily with the idea of benefiting resistance to disease.

There is also the conception that children may have their resistance increased by wrapping their throats and chests with towels wrung out of cold water. There is no good evidence in favor of this notion. Then there are the mothers who believe that they help the health of the child by baring to the wintry blasts the portion of the leg from the calf to the upper third of the thigh. It remains to be shown that any child had its resistance to colds increased by this exposure.

Certainly the biometricians have not credited such statistics as are available in favor of conditioning to cold by subjecting one's self unnecessarily to it. The reasoning in favor of the procedure is only symbolical, like the suggestion that the proper treatment of smallpox is to put the patient in a room with red velours hangings.

Germs in general succumb to sunlight. For human beings it is a pleasant measure. Hence the argument early advanced that exposure to the rays of the sun or to the rays of ultraviolet from the artificial sun lamp, using either the carbon arc or the quartz mercury vapor burner, would aid in building resistance to colds. The Council on Physical Therapy of the American Medical Association, after examining all of the evidence that could be offered in support of such measures, has withdrawn its approval from sources of ultraviolet that are advertised as beneficial in the prevention of colds. Perhaps the ultraviolet does enhance the power of the body in some generally beneficial way, but certainly it has not been proved that its effects are specific against respiratory diseases. Indeed, the exact words of the council are, "As far as normal persons are concerned, the claim that exposure to ultraviolet rays increases or improves the tone of the tissues or of the body as a whole, stimulates metabolism, or tends to prevent colds, has not been conclusively substantiated."

Vaccines Against Colds

Another measure of which much is heard in these advanced times, when people are beginning to understand medical progress and medical methods, is the use of the vaccine for the prevention of colds. The hoi-polloi refer to the use of vaccines or of any other substances administered by injection as "shots." Physicians build resistance against typhoid fever by injecting the patient with vaccine made of killed typhoid and paratyphoid germs. The injection of these killed germs stirs up the tissues of the body to resistance against the constituents of the typhoid organism. Some physicians inject mixtures of the killed bodies of germs frequently found in the noses and throats of people with colds, with the idea of building resistance to infection by these germs. There are two reasons, however, why many scientists do not approve the use of the "shots" in the cases of people with frequent colds. First, it has not been shown that any of these germs are specifically the cause of or definitely related to the colds; second, it has not been shown that the injection of these germs will stimulate resistance. Two viruses known as influenza A and B are associated with symptoms like those of a cold and vaccines against these are available. Another cold or influenza virus is called virus X. Most colds are mixed infections.

TREATMENT OF COLDS

First, everybody who knows advises rest in bed until the temperature is normal, with head of the bed elevated in order to make breathing easier. Actually, only hygienists or people who are quite serious in medical affairs go to bed when they have a cold.

The skin is usually so uncomfortable that a sponge bath with water of a temperature about 98 degrees F. is desirable, and the skin may be fairly well rubbed with a rough towel after the bath. If the bowels are inactive, it is advisable to clear them of their digested and undigested contents. The clearing may be accomplished either by washing out from below or by the usual laxatives administered above.

Fever burns tissue. Hence the diet during a cold should consist of nourishing food. Since appetite is lost in most instances anyway, food should be appetizing and enjoyable. A child should not be forced to eat what is repulsive, particularly in the presence of disturbed appetite. Let the child have what it wants. Many physicians administer sugar and fruit juices with a view to providing calories and to preventing the acid reaction which is believed to be favorable to the persistence of the cold.

The common home remedies, such as bathing the feet in mustard baths, perspiring freely under hot blankets, drinking quantities of hot lemonade and orange juice, are time-tried helps to comfort. Of a similar character are the home remedies employed to lower fever and to diminish pain. Of this type is aspirin, a widely used home remedy. Any good aspirin will do, and fifteen or twenty different pharmaceutical houses now make it available. Aspirin, like every other remedy, is a two-edged sword, capable of damage when employed improperly as well as of good when given in proper dosage at the right time. A new remedy is a mixture of codeine and papaverine that must be prescribed by a doctor.

Diets for Colds

Then there is the specific diet. Rats which have had in their food an insufficient amount of vitamin A begin to develop a breakdown of the mucous membranes of the nose and throat. Rats that are fed sufficient amounts of vitamin A do not develop such changes. From this it has been argued that human beings who eat proper amounts of vitamin A or even excess amounts should be able to preserve the integrity of their mucous membranes and thereby avoid colds. Such experiments as have been done over short periods of time not only on chimpanzees but also on human beings do not support the idea strongly. These experiments, of course, cover but a few months, whereas the entire life of the rat is but ninety days, and a week in its life may be approximately equivalent to seven years of human existence. Whether or not excess vitamin A taken over a period of seven years eventually produces an immunity to colds remains to be studied and probably will not be. Human beings do not lend themselves readily to seven-year experiments. Even presidents get only four-year terms and eight seems to be the limit. Russia seems to be satisfied with a five-year plan.

Nose Sprays for Colds

A man with an eruption wants something to put on it. A man or woman with a running nose wants something to put in it. Hence the development of innumerable antiseptics, sprays, ointments, and lotions for administration in the common cold. There are drugs which dry up the secretions, but apparently that is not the road to cure. There are other drugs which increase the secretions, but the duration of the cold still seems to average three or four days. The experts in diseases of the nose and throat feel that the discomfort when too great should be relieved by one of the sprays which diminish secretions, and which include either the old adrenalin or the modern ephedrine. For years camphor-menthol solutions and preparations of oil, camphor, menthol, and eucalyptus have been used to give relief in nasal irritation. The actual worth of such preparations in curing the cold is doubtful. Their value in securing comfort is considerable.

Most recent in the control of colds are the antihistaminic drugs, used alone or combined with aspirin or phenacetin or sprayed in the nose with camphor or menthol or privine. Such preparations are useful in colds which begin as a running nose due to allergy and these constitute a large percentage of all colds.

General Treatment

When the chest seems tight, a mustard poultice is sometimes helpful. This may be bought ready made in the drug store. If it is to be made at home, a paste is made by mixing ordinary household mustard and flour stirred together with warm water as described in the package; it is then spread between two layers of thin muslin. This plaster is put over the upper chest of the patient until the skin becomes quite red. It usually requires from fifteen to thirty minutes.

When the cough is relieved, the discomfort in the chest usually becomes less. Many remedies are used to loosen the cough, most of them being what are called expectorant remedies, containing ammonium chloride. The dose of ammonium chloride usually prescribed is eight grains to each teaspoonful. This is given every two hours. The ammonium chloride is put up with some pleasant syrup. Sometimes sodium citrate, taken in ten-grain tablets mixed with lemonade or warm water, will help to loosen the cough.

Most important in this condition is taking plenty of water. A person with a cold should take a half tumblerful every hour while awake. The water can be as is, or as lemonade or orangeade. If a more alkaline drink is desired, a little baking soda or sodium bicarbonate—usually about 10 grains—may be added to the lemonade.

There are lots of people who think they want a cathartic every time they have a cold, to clean out the system. Really the cathartic, when the cold begins, does not seem to make a great deal of difference. Somtimes it is so irritating as to induce a condition much more discomforting and worse than the cold itself.

SUMMER COLDS

Beyond the common cold there comes with the beginning of spring another type—the allergic cold, rose cold, summer cold, or hay-fever. The spring or rose cold is due to sensitivity to various protein substances derived in the spring primarily from the dandelion, the daisy, maple, and poplar, and also from various other pollens of weeds and grasses. The season and the nature of the sensitizing agent depend on the location in which the person lives and the kinds of grasses and flowers in his vicinity. The symptoms of onset are much the same as those of the common cold, but with most of the emphasis on the redness of the eyes and on the sneezing. That type of cold is a special condition prevented and treated by proper diagnosis and attempts at desensitization.

If you must blow your nose, be careful not to blow it in such a manner as to force the infected secretions from the nose through the eustachian tube into the ears. Always keep one nostril open as a safety valve. Be careful to protect yourself so as not to develop the secondary complications of bronchitis and pneumonia. The cold itself is not a fatal disorder. The complications of colds in the form of infected ears, bronchitis, pneumonia, cause long maladies and many fatalities. Try going to bed for a day, give yourself a fair chance, and get well soon!

Pneumonia

At those seasons, with increasing cold and exposure, and when epidemics of influenza strike in various parts of the country, the number of cases of pneumonia increases rapidly and also the number of deaths. The number of deaths varies from year to year, apparently related to the severity of the climatic conditions and also perhaps to changes in the nature of the germ that causes the disease.

This germ is known as the pneumococcus, a round germ which passes with the discharges from the mouth and nose of the infected person to others, and which may occasionally be carried by a healthful person who is not himself infected, and thus is distributed to others. It has been found that the germs causing pneumonia may be divided into many types. There seems to be reason to believe that the overcrowding and the innumerable human contacts associated with modern life aid in the dissemination particularly of diseases of the mouth, nose, throat, and lungs.

Since normal persons may have the germs in their breathing tracts without having the disease, there may be factors related to the person himself which are concerned with the question of whether or not he will develop the disease. Any factor which will break down the resistance of an individual will tend to cause him to become more easily infected.

A direct injury to the tissue of the lung, such as might occur from inhaling a poison gas, or such as might occur from inhaling some foreign body which would cause an irritation, will open the way for infection by the germ of pneumonia.

The disease occurs in people of all ages but is rather rare during the first year of life. It is much more serious during the earlier and later years of life than it is during the middle period. The rate of incidence and death is high during infancy, decreasing up to the age of ten, and then gradually increasing up to the age of forty, when it again begins to become exceedingly high.

For some reason pneumonia is much more serious in the colored race than in the white. It also follows frequently after such conditions as measles, smallpox, scarlet fever, and even after typhoid. There seems to be good evidence that exposure to severe fatigue, bad weather and to malnutrition give the germs of pneumonia greater opportunity to attack. For some years it has been believed that hard drinkers were more likely to suffer with pneumonia than others, but this has also been related to the fact that hard drinkers occasionally lie out in the open and are exposed to rain and freezing temperatures for long periods of time.

Modern evidence points to the fact that crowding is an important factor in the occurrence of pneumonia. The disease is more frequently found in the city than in the country and is probably more fatal in the city than in the country. The chance for infection from one person to another is much greater where people are crowded together. In trains, street cars, theaters, motion-picture houses, in tenements and under similar conditions, human beings come into contacts that are intimate for fairly long periods of time. Under such conditions germs pass directly from the mouth, nose, and throat of one to another.

When the germs of pneumonia attack the lung it becomes filled with blood, so that quite soon the person begins coughing and spitting material which contains the red streaks showing the presence of blood in the lung. This lung is, however, rather solid because of the presence of the material in it. The physician, therefore, fails to hear the air passing because of the obstruction in the air spaces. Moreover, when he thumps the chest over the lungs it gives forth the dull sound of a solid object rather than the resonant reverberation of one which is full of air.

After a time, depending on the severity of the condition, the lung begins to clear up, the breathing takes place with less difficulty. At the same time the fever goes down.

Pneumonia sometimes begins suddenly with a chill, pain in the chest, vomiting and coughing and difficulty in breathing. In other cases there may be fainting and weakness. In the serious stages of pneumonia the fever may vary from 104 to 106 degrees. Because of the difficulty in getting the blood through the lung there is great stress on the heart. Furthermore, the obstruction to the circulation causes the patient to develop a blue color which indicates that the blood passing through the lung is not receiving enough oxygen. Especially valuable is the use of X-ray to make certain of the diagnosis in pneumonia and to differentiate between lobar and virus pneumonia.

Most people know that the usual case of uncomplicated pneumonia used to last from a week to ten days and that then it cleared up by what is called a crisis; or more slowly by what physicians call lysis, or a gradual dissolving of the disease. In those cases that clear up by crisis the patient suddenly begins to get better and within a few hours is without high fever. He feels much better, his pulse is better, his breathing is slower, and in every way he is improved. In most instances the recovery is gradual. Recovery is due to the fact that the blood of the patient has developed the power to overcome the germ of the disease.

In preventing pneumonia bear in mind that contact with those who are infected is the chief source of its spread. Certainly, a baby should not be taken into a room in which someone is suffering from pneumonia. Mothers must do everything possible to prevent their children from coming in contact with other children who have running noses, coughs, colds, and sore throats. It is especially important to protect children against sharp falls in temperatures which, through centuries of experience, have been associated with the onset of fall and winter colds.

In some cities people with pneumonia are isolated, as with other serious infectious diseases. This has not yet been done on sufficiently large a scale to permit accurate estimation of the worth of the procedure, but there is reason to believe that its effect may be definitely for good.

The person attending a patient with pneumonia should wear a clean gown which is changed before contact with other people. The hands should be thoroughly cleaned with soap and water after attending the patient. The room of the patient should be kept as clean as possible and thoroughly aired, washed, and sunned after the patient's recovery.

When a person is isolated for an infectious disease the utensils, bedclothing, personal clothing, handkerchiefs, and other material in close contact with him should be sterilized. They should be kept separate from similar materials used by other members of the family.

Most important in the care of the patient with pneumonia is to keep him as quiet as possible, both mentally and physically, and to give him the best possible nursing care. The difference between good and bad nursing may mean the difference between life and death.

Because of the importance of proper care and nursing in such a case, most physicians feel that a patient with pneumonia is better off in a hospital than at home. Moreover, it is better to get the patient under good care early and not to wait until he has reached a critical stage before transferring him to a hospital.

The patient with pneumonia should have a large, well-ventilated room with plenty of access to good fresh air. This does not mean that a patient with pneumonia is to be exposed to storm and stress. In inclement weather it is much better to prevent such additional exposure. The patient himself is frequently the best judge as to when he is breathing with most ease and least distress.

The number of visitors must be kept to a minimum. The patient should not have to worry about troubles in the family or business affairs and must be kept flat on his back for at least a week after recovery has begun. Only gradually is he allowed to assume a sitting posture.

The diet in this condition, as in any serious infection, must be chiefly liquids such as soups, gruels, milk, and soft-boiled eggs. Occasionally it is well to add milk sugar to keep up the energy. Rest and quiet are more important even than nourishment in the serious stages of pneumonia. When recovery has begun, feeding is gradually extended so as to aid the improvement of the blood and the broken-down tissues.

It is well for patients with pneumonia to have plenty of water. This does not mean, however, much more than two to three quarts a day. The patient will not drink unless the water is given to him when he is quite sick. Under such circumstances it is perhaps best to give water with a teaspoon, giving small amounts frequently, or to have the patient suck small pieces of ice.

Of greatest importance in the treatment of pneumonia is the care of a competent physician. He himself must direct the nursing and determine its value. He himself must administer proper remedies at the proper time in order to support the extra work of the heart, in order to relieve stress from the circulation, in order to permit the patient to sleep, and in order to control the actions of the bowels, the skin, and of all the other organs. There is no substitute of any kind for the type of care that a well-trained physician can give in this disease.

The use of oxygen in the treatment of pneumonia has been elaborated of late and is found to be exceedingly valuable. Tents have been developed which may be placed over the patients as they lie in bed, and many large hospitals have oxygen rooms into which the entire bed may be moved and in which the nurse may remain and attend the patient. Oxygen is not to be considered an emergency measure to be applied when the patient is at the point of death, but instead one which is to be used promptly when the physician feels that it is required.

While any of the sulfonamide drugs are useful in the treatment of pneumonia, most frequently used nowadays is sulfadiazine, which is less toxic. Penicillin, chlortetracycline and oxytetracycline as well as newer antibiotics are valuable in the attack on the pneumonia germ. Large amounts of penicillin can be given by injection into the muscles and a sufficiently high level of penicillin maintained in the blood to bring about prompt control of the infection.

The former fatality rate of 25 to 30 percent in pneumonia has now dropped to 5 percent.

ATYPICAL VIRUS PNEUMONIA

The pneumonia that is caused by the pneumococcus is now recognized as quite distinctive from the atypical virus pneumonia, which is milder. Fortunately virus pneumonia is not as serious a disease as lobar pneumonia.

Deaths from virus pneumonia are exceedingly rare.

Aureomycin and terramycin are most recommended in this condition. The drug is best given in a half glass of milk.

TUBERCULOSIS

The protection of mankind against tuberculosis is based on two principles which were formulated by the famous Pasteur and Robert Koch. The first is to preserve the child against infection with the germ of tuberculosis by removing it from contaminated surroundings; the second is the isolation of the sick and the education of the well in the prevention of the disease.

Tuberculosis is a social disease in the sense that it affects groups of mankind as well as individuals. Second, it is involved with the economic status of those who are infected. For example, in Vienna in 1913 deaths from tuberculosis were five times higher in the poorer quarters than in the better class quarters.

Tuberculosis attacks all races, all ages of mankind, and indeed all classes of human society, but it is largely a disease of poverty and malnutrition. All of the available evidence indicates that the number of deaths from tuberculosis per hundred thousand of population is steadily decreasing throughout the world. There seems to be some question as to just why this trend has taken place. The decline in the death rate from tuberculosis began long before the era of bacteriologic discoveries and of modern hygiene based on such discoveries. The reason may be not only a change that has taken place in the germ of tuberculosis, but probably also a change has taken place in the nature of man.

The death rate drops among people who have had tuberculosis for many decades. The death rate rises when tuberculosis comes into a country area or into a district in which the population has previously been relatively free from tuberculosis. There seems to be evidence that the coming of the industrial era with crowding and long hours of labor produced a higher death rate for this disease. Then came the protection of labor, particularly of child labor, social hygiene, improved nutrition and improved housing, with a lowering of the rates for tuberculosis.

With the truly extensive knowledge of tuberculosis which we have, its complete prevention ultimately should be a possibility. However, perfect success in a problem of this kind is not likely in a day, a month, or even a generation.

The path to prevention seems to be clear. Young children must not be exposed to infection, or, in any event, the possibility of infection in young children must be reduced to a minimum.

Let us consider what this means in our modern civilization. Human contacts have been multiplied enormously. Today the home has largely disappeared in our great cities; instead, we have the apartment house, housing from three to fifty families. Obviously under such circumstances children are exposed not only to their own parents and relatives, but to vast numbers of other children and other families.

The child of an earlier day played in its own backyard at least until the age of six. Today it goes early to nursery school and thereafter to kindergarten. Moreover, human beings now assemble in crowds of thousands in motion-picture houses and of tens and hundreds of thousands at baseball and football games.

It is easy enough to suggest that young children be not admitted to the presence of known consumptives. It is far more difficult to establish the principle that they be kept out of all gatherings where they may be exposed to infection from unknown sources.

There are, of course, still some differences of opinion as to the proper procedure for eliminating tuberculosis. We are not at this time prepared to isolate all carriers of the germs of this disease or to exterminate them. The fact is emphasized when it is realized that practically everyone has had the disease by the time he is fifteen. Were this not the case, the mortality among adults would be terrific. The earlier infection establishes a resistance against the severe infection of later years.

The Negroes in the crowded districts in northern cities have the highest tuberculosis rate of any group in the community. The Mexican population of Chicago has eleven times the average rate of the rest of the population.

The attack on tuberculosis has been thus far an economic attack. Realizing that it is primarily a disease associated with bad hygiene, great importance has been placed on physical well being.

The treatment consisted largely of good diet, sufficient rest and fresh air. Special attention was paid to housing and types of employment, to the prices of food and wages, since it has been shown that a drop in wages is usually related to an increase in tuberculosis.

In the United States the number of beds available for patients with this disease increased from 10,000 in 1904 to more than 100,000 in recent years. Moreover, there has been a tremendous growth in open-air schools, preventoriums, clinics, and dispensaries.

With the development of new methods of diagnosis and treatment of tuberculosis the demand for sanitarium beds is decreasing. In 1954 and 1955 many sanitariums for tuberculosis were closed, including the famous Trudeau Sanitarium at Saranac Lake, N. Y. More and more patients are being treated while ambulatory with the newer drugs including streptomycin, paraminosalicylic acid (PAS), isoniazid and cycloserine.

In tuberculosis, we know the cause of the disease: namely, the germ of bacillus of tuberculosis. We know the method of transmission, which is from the patient with the disease to the person who does not have it, particularly the child, and occasionally through infected milk and food.

We know that the disease could be prevented by complete isolation or extermination of those who have it, but we cannot apply such procedures on a suitable scale, simply because social conditions do not permit the application of such stringent procedures.

Tuberculosis is a social disease because it spreads where there is poverty, malnutrition, overcrowding, bad housing, exposure to the elements and similar social disabilities. Since the disease is spread chiefly from a person who has it to those who do not, the condition could be controlled by isolating all persons who have the germs in their sputum and who spread them about. Since this is not possible, we endeavor to increase resistance to the disease by inoculating great numbers of people with BCG vaccination. We try to detect the disease in its earliest stages by the use of the X-ray and the tuberculin test. If patients are treated in such early stages, they tend to recover promptly and do not become active spreaders of the disease.

The condition requires rest in a sanatorium under controlled conditions with plenty of good food, fresh air and sunshine, and good hygiene. The ailing lung can be put at rest by artificial pneumothorax, by the operation called thoracoplasty, by suitable posture and by cutting the phrenic nerve.

Doctors know that the X-ray alone is not the only method of detecting tuberculosis. Before a final decision is made the doctor wants to obtain specimens of the sputum so that he can look for the presence of the germ of tuberculosis. He may wish to study the specimens by use of the microscope. He may wish to inject a guinea pig with the material to see if the guinea pig will become infected. Sometimes when the examination of the sputum is negative, material from the stomach (which is secured by washing the stomach with a tube) is then examined for the presence of the germ of tuberculosis. The doctor will also wish to obtain a careful record of the person's life and of his symptoms. He will wish to check the observations by studies of the chest, by **percussion or** thumping or by listening with the stethoscope.

The following hints for good hygiene in tuberculosis come from **the National** Tuberculosis Association:

"Babies and little children must stay out of your room. You must **insist on** this, because they are very likely to catch your germs. The best plan is to send them somewhere else to live while you are sick.

"Do not allow pets in your room.

"Never allow anyone or any animal to eat the food or drink that has been in your room. Left-over food should be burned; if liquid, poured into the toilet.

"Do not let visitors come close to you, shake hands with you, handle your things, or put their coats, hats, gloves, etc., on your bed.

"Never kiss or allow anyone to kiss you! This is a hard rule to obey—probably the hardest for most families. You will have to be the one to insist on it, since if you forbid kissing and remind the family of the danger, they will be less likely to think you want to be kissed, or are feeling hurt at their neglect. Kissing is a very easy way to spread your germs. Show your real affection for your family by refusing to kiss or be kissed.

"Your doctor or nurse will teach your family what to do with your dishes, linen, and other soiled articles, but the most essential thing for you to remember is this: *Protect others from your sputum!*

"Your sputum (spit or phlegm) is dangerous because there are tuberculosis germs in it. Everything your sputum soils is dangerous to others. Therefore you must catch your sputum when it comes as spit or spray from your mouth and nose in sneezing, coughing or spitting. You do this by covering your nose and mouth with paper tissues or soft old rags and burning them after use. Your supply of tissues should be placed beside your pillow or on the bedside table where you can reach them without stretching. Then do as follows:

"1. Take one or two and hold them in your cupped hand, protecting your hand and fingers. You may need two thicknesses of material.

"2. Cover both your nose and mouth.

"3. After use, drop the tissue into a paper bag (grocery bag, or one made of newspaper) pinned to the side of your bed or bedside table, where you can reach it without stretching and without missing.

"When the bag of soiled tissues is about three-quarters full, it should be taken out by your family helper and burned. Do not fill the bag so full that anyone has to touch the soiled tissues in unpinning and holding the bag.

"Never cough, sneeze or spit without using the paper tissue or rags in this way. Always turn your head away from anyone when you cough or sneeze. Later, when you are up, the doctor may let you use a sputum cup (a metal container with a paper filler), but tissues are safer.

"Try to remember that everything soiled or sprayed by the moisture from your nose and mouth is dangerous to others. Be careful! Have your set of toilet articles, toothbrush, towels, shaving kit, and, if allowed, smoking supplies. You can save your family helper many steps and much trouble by being careful about this rule of separate belongings. Your linen and dishes must be boiled before being used by other members of the family."

DIET IN TUBERCULOSIS

The diet is important in the treatment of tuberculosis. Some people simply do not get enough food. Many people are badly fed because they do not know how to select the right foods and to make the best use of what food they have. There seems to be not the slightest question but that malnutrition has an extremely unfavorable effect on the death rate from tuberculosis.

The charts of deaths from tuberculosis show a high peak in earliest infancy, then a definite drop in the rate during later infancy and school age, and a rise at the beginning of adolescence. This points definitely to the periods when children must be most closely watched for the development of symptoms and when everything possible must be done to keep up their nutrition and to see to it that they have plenty of rest and good hygiene.

CONTROL OF TUBERCULOUS CATTLE

Of special importance in the prevention of tuberculosis is the control of tuberculous cattle. The germ of tuberculosis of the type which lives in cattle is rather rare as a cause of tuberculosis of the abdomen, the glands, the bones, and the joints. There are certain methods for controlling tuberculosis in cattle which are now subject to legislation in this country.

In the first place, milk for children, unless coming from cattle free from tuberculosis, must invariably be pasteurized, and in fact it is probably better to pasteurize all milk for children—at least there is more certainty of safety. Second, it is desirable to stamp out tuberculosis among cattle. This is commonly done by testing cattle for the presence of the disease and then destroying all that are infected, at the same time compensating the owners for the loss of the animals.

CLIMATE IN PREVENTION AND TREATMENT OF TUBERCULOSIS

While it is possible for a person to recover from tuberculosis in almost any climate, climatic factors nevertheless play a considerable part in the speed of the recovery.

In considering climate one is concerned not only with temperature and humidity, but also with wind, dust, and storms, with rain, the character of the soil, the sunshine, and many other factors.

Heat or cold in great excess are dangerous to health and may be fatal to life. The effects of temperature on the body are dependent to a great degree on humidity.

Warm moist climates are generally believed to have a depressing effect. Cold, dry air is stimulating, but demands a capacity for response from the individual.

If the body is not able to respond properly to cold, dry air, as is the case with persons who have been greatly weakened by long continued illness or by old age, the effects of cold, dry air may be harmful.

Excessive moisture has a relaxing effect which may predispose to infection. The movement of the air materially influences the temperature and the humidity.

If the air is hot and moist, movement of the air will aid in elimination of heat. If the air is very cold, there will be an increased demand for heat produced from the body. If the air is both moist and cold, conditions are extremely uncomfortable and may be harmful.

There is no one best climate for tuberculosis. In other words, proper treatment under scientific conditions is more important than climate alone.

Some types of patients never should be moved in search of climate. This includes patients who are severely ill in the early stages of the disease or in the late stage of the disease. In such cases, complete rest in bed either at home or in an institution in the home city is the first step in treatment and should be continued until the patient is able to travel without risk.

The cost of invalid care almost anywhere is from $50 to $100 per week. Therefore, at least $2,500 to $5,000 per year must be available for the care of the invalid if he is to go to any health resort.

When the burden of providing for one's self in a strange land is added to those of the disease itself, the invalid has a handicap to overcome which may result in the difference between life and death. Good food and lodging are just as necessary as plenty of sunlight and fresh air.

The satisfaction of the patient's mind is of the utmost importance. A mother will not get well if she is constantly worried about the condition of the children that she has left at home.

A business man will not recover as well in a strange climate as at home if he is constantly worried about his business. It is for this reason that many institutions have grown up near all of the large cities in our country.

The routine of treatment in such instances is of greater advantage than any possible advantages to be derived from climate. The biggest advantage of an institution is the fact that the patient can be educated in the proper routine of life leading to recovery.

The second reason for treating a patient in an institution rather than at home is the advantage of a change. Wealthy people, when tired, experience a tremendous improvement in their general physical and mental tone by a complete change of environment.

This is all the more true of those with tuberculosis. People who live in apartments or tenement houses frequently do better merely by transfer to a day camp near the seashore or in the country.

The advantages of open-air life and open-air sleeping are now recognized by common experience. These increase the general tone of the body, quiet the nervous system, and favor relaxation and sleep.

Perpetual sunshine will not prevent tuberculosis, and excessive sunshine is exceedingly irksome to many people.

Dr. James Alexander Miller has drawn certain conclusions which should be borne in mind by every person with tuberculosis who may contemplate a change of climate.

Here they are:

1. The regimen of regulated rest and exercise, proper food and open-air life, is the fundamental essential in the treatment of tuberculosis. Suitable climatic environment makes this open-air life more easy, enjoyable, and beneficial.

2. When these essentials are assured, a change of climate is of definite value in a considerable number, probably the majority, of cases, but with the proper regimen many cases will do well in any climate.

3. Any change of climate involving the fatigue of travel is contraindicated in acute cases with fever or hemorrhage, or in very far advanced and markedly debilitated cases. Absolute bed rest is the one essential here.

4. No patient should be sent away in search of climate who cannot afford to stay the reasonably to be expected time and to have the necessary food, lodging and care.

5. Competent medical advice and supervision are essential.

6. One of the most valuable assets of change is the education of the patient. This may, of course, be obtained in a suitable environment without reference to climate, as in a sanatorium near home.

7. Selection of a suitable locality is an individual problem for every patient, depending upon his temperament, tastes, and individual reaction to environment, as well as the character of his disease. The advising physician should have an appreciation of these as well as a knowledge of the particular environment to which the patient is being sent. Contentment and reasonable comfort are essential.

8. There is no universally ideal climate. For each patient there may well be a most favorable environment, if we are wise enough to find it.

9. There is a reasonable amount of evidence that certain medical types of cases are more favorably influenced by certain conditions of climate, everything else being equal. For example, reasonably cold, dry, variable climate, such as is found in the mountains, for young or vigorous constitutions which will react well. Dry, sunny climates for laryngeal cases and those with marked

catarrhal secretions. Equable mild climates at low altitudes for the elderly and those of nervous temperaments, as well as for those with arteriosclerosis, weak hearts, or marked tendency to dyspnœa.

10. Successful selection of climate and environment for cases of tuberculosis requires wide knowledge of human nature, of places, and of the disease. This can only be acquired by patience, skill, and experience.

SKIN TESTS FOR TUBERCULOSIS

Many years ago it was proved that almost every human being has tuberculosis before he dies.

Indeed, the vast majority of people become infected with the disease in childhood and recover. However, a considerable number do not recover, and these represent the constant mortality from this disease. The death rate from tuberculosis has been cut tremendously through the advancement of modern medical science and modern hygiene.

In order to detect cases as early as possible and to apply as soon as possible suitable methods leading toward recovery, several systems have been established. The first is to examine all school children physically and by means of the X-ray and to give all of them the tuberculin test. The tuberculin test is a simple skin test, less painful than a pin scratch and much less dangerous.

One of the advantages of such a procedure is the fact that during the physical examination for tuberculosis, it is also possible to detect any other disease which may happen to be attacking the child.

Another method is to select from among school children those who seem particularly likely to have tuberculosis and to limit the examination to them. When a child is found to be positive to the tuberculin test, a thorough study is made of its physical conditions, then the X-ray examination is made. The X-ray reveals even small changes which may have taken place in the lungs.

If a child is found to be susceptible to tuberculosis or in a very early stage, it can be put under a course of hygiene which will aid its prompt recovery in the vast majority of cases.

One of the modern developments in the care of tuberculosis is the establishment of the preventorium to which children are taken who have very mild degrees of tuberculosis or who come of families in which tuberculosis is prevalent. There they have opportunity to recover under the best conditions.

REST IN TUBERCULOSIS

Since rest is the most important single measure in aiding recovery from minimal tuberculosis in its early stages, the provision of adequate facilities in a sanatorium is fundamental to the control of tuberculosis in any community.

Some states already have more beds than they need because of lowered number of cases.

In any ordinary year there are some fifty thousand deaths from tuberculosis in the United States. On the basis of five active cases for each death there would be about a quarter-million active cases of the disease always among us. The vast majority of people with this disease cannot be taken care of in institutions and the chief purpose of the institution may be to instruct a considerable number of people how to take care of themselves.

Rest, fresh air, and food, it has been repeatedly emphasized, are the important trilogy by which the person with tuberculosis must regulate his life. The sanatorium teaches the person how to follow this trilogy automatically and as an everyday procedure.

The person with active symptoms must have absolute rest. As symptoms quiet down the competent physician is able to tell the patient how much exercise is to be taken along with the rest to secure the best results. To most people fresh air means a lusty breeze pouring through a window or below-zero weather on an outdoor sleeping porch. It is important to realize that fresh air does not demand physical discomfort. Windows may be kept open, but the temperature should be equable, and drafts are unnecessary.

One of the chief values of the sanatorium is to teach the patient the routine facts regarding such matters as rest, exercise, diet, and fresh air. It will teach him also how to prevent the contamination of clothing, dishes, and other human beings with the organisms that are in his body. It will teach him his limitations in work and help to find work that he can do.

Thus will it have fulfilled a most useful function and when he is improved sufficiently to be on his way, the place he occupied will be filled by another pupil, and he will go out to help educate the public.

TREATMENT OF TUBERCULOSIS

For many years all sorts of specific remedies have been tried on the tuberculous, and millions of dollars have been mulcted from the people for patent medicines.

The first drug proved to be specific against the germ of tuberculosis is streptomycin. It seems to have established value in tuberculous meningitis, in miliary tuberculosis (which spreads rapidly throughout the lung) and in very severe cases of tuberculosis when there is secondary infection with pus in the chest cavity. The drug is also of value in tuberculosis of the kidney, the peritoneum and of the intestines. At present physicians do not believe that streptomycin should be used in the mild, early cases of tuberculosis because these cases are best cured by older technics which establish suitable resistance in the patient. The use of streptomycin in tuberculosis, combined with para-amino salicylic acid (PAS), and the combination of streptomycin with drugs like promin or diasone or tibione, which are sulfonamide derivatives, may bring about even more satisfactory improvement. The drugs are not a cure for tuberculosis; they supplement bed rest and specific methods of resting the lung.

Newest among drugs in tuberculosis are preparations of hydrazides of isonicotinic acid called isoniazid. It is a widely used drug and brings about improvement, aids appetite and gives a feeling of well-being. Another new drug proved efficient is cycloserine.

People with tuberculosis suffer frequently with fever and sweating at night. When these symptoms become oppressive, the doctor can prescribe drugs which will control them. An alcohol rub at bedtime or a sponge bath with lukewarm water containing about one gram of alum to the ounce is also helpful.

One of the most severe symptoms that may occur in a patient with tuberculosis is bleeding from the lungs. The appearance of this symptom is a danger signal which should cause the patient to lie down immediately and to get medical attention at once.

In the sanatorium in which the patients are treated for tuberculosis, one of the most useful remedies thus far developed is artificial pneumothorax. This involves the injection of air into the chest cavity, which serves to put the lung at rest. The same effect is also brought about by cutting the nerve which leads to the diaphragm, or by performing surgical operation on the ribs.

Tuberculosis could probably be completely controlled if every case with germs in the sputum could be isolated until freed of germs.

MENTAL ASPECTS IN TUBERCULOSIS

One of the most important factors in the care of the tuberculous is the cooperation of the patient in the handling of his disease.

In a thesis prepared in the University of Minnesota, Blanche Peterson insists that the most important single factor in the cure of tuberculosis is an intelligent attitude of the patient.

Doctors, nurses, and social workers endeavor, therefore, in every possible way to influence the patient to assume an intelligent and constructive outlook.

A questionnaire sent to a score of leading physicians who have specialized in this subject resulted in the almost universal response that reasonable and courageous attitudes are highly constructive. The worst states are those of fear, anxiety, and depression.

The patient with tuberculosis who becomes discouraged, hopeless, pessimistic, or rebellious is difficult to treat and aids in his downfall.

When a person first learns that he has this disease, he is likely to be upset and depressed. Knowing nothing of modern care, he is likely to feel that the disease will be promptly fatal.

If, however, the physician who makes the diagnosis will tell the patient that help is possible, that the disease is curable if treated sufficiently early and sufficiently long; that dozens of persons have achieved world-wide fame even though suffering from this disease, he is likely to have a different attitude and to coöperate fully in treatment.

Courage and reasonableness can come only with complete understanding of the situation. For this reason the health education of the tuberculous has come to be one of the most important factors in the control of this condition, and a vast literature has been developed for the purpose.

Practically every tuberculosis sanatorium and tuberculosis society now publishes books and pamphlets which are helpful in informing the tuberculous of the important facts relative to their condition.

The National Tuberculosis Association, 1790 Broadway, New York City, publishes much material that is useful. Such books as the guides and calendars for the tuberculous, edited by Lawrason Brown, are exceedingly helpful.[1]

Above all, the persons living with and surrounding the tuberculous must realize that it is their duty to keep the patient in a hopeful frame of mind and not treat him as a helpless invalid from the moment the diagnosis is made.

HEALTH HINTS FOR THE TUBERCULOUS

Here are some hints for people with tuberculosis. Many of these hints constitute excellent advice regarding hygiene for everyone who is slightly run down, whether tuberculous or not.

1. Never exercise to the point of fatigue. If you find yourself tired, you have done yourself harm.
2. Rest comes before exercise. By resting a surplus of strength and energy is built up and stored in the body.
3. Aim to spend as much of each day outdoors or in absolutely fresh air as possible. The air, to be fresh, need not necessarily be cold.
4. Ideal food should be appetizing, nutritious, and not too bulky. If appetizing and not nutritious, it will not nourish you; if nutritious and not appetizing, you will not eat it; if too bulky, however appetizing, it upsets your stomach.
5. Eat up to the limit of your digestion. It is the food which is digested and absorbed, and not what is put into your mouth, which will do you good. A glass of milk with each meal is advisable. Raw eggs are not as digestible as cooked eggs.
6. If your digestion is poor, tell your doctor.

---

[1] *Laws for Recovery from Pulmonary Tuberculosis.* Lawrason Brown, Saranac Lake, N. Y.

7. Eat your meals at regular hours. Do not take reading matter to the table.

8. Approach and leave each meal in a rested condition. Never eat when tired. Never exercise immediately after eating.

9. In winter, wear warm, light, or medium wool underwear; in summer, ordinary summer cotton underwear.

10. Never wear heavy underclothing or chest protectors.

11. Let your shoes be stout and warm in winter and wear warm woolen socks, by all means. Woolen socks at night are often a great comfort. In winter, a flannel shirt is much more comfortable than anything else. When sitting out in winter, have an extra wrap near by.

12. If you get overheated and perspire, change your clothing and rub dry.

13. A healthy condition of the skin is most important. A warm bath once or twice a week if ordered by your physician is advisable, and a cool sponge bath or a tub bath in the morning if your doctor permits it. The water should be cool but not ice cold. If you do not have a proper reaction after your bath, if you feel chilly or are blue, the water is too cold. Ask your doctor about it. See that your room or bathroom or wherever you take your bath is warm.

ULTRAVIOLET RAY IN TUBERCULOSIS OF THE LARYNX

Tuberculosis of the larynx has been considered, until recent years, one of the most dangerous forms of the disease, leading usually to fatality.

The drugs such as streptomycin and isoniazid are used. Tuberculosis in any part of the body demands careful treatment with the methods that are used for tuberculosis of the lungs and special methods designed for kidneys, skin, larynx or other part that may be involved.

With the discovery of the apparatus which yielded ultraviolet rays, in the form of the carbon arc and the quartz mercury vapor lamps, it became possible to apply concentrated sun's rays directly to the larynx. In order to get the rays directly to the laryngeal cords, various systems of mirrors have been devised, and also quartz stems along which the ultraviolet rays pass.

It has been found that people who are very frail, those with advanced tuberculosis of the lung, and those who have very severe lesions in the throat are treated better by means of the mirror reflection than by other methods.

A steel mirror will reflect about 44 per cent of the valuable rays into the larynx whereas ordinary glass mirrors absorb these rays and reflect only about 9 per cent. It has been found that practically all of the patients treated by direct sunlight to the cords tend to heal.

CONCLUSIONS

Particularly of importance in controlling the spread of tuberculosis is the use of dispensaries in which the disease can be diagnosed in its earliest stages and properly controlled. Experimentation with the method of vaccination against tuberculosis by Calmette has not yet gone sufficiently far to warrant its general adoption in this country.

The most powerful social factors in controlling the disease are housing, nutrition, and education. In educating people it is desirable to educate them not only in general hygiene but also especially as regards the prevention of tuberculosis. The regular examination of school children and teachers, studies of the nutrition of the school child, and education of those who are infected in methods of preventing the spread of the disease are significant factors.

The preventive institutions against tuberculosis today include holiday camps, open-air schools, preventoriums for children who are perhaps not certainly infected with tuberculosis but in such poor state of nutrition and general health that they offer easy prey to the disease, and certainly removal of children as soon as possible from contact with adults who are infected.

RESPIRATORY TRACT See *Colds, Rhinitis,* et cetera.

RESPIRATORY TRACT, UPPER—defined: See HEART, article DISEASES OF THE HEART AND CIRCULATION.

RESUSCITATION The human being can do without food for about forty days, without water for about four days, and without air for about four minutes.

Whenever people become unconscious due to inhaling carbon monoxide, because of electric shock or drowning, the first essential is to restore the breathing. This fact was recognized as long ago as 1633, when an English doctor named Stephen Bradwell described a method for taking care of people who were apparently drowned. He wrote, "Turn the feete upward, head and mouth downward and so hold by the heels that the water may come out. Let others help forth the water by stroaking, crushing, and driving his belly and stomach reasonably hard, from the bottom of his belly toward his throat. If it be cold weather let all this be done in a warme roome before a good fire."

The average person breathes from sixteen to twenty times a minute. Most experts believe that the movements for artificial respiration should be given more rapidly than this, since sufficient air will not be taken in at that rate to comfort the patient. Some recommend that the rate be between twenty-four and forty movements per minute.

Among the most serious of emergencies which may occur, demanding first aid, is resuscitation after asphyxiation, which may result from drowning, from electric shock, and from exhaust-gas poison. Occasionally also there may be asphyxiation from other sources, such as gas escaping from electric refrigerators.

It has been estimated that 25 per cent of men and boys past twelve years of age do not know how to swim, and there are few women who would be capable of swimming long enough or far enough to save themselves in an emergency. When a person has been under water long enough to become unconscious—about four or five minutes—first aid measures are of greatest importance to save life. The practice of resuscitation by the manual method is important because it is the quickest and most readily available. There are numerous devices for artificial resuscitation, but it is usually not well to wait until these come. Until 1952 the most commonly practiced method was the Schaefer technic. Then the American Red Cross, the American Medical Association and other agencies after extended research adopted a new method called the Holger. The Holger method and a few of its variations are described below.*

The Holger: The unconscious person is placed face down with the hands on top of each other, the forehead resting on the hands with the face turned slightly to one side. His elbows are extended toward the side. The operator kneels on one or both knees in front of the head of the unconscious person. The operator places his hands under the victim's arms above the elbow and rocks backward drawing the arms upward and toward himself. The arms are elevated until firm resistance is met, then replaced on the floor. The operator then moves his hands to the back just below the shoulder blades and rocks forward exerting pressure on the back. The operator's thumbs lie close to the spine and the fingers are separated extending backward

---

*The description of the Holger method and its variations is reprinted by permission of the *Journal of the American Medical Association,* from the article "Critical Survey of Manual Artificial Respiration," by Dr. Archer S. Gordon, et al., 1951, 147–15:1445–47.

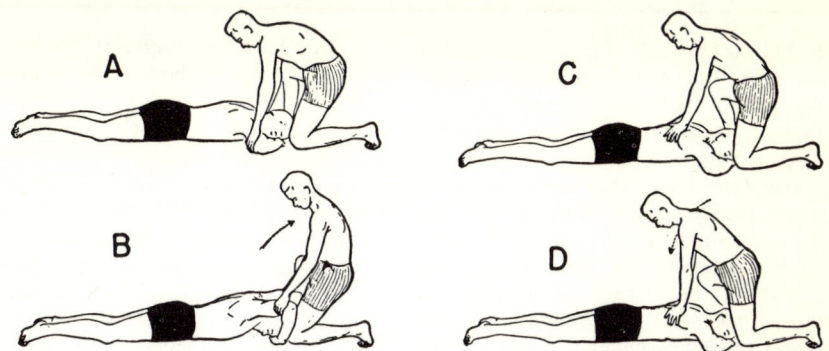

Arm lift-back pressure method of manual artificial respiration (after Holger Nielsen). A, placing hands for arm lift. B, arm lift. C, placing hands for back pressure. D, back pressure.

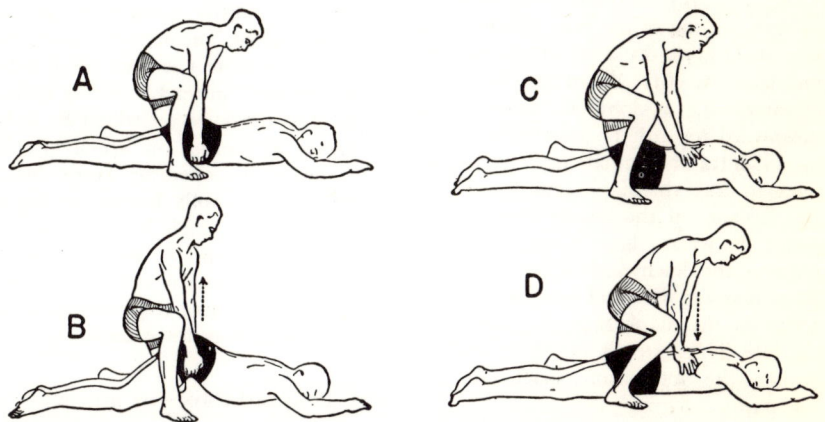

Hip lift-back pressure method of manual artificial respiration. A, placing hands for hip lift. B, hip lift. C, placing hands for back pressure. D, back pressure.

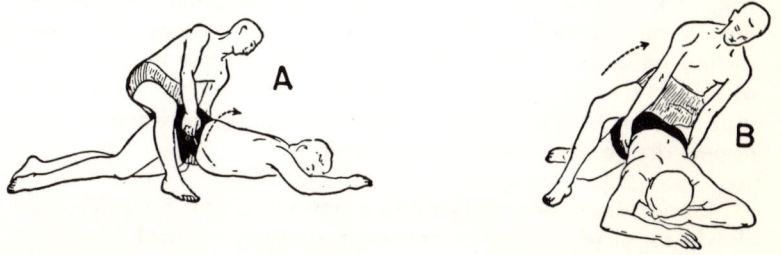

Hip roll-back pressure method of manual artificial respiration. A, side view of hip roll. B, front view of hip roll.

and toward the side. The operator's arms are kept straight during both the lift and the pressure phases and the complete cycle is repeated about ten to twelve times a minute.

Hip Lift: The victim is placed in the prone position, face down, as for the Schaefer method. The operator kneels on one knee at the level of the hip, straddling the victim and placing the other foot near the opposite hip. He places his hands under the hips (at the anterior superior iliac spines) and raises the pelvis vertically upward 4 to 6 inches. The hips are then replaced on the ground, and the cycle is repeated. The hip lift is performed at 12 times per minute. Lifting of the hips produces active inspiration as a result of several mechanisms: (a) When the hips are elevated, the abdominal contents sag downward toward the floor; this results in an intra-abdominal negativity that tends to draw the diaphragm downward. (b) Because of the ligamentous attachments between the viscera and diaphragm, the downward movement of the abdominal organs is followed by a similar action of the diaphragm. (c) Elevating the hips hyperextends the spine and increases the intercostal spaces of the lower ribs.

Hip Lift-Back Pressure: The hip lift-back pressure method combines alternate lifting of the hips, as described, with pressure on the midback (just below the scapulas) with the fingers spread and the thumbs about an inch from the spine. As the operator lifts the hips he rocks backward, and as he exerts back pressure he rocks forward. In each phase he keeps the arms straight, so that the work of lifting and pressing is distributed over the shoulders and back, rather than being imposed primarily on the arms.

Hip Roll-Back Pressure: This is a modification of the hip lift-back pressure method in which a roll is substituted for the lift in order to increase the ease of performance. The operator kneels astride the prone subject as described for the hip lift method; instead of lifting both hips, he uses the knee on which he is kneeling as a fulcrum on which to roll the victim. The operator keeps his arms straight and rolls himself in the same direction in which he rolls the victim. Great care must be exercised to insure that the victim is rolled up onto the operator's knee or thigh so that both hips are raised from the ground.

RESUSCITATION—See article FIRST AID.

The back pressure-arm lift method of resuscitation. (A) Victim is placed on stomach with arms folded under head and cheek resting on crossed hands. Operator kneels on one or both knees at subject's head. Hands are placed on back with thumbs touching; heels of hands are just below line running between armpits, fingers are spread down and outward.

(B) Compression phase. Keeping elbows straight, operator rocks slowly forward until arms are approximately vertical. Weight of upper part of body exerts steady, even pressure downward on victim's back. This forces air out of lungs.

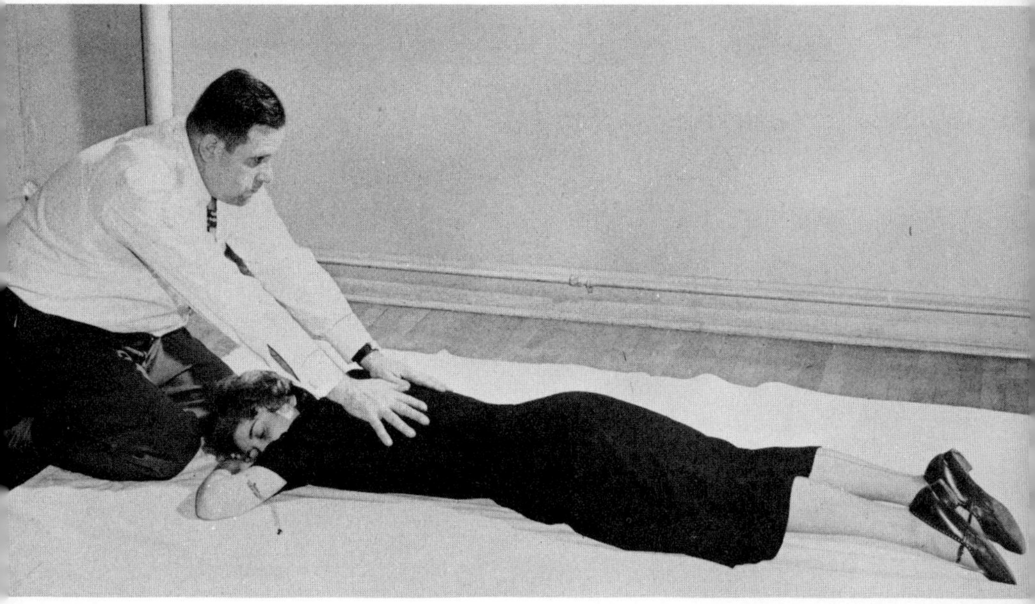

(A)
(B)

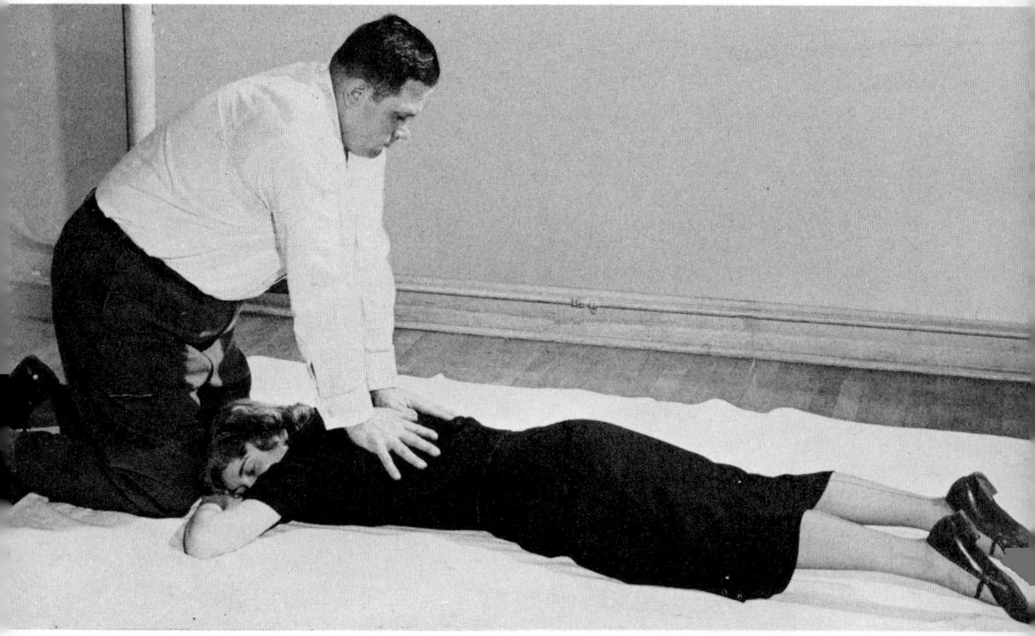

1723

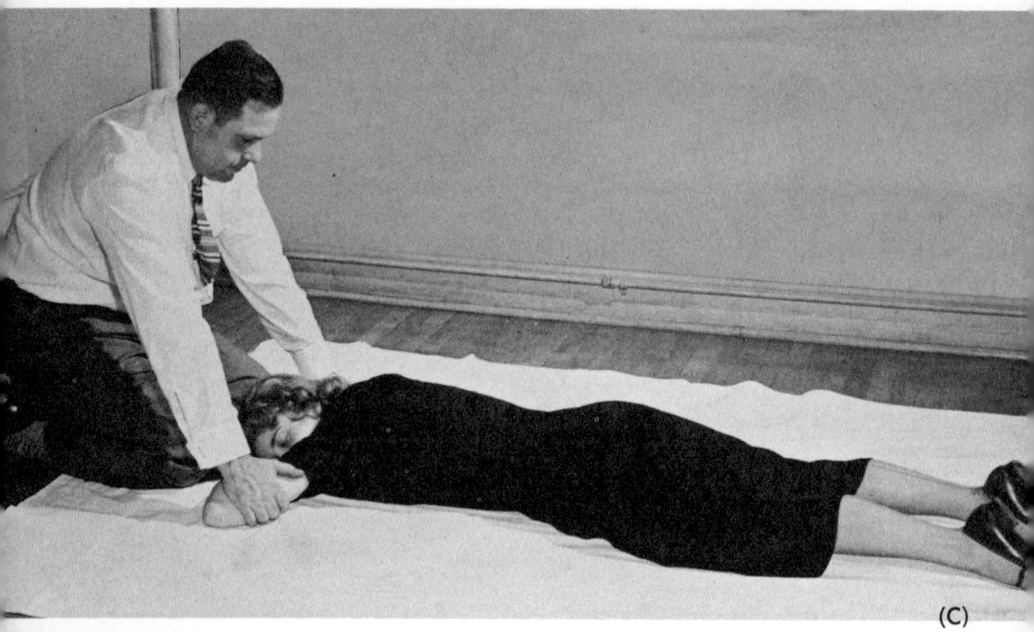

(C)
(D)

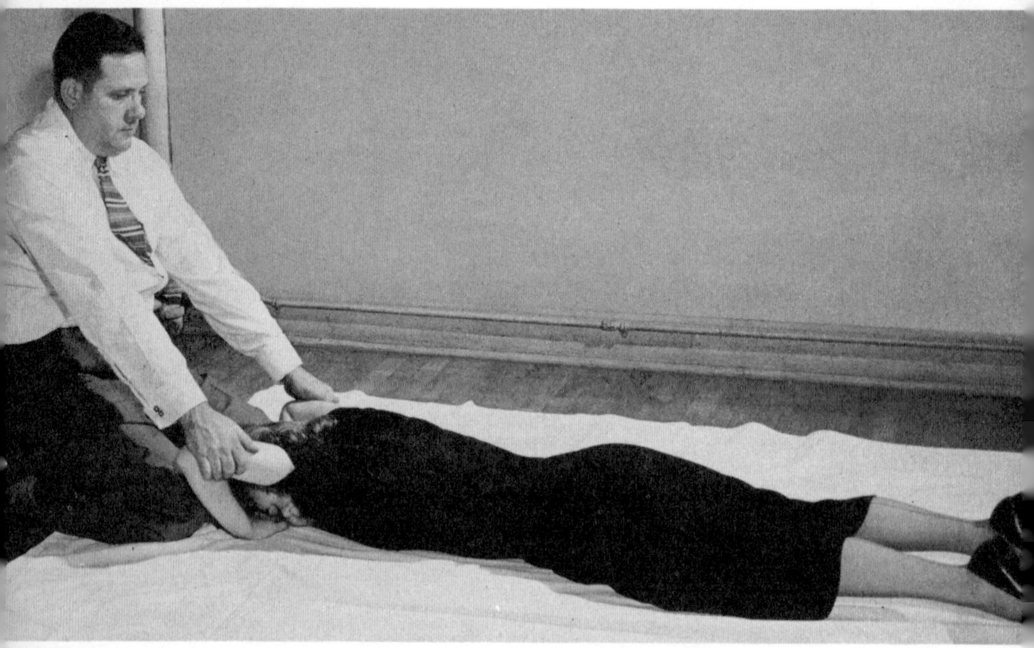

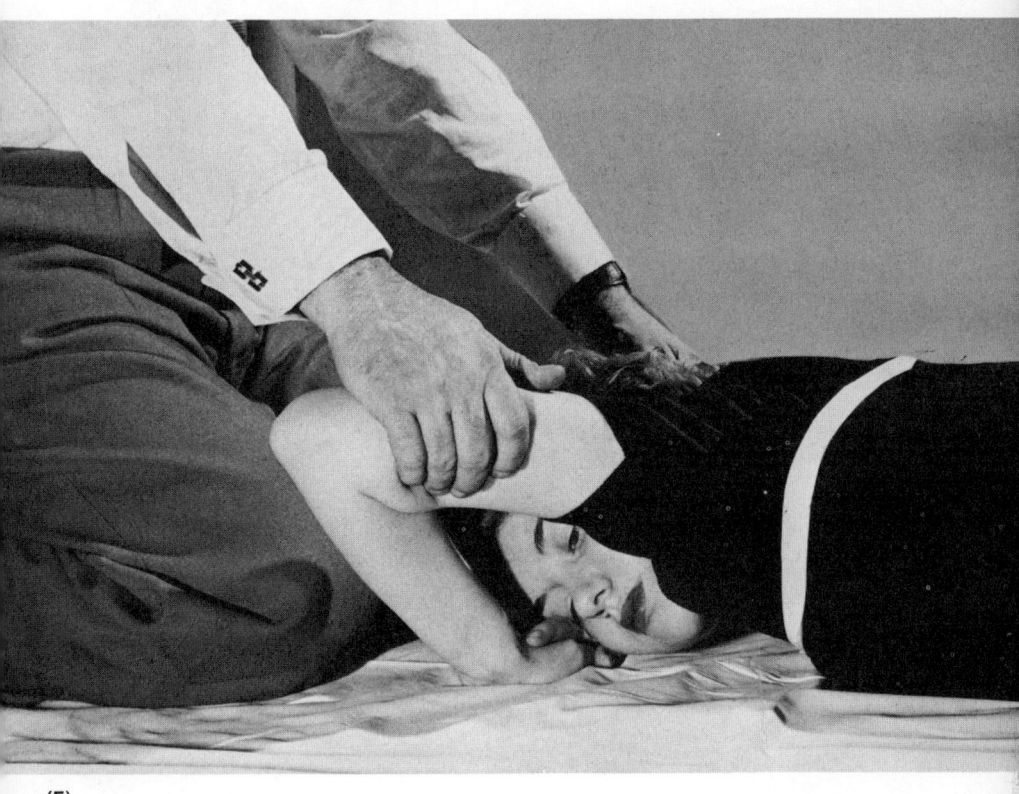

(E)

(C) Release phase. On releasing pressure, operator rocks back slowly, sliding hands to position on victim's arms just above the elbows. Operator should avoid a final downward thrust on back before releasing pressure. Release phase should be of minimum duration.

(D) Expansion phase. Continuing backward rock, operator draws subject's arms upward, applying just enough lift to feel resistance and tension at victim's shoulders. Arms then are dropped to complete the cycle, which should be repeated 12 times a minute at uniform rate. Arm lift, by expanding chest through pull on chest muscles, forces inhalation of air.

(E) Close-up view of position of victim's head as arms are lifted. Mouth is lower than throat to permit drainage of fluid from respiratory passage. Operator should make certain tongue or foreign objects are not constructing air passages of person being worked on.

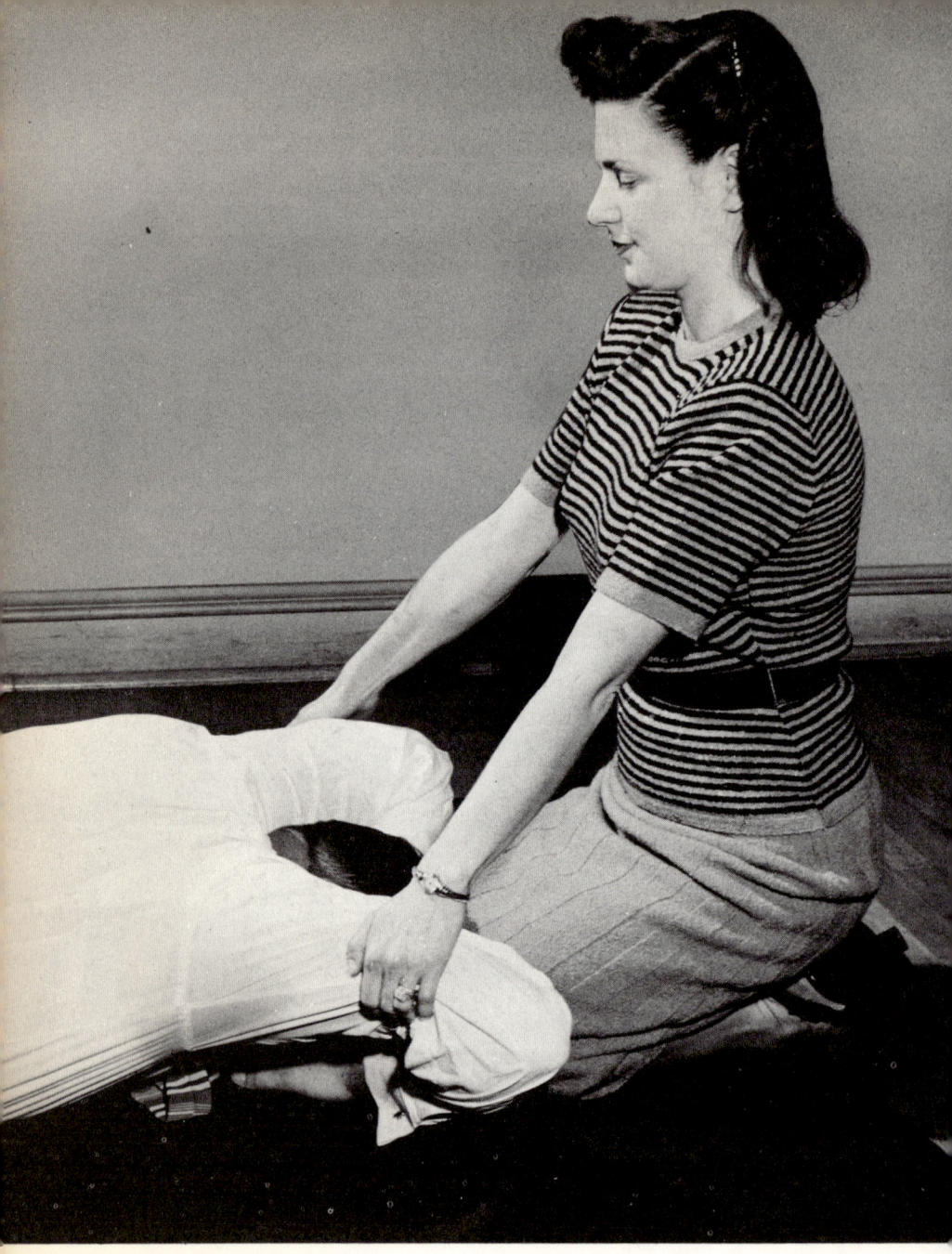

(F) Operator who weights 98 pounds applies arm lift on 220-pound subject to demonstrate ease with which a small person can carry out the method on a larger victim. The method is effective in resuscitating victims of asphyxia caused by near drowning, electric shock, nerve gas. Post Dispatch Pictures from Black Star

RETINA Vision in the human being is brought about through the passing of light rays through the eye to the nervous tissue at the back of the eye called retina. A serious condition is detachment of the retina. An operative procedure has been developed which is helpful in such cases. The doctor can see the retina at the back of the eye by the use of the device called the ophthalmoscope. An inflammation of the retina is called retinitis. This may be due to either infection, hemorrhage, or other types of injury. Sometimes it is associated with inflammation of the kidneys or hardening of the blood vessels.

RETINA—See EYE, article THE EYE.
RETINA—detachment: See EYE, article THE EYE.
RETINA—inflammation: See EYE, article THE EYE.

RETROLENTAL FIBROPLASIA (See also *Eye, Premature Babies*) Recent investigations of retrolental fibroplasia—the newly recognized scarring behind the lens of the eye, which causes blindness to develop in premature babies after birth—indicate that concentration of oxygen available to the tissues may be a causal factor. Doctors are now cautioned against giving too much oxygen to prematurely born babies in view of the danger of the development of an oxygen deficiency when the infant is returned to normal concentration. For this reason special attention is being given to the amount of oxygen available in different forms of modern incubator. In experiments with the offspring of mice previously subjected to an oxygen deficiency, one group of investigators produced changes in eye tissues similar to those that occur in retrolental fibroplasia.

A disease of premature infants which causes blindness is called retrolental fibroplasia. The disease is fully developed in this 2-year-old child. Note the white membranes in the pupils of the eyes. Retrolental fibroplasia appears most prevalently in premature infants of low birth weight. The eyes appear normal and do not differ from the eyes of other premature infants who do not develop the disease. But at one month to six weeks of age the blood vessels in the eyes enlarge and the first stage in the development of retrolental fibroplasia begins. The cause of retrolental fibroplasia is believed to be the injudicious use of oxygen during the early weeks of postnatal life. Postgraduate Medicine

RHEUMATIC DISEASES (See also discussion under *Arthritis, Climate, Osteoarthritis, Rheumatic Fever*) First among the causes of chronic disability in the United States are the rheumatic diseases. Estimates indicate more than 7,500,000 persons or approximately one in every twenty of our population suffer from such disorders. The economic cost of this disability in terms of lost wages, absenteeism from work, and expenditures for medical care would seem to come close to a bililon dollars annually.

The discovery of cortisone in 1949

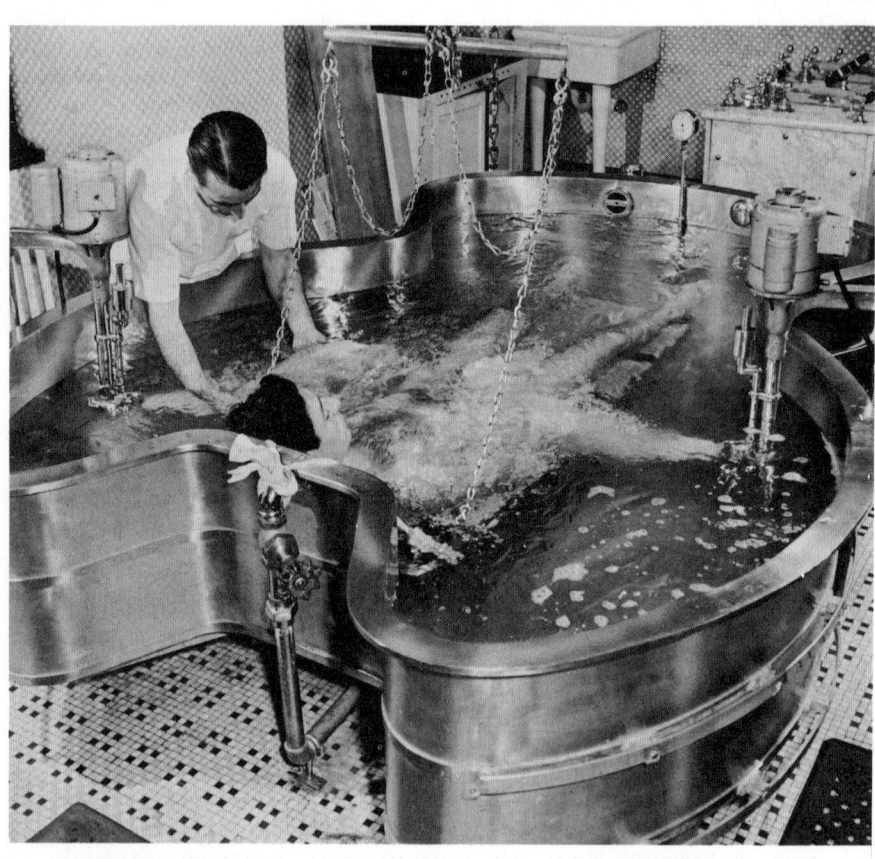

Hydrotherapy in the treatment of rheumatic diseases was used by the Romans and is still probably the most universal if not the most effective form of treatment. This modern tank directs a constant flow of whirling aerated water maintained at about 100 degrees Fahrenheit over the patient's body. The process exercises painful joints, stimulates circulation and is beneficial to the patient's morale.
Three Lions, Inc.

led to renewed interest in the rheumatoid disorders. Here were new tools for research and news ways of estimating the nature of the disease.

The rheumatoid disorders include rheumatic fever and also rheumatoid arthritis and osteoarthritis as well as other conditions which have been included by medical scientists in a group of collagen disorders involving a certain type of connective tissue in the human body.

RHEUMATIC FEVER (See also discussion under *Heart*) Rheumatic fever has come to be recognized as one of the most important public health problems of the country. It is important not only as a cause of death but as the chief disabling heart disease.

Fortunately, research has established a method of controlling rheumatic fever and relapses by treating sore throats promptly with sulphadiazine and penicillin. This eliminates the hemolytic streptococcus and its toxins.

Apparently infections coming into the body by way of the nose and throat and lungs are followed not infrequently by attacks of rheumatic fever. Nevertheless, great numbers of children with infected tonsils and adenoids do not get rheumatic fever, so that some additional factors must be concerned.

Studies have been made to find the part played by crowded, unhygienic living conditions and poor nutrition, but the occurrence of cases not infrequently in families that are well to do and in which the children are well nourished causes skeptics to doubt that the social-economic factors are primarily responsible. For a long time it has been thought that climate was one of the most important factors. Yet we now know that the disease may occur in warm as well as in cold, damp climates.

When rheumatic fever gets in the heart, it produces changes in the muscles of an inflammatory character, damaging the strength of the heart and permitting it to dilate, making it impossible for the heart to do its work. Often rheumatic fever comes on insidiously. Occasionally the so-called rheumatic lesions affect the joints, giving symptoms like those of growing pains, and these seem to be of great importance. Sometimes there are severe attacks of pain in the abdomen related to infections of lymph glands. Sometimes there are mild, fleeting pains in the tendons or muscles. Pains in the heels are not infrequent. Also associated with this condition are symptoms like those of St. Vitus' dance, which may be the first sign of rheumatic fever. The attack on the heart, however, is the fundamental problem and the one that deserves greatest consideration.

Any infectious disease is a grave risk for children who have had rheumatic fever. The secondary infection brings on a recurrence of the attack on the heart. Yet this seriousness need not cause despair, for more attention is now being given to the disease. Hospitals and sanatoriums are being developed in which everything possible is done that can be done. The outlook seems brighter every day for the appearance of new knowledge which will permit proper control of rheumatic fever.

The doctor who studies the patient with rheumatic fever will find signs and symptoms which are not easily apparent to the non-medically trained person.

Over half of the patients with rheumatic fever have tonsillitis or sore throat from one to four weeks before the rheumatic symptoms appear. The rheumatic symptoms may come on gradually or suddenly, usually associated with overexertion or chilling. Then the fever rises to 102 or 104 degrees, the pulse becomes rapid, there is profuse sweating, pains in the joints, and prostration. Seldom do the pains begin in all of the joints at once. Those most subjected to stress and strain are first affected. Sometimes the joints swell because of the accumulation of fluid in the joints. It is quite possible for the doctor to control the pains in the joints and the symptoms of the rheumatic type with drug preparations that are now available and with other methods of treatment.

The detection of the first signs of the disease in the heart is somewhat more difficult. In cases in which these patients come early to the hospital, the electrocardiogram shows transient abnormalities in the heart early in the condition. The obvious signs of damage to the heart, like irregularity, rapidity, pain, changes in the size of the heart, and the accumulation of fluid in the heart sac, come on somewhat later and are easily detectable by the physician. Just as soon as the heart enlarges and becomes incompetent, there are changes in the sounds of the heart as they are heard by the doctor with the stethoscope. The pulse generally reflects the condition of the heart, and the physician trained to detect changes in the pulse will find these early. In rheumatic fever there are also changes in the skin, with the appearance of eruptions. There are also nodes which appear under the skin and which are typical of rheumatic conditions.

When the blood is examined, it is found that the white blood cells increase with the infection. Especially important, however, from the point of view of laboratory study, is the sedimentation rate of the red blood cells. This is considered, in general, to be a good index of the activity of rheumatic disease. The sedimentation is high when the disease is active and low as improvement occurs.

Sometimes infections of the kidney and of the intestinal tract will accompany the rheumatic condition. Such conditions may also give severe pain in the abdomen like an attack of appendicitis. In some instances these attacks have been so severe that operations have been done when the condition was actually due to involvement of the heart with rheumatic fever.

When a child has been attacked by rheumatic fever, there comes a time in many cases when the acute disease becomes chronic or, in other words, when the activity lessens and the infection becomes relatively inactive. For that reason any improvement is welcomed by the doctor because it means that the condition may be tending toward the quiescent stage.

When the condition finally becomes stabilized, the doctor will usually want to make another complete examination, testing the blood for the white blood cell count and the red blood sedimentation rate, determining the function of the heart with the electrocardiograph, measuring the vital capacity of the patient to see if his lungs are working efficiently, perhaps getting a measure of the ability to respond to mild work. If the rate of the pulse of the patient continues high while he is asleep or if the pulse does not come back fairly promptly to its normal rate following slight activity, the doctor knows that it is too soon for the infected child to begin work and exercise. On the basis of these tests the doctor can tell what the likelihood is of partial or complete recovery.

The chance of complete recovery is less if the condition comes on very early in childhood. Obviously also the condition is not good if there are repeated attacks of fever with inflammation of the heart. In general doctors are inclined to believe that the worst side of this disease has received too much emphasis. There are now great numbers of people alive and active in this country who had rheumatic fever when they were children and who in adult life carry on vigorous activity, although perhaps they are unable to submit themselves to excessive exposure or stress.

As I have already said, the child with rheumatic heart disease or with any congenital heart disease is especially susceptible to secondary infection and must be guarded against dangers of this kind. Nevertheless, a significant proportion of children with rheumatic fever escape fatal damage to the heart. The life insurance studies show that young adults who have had a single attack of rheumatic fever without too much damage to the heart have an almost usual life expectancy. All this means, therefore, that the child with rheumatic fever must be given special care for a long time not only when the disease is active but also when it has become inactive.

At present children with rheumatic fever and adults as well are treated during the active stage of the disease with a variety of treatments few of which are known, however, to be absolutely specific against rheumatic fever.

All sorts of treatments have been tried, including the sulfa drugs, penicillin, heat, vitamins, and blood transfusion, but it cannot be said that any of these methods has shown ability to conquer rheumatic fever. The failure to have as yet a specific treatment for rheumatic fever means that the general care of the patient, the kind of nursing he receives, and the regular watchfulness of the doctor to meet every change as it develops are of the utmost importance in controlling the progress of rheumatic fever.

For many years it has been shown that drugs of the salicylic acid type are especially useful in controlling the fever, the pains, the swelling in the joints, and such symptoms. These are called symptomatic drugs, however, because they do not cure the disease.

They do relieve the painful symptoms.

When the heart is especially involved, extra attention must be given to supporting its work so that every possible strain can be kept from the heart. Continuous rest in bed for the duration of the active stage of rheumatic fever is the one technic of which we are certain. The rest may involve weeks, months, or even more than a year in bed. As the condition improves, the doctor begins to permit a certain amount of physical activity, first from the bed to a chair, then walking, and finally return of the child to school. Nevertheless, I have just heard of a case of a child fourteen years old who had recovered from the acute stage of rheumatic fever. On the second day that the child was home from the hospital the father called the doctor and asked if the child could go swimming in the lake. Parents must simply learn that the child with rheumatic fever must be carefully guarded by those responsible for him until he reaches the age when he is able to make wise decisions for himself. The gradual resumption of physical activity must be most carefully controlled. For instance the child is allowed to sit in a chair half an hour twice a day for one week. Then the next week this allowance may be increased by fifteen minutes a day if there have been no untoward symptoms. At the end of two weeks the child may perhaps be permitted to go to the bathroom himself. Then moderate exercise may be allowed for fifteen minutes a day for two or three weeks. Perhaps after five or six months the child is able to have physical activity.

The most disappointing part of the treatment of rheumatic fever is the fact that it tends to come back again after it has apparently gone. This means that the doctor must determine, after the active stage has passed, that the heart has either been permanently damaged or not damaged. It means also that the child must come back for examination at regular intervals for a fairly long period of time to make certain that new activity has not begun and to make certain also that everything possible is being done for improvement of personal hygiene.

There is no doubt that children with rheumatic fever are best cared for in special institutions like Irvington House, Irvington-on-Hudson, New York, or La Rabida Sanitarium, Chicago, where the child may remain for weeks or months under the best possible conditions of ventilation, rest, sunshine, and nutrition. If it is found while the child is in the sanitarium that the conditions at home are not suitable, everything possible must be done to improve those conditions so that the child will return to a better place.

If the child with rheumatic fever has blood that is not up to normal, the anemia must be improved with suitable foods and drugs. Infected tonsils and adenoids are removed during the quiet periods. Nowadays we know that secondary infections with the streptococcus are fatal to such children. It becomes possible by the use of the sulfa drugs or penicillin to prevent any secondary streptococcus infection at the time when the tonsils and adenoids are removed.

The vast majority of children with rheumatic heart disease can and should attend regular schools and engage in a normal school life. In many of our large cities there are special schools for children with handicaps related to the heart or other parts of the body. The program for these children should be planned, however, not to make them invalids with rheumatic heart disease but rather toward teaching them that they can lead a reasonable and well-regulated life and be useful members of society.

In climates that are warm and dry there is less chance of secondary infections of the nose, throat, and lungs, which are so fatal in rheumatic fever. Probably for that reason the warm, dry climate is better for children with rheumatic fever than the chilliness and dampness that sometimes prevail in more northerly climates.

In a recent report by experts in the care of rheumatic fever there were six definite directions given to be followed while the disease is inactive:

1. Take measures to improve the general health and resistance of the child.
2. Observe the patient regularly for signs of recurrence and alterations in cardiac status.
3. Encourage physical activity, to the limit of the child's capacity. Only a small percentage of children at adolescence are found to have sufficient permanent heart disease to preclude normal activity.
4. Provide vocational guidance and occupational training for the relatively small group who cannot engage in normal physical activity.
5. Discourage parents and teachers from making a chronic invalid of the child. Educational authorities need to know that the vast majority who attend regular schools when the disease is inactive can and should engage in normal school life.
6. Minimize exposure to upper respiratory infections, if possible, by improving unfavorable living conditions—for example, overcrowding in the home, particularly in bedrooms—and by controlling the spread of infection through school and family contacts.

Newest in the treatment of rheumatic fever as in rheumatism is the use of Cortisone (compound E) or the adrenocorticotropic hormone (ACTH). These new substances seem to be able to control the inflammation in this condition.

When CORTISONE and ACTH were first developed they were hailed as the final answer to rheumatic fever. A cooperative study has been made by clinics throughout Canada, England and the United States and their joint report indicates that both ACTH and cortisone are extermely valuable in relieving immediately the severe inflammation of rheumatic fever which frequently destroys a child within a few weeks of the onset of this disease. They are not however the cure for rheumatic fever. In fact salicylates which used to be largely depended on for this purpose are still found to be beneficial in relieving the severe symptoms. During the healing process which sometimes seems to occur almost spontaneously the dilated heart may shrink back toward normal size and the murmur of the injured heart may disappear. In overcoming the after effects of rheumatic fever, surgery is now of the greatest importance. Suffice here to say that narrowing of the mitral valves is now overcome by the use of surgical operations first done by Cutler, professor of surgery at Harvard University, and now widely extended not only throughout the United States but also elsewhere in the world. When the narrowed valve is opened, the shortness of breath and the swelling of the body associated with this difficulty is relieved.

A British clinic reports having performed this operation on 150 patients (31 men and 119 women, with ages ranging from nineteen to fifty-seven years). Only 4 of the 150 patients died as a direct result of the operation. Results of the operations have been followed in 111 of the patients for as long as two and a half years; good results were obtained in 81 of the patients, only fair or poor results in 22 of them. The operation is not performed when a patient has active rheumatic fever, severe damage to the heart, or infection of the lung.

Among other conditions related to rheumatic diseases are lupus erythematosus, periarteritis nodosa, scleroderma, dermatomyositis and a kidney condition called nephrosclerosis. These are rather peculiar conditions which have the common feature of widespread degeneration of connective tissue in the body. Early research with the cortisone drugs has shown a definite influence on all of these diseases exerted by cortisone and ACTH. The immediate results are often excellent and during the acute phases of these diseases, the hormones may be life-saving.

RHEUMATIC FEVER—See HEART, article DISEASES OF THE HEART AND CIRCULATION.

RHEUMATIC FEVER—adenoids: See HEART, article DISEASES OF THE HEART AND CIRCULATION.

RHEUMATIC FEVER—annual variations: See HEART, article DISEASES OF THE HEART AND CIRCULATION.

RHEUMATIC FEVER—attack: See HEART, article DISEASES OF THE HEART AND CIRCULATION.

RHEUMATIC FEVER—baffling: See HEART, article DISEASES OF THE HEART AND CIRCULATION.

RHEUMATIC FEVER—causes: See HEART, article DISEASES OF THE HEART AND CIRCULATION.

RHEUMATIC FEVER—childhood, manifestations in: See HEART, article DISEASES OF THE HEART AND CIRCULATION.

RHEUMATIC FEVER—chorea: See HEART, article DISEASES OF THE HEART AND CIRCULATION.

RHEUMATIC FEVER—collagen disease: See HEART, article DISEASES OF THE HEART AND CIRCULATION.

RHEUMATIC FEVER—compounds E and F: See article ENDOCRINOLOGY.

RHEUMATIC FEVER—dampness as

cause: See article OCCUPATION AND HEALTH.

RHEUMATIC FEVER—effect of climate: See HEART, article DISEASES OF THE HEART AND CIRCULATION.

RHEUMATIC FEVER—endocarditis occurs frequently in those who have had: See HEART, article DISEASES OF THE HEART AND CIRCULATION.

RHEUMATIC FEVER—epidemics: See HEART, article DISEASES OF THE HEART AND CIRCULATION.

RHEUMATIC FEVER—family predisposition: See HEART, article DISEASES OF THE HEART AND CIRCULATION.

RHEUMATIC FEVER—heart changes: See HEART, article DISEASES OF THE HEART AND CIRCULATION.

RHEUMATIC FEVER—name not apt: See HEART, article DISEASES OF THE HEART AND CIRCULATION.

RHEUMATIC FEVER—not contagious: See HEART, article DISEASES OF THE HEART AND CIRCULATION.

RHEUMATIC FEVER—prevention: See HEART, article DISEASES OF THE HEART AND CIRCULATION.

RHEUMATIC FEVER—resistance reduced by chronic disorders: See INFECTIOUS DISEASE, article THE PREVENTION AND TREATMENT OF INFECTIOUS DISEASE.

RHEUMATIC FEVER—seasonal variations: See HEART, article DISEASES OF THE HEART AND CIRCULATION.

RHEUMATIC FEVER—subsequent progressive damage possible: See HEART, article DISEASES OF THE HEART AND CIRCULATION.

RHEUMATIC FEVER—symptoms: See HEART, article DISEASES OF THE HEART AND CIRCULATION.

RHEUMATIC FEVER—symptoms produced by an allergy: See article ALLERGY.

RHEUMATIC FEVER—tonsils: See HEART, article DISEASES OF THE HEART AND CIRCULATION.

RHEUMATIC HEART DISEASE—high systolic pressure: See article BLOOD PRESSURE.

RHEUMATIC HEART DISEASE—irregularity of pulse: See HEART, article DISEASES OF THE HEART AND CIRCULATION.

RHEUMATOID ARTHRITIS (See also discussion under *Osteoarthritis, Rheumatic Diseases, Rheumatic Fever, Pemphigus*) Many theories have been proposed to explain rheumatoid arthritis but the exact nature of the condition is still not established. Currently popular is a view that the fundamental fault is in the constitution of the person concerned. Because of his nature he reacts abnormally to various types of injury, the reaction appearing chiefly in the connective tissue elements of the body. Among the various substances or stimuli that may produce these inflammatory reactions are infections, emotional stress, bruises and wounds, exposure, fatigue, nutritional disturbances and psychogenic factors. Most people have observed that arthritis becomes worse in response to heightened emotions, often related to the loss of security. The dominant changes appear in the joints and related structures but also in muscles and in nerves.

For many years rheumatoid arthritis has been treated by a variety of methods including physical therapy with the application of heat, the salicylate drugs, the changes in diet and psychologic methods. Gradually a system of treatment is being developed which is more effective than anything previously known and which arose through the basic studies that were made when cortisone appeared upon the scene. Scientists are still searching for drugs that will be better than cortisone or ACTH or even the improved prednisone known also as metacortin.

Some patients who have ceased to benefit after prolonged treatment with hydrocortisone and cortisone react favorably to the new drugs. The side effects are apparently less frequent with the new products, although adverse reactions, such as digestive complications, vasomotor symptoms and lesions affecting the skin, have been reported. Forsham found that the excretion of hydrochloric acid is considerably increased in amount during administration of prednisone over that occurring with hydrocortisone.

The newer drugs have been used largely, as might be expected, in the treatment of rheumatoid arthritis. In this condition practically all investigators agree that the superiority of prednisone to cortisone and hydrocortisone as an antirheumatic agent has been clearly demonstrated. The therapeutic effects are enhanced as evidenced by increased functional capacity and reduction of inflammation of the joints. Moreover, these effects are achieved with lower dosages and with less side effects. The time has been too short to say anything with certainty as to the permanence of the effects.

In addition to the use of these drugs in rheumatoid arthritis, they have had extensive trial in intractable bronchial asthma and in several instances have made injections of epinephrine unnecessary. Among other conditions in which the drugs have been tried are nephrosis, disseminated lupus erythematosus, periarteritis nodosa, pemphigus vulgaris, erythema multiforme and various disorders affecting the eye. The reports thus far available indicate that prednisone may be substituted for hydrocortisone in these conditions as a preferable preparation. No doubt, as time elapses, experiences with prednisone in other conditions will be broadened and a more thorough knowledge of its effects on various functions of the body more definitely determined.

The development of these drugs and their availability through a number of excellent sources, at costs which are quite reasonable even for long-continued treatment, constitute a major advance in the care of rheumatoid arthritis and other collagen disorders.

Coming into view is the concept that a single drug is not going to be the answer but that the total approach involving rest, prevention and correction of deformities, restoration of function by physical therapy and graduated exercises, avoidance of emotional stress and a sensible well balanced diet cannot be neglected. The drugs that have been mentioned including the various modifications of cortisone and ACTH as well as the salicylates are potent remedies which should never be taken except under the advice and control of a physician. New drugs have been developed which are anti-inflammatory in character. One of the most important of these is phenylbutazone also known as butazoladine. This drug also is a valuable tool in the hands of the specialist.

RHINITIS Any inflammation of the mucous membranes that line the nose is called rhinitis. This is of various forms, chief of which are those that are due to infection and those due to sensitivity to various substances. The infections are described according to the name of the infecting germ. A condition called ozena (see discussion under *Ozena*) is also known as atrophic rhinitis.

RHINITIS—acute catarrhal: See RESPIRATORY DISEASES, article THE RESPIRATORY DISEASES.

RHINITIS—allergic: See article ALLERGY.

RHINOPHYMA Occasionally, due to changes in the blood vessels, the nose becomes swollen with great nodules. This change in the nose is called rhinophyma, which merely means a nose that grew. There is not much that can be done for this condition except by what is called rhinoplasty, or plastic surgery of the nose.

RHUBARB Rhubarb used to be much used in medicine as a laxative and particularly in that form of constipation which was related to the intestine. The product is still included by many physicians in prescriptions for purgatives.

RIBOFLAVIN DEFICIENCY (See also, *Vitamins*) The Vitamin B complex includes not only niacin and thiamin but also riboflavin and other substances. When riboflavin is deficient the symptoms noted include principally fissures and soreness at the corners of the mouth, redness of the white portion, or cornea, of the eye with pain on seeing strong light, and also some changes in the tongue and skin.

Seldom is a deficiency of riboflavin observed alone since it is so closely associated with other portions of the Vitamin B complex. Most of the symptoms are regularly associated with pellagra which is chiefly the result of lack of niacin.

Dr. William Darby has described the appearances around the corners of the mouth which are typical. First the lips get pale at the corners and then they seem chewed or softened after which the fissures appear. As these heal pink scars appear. The sore spots may become covered with crusts. The surface of the tongue gets a mushroom-like appearance and the color has been described as magenta.

Patients with ariboflavinosis complain of a sandy feeling of the eyelids with blurring of vision and burning on exposure to strong light. As in pellagra these patients have a record of failure to include in their diets such substances as lean meat, green leafy vegetables, milk, eggs or liver.

Once the diet of the patient is supplemented with adequate amounts of the food mentioned the symptoms disappear. In difficult cases doctors prescribe a normal dosage of riboflavin itself. Since, however, few patients have an uncomplicated shortage of riboflavin but rather a shortage of all of the Vitamin B complex and since B complex is so easy to secure and administer, the whole B complex is given.

RIBS There are twenty-four ribs in the human being, each of which extends from the bones of the back around toward the front. Because they act as a protective case for the organs of the chest, they are subjected to injuries so that they become bruised or broken. Frequently a broken rib heals simply by having it properly strapped in place. Whenever there is a suspicion that a rib has been broken, an X-ray picture should be taken. Sometimes there is an extra rib high up in the chest which may cause disturbances by pressure on tissues. This is called a cervical rib. Sometimes the lower pairs of ribs do not make connections except at the back. They are called floating ribs.

RICKETS When lime salts fail to be deposited in sufficient amounts in growing cartilage and in newly formed bone in the body, deformities result which, taken together with the other symptoms that occur, make the disease called rickets.

Once rickets was a disease little understood, but today the condition is recognized to be a deficiency disease caused by insufficient amounts of vitamin D, calcium, and phosphorus during the age when growth is rapid. Incidentally, with rickets, as with every other deficiency disease, the failure to receive sufficient amounts of one vitamin is likely to be associated with the failure to receive sufficient amounts of other vitamins and minerals.

Human beings once spent much of their time in the sunlight and developed vitamin D in their own bodies by the action of the sun on a chemical substance in the skin. Then mankind moved into tenements and apartment houses; playgrounds disappeared; smoke poured over the sky, and sunlight became absent from the human environment. As a result it became necessary to supply children with their vitamin D from artificial sources or otherwise provide them with artificial sunlight.

As far back as 1905 there were from 94 to 98 per cent of children in cities who had rickets. As recently as 1920 from 44 to 60 per cent of children in Baltimore were found with symptoms of rickets. Today the percentage is much less because of the provision of cod-liver oil, cod-liver oil substitutes, vitamin D milk, artificial sunlight, or similar dietary accessories.

Rickets is diagnosed with certainty by the use of the X ray, which shows the failure of the skeleton of the body to develop as it should. There are, however, other symptoms which result from the failure of the bones to develop properly, including beading of the ribs, the development of potbelly, bending deformities due to the fact that the bones are soft. Commonly the child with rickets sits with his thighs slightly spread apart and with one leg crossed over the other; the hands are placed on the floor or on the thighs to assist the backbone in holding the body erect. The pull on the tissues by the muscles and ligaments and the softness of the bones cause bending, so that the bowlegs and knock-knees of rickets are characteristic. Rickets also leads to delayed eruption of the temporary teeth and to deformities of the unerupted permanent teeth.

It is much better to prevent rickets than to try to cure it. Parents should make certain that children, even in the nursing period, receive sufficient amounts of vitamins A and D and vitamin C as well, also adequate amounts of calcium in the diet, best taken perhaps as milk, to insure proper and healthful growth. The dosage of the vitamins and of calcium received through the diet and in other ways will be determined by the doctor.

RICKETS—See articles SEX HYGIENE; DEFICIENCY DISEASES.

RICKETS—caused by deficiency of vitamin D: See INFANCY, article CARE AND FEEDING OF THE CHILD.

RICKETS—childbirth affected by: See article SEX HYGIENE.

RICKETS—infants: See INFANCY, article CARE AND FEEDING OF THE CHILD.

RICKETS—United States: See article DEFICIENCY DISEASES.

RICKETS—vitamin D: See SKIN, article THE SKIN.

RICKETTSIAL INFECTIONS (See also, *Infections and Immunity*) The Rickettsia are minute infectious agents, smaller than most germs and larger than most viruses. Most classifications put them midway between the bacteria and the viruses. Rickettsia are too large to pass through a bacterial filter and are visible with an ordinary microscope. Like the viruses, they multiply only in the presence of living cells and many of them live inside living cells. They usually are transferred from animals to men by ticks, mites, fleas, or lice. Many of the rickettsial diseases of man have been identified as such only during the last fifty years. The word "Rickettsia" comes from the name of Howard Taylor Ricketts, a physician of Chicago who was one of the first to observe these organisms and determine their nature.

A form of typhus fever called murine typhus is an acute infectious disease caused by an organism of the rickettsia. The disease usually begins with a sudden fever that lasts two or three weeks; the rash is located mostly on the trunk. The disease was first described in the United States by James Paullin of Georgia in 1913. The chief mammalian carrier of murine typhus is the rat. The infection is transmitted from rat to rat by fleas. The rat louse will not feed on man but the flea will if given opportunity. The flea bite is not infectious but when the flea bites a man, the flea may deposit its excretions; then the human being scratches himself and thus may force these excretions of the flea into his skin.

About six to fourteen days after such infection has taken place, illness begins with a chill and muscular aching, headache, fever, loss of appetite, and cough; with this comes a feeling of severe illness. A skin eruption helps make the diagnosis. This eruption is present in 90 per cent of the white patients, but of course is difficult to see on patients with a colored skin. The lesions of the skin are not hemorrhagic. In many patients the spleen is enlarged. Usually after eight to ten days the symptoms lessen and diminish—the condition clearing up in about three weeks.

Fortunately two of the new antibiotic drugs—aureomycin and chloromycetin—have been established as valuable in controlling the symptoms of this virus infection. Most of those with murine typhus need lots of fluids while they are ill; if they cannot drink water, it is gotten into the body in other ways.

About one out of every one hundred people with the disease may be so severely sick as to die of it. The ones who die are usually the very old or sick people.

The extremely severe epidemic typhus that is seen in Russia is exceedingly rare in the United States. A form of typhus which occurred to our soldiers in the Far East is called scrub typhus and known to the Japanese as tsutsugamushi disease. In these conditions modern treatment involves the use of aureomycin, chloromycetin and sometimes para-amino benzoic acid which is effective in interfering with the nutrition of the virus in the body.

RINGING IN THE EARS (See also discussion under *Dizziness, Ear, Senescence*) Ringing in the ears, called tinnitus—just about the most common complaint of older people—is sometimes associated with loss of hearing. Some people say that the loudness of the tinnitus is so great that it interferes with their ability to hear. Some people have found that they can mask the ringing in the ears when they try to fall asleep by playing the radio softly. Occasionally people without any loss of hearing or without any trouble in the ear whatever will have sudden sensations of head noises, high pitch, which last just a moment. These are apparently without seriousness as are occasional flashes of light to the eye. Specialists have classified various forms of tinnitus associated with almost 30 different varieties of disorders such as loss of hearing, Meniere's disease, disturbances of blood pressure, glandular changes, allergic reactions and even psychoses. When a definite cause can be found, treatment is applied to the cause. In other cases, sedative drugs are used and with that psychotherapy. Many different techniques are known by which the noises may be lessened in frequency and intensity. People who have this condition should recognize that it is a symptom and not a disease and that it often occurs with advancing years but without any serious effects on longevity.

RINGWORM In addition to the infection of the feet called athlete's foot, ringworm may affect any portion of the body. One form of ringworm produces coffee-colored scales on the inner side of the thigh. Associated with this infection there is irritation of the skin and itching. Ringworm of the groin is apparently more easily controllable than ringworm of the foot.

In the treatment of ringworm of the groin physicians usually recommend that underwear be boiled so as to prevent reinfection of the area by the clothing. The specialist prescribes a variety of treatments depending on the nature of the infection. Often weak ointments of sulfur or salicylic acid and lotions containing such substances are prescribed for the condition and bring about healing. The dryness of the area is also important for the prevention of reinfection.

Another form of ringworm attacks the skin of the body away from the hair and produces spots of infestation like circles. Ordinarily this form of infection is treated with ointments of salicylic acid. If this ointment is rubbed well into skin in the infested area, the skin will peel and the infection will be eliminated.

In addition to treatment with salicylic acid, several different dye substances like gentian violet, crystal violet, and brilliant green have been used against ringworm.

Ringworm which attacks the scalp may be still a different variety and may be much more difficult to control because of the necessity of removing the hair. There is no single salve or ointment that can be placed on every case of ringworm with a useful result. Because the ringworm gets into the hair follicles, repeated infection may occur. In such cases it is necessary to cut the hair, to shampoo it daily with tincture of green soap, and to apply an ointment capable of destroying the ringworm. Sometimes it is necessary to cause the hair to fall out by other technics.

Ringworm of the scalp has always been considered primarily a disease of childhood which usually disappears about the time when puberty arrives. Nowadays considerable numbers of cases of ringworm of the scalp have appeared around the country, apparently even in epidemic form. Some suggestion has been made that motion picture houses put fresh paper on the backs of seats occupied by children so that a child will not become contaminated from the child who has sat in the seat previously. An outbreak of 57 cases of ringworm of the scalp occurred among adults in Texas. The infections produced scaling and crusting of the scalp. Under modern conditions the proof of the presence of this condition is made by using a special ultraviolet light, and a special form of ringworm has been found to be associated with such cases. In the treatment it becomes necessary often to eliminate the hair and to treat the ringworm with preparations capable of destroying the infestation.

ATHLETE'S FOOT—See SKIN, article THE SKIN.

ATHLETE'S FOOT—eczema may be complicated by: See SKIN, article THE SKIN.

RINGWORM—See SKIN, article THE SKIN.

RINGWORM—nails: See HAIR, article THE HAIR.

RINGWORM—scalp: See HAIR, article THE HAIR.

RINGWORM—Wood's filter: See HAIR, article THE HAIR.

ROCKY MOUNTAIN SPOTTED FEVER

Since the first settlement by white men the disease known as Rocky Mountain spotted fever has been prevalent in Idaho and Montana. Now we recognize that this condition prevails throughout the world, and cases have been found in many of the states of the United States; the only ones escaping have been Maine, Michigan, Mississippi, New Hampshire, Vermont, and Wisconsin.

Rocky Mountain spotted fever is an infectious condition which is transmitted by wood ticks in the Rocky Mountain Pacific coast states and by dog ticks in the Southern and Eastern states. The time when spotted fever appears is usually the time when the ticks are prevalent. Not only the ticks that have been mentioned carry the disease but almost any kind of tick. In the mountain states where the rabbits may be infected by the virus of Rocky Mountain spotted fever, the rabbit tick can carry the disease. In the United States for a period of four years, 1933–37, 2190 cases were reported with 420 deaths.

After a person has been bitten by an infected tick, there are a few days of moderate illness accompanied by chilly sensations and loss of appetite. Then come the chill, with pains in the bones, muscles, back, and joints, headache, and general illness with not infrequently a short dry cough. A fever develops, which may go as high as 105. About the third, fourth, or fifth day of the fever there is a rash which appears first on the wrists, ankles, and back and then spreads over the body. This takes about twenty-four to thirty-six hours. People with this condition sometimes also develop restlessness and insomnia, occasionally delirium and convulsions.

In general one attack of this disease will protect the person against future attacks of the same disease, although second attacks have been reported in

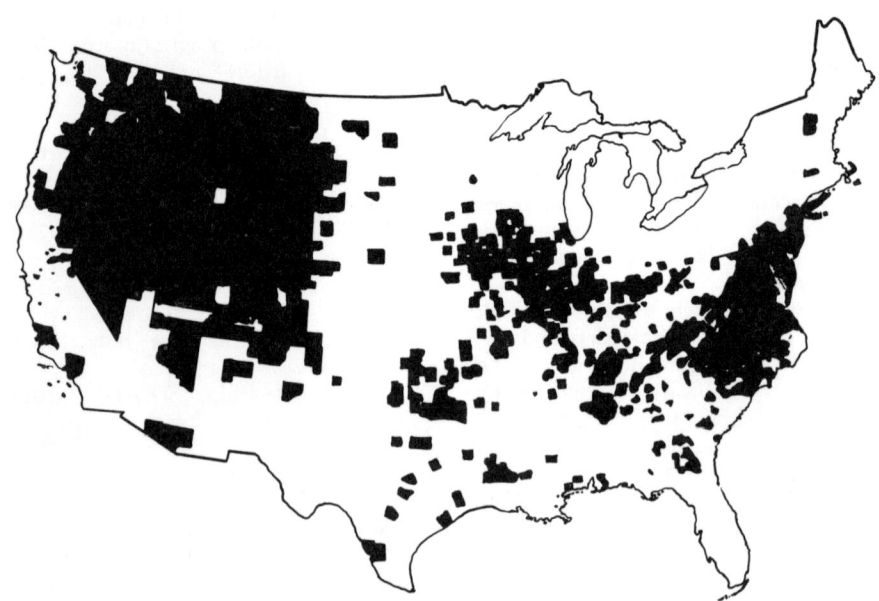

The shaded areas are regions where Rocky Mountain spotted fever has been detected during the past seventy-five years.

ROCKY MOUNTAIN SPOTTED FEVER

some cases eight or more years after the first attack.

A vaccine has been developed which protects people against the disease. Of course the best way to control Rocky Mountain spotted fever is to reduce the number and limit the distribution of ticks. In the Bitter Root Valley this is done by destroying the small animals and dipping the cattle. Clearing and cultivation of land also make it impossible for the ticks to thrive. People themselves can avoid tick bites by wearing a specially designed working costume with the trousers worn inside of heavy woolen socks and high

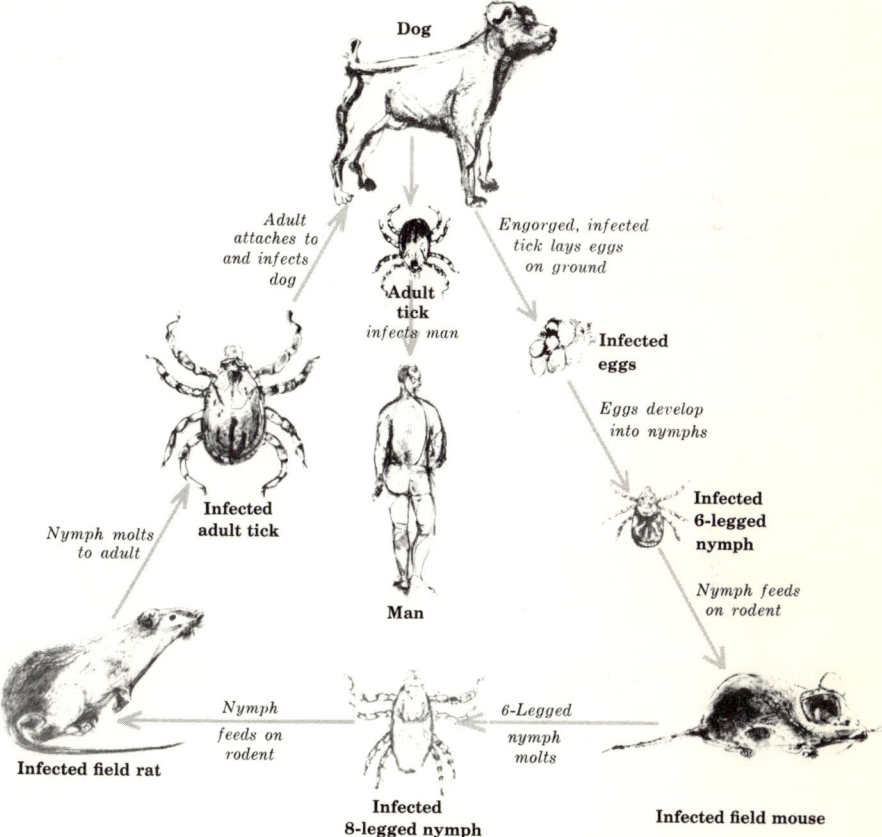

Rocky Mountain spotted fever is transmitted through the wood tick. The female tick transfers the organisms to the offspring through her eggs. The nymph feeds on the blood of rodents, and the adult tick infects dogs and man. Care should be taken to protect pets from ticks.

Chas. Pfizer & Co., Inc.

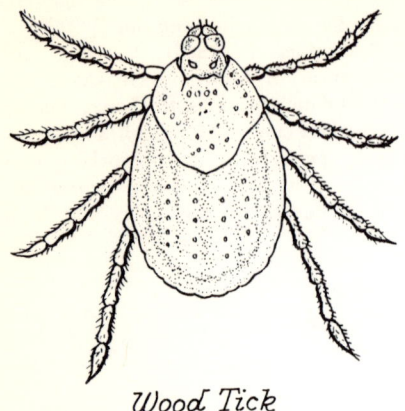

Wood Tick

The wood tick, which may carry a variety of virus diseases, including Rocky Mountain spotted fever.

laced boots. It is also customary to interpose strips of felt or other absorbent material in the neckband and wrists to prevent the ticks from getting under the clothing.

Arrangements should also be made to be certain that dogs, cats, and other pets are free from ticks.

Children are examined twice a day to make certain that the ticks are not on their bodies.

When a tick is found on the body, it should be removed by gently pulling it off with the fingers. Crushing of the tick should be avoided.

Because of the severity of this infection, every necessary supportive treatment is used by the doctor to bring the patient safely through to recovery.

A new antibiotic drug especially valuable in this condition is chloromycetin or choramphenicol.

ROCKY MOUNTAIN SPOTTED FEVER— See article TRANSMISSIBLE DISEASES.

RUBELLA Another name for *Measles, German,* which see.

RUPTURE See *Hernia*.

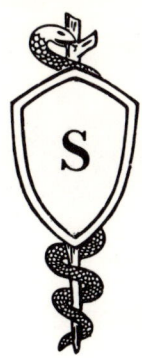

SACROILIAC See *Backache*.

SACRUM At the lower end of the spine there is a triangular bone which is formed of five united bones of the spine. This is called the sacrum. Many a case of backache is ascribed to a disturbance of the joint between the sacrum at the back and the bones of the pelvis in front.

SALIVA The saliva is a fluid put out by the salivary glands, of which there are some under the jaw in front of the ear and under the tongue. It contains a starch-digesting ferment. It serves also to moisten and soften food and to keep the mouth moist.

SALIVA—dyspepsia frequently accompanied by increased salivation: See article DIGESTION AND DIGESTIVE DISEASES.

SALIVA—germ carrier: See INFECTIOUS DISEASE, article THE PREVENTION AND TREATMENT OF INFECTIOUS DISEASE.

SALIVA—germ identification: See INFECTIOUS DISEASE, article THE PREVENTION AND TREATMENT OF INFECTIOUS DISEASE.

SALIVA—mumps carried by: See CHILDHOOD DISEASES, article INFECTIOUS DISEASES OF CHILDHOOD.

SALIVA—oversupply in epidemic encephalitis: See article TRANSMISSIBLE DISEASES.

SALIVA—rabies transmitted by: See article TRANSMISSIBLE DISEASES.

SALIVARY JUICES—See DIET, article ADVICE ON THE DIET.

SALK VACCINE (See also discussion under *Infantile Paralysis*) For

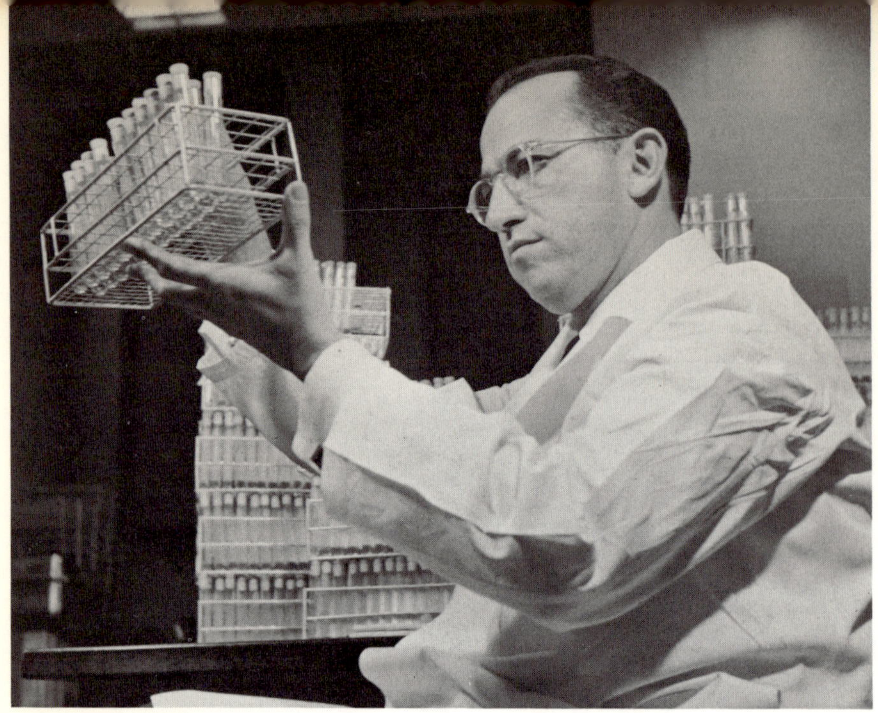

Photographs show Dr. Jonas E. Salk, discoverer of the polio vaccine, with his assistants at work in the laboratory. In one of the pictures Dr. Salk is seen giving a youngster the vaccine during polio vaccine trials held at an elementary school.

The National Foundation for Infantile Paralysis

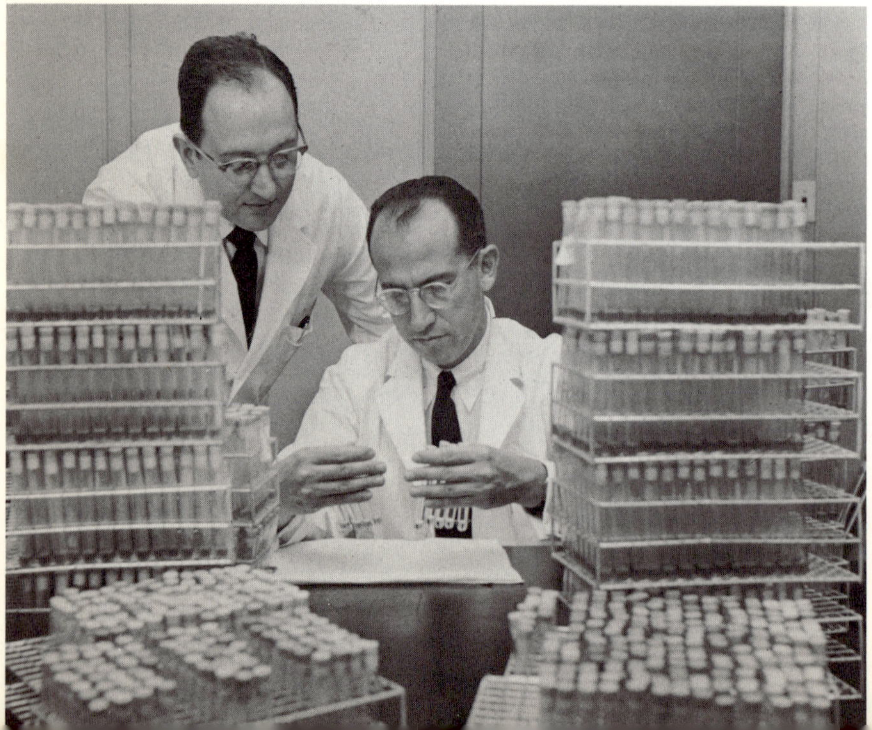

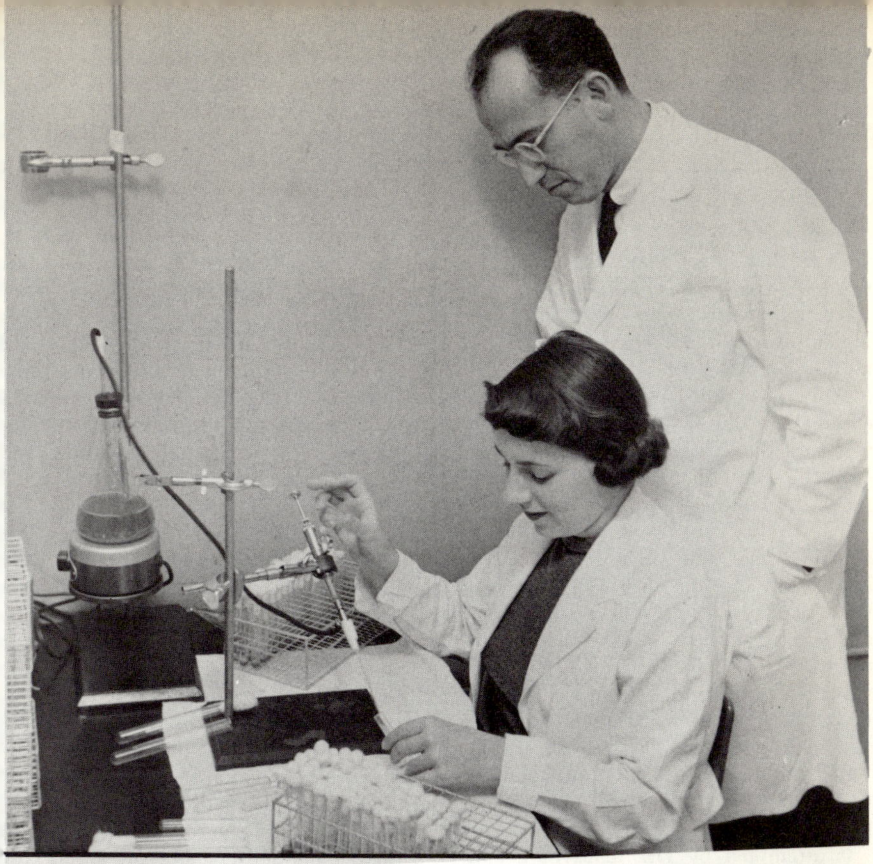

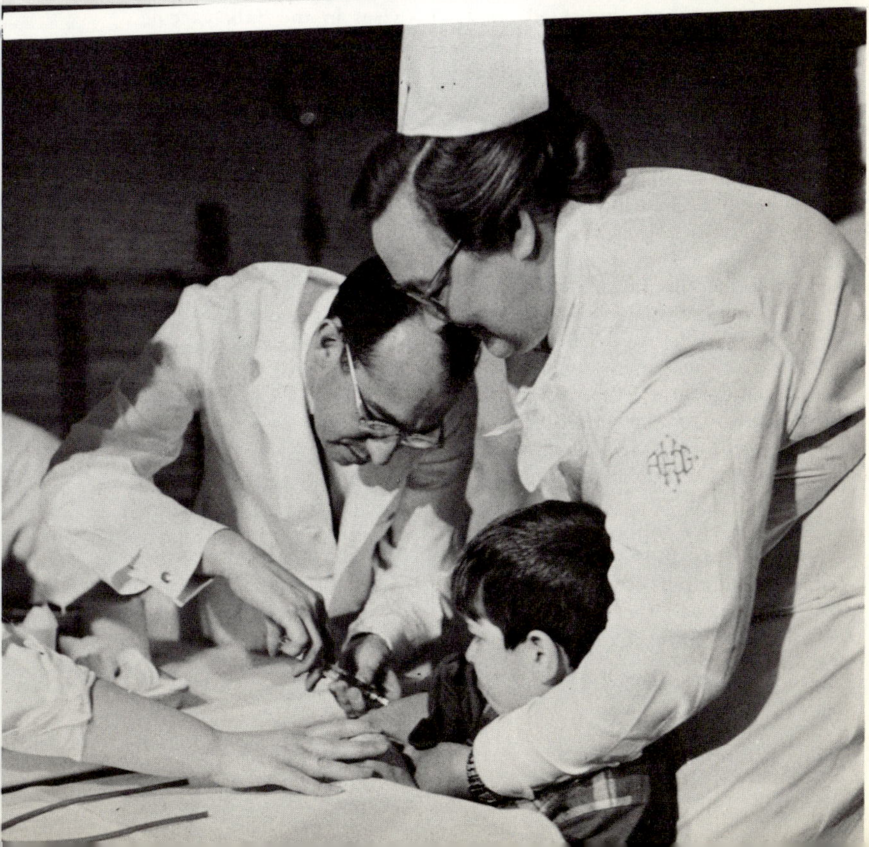

many years infantile paralysis has been the most feared of all the crippling diseases that affect mankind. Today as we look back on the year 1955 we stand on a new front where we can predict the ultimate elimination of infantile paralysis as a threat just as typhoid fever and smallpox have been eliminated. This has resulted from the work of the National Foundation for Infantile Paralysis which began raising funds for research on this disease in 1937. Up to that time the suspicion prevailed that this disease was caused by a virus but the virus was not isolated. Today the viruses, because there are several of them which cause infantile paralysis, have been isolated and grown in pure form outside the human body. For this work Enders and his associates received the Nobel Prize. When the virus could be grown outside the human body on monkey kidneys in pure form, the preparation of a vaccine was attempted by Dr. Jonas Salk and early experimentation indicated that the inoculation of a mixture of killed viruses would produce in a child resistance against infection with this disease. After pilot experiments a vast experiment was undertaken under the auspices of the National Foundation for Infantile Paralysis in which great numbers of children were inoculated and compared with a similar number who did not receive the inoculation. Once this effective experiment was reported on April 12, 1955 at Ann Arbor, Michigan the vaccine was made available by various manufacturers throughout the United States. In the latter part of 1955, Dr. Alexander D. Langmuir of the United States Public Health Service surveyed the results. From New York State comes the report that the paralysis rate was four per 100,000 for vaccinated children contrasted with 20.9 for 100,000 for unvaccinated. From Minnesota the report indicated 2.7 for vaccinated compared with 30.1 for unvaccinated children. In children ages 7 and 8 years the attack rate was much lower than in younger and older children. The poliomyelitis vaccine was most widely used in children of 7 and 8 years. From other countries also came reports of the effectiveness of the vaccine. In Canada the rate was 1.07 for 100,000 for vaccinated children and 5.39 for 100,000 among unvaccinated children. In Denmark there was not one case of paralytic poliomyelitis among over 400,000 children who were vaccinated. Here is a situation of great hope because over a period of ten years greater and greater numbers of children will be vaccinated. The vaccine in the meantime will be continuously improved by new techniques which are being studied in laboratories. Among these new techniques is a combined method of killing the virus using ultraviolet rays and the formaldehyde which is the substance used for killing the virus in the Salk vaccine.

As 1955 ended, a survey revealed that the number of admissions of children to hospitals for infantile paralysis had dropped 52% among the 8 year old children and 40% among 7 year old children. These were of course the principal age groups that received the Salk vaccine. Children from 15 through 19 years of age who had not received the vaccine had a decrease in hospital admission rates of only 12% as contrasted with a decline in the general population of 17%. All of this is taken as good evidence of the virtue of this vaccine. Estimates by epidemiologists indicate that some 1700 cases of paralytic poliomyelitis were prevented in 1955 by the use of vaccination.

SALPINGITIS (See discussion under *Fallopian Tubes*) Infection of the fallopian tubes is called salpingitis.

SALT Pure sodium, which is one of the two elements in sodium chloride or common salt, is seldom found except in chemical laboratories. Many combinations of sodium with other elements are used in diet and in industry. Table salt is sodium chloride. Baking soda is sodium bicarbonate.

The average man takes in his diet about half an ounce of sodium chloride every day. It is easy, on a low salt diet, to reduce this to about one fifth as much. This is done particularly when excess of fluid accumulates in the tissues as in dropsy. No one knows exactly the minimum or maximum of sodium chloride that any one person ought to have, but fortunately the human body is equipped with factors of safety so that it can get rid of excesses of various substances. The average human body contains at all times about three ounces of sodium chloride. The use of salt by the body and its elimination by the kidney are apparently controlled by the cortex or outer layer of the adrenal gland.

Many vegetables contain another salt with an element similar to sodium, namely, potassium. A person who subsists on a vegetable diet craves salt because vegetables contain less sodium than meat. The moment the salt in the human body falls below the amount necessary, a craving is set up.

Salt is also important for supplying the chlorine element since hydrochloric acid is secreted by the stomach regularly as an aid to digestion. Pepsin works as a digestive substance only in the presence of hydrochloric acid. However, hydrochloric acid should not be taken by the average person in that form except on the advice of a physician.

Various diets free from large amounts of sodium chloride have been developed. Most physicians are convinced that there is a definite relationship between salt in the diet and the occurrence of various conditions affecting the blood pressure and the kidneys. However, in the presence of unusual craving for salt, or, in fact, in any disease condition, it is well to be guided in such matters by competent advice.

SALT—blood pressure affected by: See article BLOOD PRESSURE.
SALT—daily requirement: See DIET, article ADVICE ON THE DIET.
SALT—dropsy: See KIDNEY, article THE KIDNEY: ITS DISEASES AND DISTURBANCES.
SALT—food value: See DIET, article ADVICE ON THE DIET.
SALT—heat stroke prevented by: See article FIRST AID.
SALT—iodized: See article ENDOCRINOLOGY.
SALT—kidney disease: See KIDNEY, article THE KIDNEY: ITS DISEASES AND DISTURBANCES.
SALT—substitutes: See article BLOOD PRESSURE.
SALT—urine contains: See KIDNEY, article THE KIDNEY: ITS DISEASES AND DISTURBANCES.
SALT-FREE DIETS—See article BLOOD PRESSURE.
SALTS—deficiency will produce disease: See article DEFICIENCY DISEASES.
SALTS—metallic: See SKIN, article THE SKIN.
SALTS—mineral: See INFANCY, article CARE AND FEEDING OF THE CHILD.
SALTS—silver: See article OCCUPATION AND HEALTH.

SARCOMA Tumors which are malignant but not made of epithelial tissue (like cancer) are usually of the sarcoma type. They may involve cartilage or bone or fibrous tissues. The diagnosis is made by the doctor, who takes a piece of the tumor and examines it under the microscope.

SARCOMAS—See article CANCER.
SARCOMAS—bone: See article CANCER.
SARCOMAS—outnumber carcinomas in children: See article CANCER.

SCABIES Scabies, also called seven-year itch, Cuban itch, prison itch, and similar names, is caused by the itch mite. It spreads amidst poverty, overcrowding, and uncleanliness. Usually scabies is transmitted by body contact.

The itch mite does not have the same habits as the body louse. The body louse lives in the clothing and feeds on the body, but the itch mite lives in the body under the skin. Any infestation of clothing or bedding by the itch mite is accidental. Only about 3 per cent of all cases are infested from clothing or bedding.

The itch mite tunnels under the skin. If the skin is cleaned and is free from crusting and secondary infection the little spots of invasion can be seen. The female mite burrows into the skin through the hair follicles and travels along a tunnel, which she creates. At the inner end of the tunnel she lays her eggs. After three to five days the eggs hatch and the larvae burrow along new tunnels or come out of the old one.

The most common areas of infestation are between the fingers, on the backs of the hands, elbows, under the arms, in the groin, under the breasts, around the navel, the sex organs, the shoulder blades, and the back.

During World War II several new treatments were developed for scabies. Emulsions of benzyl benzoate, 23 per cent, is most frequently used. Several proprietary preparations like Kwell and Eurax embody this principle. After the body has been thoroughly scrubbed with hot water the emulsion is applied with a brush or with an insecticide gun and the whole body is covered from the neck down. The emulsion is allowed to dry, and then after ten or fifteen minutes a second application is painted on. The patient then puts on his clothing and refrains from bathing for twenty-four hours. Then he is given another painting with the benzyl benzoate emulsion. After a second twenty-four-hour period he is instructed to bathe and put on all clean clothing. If these instructions are carried out carefully 95 per cent of patients are cured. The failures are given another course of treatment. The ointment called Gammexane, which is hexachlorocyclohexane, is also used effectively against scabies. The new treatments tend to replace the older use of sulphur ointment, pyrethrum ointment, and rotenone ointment.

SCABIES—See article FIRST AID; SKIN, article THE SKIN.

SCABIES—allergy mistakenly diagnosed: See article ALLERGY.

SCARLET FEVER The story of an attack of scarlet fever is rather typical. From two to four days after a person has been in contact with someone who has scarlet fever, a chill occurs. Then there is sore throat with some nausea and vomiting. Promptly the pulse becomes rapid. The fever rises as high as 102 to 104 degrees. Bright red spots about the size of a pin point begin to appear, usually first on the neck and chest. This eruption spreads rapidly over the rest of the body. The face appears red, usually because of the fever and not because of the eruption. After a few days the rash begins to fade, and in about a week the skin is normal in color.

There is usually a severe sore throat and an intense redness of the inside of the mouth. The tonsils are swollen. The tongue develops a peculiar appearance which has given it the name of strawberry tongue. Sometimes the glands in the neck enlarge because of the infection.

Infection with scarlet fever varies in severity. There have been times when exceedingly severe forms of scarlet fever have attacked whole communities. More recently scarlet fever seems to have become a relatively mild disease, and the number of deaths has greatly decreased. Each winter brings an increase in scarlet fever, as does also late spring.

Many people believe that scarlatina and scarlet fever are different conditions—one milder than the other. Actually there is just one disease of this type, although from time to time cases of German measles and eruption due to sensitivities of various kinds are mistaken for scarlet fever.

Scarlet fever seldom occurs during the first year of life, probably because babies inherit from their mothers some resistance to the disease. Most cases occur in children between six and ten years of age. Incidentally these are the ages when children first begin to have contacts with other children in schools and on playgrounds. Scarlet fever is not, however, exclusively a disease of childhood. More than 15 per cent of those who have scarlet fever are more than sixteen years old.

The height of infectivity in scarlet fever occurs when the nose and throat are filled with discharges contaminated with the germs that are now recognized as being responsible for scarlet fever. Most people are now convinced that the cause of scarlet fever is a special type of streptococcus. In most cases the infected person has the germs in the discharges of the nose and throat for from ten to fourteen days.

Since 1924 great advances have been made in our knowledge of scarlet fever. Among these has been the development of a test of the skin called the Dick test (like the Schick test in diphtheria), which shows whether or not a child is likely to have scarlet fever if exposed to the disease. This is known as susceptibility.

In the skin test for susceptibility to scarlet fever the toxin is injected under the skin, and a simple salt solution is injected as a control. Reddening in the area in which the toxin was injected is taken as a positive test. There is also available an immunizing toxin which, when injected into the body, causes the child to develop resistance against scarlet fever. In times of epidemic immunization with the scarlet fever streptococcus toxin is recommended for any person who shows a positive reaction to the Dick test.

Sometimes there is a local reaction to the injection of the toxin, but this usually disappears within forty-eight hours. In other instances there may be a general reaction, with pain, some fever and nausea, sometimes even a slight rash. However, immunization against scarlet fever avoids long isolation, serious complications, and makes the disease much milder.

Various communities in the United States differ as to the length of time children with scarlet fever should be kept at home. The recommendations vary from a minimum period of twenty-one days to a maximum of six weeks. The decision as to whether or not schools shall be closed during an epidemic of scarlet fever depends on the extent to which the closing of the school helps or interferes with the spread of the disease. In country districts, where children go to widely separated homes, closing of the school may be of value. In cities, where children mingle much more closely at home and in the neighborhood than they would in the school, it is customary to keep the schools open.

Children in families where there are cases of scarlet fever will stay home during the time of the infection. Every person who has scarlet fever should be isolated and remain isolated until the doctor declares that it is safe for that person to mingle with other people.

If every case of scarlet fever is diagnosed promptly, if the patient is put to bed, and if proper measures of disinfection are carried out in relation to discharges from the nose and throat and in regard to contaminated materials, and if, in addition, we apply all that we now know about the specific prevention of scarlet fever, this disease may someday soon be eliminated as an infection threat to human beings.

From ten days to two weeks after scarlet fever first appears the skin begins to peel or scale. Great patches of skin may come off the hands and feet. Over the rest of the body the skin usually comes off in small scales. The scales of the skin and the skin that peel off are not important in spreading the disease except when they are contaminated with secretions of the nose and throat. These secretions do contain the germs and will themselves spread the disease or do so by contaminating the skin, the patient's dishes, or anything else which he soils.

Since infection with scarlet fever is a menace not only because of itself but particularly because of the secondary complications, special attention is given in scarlet fever to protecting the kidneys and the heart during the time when the person is sick. Every patient with scarlet fever should remain in bed for three weeks.

The severe inflammation and swelling in the throat may extend into the Eustachian tubes, which pass from the back of the nose to the ears. Thus the scarlet fever infection may spread into the ear and bring about a serious complication, even mastoiditis, with permanent damage to hearing.

The antitoxin for scarlet fever is successful in controlling the disease and in greatly decreasing its severity. The decision as to whether or not the antitoxin is to be given in scarlet fever must, of course, rest with the physician. New methods of treatment, including the sulfonamides and antibiotics like penicillin and tetracyn make scarlet fever a much milder disease than it used to be. The antitoxin for scarlet fever is given particularly in those cases in which the disease is severe. The antitoxin of scarlet fever does not affect the germs themselves but does affect the toxin, which is responsible for the symptoms of scarlet fever. The drugs of the sulfonamide type act directly on the germs, preventing their growth and thus decreasing the menace of the infection and the amount of toxin that develops. Deaths from scarlet fever are now exceedingly rare.

The doctor who takes care of the patient with scarlet fever will prescribe remedies which prevent headache and other pains, also lotions to take care of itching and irritation of the skin. He advises the family as to the cleaning of linens, utensils, and other materials used by the patient, in order to prevent the spread of the disease. After the patient has recovered, the bed and body linens and any other material that may have come in contact with discharges from the patient and all objects, such as thermometers, spoons, cups, and toys that have been used by the patient, should be boiled, steamed, or soaked in a suitable germicidal solution. The permanent furniture should be thoroughly washed and cleaned, and the room aired and sunned for at least one day as a means of eliminating infection.

SCARLET FEVER—See CHILDHOOD DISEASES, article INFECTIOUS DISEASES OF CHILDHOOD.

SCARLET FEVER—albuminuria: See KIDNEY, article THE KIDNEY: ITS DISEASES AND DISTURBANCES.

SCARLET FEVER—childhood disease: See CHILDHOOD DISEASES, article INFECTIOUS DISEASES OF CHILDHOOD.

SCARLET FEVER—confused with German measles: See CHILDHOOD DISEASES, article INFECTIOUS DISEASES OF CHILDHOOD.
SCARLET FEVER—confused with measles: See CHILDHOOD DISEASES, article INFECTIOUS DISEASES OF CHILDHOOD.
SCARLET FEVER—contagious disease: See INFECTIOUS DISEASE, article THE PREVENTION AND TREATMENT OF INFECTIOUS DISEASE.
SCARLET FEVER—deaths annually: See CHILDHOOD DISEASES, article INFECTIOUS DISEASES OF CHILDHOOD.
SCARLET FEVER—diet: See CHILDHOOD DISEASES, article INFECTIOUS DISEASES OF CHILDHOOD.
SCARLET FEVER—hair fall may follow: See HAIR, article THE HAIR.
SCARLET FEVER—hypertension may result: See article BLOOD PRESSURE.
SCARLET FEVER—immunity induced: See RESPIRATORY DISEASES, article THE RESPIRATORY DISEASES.
SCARLET FEVER—incidence: See INFECTIOUS DISEASE, article THE PREVENTION AND TREATMENT OF INFECTIOUS DISEASE.
SCARLET FEVER—incubation period: See INFECTIOUS DISEASE, article THE PREVENTION AND TREATMENT OF INFECTIOUS DISEASE.
SCARLET FEVER—measles frequently precedes: See CHILDHOOD DISEASES, article INFECTIOUS DISEASES OF CHILDHOOD.
SCARLET FEVER—measles spreads more rapidly: See CHILDHOOD DISEASES, article INFECTIOUS DISEASES OF CHILDHOOD.
SCARLET FEVER—mental defectiveness may result: See MENTAL, article NERVOUS AND MENTAL DISORDERS.
SCARLET FEVER—nephritis: See KIDNEY, article THE KIDNEY: ITS DISEASES AND DISTURBANCES.
SCARLET FEVER—pneumonia frequently follows: See RESPIRATORY DISEASES, article THE RESPIRATORY DISEASES.
SCARLET FEVER—prevention: See CHILDHOOD DISEASES, article INFECTIOUS DISEASES OF CHILDHOOD.
SCARLET FEVER—skin reaction: See SKIN, article THE SKIN.
SCARLET FEVER—streptococcus-like organism causes: See article TRANSMISSIBLE DISEASES.
SCARLET FEVER—symptoms: See CHILDHOOD DISEASES, article INFECTIOUS DISEASES OF CHILDHOOD.
SCARLET FEVER—tongue inflammation: See EAR, article THE EAR, TONGUE, NOSE, AND THROAT.
SCARLET FEVER—treatment: See INFECTIOUS DISEASE, article THE PREVENTION AND TREATMENT OF INFECTIOUS DISEASE; CHILDHOOD DISEASES, article INFECTIOUS DISEASES OF CHILDHOOD.

SCIATIC NEURITIS A long, large nerve known as the sciatic nerve passes from the lower part of the spinal column out of the spinal canal through some openings between the bones, then down to the back of the thigh and onward to the leg. Whenever this nerve becomes irritated or inflamed, there is pain in back of the thigh and in other portions of the body through which this nerve passes. The sciatic nerve is the longest nerve in the body. Frequently the pains that result from inflammation of the sciatic nerve are confused with rheumatic pains. Pain develops in this nerve as a result of pressure on it due to changes in the blood vessels, by disturbances of the spinal cord in the area in which the nerve arises, as a result of falls or strains, by exposure to rain, wading in cold streams, working in damp places, or similar experiences. Sometimes pain in the sciatic nerve is associated with severe constipation either from pressure of material in the loaded bowels or from absorption of toxic materials from the body which affect the nerves.

When the doctor studies the patient

SCIATIC NEURITIS

for the presence of sciatic neuritis, he will make a number of tests to determine whether the pain is due to the sciatic nerve or to some other cause. He will examine the back for any unusual curvature of the spine or any pressure that might result from bones in the wrong position. He will study the legs for signs of spasms of the muscles or for wasting. He may test the effects of raising the leg in a straight position while the patient lies flat on the back. This puts a strain on the large hamstring muscles which, in turn, refer the strain to the nerve. It is also important to determine whether the pain is the result of difficulty with the nerve or with the sacroiliac joint.

In treating a sciatic neuritis the doctor must overcome any unfavorable conditions of work or climate which may be contributing factors. He studies the diet to make certain that there are adequate amounts of such nutritional substances as thiamine. He prescribes rest and arranges the bed so that there is relief from tension and support to the inflamed tissues. Heat is helpful in relieving the pain.

After the pain has subsided, the patient must continue to avoid strenuous exercise, which is often followed by twinges in the nerves.

There are a variety of methods of special treatment, including injections of various substances in and around the nerve.

Finally, there are surgical processes involving work on the bones and muscles or on the nerve. In a severe case of sciatic neuritis determination of the causative factors and treatment applied specifically to control these conditions involves the highest art of the physician.

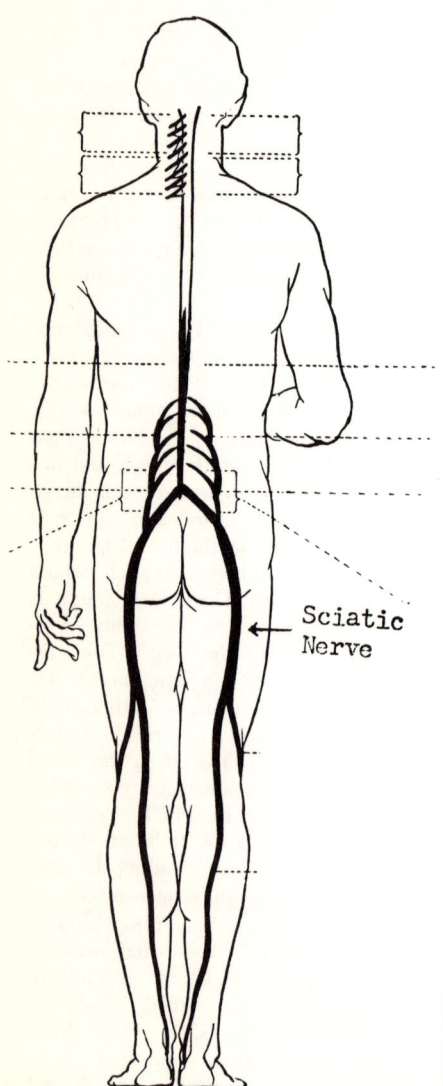

Diagram shows the sciatic nerve passing out of the spinal column, down the back of the thighs and onward to the leg. The sciatic nerve is the longest nerve of the body. Pains from inflammation of this nerve are usually felt in the back of the thigh.

SCLERODERMA Sometimes the skin of a human being becomes altered in its consistency and color, so that there are large or small areas of the skin that become hard and yellow, occasionally hard and white. No one knows the cause of this condition. Women are far more commonly affected than men, and most often between twenty and forty years of age. It has been thought from time to time that glandular changes have been responsible. Many physicians are convinced that the disturbance is definitely related to some condition in the nervous system because changes in certain areas of the spinal cord have been found on post-mortem examination. There are many methods of treatment, including the use of the electric needle for removing the area or various ointments for softening the tissue. In general, however, treatment is unsatisfactory in stopping the progress of the disease or in curing it.

SCLERODERMA—See SKIN, article THE SKIN.

SCLEROSIS This is a scientific term derived from a Greek word meaning hard. It is used to describe a hardening of any tissue of the human body. There are many different forms of sclerosis, involving tissues of the eye, tissues of the spine, tumors of the breast, and other tissues.

SCOLIOSIS See *Spinal Curvature*.

SCURVY (See also, *Vitamins*) The discovery that the lack of certain essential substances from the body—either because they were not in the diet or failed to be absorbed and utilized—would cause serious disturbances of growth and health, was one of the most startling in all the history of medicine. Now these substances are called vitamins—a word coined by Casimir Funk around 1910.

Scurvy—a disease known for centuries—is now definitely established as resulting from a lack of Vitamin C, also called ascorbic acid. The chief sources of Vitamin C are the citrus fruits, the leafy green vegetables, Irish potatoes, and tomatoes. Milk contains a little Vitamin C but even this little is lessened by pasteurization, or boiling, or any form of treatment that results in oxygenation.

Physicians see few cases of scurvy nowadays. Such cases as are reported affect chiefly people who live alone on greatly restricted diets, or people addicted to strange eating habits which interfere with normal nutrition. Sometimes the condition is seen in babies fed artificially when mothers or nurses have failed to make certain that proper amounts of Vitamin C containing substances are included in the diet.

Among the chief symptoms of scurvy are bleeding from the gums and black and blue spots over the body showing easy bleeding. Wounds of the skin heal slowly in those with Vitamin C deficiency.

Scurvy can be controlled by taking plenty of Vitamin C which is now available in several medicinal forms. The material need not be injected into the blood but can be taken by mouth, after which the condition usually clears up promptly. Much better is the prevention of scurvy by the daily taking of some citrus fruit juice, tomato juice, or by eating leafy green vegetables, which add other important factors to the diet.

SCURVY—See BLOOD, article THE BLOOD AND ITS DISEASES; article DEFICIENCY DISEASES.

SCURVY—cause: See INFANCY, article CARE AND FEEDING OF THE CHILD; SKIN, article THE SKIN.

SCURVY—cured among Dutch and

SEASICKNESS

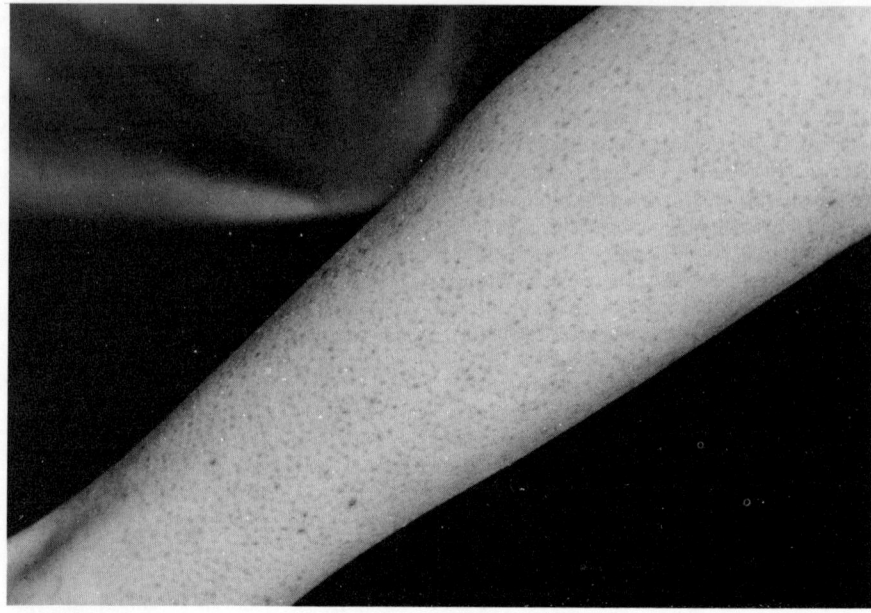

Perifollicular hemorrhages of early scurvy. Scurvy results from a deficiency of vitamin C. Fresh cabbage and citrus fruits contain large amounts of vitamin C. Much of the vitamin C content in foods is destroyed when the foods are cooked or exposed to the air.

Chas. Pfizer & Co., Inc.

British seamen: See DIET, article ADVICE ON THE DIET.

SCURVY—nosebleed: See EAR, article THE EAR, TONGUE, NOSE, AND THROAT.

SCURVY—pellagra related: See article DEFICIENCY DISEASES.

SCURVY—rheumatic complications: See article ARTHRITIS, RHEUMATISM, AND GOUT.

SCURVY—vitamin C deficiency: See INFANCY, article CARE AND FEEDING OF THE CHILD.

SEASICKNESS The immense amount of ocean transportation during the war has kept attention focused constantly on seasickness, a condition which, of course, must be considered in relation to carsickness and airsickness.

The investigators are convinced that there is some relation between the eye, the ear, and the sensation of air-, car-, or seasickness. The exact cause of seasickness has not yet, however, been determined—at least not to the extent that there is a specific remedy related to the cause.

People in trains, ships, and airplanes who are confined in stuffy rooms and who are unable to move around are more likely to become sick than those who are comfortably located. People who travel on trains and who get carsick in a compartment or room may not be carsick if they sit in the open car. Overloading the stomach increases the tendency to seasickness or airsickness. Small amounts of food taken frequently are sometimes helpful.

People who become nauseated easily have their symptoms of seasickness intensified when there is an oily smell from the engines. Sometimes people become nauseated when the odor of food spreads through a plane as the stewardess begins serving dinner.

The semicircular canals in the internal ear, which are associated with balance, seem to have a definite part to play in the symptoms of seasickness. It has been found, for instance, that quick vertical movements of an airplane are a factor in producing airsickness. Many people become airsick or seasick when noises and vibration are excessive. Some people become sick in trains while riding backward but not while riding forward. People who have chronic infections of the sinuses and of the ears are more likely to be airsick than those who are without such infections.

Among the various remedies that have been offered for seasickness are the following:

1. A tight belt.
2. Champagne before sailing.
3. Hold a bag over the nose and breathe into the bag.
4. Stuff cotton wool in the ears.
5. Keep a bandage over the eyes.
6. If you are smoking, don't stop smoking.
7. If you are smoking, stop smoking.
8. Lie flat on the back.
9. Dance in rhythm with the ship's movements.
10. Eat heavily of fruits and alkaline foods.
11. Take baking soda.

In general, however, it is well to be advised by a doctor such as the one who for years traveled on the *Aquitania* and who made a record of some of his experiences with seasick passengers. He says that seasickness, when not complicated by a hangover from too much celebration before going on board, is due to unusual reactions that occur in the nervous system because of excessive stimulation reaching the parts of the body that are concerned with balance. This means particularly the semicircular canals in the internal ear. For the prevention of seasickness he has recommended fresh air with bodily warmth. Have plenty of sleep before going on the boat. Because of uneasiness around the center of the abdomen, many people find the wearing of a firm abdominal binder comfortable and helpful. Be moderate in drinking and eating before going on the boat and make sure that the bowel is working satisfactorily. Alcohol tends to take the edge off the apprehension but will not itself prevent seasickness. Take such sedative drugs as the doctor may prescribe.

Up to recent times medicine has not had information concerning any drug or method of treatment that has been quite satisfactory in preventing, relieving, or curing motion sickness. The United States Navy during World War II made extensive studies and proved that psychosomatic factors are unimportant in seasickness. Studies were made of keeping sailors in different positions from lying down to crouching and standing. Almost by accident a discovery was made in 1947 that seems to be the answer to the problem of motion sickness. It is a drug called dramamine, one of the antihistaminic products similar to those that are used against hay fever and food sensitivities. It was sent to the clinics for experiments in these conditions. In the course of the trials the drug was given to a pregnant woman who was sensitive to foods and who all her life had been sensitive to carsickness. When she took this drug for food sensitivity, she was completely relieved of carsickness. Repeated tests using the new drug and using a simple capsule of milk sugar proved that only the new drug gave her relief. Later the drug was used on other people who suffered from airsickness and they too obtained relief.

Extensive studies were then made on sailors on one of the large ships and proved again that the drug was excellent. Dramamine is now recognized as being effective for both preventing and treating motion sickness. The drug may be taken by mouth or given in other ways. It is supplied on prescription of doctors and is worthy of trial by people who look on ocean voyages with dread because of invariable seasickness. The drug is also successful in airsickness and carsickness and possibly in some cases of Menière's disease and migraine.

MOTION SICKNESS—A combination of Benadryl and hyoscine that overcomes motion sickness is now on the market. The manufacturer claims that the mixture of the two drugs is more effective than either of the drugs individually. The company made tests on students taking routine training flights and found that those who had taken a combination of Benadryl and hyoscine fared better than did those who received hyoscine alone or who received placebos. None of the subjects who took Benadryl with hyoscine experienced nausea or vomiting. All but 10 per cent of the students had flown before.

SEBACEOUS CYST See *Wen*.

SEBORRHEA (See also discussions under *Dandruff* and *Hair*) Some people perspire more than others. Some people have more dandruff and peeling of the skin than others. Many specialists in diseases of the skin are convinced that seborrhea or dandruff is an infectious condition which arises from germs which are normally on the skin but which are especially prevalent on a greasy skin.

Some physicians are convinced that seborrhea represents a special type of constitution in which there is an increase of the secretion from the glands in the skin, an overgrowth of such glands, and an enlargement of the pores. Associated with this there is usually a thickening of the skin and also an increased activity of the sweat glands.

One British physician is convinced that seborrhea is associated with similar activities which affect the mucous membranes of the mouth and the other orifices of the body, and that sometimes there is also change of the mucous membrane of the nose in conditions like hay fever and asthma.

For this reason it has been suggested that the person who has an unusually greasy skin with excess secretion might well take a diet which is rich in proteins but restricted as to sugars, fluids, and salt. It should also be a diet that is high in vitamins, particularly leafy green vegetables and fresh fruits. Irritating foods and highly seasoned foods like fried foods and pork are also to be avoided.

In the worst types of seborrhea it is obviously necessary for the physician to treat the entire body from the point of view of rest, exercise, and hygiene generally. In certain cases, however, where the condition is largely confined to scurf on the scalp, treatment applied directly to the dandruff is itself sufficient to bring about a successful result.

Certainly anyone with dandruff ought to wash the hair at least once a week, bathe the body regularly at least once a day, and avoid the wearing of clothing that produces heat next to the skin with maceration and softening caused by the fluid.

Dandruff of the scalp is, however, only one manifestation of the seborrheic constitution. The regular washing of the hair and the application of suitable scalp treatments can keep dandruff under control week by week. When, however, there is an eruption of pimples on the face with a greasy complexion and enlarged pores, when there is scaling and inflammation of the skin behind the ears and in the groins, the condition demands much more serious attention.

Patients of this type must be kept in a good mental frame of mind, must get plenty of sleep, must be given proper treatments to avoid itching and irritation. They must have their blood brought up to par by the suitable administration of the necessary vitamins, iron, and similar substances.

A new drug specifically against seborrhea is called Selsun. This is used as a shampoo, left on for ten minutes, and then rinsed away.

Seborrhea—See Skin, article The Skin.

Seborrhea—baldness blamed on: See Hair, article The Hair.

Seborrheic Disorders—See Hair, article The Hair.

Seborrheic Keratoses—See Skin, article The Skin.

Seborrheic Warts—See Skin, article The Skin.

SENESCENCE Old age can be divided into two periods—senescence, which is the gradual aging of the body, and senility, in which the aging process is complicated by a variety of conditions.

Unfortunately uncomplicated old age is exceedingly rare. As people get old, the cells of the body lose their power of repair. When this happens, tissues become fibrous, occasionally even calcified. The rareness of uncomplicated old age is shown by the fact that one famous pathologist reported that he had never seen a case of a completely natural death in an experience of thirty-eight years, during which he had examined by post-mortem examination many thousands of bodies; another pathologist, who had examined post mortem more than 20,000 bodies, said that he had seen only twenty-five which could be called examples of healthy old age. In these twenty-five death occurred simply through a gradual wearing out of the heart.

Normal old age comes on gradually and is usually well established by the age of sixty-five, although there are exceptions. For that reason the age of sixty-five is usually set up as the age for retirement from public office or positions of administration. Longevity and the postponement of senility depend on several factors, the first of which is the influence of heredity. In many families youthfulness persists much longer than in others. Much can be done to prevent the development of the changes associated with old age by practicing temperance in food and drink, by relaxation of the mind through hobbies and vacation periods, by healthful but moderate exercise and other practices in the field of good hygiene.

Unquestionably the condition of the blood vessels is the most important single factor in the aging of the human body. Hardening of the arteries is likely to be associated with more rapid degenerative changes, since the tissues depend on the blood vessels for their supply of nutriment, especially oxygen. Associated with rapid old age also is the wearing out of muscular tissues in the bowels and in the walls of blood vessels.

The diseases most likely to occur in old age are enlargement of the prostate gland, which is said to occur in at least half of all men over the age of seventy; cancer, which is especially a disease of old age, although cases do occur in the young; and arthritic changes in the bones and joints.

Pediatricians say that the first year of life is the most critical. Others insist that the first ten years are the hardest. Some call adolescence, with the transition from childhood to adult life, the most critical period.

The great control that is now asserted over infant mortality and the elimination of many of the diseases that used to affect youth make the majority of doctors today think that the most serious age is the period of transition from maturity to old age. Men enter the most critical period of their lives at fifty. This is the time when they begin to need glasses to read the print in the telephone book. Now they begin to get tired a little earlier in the afternoon.

Occasionally the onset of these conditions induces resentment. Many a physical-culture expert or the proprietor of a health institute or gymnasium has earned an excellent livelihood from the fact that these men take up exercise and try to prove to themselves that they are better than they really are. The wise man will realize that aging is a natural process and that the conditions that come with advancing years must be treated with respect. If the thyroid gland, the sex glands, and the pituitary are less efficient, the deficiency will be reflected in the body generally. A doctor can prescribe glandular substances to overcome such deficiencies in part.

Hardening of the arteries and high blood pressure are two of the most important symptoms. Many years ago a wise physician said that a man is as old as his arteries. Incidentally, men are more frequently affected with hardening of the arteries than women.

Arthritis is another condition especially frequent in people after the age of forty and which cripples and disables a good many older people.

Medicine can do a great deal for these disturbances if they are brought soon enough to medical attention. But man is not immortal and the wise man will recognize the aging process and conduct himself accordingly.

Eyes of the Aged—The aging process is continuous from the time of birth to the time of death. Some human beings age more slowly than others.

Many of these changes in the vision of older people are associated with changes in the circulation, including hardening of the arteries. The eyelids of old people develop wrinkles.

Old people seem to cry easily and sometimes suffer from an overflow of tears. This is often due to relaxation of the tissues of the eye, which do not hold the material as do the elastic tissues of the young. Surgeons have developed technics for maintaining the normal relationships between the tissues, overcoming this overflow of tears when it becomes a nuisance.

Elderly people often complain of heaviness of the eyelids and inability to raise them, especially in the morning. The weakness may be due to a gradual disappearance of the elastic tissue from the eyelids.

In the old person the pupil of the eye becomes smaller and less movable, and the color of the eye becomes lighter. The lens of the eye grows and increases in weight throughout life. Sometimes a ring seems to form around the colored center of the eye. This is called an "arcus senilis" and is characteristic of aging.

Cataract is typical of the aged, and the exact cause is not known. The decision as to whether or not a cataract is to be removed by surgical operation depends on many factors having to do with the patient's physical and mental condition as well as the actual condition of the eye.

Old people need much higher intensities of light than young persons. In fact, improvement of the light often decreases the need for stronger eyeglasses.

What Old People Remember—With

the improvement in health our life expectancy at birth has gradually risen. The ancient Greeks apparently lived to an average age of just under thirty years. In 1900 the average age at death in the United States was forty-five. Now we have raised the average life expectancy at birth to almost seventy years and for white girl babies to more than 70 years.

Our mental activities are dependent to some extent on our physical condition. The more any mental activity is dependent on some physical activity of the body, the more that activity is likely to decline with age.

From birth to fifteen years the growth of the human being is rapid. At around twenty-five years of age the human physique reaches its maximum in strength and skill. Most human beings descend slowly from this level until the age of forty-five, when the momentum of decline increases. Then at about fifty-five years of age the rate of decline again increases until the age of seventy.

Intelligence, which is the effective organization of mental abilities for a certain purpose, matures quickly, so that by sixteen years of age the intelligence of the human being is about at its peak. It remains on this level until the early twenties. From twenty years on, the intelligence decreases. By the age of fifty-five many human beings have receded to the fourteen-year-old level. Not all of the factors involved in intelligence are lost at the same rate. The voice and the hearing remain efficient until well along in life. The reaction time is, however, likely to decrease more rapidly.

Memory reaches its peak in the late teens and early twenties and declines rapidly with age. The inability to remember recent events is always a telltale sign of senescence. Old people remember happenings of their childhood and forget what happened yesterday. With senescence they become careless of accuracy, but some youngsters never learn accuracy.

LEARNING AND OLD AGE—"Never too old to learn" is a trite phrase; also "some people never learn." The ability to learn reaches its maximum in the late teens and early twenties and then declines slowly. One psychologist found that there is a 1 per cent loss in learning ability every year from the age of twenty-five on.

Few people develop new interests after fifty. Most people tend to dislike change as they approach old age. The interests of people after middle age are reflected in the physical condition of their bodies. As people get older they enjoy sedentary pursuits and dislike strenuous physical or mental activities. Television has proved to be a wonderful medium of interest and enjoyment particularly for old people.

As people get older their love of amusement declines in the majority of instances in favor of distinctly cultural pursuits. Older men are likely to prefer forms of amusement and relaxation which they can do alone rather than the gregarious types of amusement which interest younger men. Of course there are exceptions to every rule, and some older people possess the ability to renew their minds continually. Thus many old people find their chief delight in reading history and biography.

The world tends to reject the older individual and to make less opportunity for him to take up new jobs or new interests. The man who takes up a new job or profession or returns to school at sixty-five or seventy is rare.

Some men who take up amateur gardening or collection hobbies exhibit surprising skill. Wars give the old people opportunities far beyond those of peacetime.

The suggestion has been made that our recreation experts and our adult education groups ought to plan particularly for the special needs, interests, and abilities of men and women who are more than sixty years old. The mental stimulation which they would receive in such courses would not only help them to live longer and more healthfully but would also be exceedingly productive for the world as a whole.

Old Age—See article Old Age.
Old Age—beauty of: See article Sex Hygiene.
Old Age—cancer: See article Old Age.
Old Age—changes: See article Old Age.
Old Age—diabetes: See article Diabetes.
Old Age—diseases: See article Old Age.
Old Age—emotional problems: See article Old Age.
Old Age—employment: See article Old Age.
Old Age—exercises: See article Old Age.
Old Age—hygiene: See article Old Age.
Old Age—psychoses: See Mental, article Nervous and Mental Disorders.
Old Age—sex hygiene: See article Sex Hygiene.
Old Age—Warthin (A. S.) on: See article Sex Hygiene.
Senile Cataract—See Eye, article The Eye.
Senile Freckles—See Skin, article The Skin.
Senile Keratoses—See Skin, article The Skin.
Senility—natural process: See article Sex Hygiene.
Senility—premature: See article Deficiency Diseases.

SEPTICEMIA Whenever infection invades the blood, the condition is called septicemia. Such infection is always accompanied by chills, profuse sweating, and prostration. The appearance of these symptoms indicates that the doctor should be called immediately because every moment counts in controlling the spread of such an infection.

SEPTIC SORE THROAT A germ called the *Streptococcus hemolyticus*, which is one of the many different forms of this organism, is responsible for a condition called septic sore throat. Of all the sore throats, septic sore throat is the worst. Usually the condition begins with a severe chill and a rapidly developing fever which may reach as high as 105 degrees Fahrenheit. Occasionally, however, the infection takes place more slowly, with some sore throat, headache, and slight fever for a day or two, intensifying as the disease progresses. Soon the swelling in the throat makes swallowing difficult. The head and neck are held stiffly because movement is painful. As the infection extends downward, the voice becomes hoarse, coughing occurs, and there may even be shortness of breath.

When the doctor looks at the throat, he discovers that it is dark red and that there are patches of grayish material. This inflammation may extend even to the point of ulceration. Because of the extent of the infection the glands in the side of the neck become greatly enlarged and this type of inflammation may go on to the formation of abscesses.

The number of fatalities from septic sore throat is not exceedingly great because the location of the infection makes it possible for the doctor to attend to it promptly. However, many instances occur in which the infection may extend to the heart, causing heart disease, or to the abdominal cavity, causing peritonitis, or indeed to any other portion of the body.

SEPTIC SORE THROAT

Fortunately we now have a remedy which is practically specific in the control of septic sore throat. The various sulfonamide drugs are known to have a definite effect on the streptococci and particularly on the *Streptococcus hemolyticus*. Therefore the doctor gives large doses of this drug at once and continues until the infection is under control. Anyone with septic sore throat should go to bed immediately.

As an aid to causing the infection to break up, hot wet packs are applied to the neck. Little is gained, however, by using gargles or sprays or washes of any kind applied to the surface of the throat.

In severe cases when the obstruction in the throat becomes so bad as to interfere seriously with breathing, the administration of oxygen may be used. Naturally any secondary infections such as abscesses or inflammations elsewhere in the body are given immediate attention.

SEPTIC SORE THROAT—See EAR, article THE EAR, TONGUE, NOSE, AND THROAT.

Sex Hygiene

BY

THURMAN B. RICE, M.D.

Professor of Bacteriology and Public Health, Indiana Univ. School of Medicine, Indianapolis, Ind.

Introduction

THE INVESTIGATIONS *of recent years indicate how profoundly various aspects of sex hygiene affect our lives not only from the physical but also from the mental point of view. The chief contribution of the Freudian psychology has been the emphasis which it has placed on the extent to which the inhibitions of previous generations have operated to establish many neuroses and sexual disorders. Certainly, there is good evidence that some conditions which were formerly thought to be wholly physical in character have a mental basis, and that this mental basis is established by failure to develop proper relationship between the sexes.*

Much of the background of these disorders is established in childhood and in adolescence. It is therefore important to recognize the significance of proper education in the facts of sex early in life. In the section which follows, the whole problem of sex education beginning with the instruction of the child in these important matters and carrying his subject through to relationship during courtship, marriage, and wedded life is considered.

A proper appreciation of the relationship of sex to health and to daily life is essential for satisfactory living.

The continuation of our basic culture and the propagation of life itself is directly dependent on the functioning of the fundamental instincts which bring men and women together in an infinitely important relation known as the family or the home, and into which are born other human beings like unto themselves. Sex is everywhere about us. We see it in the clothes we wear, in the occupations we serve, and in the sports and games by which we seek relaxation. Short stories, novels, poetry, art, sculpture, music, and the drama constantly remind us of the fact that men and women are different but closely interrelated and that they behave as they do largely because of this difference. If we would know what it is that motivates men and women and boys and girls; if we would understand the psychology, the hopes, the fears, the desires, the lusts, the passions of our neighbors; if we would know what it is that makes one man a hero and another a beast, we will do well to look into this matter of sex.

Is it not strange, then, that there should be so much misunderstanding of this vital subject? Is it not rather amazing that intelligent men and women should be in so many instances utterly ignorant of the true significance of this, the basic fact of life?

The Ideals and Purposes of Sex Education

There are many reasons why every child and every adult should understand, as well as he may or can, the various complicated functions by which the race reproduces itself and by which the family comes into existence and is held together as a unit. How this information may be transmitted correctly and decently to the younger generation is a problem of the utmost consequence to the success of the family and the nation.

The layman needs comparatively little detailed information concerning the minutiæ of the process of reproduction. He needs rather a broad understanding of the general principles involved. He should regard the understanding of sex as being of the nature of an art rather than a science, the science being needed only that he may practise the better the fine art of living broadly, deeply, and well. Sex and life are inseparable; each is the origin and the end of the other.

Happy is the man or woman, the boy or girl, in whom sex is a well integrated part—*and nothing more*—of the whole purpose and philosophy of life.

Sexuality has been confused with sensuality. A mere incident in the program—an incident that corresponds to the carrying of the pollen by the bee—has been regarded as the *whole* program. It has been supposed that sex is selfish and seeks only its own self-gratification when actually nothing is so unselfish as the love of a mate for a mate or a parent for a child. It has been said that sex has ruined many a man or woman, but it has been forgotten that it has brought out the best that was in countless millions of others. It has made men and women of foolish boys and giddy girls. Sex can inspire an ordinary swain to poetry; it can make heroes of us all when our children or loved ones are in danger. Sex endangers us only when it is misunderstood or misused.

Our young people are demanding a positive education. They will not take "don't" as a rule for conduct. If "mother knows best," they think that mother should be able to give a reason for thinking that she knows best. Negative education tends to produce a pedagogic vacuum which will speedily be filled with something, be it good, bad or indifferent. When the minds of children—and adults—are loaded high with positive facts and principles based on the assumption that sex is natural, good, beautiful, and entirely proper when in its proper place, there will be little to be feared from the untruths and half truths which may otherwise be so disastrous. Once the mind is filled with pertinent facts it is satisfied and goes about its legitimate business untempted by morbid or lascivious curiosity. We much prefer to have our children turning toward the beauties of virtue rather than fleeing from the ugly face of sin. It is most unfortunate that virtue has so often been made to appear dull and prosaic while dangerous and immoral practises have been made most enticing.

Particularly is it important that the child should never be frightened when this subject is discussed. The method of imparting sex education whereby the mother calls the child to her side and tells him or her that she went down to death's door in order that the child might be born is most vicious. Children cannot understand the fact that suffering and sacrifice may make a thing precious. The normal child may be told that the benefits of a dental operation are immeasurable, but, just the same, the fact that "it will hurt" when he goes to the dentist outweighs, to him, every conceivable gain. The mother who associates sex with pain and danger is often laying the foundation for an unsatisfactory or even destructive attitude toward life. Likewise, the parent who makes the subject ugly or disgusting or vulgar is injuring the child instead of helping him. Some suppose that it is necessary to do this in order to guard the virtue of the unmarried young person. Virtue is far better guarded by those who have a thorough understanding and appreciation of its worth.

Sex is a red-blooded thing; it throbs with high passion; it lives, and loves, and fights. It is a giant who constructs or destroys, makes or breaks, according as it is understood or not. Pink pamphlets for pale people will hardly serve the needs of the robust men and women who make the world go around. As well say "naughty, naughty" to a hurricane as to prescribe certain anemic books as a means of helping young people to control the powerful forces which surge within them. Most publications of this sort have been written by persons who have never known *la grande passion* or who, having seared themselves in its flame, are now devoutly wishing "to save the young people from what I have gone through." The services of such are not needed in the present purpose. This is a task for men and women who have felt the divine urge to create, have gladly accepted the challenge, and have not betrayed the trust.

We shall make no attempt to anticipate the questions which some bright-eyed child may ask, but are merely hoping that we may be of aid in preparing the parent so thoroughly in the basic principles of the subject that he or she may be able to feed and to satisfy the perfectly natural childish curiosity which brings a child to his parent with vital questions. Possibly the choice of words which we use may be of value, inasmuch as the lack of the proper word to use is often a serious difficulty. The method of approach may be of value to some who know well enough the subject matter but not the pedagogic methods for putting it across. The parent need not expect to learn or build up a philosophy of sex and life in a moment. Nor can he acquire one second hand by reading a book on the subject. He will need to study long and seriously before he will be skillful in the handling of so delicate a matter. Unless the parent has had a reasonably satisfactory understanding of, and attitude toward, the subject, he need hardly expect to become expert in teaching his children concerning it. This is particularly a subject to be taught by example as well as precept. The man who treats his wife as if she were an inferior creature will have difficulty in instructing his boys, and the nagging wife will fail utterly in leading her offspring to a beautiful conception of sex life.

Reproduction in the Plant and Animal Kingdoms

Those who would understand the marvelous process by which plants and animals may produce other plants and animals of the same sort, and, in particular, would like to understand the matter of sex as it is manifested in the reproduction of the human race, can do no better than to study the phenomenon as it is manifested in simpler forms of life. The process as it is observed in man is so complicated as a result of various social, moral, and ethical relations that it is necessary first to study the subject in some easier form. As a matter of fact, every phase of the process may be scrutinized in this way without arousing the various prejudices and suspicions which have so clouded the issue. Many parents are anxious to initiate their children into the mysteries of the subject, but are deterred by the lack of suitable means of expression. They need elementary examples of sex life before attempting to instruct in the extremely complex relations of modern human society.

A fairly complete understanding of the phenomenon in lower forms of life will give the parent or teacher poise and resourcefulness which will be greatly needed in teaching the subject and in developing a satisfactory philosophy of life. Not infrequently the parent or teacher needs more than anything else concrete illustrations for the explanation of the various difficult points. Very frequently an accurate and dignified vocabulary is needed. It is impossible to suppose that the vulgar words of the alley can be used in good sex instruction. We insist that he or she who teaches must himself or herself have reached some degree of mental poise and decision on these matters. There is no better way to do this than to become acquainted with the elementary biology of sex as it is manifest everywhere about us.

Obviously each species must have some adequate way of reproducing itself, otherwise it would long since have perished from the earth. The continuation of the species is the most fundamental instinct of every plant and every animal species. Most plants begin to die as soon as the seeds are well along toward maturity, and all animals except man are ready to die as soon as the end of the reproductive cycle has been reached. It is sometimes supposed that the self-preservative instinct is strongest in man and beast, but everyone must have seen men and women risking life, reputation, health, social standing, wealth—everything—in order that they might express themselves sexually or take care of their offspring. In such case we must conclude that the instinct for reproduction is really basic.

Two general methods by which the species may be reproduced are observed in nature: the sexual and the asexual. Animals, except in the very lowest forms, use the sexual method. The same is true of most plants, but there are a considerable number of them which have dispensed with sex as a means of procreation. The bacteria, for example, merely divide in the middle, making two new individuals which are exactly alike and like the parent cell. In a sense the different individuals in a bacterial culture are really different fragments of the same original germ. Even high in the plant kingdom we see essentially the same thing. A twig from a willow tree becomes itself a willow tree. It is like the parent tree for the good reason that it is a detached part of the parent tree. A number of cultivated species of plants are propagated by tubers, roots, bulbs, cuttings, and grafts, which are all asexual means, though these plants have sexual organs as well. Seed *potatoes* represent a use of the asexual method, while potato *seeds* (occasionally found in small pods where the flowers have been) are of sexual origin. Several of the very low forms of animal life can reproduce themselves merely by dividing or being divided. We need not discuss this phase of the subject, however, for the good reason that we are wishing as quickly as possible to make the application to the human race.

Even though some forms of life may use the asexual method of reproduction, it is now believed that all of them have some sort of sex, rudimentary though it may be. Bacteria, until recently, have been considered as being exceptions to this general rule, but now a great many authorities believe that even they manifest an extremely primitive activity which is to be regarded as being essentially sexual. Inasmuch as Nature has used this particular plan in the life of every one of her products, the conclusion is inevitably forced upon us that there must be some most excellent reason for the phenomenon. Let us suppose that every individual of a given species were free to reproduce himself by asexual means for an unlimited number of generations. It is easy to see that a given strain might come rather soon to be quite different from the original species. In this way there would arise an enormous number of varieties, and a condition approaching chaos would result. This is, indeed, exemplified by the fact that those plants which are reproduced by bulbs, cuttings, and tubers commonly have a great number of varieties: roses, dahlias, gladioli, etc. Nature seems, however, to hold the majority of species more constant, and so each time the act of reproduction is repeated it is necessary that a given individual fuse his heredity with that of another individual of the same species. In this way each separate drop of living matter is merged with the great ocean of related living matter, and wide deviations from the type species are rendered much less likely to occur.

However that may be from a theoretical standpoint, it certainly is a practical fact that sex is fundamental to the continuation of all higher forms of life. It is the warp of life into which an infinite variety of patterns may be woven by manipulation of other factors which may be called the woof. Sexual reproduction is the masterpiece of Nature. Into this process she has poured her sweetest perfumes: the flower, for example, is the sex organ of the plant. About it she has drawn her most beautiful patterns. Into it she has dumped her paint pots, as witness the colors of the mating bird, the butterfly, and the flower. On the human level music and poetry are called upon to adorn it. Sex is motivated by the most precious of all passions, conjugal and parental love. Young girls are as enticing as it is possible to be; young men are handsome and valiant. The young of most species are charming—or, if not that, are at least interesting. Everyone loves the puppy, the colt, the kitten, and most of all, the baby. Who can be so blind as to fail to see in this thing the very essence of life itself? If life be good then this is the very best thing in life—or the worst when it has gone sour.

If we look into even the simpler and most familiar forms of sex, we may discern opportunities for the teaching of human problems to children. There is the flowering plant; for example, the bean. Every child is familiar with the seed of the bean, and if not accustomed to seeing the growing plant, it is quite a simple matter to plant a few beans and see them grow. (Beans bought for food purposes have often been heated so that the germ of life has been killed; therefore beans intended for planting should be used for this purpose.) A flower pot in the window will serve if there is no room for a garden. The child will be much interested in planting the seed and in seeing it grow. Finally the buds and then the flowers will appear. They are the most beautiful part of the plant. Insects will visit the flowers and will go from one to another sipping the nectar and transferring the pollen as it sticks to their legs. Even a crude dissection of the flower will reveal two sets of organs in the heart of the blossom. The one set, the stamens, carry at their tips a yellow powder (pollen) which is the male element; while the other, the pistil, is the female portion of the plant and has a sticky spot on the end to which pollen will adhere if it touches.

The insect, in visiting one flower after another, carries the pollen of one plant to the pistil of another. The pollen grains sprout and grow down the entire length of the pistil and carry the tiny cells which unite with the egg cells to form the seeds which are essentially new individuals. The growth of the seeds in the pod—the body of the mother plant—may be easily followed. Essentially the process is the same as is observed in the higher animals, except that the points that are hardest to get across to children are much more simply explained. Most important is the fact that the part of the process which corresponds to the mating of the sexes is the apparently trivial visit of the bee who carries the male element to the female organ of the next flower. In teaching children it is usually this point that puzzles and deters most parents. Possibly the use of the bean plant as an example may make it easier to explain this part of the process. Emphasis must, of course, be put upon the significance of *the whole program* and not upon this particular episode. The purpose of the process is the reproduction of the species—a very important matter indeed—rather than the making of an opportunity for the bees. The whole process is magnificent while the transfer of the pollen—except as it is part of the whole—is trivial.

Other plants may be used in somewhat the same way. For example, the flowers of the members of the melon family—muskmelons, pumpkins, cucumbers—are not all alike. Some of them have only the female organs, while others have only the male. In this respect they are more like the higher animals with which we are particularly concerned. In the case of strawberries and certain fruit trees there are some barren plants which are male. These plants never have fruit, but if they are all pulled out the other plants will be worthless as well.

The nesting habits of fish furnish an excellent example for teaching purposes. The females lay their unfertilized eggs over a clean spot on the bottom of the lake or stream. The male then comes to the nest and pours over the eggs a secretion known as "milt," which consists of millions of the sperm cells. When one of these sperm cells unites with an egg cell a new individual life begins. Obviously the method is exceedingly wasteful, but it is the best that fish can do. The young are compelled to get along as best they can after they are hatched, and, as a matter of fact, great numbers of them perish. In consequence, it is necessary that thousands or even millions of eggs be laid. By paddling slowly in a boat about the edge of a lake during the spawning season, the nests of sunfish may easily be found as clean round spots on the gravelly or sandy bottom, over which the parent usually hovers. The parent fish keeps the area clean and will chase away enemies who may come to destroy.

The mother frog does somewhat better. Her eggs are put out in a gelatinous material that protects them considerably. Then, too, they are black above and light below, making them harder to see. The dark color absorbs the heat of the sun and hastens the hatching process. The male fertilizes the eggs at about the time they leave the female's body. When the young tadpoles are finally hatched they are usually compelled to get along as best they may in a cruel world and many of them serve as juicy tidbits for birds, fish, and other animals.

The turtle illustrates a marked step in advance. The eggs are fertilized before they are laid and are held in the body of the female until a considerable quantity of food has been stored up in them and a firm shell is built about the food and the living portion of the egg. The eggs are then laid in and covered with the sand near the water's edge. There the heat of the sun stimulates growth. They will not be hatched until they are in a rather advanced state of development as compared with the young of the fish and the frog. Far fewer eggs are laid, for the good reason that the few that are laid are better equipped for survival. Even so, there is no further care on the part of the parents, and the young have strenuous times finding food and escaping the myriad dangers which beset their paths.

Birds do still better by their young. The parent birds mate and build a home—a most interesting home, indeed, as may be found by the simple expedient of sitting quietly and watching. The egg is retained in the mother's body until it is large and loaded with food for the young bird. It is then laid in the carefully prepared and concealed nest, where it is faithfully guarded for days by the mother, who hatches it with the heat of her own body. In the meantime, the father bird has protected the nest by driving away enemies, or has attracted attention and danger away from the nest and to himself by flashing his bright colors and brilliant song from a tree safely remote from the nest. When the young are hatched, the parents bring food, the mother keeps the nest clean and picks lice and other vermin off the young. She hovers over them when they are cold or when it is storming; she powders them with dust from the road, thereby discouraging insect pests; she never rests in her untiring efforts to feed and protect them; she teaches them to fly and to find food for themselves.

A most interesting subject for children to study is the nesting habits of the birds. City children need not often be at a disadvantage in this respect, for robins nest everywhere, and canaries can be had for a small sum. The larger cities may have fewer natural facilities, but such cities have zoölogical gardens and museums where there are unusual opportunities for such study. Parents who are awake to the possibilities can always find opportunity for such instruction in nature.

Higher in the scale the mammal takes even better and longer care of the young. The egg is developed as in the case of the other animals mentioned, but is never entrusted to the dangers of the outside environment—being far too precious—and so the young develop in the body of the mother. When the time comes that they must be delivered, Nature has provided for them a food which is taken from the mother's body and is the perfect food for the growing baby animal. The protective instincts of the mother are easily observed. Here is an example of parental love which is easily recognized even by a young child. Unfortunately, the function of the father is often much less inspiring, inasmuch as the male of the most easily studied mammals is generally apparently little interested in his offspring. There are, to be sure, instances in which the mammals have something somewhat like a human family, but most of these are in animals not easily observed by the child.

It is for this reason, in our opinion, a mistake to say too much about the male parent when referring to mammals. The example of the birds is better and more easily observed. By this we do not mean that the act of fertilization is any the less proper, but as we are teaching human children it is better to use examples which are more nearly like human customs. It is not that we would attempt to conceal the facts, but only that we would not call attention to them as they may be observed in the polygamous animals. There are authorities on sex education who advise that children be deliberately shown every phase of reproduction, as may be easily shown in dogs, for example. Personally, we are inclined to think that it must be rather hard to make the demonstration edifying. We believe that this is a phase of mammalian life that had best be left to accidental observation. If the child, after having been properly instructed in such matters as indicated above, asks questions about the more obvious facts of mammalian life, the whole matter should be discussed with him, and the social need for discretion in the mentioning of such matters should be explained. The subject is not of itself improper, but it has been treated in such a way that the child might easily get the wrong impression if he talks about it outside his own family.

Even a child must have observed that the human being is an animal, and as such has many of the ways of an animal. Even a child must learn early that the human being is *much more than a mere animal,* however, and should conduct himself or herself accordingly. Human children are precious. They must be given tender care over a long period of time. In this way the child can be made to see the reason for the family as we have it. In this way he comes to appreciate the rôle of the father and the mother, who have built about him a home that is stable, safe, and the very core of his existence. The functions of the father and the mother in that home seem widely different, but each is equally important and each has for its purpose the preservation of the child himself. The child sees his father working, bringing home food, paying for coal, furnishing a house in which to live, protecting him from injury, giving elemental care, playing and romping with him, planning with him, helping him, and advising him in ways that help tremendously. Every boy and girl should believe that his or her father is of the nature of a god, and so in this way the human father lifts himself above the level of the father of a puppy. The child sees—or should see—the father and mother exchanging embraces and words of affection. He realizes that sacrifices are being made, and so he comes to the way of thinking that anything that his father does must be quite all right—and as a matter of fact the father's position in the family will be much easier taught when everything that the father does *is* quite all right.

We are here giving much attention to the father for the reason that his rôle is commonly considered to be the hard part to explain. It is hard to explain, probably, for the reason that the male of most of the lower species have so little to do that is exemplary in terms of human conduct. Unfortunately, for one reason or another, a considerable number of human fathers also do little that is exemplary by the same standards, and so their purpose is rather hard to explain to the innocent child.

The function of the mother is much more obvious and needs no particular elaboration here. One point is important: The actual deliverance of the child from the body of the mother is usually a considerable ordeal and may easily become a family catastrophe. It is hard to make the child understand why such a process is necessary if he knows all of the sordid details. For that matter, it is hard to make adults understand why the bearing of children should be so difficult. We are happy to report that a great deal has been

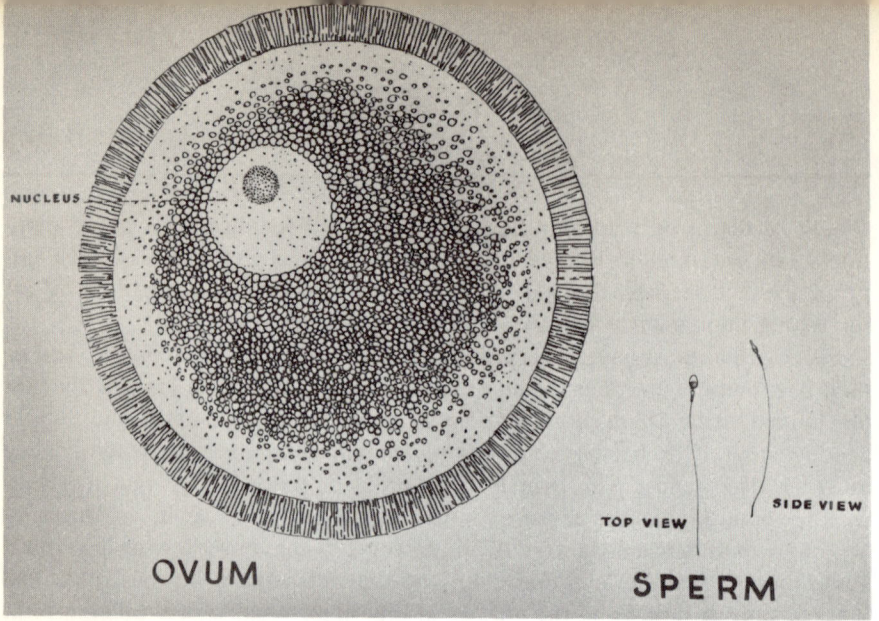

The sex cells. The ovum (egg) is much larger than the sperm. The inherited characteristics of the individual are carried in the head of the sperm and nucleus of the ovum. One sperm will attach itself to the egg wall; it loses its tail and its head penetrates into the interior of the egg. When the head fuses with the nucleus of the egg, fertilization is said to have taken place and the first cell of a new individual is formed.

Cleveland Health Museum

Early stages of development. We begin to grow into a new human being as soon as the egg is fertilized (1). Development takes place by repeated cell divisions into two cells (2), four cells (3), eight cells (4), until a stage is reached that resembles a mulberry (5); this is the morula stage. A hollow ball of cells results a few divisions later (8), known as the blastula. One side of this begins to push in (9) like denting the side of a tennis ball, and eventually the whole mass begins to elongate (10), with the "dent" growing into a hollow tube which later forms the digestive tract.

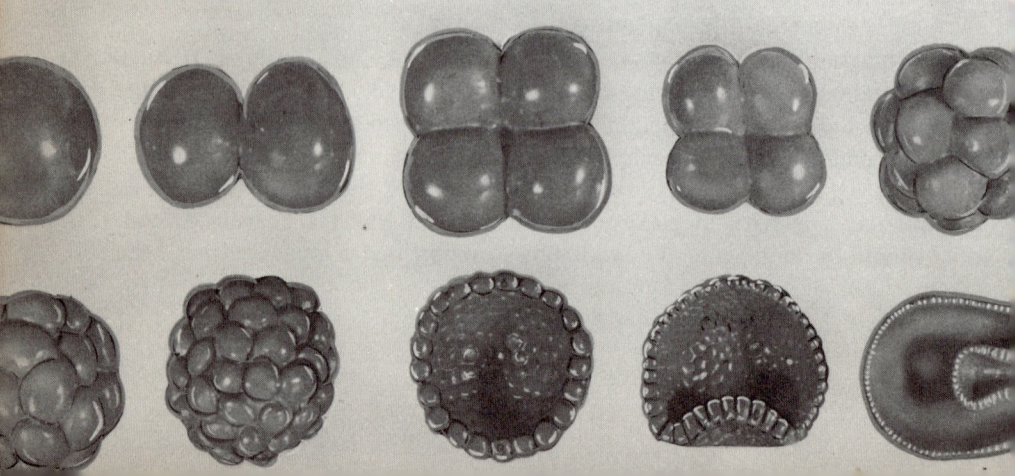

done by the medical and nursing professions to relieve that difficulty and danger.

Why must childbirth in the human be so much more difficult and dangerous than in the lower animals? The reason is to be found in several relations which are not very obscure. In the first place, there is the matter of the erect posture, which has done so much to change the configuration of the pelvis in many women, and particularly in those who may have suffered as children from the disease known as rickets. This disease allows the abnormally soft bones to be excessively distorted by the weight of the body, and, in consequence, the birth canal is made too narrow. Erect posture is, however, a fundamental advantage to the human race and is not to be lamented. Secondly, the nervous development of the human mother makes her much more susceptible to pain than are the lower animals. Human beings are not clods, and so they feel more keenly. Frankly, we would not have it otherwise. In the third place, the human child is so precious that Nature strives to hold it as long as possible in the place where it is safest. The newly born human infant is exceedingly helpless even then, and would be dangerously so if it were born any sooner. For this reason the mother must carry the child a relatively longer time. Finally, the development of the head which is made necessary by the large size of the brain enormously complicates the act of delivery. But that marvelous brain is the one really great characteristic of man, and we must not find fault with that which makes us great among the creatures of Nature. Thousands of those brains are now actively engaged in devising means of making childbirth easier and safer, and they are succeeding, too.

We are presenting these facts for the enlightenment and instruction of adults, but *for the sake of the child*. As mentioned previously nothing is gained by telling the child of Mother's travail and sacrifice. The child knows nothing, and can understand very little, of sacrifice and suffering. He does not know that things that are precious are also expensive. He is often shocked and frightened. Pain is always bad to the child and to be avoided. Entirely too much has been said about the *sacrifices* of motherhood, and far too little about the *privileges* and compensations. No parent worthy of the name begrudges a reasonable personal sacrifice which he or she has been compelled to make for the sake of a bright and healthy child. Then why talk about it? Particularly is it bad to throw the matter in the face of the child itself, as if he or she were somehow to blame.

We are in great need of an understanding of sex as a *normal* physiological function of the greatest consequence to the perpetuation of life on the earth. When assigned to its proper place in the scheme of things, and when interpreted properly, the understanding of this subject adds enormously to the meaning of life. Unfortunate, indeed, is the child—or adult—who is led to believe that sex is a *risqué* or low experience that lies out on the edge of things—a subject to be hushed and covered at every turn. Fortunate is the child whose parent so understands the subject that he may lead the child by gradual steps to a realization of the importance and beauty of sex and who arouses in him a determination to protect and conserve this vital force which unites in him the glorious past and the still more glorious future. There is no better way to attain such a position of wisdom and understanding than by studying the manifestations in those species which represent the steps by which we have attained our present position of eminence in the world of living things.

The Anatomy and Physiology of the Reproductive System

Before one may expect to teach the subject of reproduction to his or her children, he or she should be thoroughly grounded in the elemental principles of anatomy and physiology by virtue of which the miracle of life begins. It is not at all necessary that the layman should know all of the great Latin names for every little part, or that he should hope to understand the chemistry and physics of the whole process, but he does need to know something of the amazing things that take place in the months preceding the birth of a child, and he needs to understand the system well enough to be able to give it the care that hygiene demands. Very badly indeed he needs a vocabulary by means of which he may discuss these matters without the faintest taint of vulgarity or obscenity.

The generative system in either of the two sexes consists of two portions: 1. The sex glands themselves (ovaries in the female, testicles in the male). 2. A system of tubes which carry the sex cells, and later in the female, protect and nourish the developing child. Strange as it will seem to the layman, the organs of the two sexes are really much alike, each organ of the one sex having its exact but poorly developed homologue in the opposite sex.

The sex glands of the male, the *testicles,* consist of a great number of microscopic tubules which are lined with cells which are constantly undergoing cell division after the individual has attained sexual maturity. These cells become the *spermatozoa* or sperm cells, which are tiny little living bodies with long slender tails which whip about and in this way propel the sperm in its search for the egg cell. These sperm cells carry the entire inheritance which a given child will or can get from his father. The spermatozoa may live for several days in the tubes of the male, or may even live for a day or two after they have gained access to the female organs. They begin to be produced when the boy reaches puberty (about fourteen years of age), and continue to be formed until senility has been reached. During the period of sexual maturity they are commonly produced at the rate of millions per day.

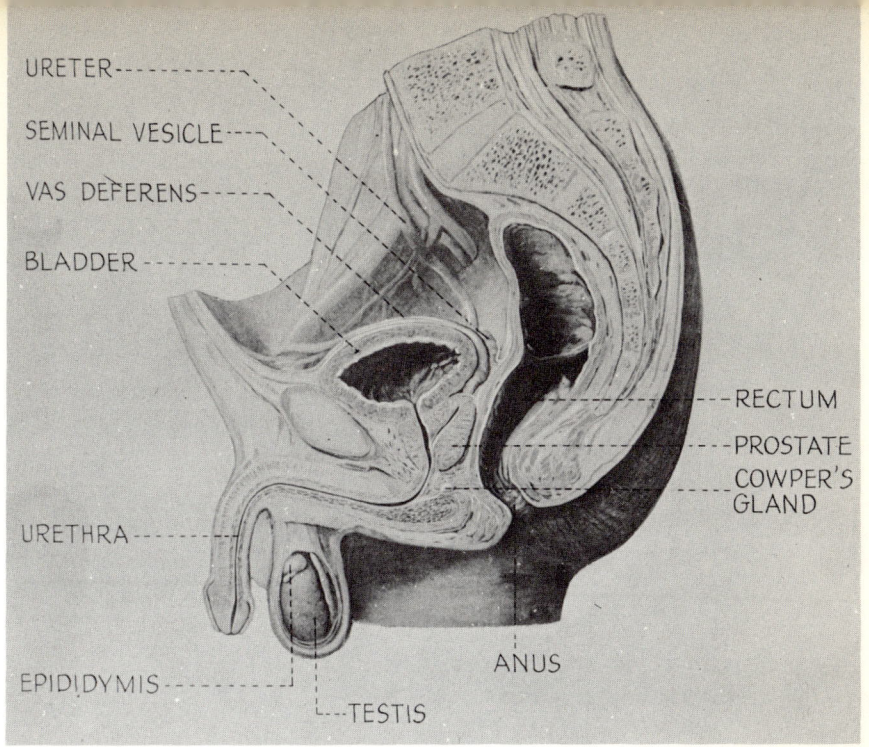

The anatomy of the genito-urinary system in the male.
Cleveland Health Museum

In addition to the above function of the testicles, there is another that is nearly or quite as important as the production of the sex cells. Between the tubules which produce the spermatozoa there lie certain cells which are called the *interstitial* cells. They secrete a substance which is absorbed by the blood and is responsible for the development of the secondary sex characteristics of the male. Every one is familiar with the fact that the body of the man differs from that of the woman in other respects than the appearance of the sex organs themselves. The beard of the male, the deeper voice, the heavier bones, the narrowness of the pelvis, the texture of the skin, the scantiness of the subcutaneous fat, the lack of development of the breasts are all the results of this secretion. Unfortunate, indeed, is the man who does not have enough of this secretion to cause such a differentiation of his body that he may be immediately recognized as being definitely masculine in appearance. It is because of the loss of this substance that the castrated male (known as a eunuch) loses the characteristics of a manly man. Such individuals are commonly held in contempt by normal members of both sexes.

The *ovaries* of the female serve a purpose in the female exactly comparable to that of the testicles in the male, though there are, of course, differences in the details. The egg cells are already pretty well formed in the ovary at the time of birth, or shortly afterwards. They need to be matured, and

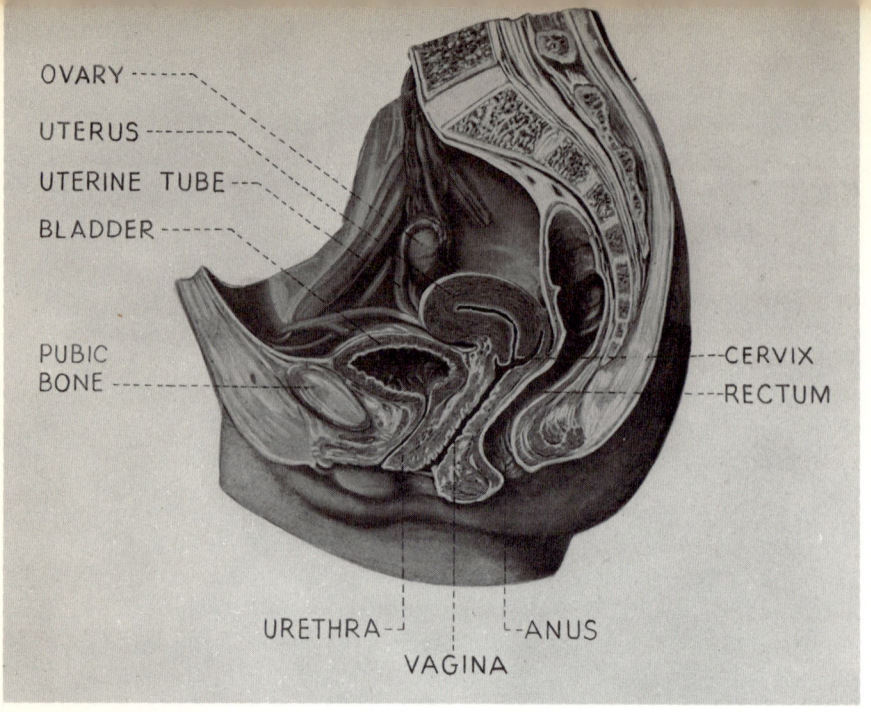

The anatomy of the genito-urinary system in the female.

stocked with a small supply of food, and then are ready to be extruded from the ovary. At the age of *puberty* (age twelve to thirteen years) the girl begins to produce mature egg cells at the rate of one (occasionally more) per menstrual month (usually twenty-eight days). This is continued until the *menopause* (change of life) is reached. This means that, on the average, less than five hundred egg cells are actually released in a lifetime.

As in the testicle, the ovary contains *interstitial* cells which produce a secretion that is responsible for the secondary sex characteristics of the female. The soft skin, the abundant subcutaneous fat, the development of the breasts, the higher pitched voice, the wider pelvis, and a great many other typically feminine attributes are too familiar to need enumeration. Women, because of loss or atrophy of the ovaries, or because of some other glandular disturbance, occasionally lose much of their femininity and may develop a beard or coarse, man-like features. Such a misfortune is distressing, indeed, to the individual herself, and greatly disfigures her in the eyes of others.

The *testicles* and the *ovaries* are the essential organs of reproduction. Indeed, as we have seen, many of the simpler animals and plants have hardly any other organs of reproduction than just these. Even in somewhat higher animals, as the fish and the frogs, the eggs are simply turned out into the water, and the spermatic fluid is spread over them there. The accessory organs of reproduction in such a case are exceedingly simple, and sex, as we commonly think of it, can hardly be recognized by examination of the exterior of the body. The episode *coitus* which is considered by the thoughtless person to be the whole of the process becomes a trivial part of the program—merely the spreading of the milt of the male over the eggs laid in the water by the female.

As the higher forms of life are studied, it is noted that more and more care is given the fertilized egg. The reptiles and the birds lay large eggs containing abundance of food so that the young may attain considerable size and development before they need to begin to fend for themselves. The mammals give their young even better care, and for weeks and months the female carries the young in her own body, and then, after releasing them, suckles them for another rather long period. Obviously such an arrangement has necessitated an enormous increase in the complexity of the system. The entire body of the female is modified to take care of the fertilized egg, to expel the developed fetus and to nourish the young after it has been born. The body of the male is likewise modified so that it may be able to impregnate the female and protect her and the young during the critical months before and after the birth of the young. Sex as we commonly think of it is highly developed in these animals.

The human species is characterized by the fact that the infant has an unusually long period of gestation, infancy, and dependency. It is this long period of comparative helplessness that allows the child to develop countless possibilities which would have been quite out of the question had he been compelled to look after himself from the first. Likewise it is this which has made necessary the tremendous changes in body structure of the two sexes, and the even more complicated development of the human family life, upon which the happy and efficient functioning of so much in the life of the child depends.

The accessory sex organs of the male consist of the *scrotum*, a baglike sac or pouch, containing the two testicles which produce the spermatozoa or male sex-cells; a long tortuous tube from each of the testicles to the corresponding *seminal vesicles* or reservoirs, where the spermatic fluid and the sperm cells are stored until such time as there may be opportunity for extrusion (ejaculation); the *prostate gland,* which secretes a mucus-like fluid which carries the seminal secretion and makes a medium which will permit the spermatozoa to live and reach their objective; and the *penis,* which is an erectile tube capable of depositing the mixture of spermatic and prostatic secretion into the vault of the *vagina* near the mouth of the *womb.*

The accessory organs of the female are necessarily much more complicated for the reason that they must not only protect the egg cells but must provide a home for the developing child for nine long and eventful months. Essentially they consist of two tubes (*Fallopian tubes* or *oviducts*) which are open at the upper end and receive the egg cells when they are extruded from the ovaries.

These tubes open into the *womb,* which is a thick-walled, muscular, hollow organ capable of enormous expansion. The womb in turn empties into the *vagina,* which is for the purpose of receiving the seminal secretion, and later of serving as a passageway for the child at the time of birth. The external female organs are called collectively the *vulva.* The breasts nourish the newly born child until it is old enough to eat other food.

The egg cell, after being released by the ovary, passes into the *Fallopian tube,* where it may or may not be fertilized by coming into contact with sperm cells. In case it does not make such a contact it lies there for a few days and then passes down into the womb and finally to the exterior. If it is fertilized it begins at once to divide rapidly and grows apace, utilizing the food that is stored in the egg cell and probably also some food absorbed from the surrounding tissues. It now migrates down into the womb and attaches itself to the inner wall of the womb (*uterus*) much as would a parasite. After a time a *placenta* is formed. This organ is the point of contact between the mother and the child. The bloods of the two individuals remain separate, both the mother and child having a set of closed vessels in the placenta, but fluids and gases can freely pass from the one to the other through the vessel walls by the process of *osmosis.* The mother furnishes food, water, oxygen, and other requirements; the child gives off waste materials of various sorts to the mother. No nerves pass from the one to the other. Various membranes for the protection of the child are also produced. These membranes and the placenta are delivered after the child is born and are collectively known as the "afterbirth." At the time of birth the walls of the womb contract strongly and expel the child and after a time the "afterbirth."

The life of a new individual begins when the living egg cell of the mother is fertilized by the living sperm cell of the father. Really, then, the human child is approximately nine months old when it is born, and more has happened in the development of the individual during that nine months than will take place in the next nine years. There are many who suppose that life begins in the child at about the time that the mother may feel the movements of the child in the womb. Indeed, it is customary to refer to these movements as the "beginning of life." This phenomenon is usually observed at about the middle of the pregnancy. Actually, however, the child is alive from the time of the union of the egg and the sperm, and as a definitive human being has certain recognized human rights.

As soon as it is known that a baby is expected, parents are usually greatly interested in the speculation as to whether it is a boy or a girl. There is good reason to believe that the sex of the child is unalterably determined at the time of fertilization. To date there is no realiable means of controlling the sex of the offspring, and there is no accurate way of knowing until the child is born whether it is male or female, though the physician may make shrewd guesses which will be correct in a high percentage of cases. According to the most widely accepted theory of sex determination, each cell in the body of the female contains two determiners for sex (*chromosomes*), while each cell in the body of the male has but one such determiner. When the egg cells are produced, each cell contains one of these determiners; when the sperm cells are made, half of them have one sex determiner and the other half have none. If, then, the sperm with one sex chromosome meets an egg cell which always contains one, the fertilized egg cell will have two and is therefore female. If the sperm cell has no sex chromosome, then the fertilized egg cell will have but one—the one from the egg cell—and the sex is then male. If this theory is correct, and there is little doubt about its being correct, it would seem that the control of the sex of the unborn child by any practical means is probably quite outside the range of possibility. Many attempts to control sex have been tried, but none have as yet succeeded.

Even though the sex of the child is determined from the very first, it will be weeks before the differentiation of the organs is such that the sex might be recognized, even if the child could be examined closely. By such careful examination it is possible during the third month of fetal life to determine whether or not the child would have been male or female if it had lived. Previous to this time, the sex organs appear exactly alike, and, even in adult life, it is possible to find in each sex the exact homologue of the organs of the opposite sex. In the early months of fetal life the one or the other set of characteristics begins to be accentuated, and the opposing organs begin to atrophy.

Obviously the matter of reproduction is of the utmost consequence both to society and to the individuals concerned, and for that reason it is extremely important that every person of mature age should understand something of the complex phenomena which take place during the months of pregnancy, the hours of actual confinement, the days of the lying-in period, and the months of lactation. It is, furthermore, most essential that this information shall be highly authoritative. If these relations were well understood, a vast amount of suffering, distress, and danger to the mother and child might be avoided. These matters have been well covered in another part of this book. The race must go on, and there is positively no other way by which it may do so.

There are three proper functions of the reproductive system in the human species: 1. The production of and the bringing together of the sex cells. 2. The production and the protection of the child, whether it be before, during, or after birth. 3. A means whereby a man and wife may express affection for each other, and on that solid foundation build a home which is, in turn, the foundation of society. All of these functions are absolutely legitimate, proper, and respectable when exercised according to the laws, customs, and ethics of the time and domain.

The Teaching of Sex to the Young Child

We need hardly point out that the process which brings an innocent child into the world and reproduces the species is inherently clean and decent. The parent who attempts to instruct a child in the marvels of sex must thoroughly convert himself to a firm belief in this fact, self-evident though it may seem. The process is right, and the child is pure. If, then, there is anything wrong about it, the difficulty must be in the parent or his understanding of the situation.

It is most unfortunate, for the sake of the child, that we cannot assume that persons about to become parents have become familiar with the fundamental facts concerning the process which has brought the child into existence. Even before marriage they should have talked over these matters and should have sought to learn through legitimate channels the facts about so important a matter. Surely there is no further excuse for hesitancy after marriage. During the months between conception and the birth there are many reasons why intelligent persons will wish to know something of what is going on. Between the time of birth and the asking of the first question there is a period of two to four years, during which time one might be expected to prepare himself or herself for the time when the child will want to know something of vital matters, and yet a large percentage of parents find themselves utterly unprepared for the inevitable time when the intelligent child begins to ask questions. Mothers are shocked when the first question is asked. They seem to think that the child is still a babe in arms. Fathers tell the distressed mothers to explain matters to the children, but usually have no suggestions as to what to tell or how to tell it.

Long before it is time to begin to teach the child by word of mouth about these matters, there are other responsibilities which must be met. Within the first few days of life the genital organs of the baby should be carefully examined for evidence of defects or abnormalities. In case such defects are found they should be corrected when possible, inasmuch as such peculiarities are often responsible for irritations or abnormal stimulations which may greatly complicate the sexual life of the child when he or she is older. The tissues of the infant are still highly plastic, and it frequently happens that corrections made early are surprisingly successful for this reason.

The boy baby should be carefully examined to see if he needs circumcision. If the foreskin can be completely and easily retracted most authorities think that circumcision should not be done, but when there is the least doubt about the matter decision should be made in favor of the operation, which is a trivial one when done within the first week or two of life. When the foreskin is tight or adherent there will accumulate under it secretions which will produce bad odors and cause pain and itching. Such a child is likely to get into the ugly habit of pulling at and handling the genitals and may develop habits which are harmful and unsightly. In case circumcision is not done, the mother or nurse should carefully retract the foreskin each day and see that the organ is thoroughly clean. Many "nervous," restless, and "fidgety" boys can be helped by circumcision, provided there is real reason to think that they need such care.

At an early age boys should also be examined to determine whether or nor the testicles have descended into the scrotum. These essential organs of sex are developed in the abdominal cavity, but at the time of birth or rather soon thereafter they should have descended. If they can be felt in the scrotum or can be gently pressed down into the scrotum there is no need for apprehension. If, on the other hand, they cannot be found, attention should be given to the matter—without causing too much curiosity on the part of the child—and the advice of a physician obtained. If descent does not take place, an operation to transplant the testicle into the scrotum should be performed before the boy reaches puberty. Undescended testicles commonly atrophy, and if both are in this condition sterility may result. The proper development of the testicle is important also from the standpoint of the proper secondary sex characteristics.

The girl baby also should be carefully examined for abnormalities. In not a few instances she may be in need of an operation which is essentially the same as that of circumcision in the male, i.e. the clitoris may be tied down by adhesions. Other defects may be present. In the washing of the female infant, care must be taken. Sometimes the hymen may be ruptured by rough handling. While it is true that the presence of an intact hymen is by no means proof of virginity, or the absence of it proof of sexual experience, there is still a large percentage of people who believe that such is the case, and so care must be taken to prevent an accident which might later put the babe, grown to womanhood, in an embarrassing position. Washing of the parts should be done in such a way that the friction will not cause erotic stimulation and in this way lead the child to the habit of playing with herself.

It is well known that crying babies, male and female, will nearly invariably hush when the genital organs are manipulated. This is an old, old trick of careless nurses and ignorant mothers. Under no circumstances must it be practiced, as it may lead promptly to the practice of masturbation in some form. Masturbation is probably far less harmful than has been supposed. Still, it is certainly an ugly habit, and every reasonable means of preventing it from establishing itself should be taken. It is doubtful if *mothers* have often practised such means of quieting their babies, but others to whom the child may have been entrusted have been less conscientious. The routine care of a child should never be delegated to someone else when it is physically possible for the mother to see to it herself.

During the period when the child is too young to be given definite instruction, much can be done to lay the foundation for sound health and useful habits. The child who learns cleanliness and regularity of body function will be much more likely to respect the purposes of the reproductive system when grown than will a person who as a child was permitted to abuse or neglect the various bodily functions. The strictly normal individual is less likely to develop improper habits or perversions than the one who suffers from various biases or abnormalities. Childhood is the time for health training, and health is the sound base upon which rest normal reactions with regard to sex.

Much of the difficulty in teaching and training children in these matters concerning sex is due to the mistaken idea that children do not manifest interest in such subjects until they are several years old. Sex is far too fundamental a thing to lie dormant for so long a time. The excretory organs are inseparably related to it, and indeed, it has its effect upon the entire body. Regularity in sleep, in eating, and in going to the toilet; pleasant manners and polite speech; love of beauty, truth, and decency; play in the open air; development of a natural attitude toward other children; modesty and respect for one's self are every one of them developed in large measure—if they are well developed at all—before the child is four years old. Every one of these traits is of the greatest value in the development of an admirable sex life. It is hard to see how the child that hears and sees vulgarity and lives as a waif can get a fair start in the understanding of so pure and chaste a subject.

Great care will be needed in teaching the child that the social conventions are necessary without instilling in him or her the idea that the sexual organs are inherently ugly, unclean, or sinful. The nude baby is proudly exhibited to admiring relatives and friends, the nude child of four is to be seen by the family only, and the boy or girl of eight is expected to be careful about such matters even in the bosom of the family. A fine sense of modesty is of the utmost consequence in the social training of the child. On the other hand, there are times, as when medical examinations must be made, when what has been called modesty is really prudery. The development of poise in these fine qualities is of the utmost consequence. It can be taught only when the child has been led to regard the sexual apparatus with respect rather than shame. Dignity and modesty are closely allied here as elsewhere. The child is made to understand that there are some things that are sacred and for that reason not to be cast before swine; there are some things so fine that they must not be permitted to become common. The child is shown that grown-ups, men and women, cover themselves, and that if he or she would be like them he or she must do so as well. Reserve rather than shame, pride in something that is too important to be left lying around, is the motive to be emphasized.

Many of the difficulties attendant to the teaching of sex are immediately solved when the child is taught the proper, the dignified names for the parts of the body. It would be hard to understand how a child could use the vulgar names which are commonly heard without deterioration of dignity and respect. Hardly better are the baby names and the meaningless terms which are often given them in the vain attempt on the part of the mother to save the child from what she supposes to be vulgarity. The child must acquire a dignified vocabulary if he is to keep the subject clean. It is hard to see why it should be more embarrassing to the mother to have the child come to her saying that he wishes to go to the toilet than to have him use some of the other expressions which are equally evident in their meaning under the circumstances. A frank acknowledgment of these things and their meanings is the very basis of future understanding of them. Hypocrisy and prudery have had their day and have made a mess of it.

During this impressionable period of life the attitude of the father and mother toward each other will have a profound effect on the character and sexual behavior of the child in later life. The child who sees his father treat his mother with chivalry and respect is much more likely to treat girls and women in the same way. The little girl who sees in her own mother a beautiful character is unconsciously receiving an education in these matters which is infinitely more effective than all the carefully planned precepts which might be memorized from books or articles on sex education.

But while it is really the generalities which count in the training of the child it is the details which are more perplexing to the parent in charge. This is because the details have a way of demanding immediate attention. What shall the mother or the father tell the child when he asks the highly pertinent and searching questions which have perplexed parents for so long? There is but one thing to tell him. It is the *truth*. By this I do not mean that it is necessary to tell a child of four the *entire* truth, or that it is necessary to give him the *detailed* truth. As a matter of fact, that would be impossible for the good reason that not even the wisest man knows the entire or the detailed truth about these matters. When the child asks a question he does not expect the scientifically complete answer, but in later life he will greatly appreciate the fact that he was told the truth in so far as he was able to understand it at the time.

When the child notices the difference between his or her body and that of the opposite sex it is an easy matter to explain that there are two sorts of people, and two sorts of everything else that is alive. That is so that each little child and each little baby animal may have a father and a mother to care for him and make a home for him. It is pointed out that birds of certain kinds are different in color and appearance, and that there are differences in function which correspond to this difference in appearance. By all means arrange for him to see a bird's nest, if possible, and understand something of what goes on there. He will have observed that fathers and mothers have different purposes in life, and there are marked differences in dress, in habit, and occupation. The whole process is perfectly natural, and when naturally told to a normal child will give rise to no morbid curiosity whatsoever. It is merely an interesting fact about the most interesting thing in the world—life.

A momentous question is that concerning where the baby came from. It is a question that every child should have asked by the time he is four or five years old or even sooner if he is interested. The most ridiculous substitutes for the beautiful truth have been given him—most of them extremely unconvincing. What a pity that mothers have seen fit to tell children that babies—they themselves, indeed—are found in garbage pails, in the straw pile back of the barn, under the leaves in the woods, in a hollow log, in the doctor's satchel, and in other monstrous places. Hardly better is the "made in Germany" story of the stork, except that it is somewhat more dignified. The children of Germany love and respect the stork, but the small children of this country know nothing of such a creature.

Children are invariably tremendously interested in babies and commonly are asking their parents if they may have a baby brother or sister. They see no evil in the possibility, as, indeed, there is none.

The question that is most dreaded is, "How did the baby get in the mother's body?" Here is something that is supposed to be hopelessly vulgar. Well, for those who think it is so we can understand that the problem is difficult. When, however, the father and the mother have loved each other as they should and are legally married, the act that is the expression of that love and the act that enables them to bear beautiful children is not vulgar in any sense. The child—bear in mind that this is a young child—can be told that as a result of the love which the parents bear for each other and for the child the baby began to grow in the body of the mother. An older child will need more information, to be sure, but this is as essentially the truth as the most tediously accurate and scientific account of the union of egg cells and sperms, such as he or she will need at a later stage of development.

The difficulty of explaining the role of the father will fade into nothing at all if the child believes that his father is a great hero who can do no wrong. When the child has seen his father caressing his mother nothing could be more natural—as indeed nothing is more natural—than that they should desire and have children. It is most unfortunate that so many fathers live and treat their families in such a way that the children may learn to know that their acts are commonly selfish. In such case the teaching of sex will be difficult. In the main, however, small children believe that their fathers are great persons, indeed, and that whatever they do is just right, and in such case nothing could be easier than proper instruction in these matters. The role of the mother is easily taught. As it is perfectly natural for the child to develop in the mother's body, it is perfectly natural that the child should accept the method as the ancient and honored way of life, and that is all there is to it.

After the child is old enough to understand the simple anatomy of the two sexes, it may be explained that the sperm cells of the male are introduced into the body of the mother and there combine with the egg cells somewhat as the pollen of the male plant fertilizes the female. It should then be explained that such transfer of the male to the female must take place only between married persons, else a child may be born when the parents cannot make a home for it. Even a little child can understand that illegitimacy is a pretty serious thing, in as much as every child needs *both* a father and a mother as he grows up. It may easily be explained that the process is one that is perfectly proper when the man and woman are married and much in love with each other, and that it is an act of the utmost intimacy and delicacy.

When the child asks the *details* of birth—as he or she rarely will—care must be taken that he or she is not frightened by morbid details. No small child can understand the forces which come into play in such an event. It is a serious mistake to worry him with the harrowing details in such a case, then. It is enough to know that when the time came, the mother worked hard and was very tired. After such an experience she will need to rest in bed for several days and must be shown every possible deference and affection. She is not *"sick"* in the usual meaning of the word, but is merely *resting* after a tremendously important and vital contribution to the beloved family.

The most important principle in the training of a child in these matters is that the native curiosity of the child should be satisfied, and satisfied with something that can serve as a basis for subsequent teaching. The child must learn that it can depend *absolutely* upon the father and mother as a source of honest and authentic information on this subject, just as he can go to the same source for food, for shelter, and for help of any sort. The child should never be repressed when asking honestly concerning such matters. Once the demand for the truth is filled, the child can then go about his or her normal activities without being bothered with things he or she is too young to understand thoroughly. At this age interest may be keen for a moment, but when satisfied will soon turn to other things more closely related to the development of the child. There is not the least reason for the artificial stimulation of an interest in the subject, but there is good reason for quieting the natural interest by satisfying it. Questions put by the child should be answered when possible, but they need not be provoked. Generalities are sufficient for small children. Mention of pain, danger, or sacrifice should never be made, for the good reason that they cannot be understood by a child of tender years.

In case questions which cannot be answered are asked, the parent must make it clear that the question is perfectly proper if it is honestly asked. If the subject is one that cannot be answered but can be looked up, it is the duty of the parent to tell the child that he will investigate the facts and inform him later. If it is one that cannot be answered, the point should be explained as well as may be and the incident used as an example of the greatness and intricacy of the whole marvelous process. Frequently the ingenuity of the parents will enable them to restate the question so that the child can be satisfied though the direct question was not really answered. Always the teaching and the example set should be on the highest possible plane that the child can understand and appreciate. Parents who understand the process and live the part joyously will have no difficulty. They must not seem to apologize for normal sexual behavior or to make of it some sort of weakness in which they have indulged because they have not had the strength to refrain. Sex is good—in its proper place, of course—and must not be treated as a weakness or in any way sinful when kept in legitimate family circles.

The imagination and resourcefulness of the parent will do better than any "canned" information. It is not necessary that every bit of the information be absolutely scientifically up-to-the-minute provided it is earnestly and truthfully set out as the best that the parent knows on the subject. The development of a sound philosophy of life and living is much more needed than are the latest scientific details.

Whatever is done or taught, the idealism of the child must be preserved. The rôle of the father as hero, provider, and protector; the part of the mother as one who will love and protect whatever may happen, cannot be too strongly emphasized. The child easily understands such teaching and responds eagerly to idealism of this sort. The love of the father and mother for each other and for the child is the means by which the child came into existence and is as essentially the truth as if every detail were explained in full. It is the broad base upon which the family and all modern culture rests. For that reason it should be a real rather than a furtive thing in the every day family life. How reassuring it is when a child sees his parents making love and manifesting close loving attitudes. Such a child is safe. A quarrel between his parents is terribly disturbing to children of every age.

The School Child

The school child is no longer under the eye of his parents. He will hear and learn of sex. The pertinent question is not "Will he learn?" but, rather, "Where and of whom will he learn?" It is a foolish parent who thinks that a boy or girl in school will remain ignorant of these matters, and it is, indeed, a trusting parent who is willing to turn the instruction of his son or daughter in these matters over to ignorant companions. The child of this age is getting started to school and is beginning to feel that he knows something of life. Quite naturally he wants to understand things as they are. Fortunately he has not yet reached the age of puberty with its many perplexing problems and disturbing urges which will furnish an additional motive for sex interest.

Except that it will be necessary to give these children more information than was given the pre-school child, the problems are not greatly different from those that have just been discussed, for the good reason that the sexual system is still relatively undeveloped, and the child has only a passing interest in such matters. The teaching is still indirect and should consist of principles rather than details. It is a matter of ideals and of idealism. Questions should be answered fully and frankly—in so far as the child is able to understand or is interested—but disturbing questions are not to be raised in the mind of the child.

This is the time when children are so tremendously interested in nature, and it is easy, indeed, for them to have observed most of the essential phenomena of sex before they have become involved in the complex social phenomena which so muddle the issue in the human race. The parent who understands the fundamentals of sex and life as they are manifested in plants and animals and has the language to transmit such information will have an enormous advantage in the teaching of his children.

An important matter during this period is the teaching of a sense of modesty without at the same time teaching shame. Parents all too often shame their children into a state of mind that is mistaken for modesty. Shame, except for some improper act, is an emotion that should never be utilized in teaching. There is nothing about the reproductive organs for which a child need be ashamed. He learns to cover himself because it is the custom to do so, and because the older persons whom he wishes to emulate do so. There is nothing wrong about the genitals, but rather they are so important that they must be protected. They are so intimately one's real self that one must not go about exposing in a cheap and common way that which is so essentially private. Nice manners prescribe that care must be taken in these matters, and the child soon learns to take this view if he has a good example set before him.

Nearly all normal children have their little love affairs during the first years in school. Since it is so obviously true that one of the most important tasks in later life is the selection of a worthy mate, it is well that even children should be gaining a little proficiency in so vital a matter. Just as the kitten playing with a ball is really learning to catch mice, so these children are practising the greatest of all arts. It is a grave mistake for parents or others to tease children about their love affairs. Such teasing puts the idea into the head of the child that there is something inherently wrong about the whole matter and that he or she has done something that is improper. When, subsequently, a real affair is developing, it will be carefully concealed from the parents, and in this way the parent loses his opportunity to be of service in teaching the child how he or she may select the best companions. Furthermore, the curiosity of the child teaches him to seek the evil which he has been led to believe is in the apparently harmless relation which he or she has with another of the opposite sex. With such stimulation he will all too soon find the evil. The truth insofar as he can understand it is far safer than some silly tale which seeks to give a superficial explanation of the facts of life. "Ye shall know the truth and the truth shall make you free."

Parents who tease their young children about their beaux and seek to deter them from making dangerous alliances should look about them and learn that the best way to insure against these play love affairs going too far is merely to let them run without resistance. Children are far too fickle as a rule to do more than toy with a passion which they are much too young really to understand. Soon it will be forgotten. On the other hand, the parent who attempts to break up such an affair is assuming a grave responsibility. He will be almost sure to intensify it. There is no more certain way to drive a young—or older—couple into each other's arms than for a persistent parent to personify the well-known bull in a china shop and "set his foot down on the whole business." The reason for this is easily seen. We naturally tend to protect our friends when they are attacked, and we invariably learn to love those whom we protect. Not only are the children being set into mischief when they are teased, but the parents are accomplishing exactly the opposite result from that which they desire when they indulge in so low a form of correction —or amusement.

The parent who allows his or her children to assume natural relations with other children of the same or opposite sex need rarely fear that mischief will be done. The child, being still undeveloped sexually, gives no thought to the grosser manifestations of the subject unless they are suggested to him by his elders. When the relation is perfectly natural and the parent has abstained from teasing, the child will be free to talk about the matter, and so the parent may keep himself informed concerning the course of events. In case, then, the child gets on dangerous ground, a frank discussion of the matter is possible and will not be resented if skillfully handled. The parent may be able to point out in a kindly manner the good and bad traits in the favored friends, and in this way may be of real service in the important matter of picking the permanent mate a few years later.

Boys and girls will frequently play "father and mother" games. Though it may seem far-fetched to some, they are actually gaining much experience which may be of great benefit to them in later life. It is not at all unusual to hear children of this age express themselves as to what they will do when they are men or women, as the case may be. For the most part they will do well if they later come up to these expressed ideals. It is also common to hear children say what they will do when they have children of their own, or what their children will or will not do. The wise parent at such a time may well listen and note. It is possible that he or she may learn something. Under no condition may the children be ridiculed or teased at such a time. Here is manhood and womanhood in the making, and it is mighty serious business.

Much worry has been needlessly suffered by devoted parents who have failed to understand children of this age. Boys and girls are curious. They will naturally examine their bodies, or, if the opportunity presents itself, the body of another of the same or opposite sex. The misguided parent thinks that this is exactly the same as if an adult should do so and gets all excited about it. Frankly, we would be inclined to question the mentality of a child who has not done so. The best way to draw the teeth of such a possible menace is to allow the child to satisfy that fine sense of curiosity which impels him to try to find out how things are made, and, having found out, lets him go on to something else. Two little girls in a closet were caught discussing these matters, and the mother was needlessly alarmed. It was explained to them that such conduct is not considered to be good social form, and no more was said about it. They had satisfied their curiosity, and the episode was ended. It is likely that they rather soon forgot about it. If they had been severely punished, however, they would have had good reason to remember and to wish to continue the experience when the opportunity to do so without being caught presented itself.

Frequently children will get into the habit of playing with or pulling at the genitals. Such children—both boys and girls—may be in need of a thorough examination by a competent physician. It is not unlikely that circumcision or other special corrective measure is needed. If there is no pathologic basis for the habit, the child should be taught that it is bad manners to behave in such a way and that an ugly habit may be formed. With help, rather than scolding, he may soon correct the ugly practice. Parents should remember that no one can break a bad habit except the person who has it, and that the task is one that sometimes requires patience and perseverance beyond that which a child may be expected to have. Little boys and girls are occasionally found to have developed the practice of masturbation. Normal children of this age will rarely go to excess unless they are being stimulated by some older person. If a child of this age masturbates frequently, a careful watch should be made, not so much of the child as of its older associates. The reason for this is evident, as the child is not often sufficiently developed for the habit to have arisen from within.

Children of this age should be interested in many things, and when they are so, one need not worry about their being too much concerned about an instinct which is still far from being mature. All sorts of healthy activities are to be encouraged. Exercise in the open air is far more conducive to good results than excessive poring over books. Regular habits in matters pertaining to health will lay the best possible foundation for a normal sex life in later years. The child should grow in "wisdom and stature" during this time. He or she should develop the body as it was intended to be developed. School interests, play, club work of all sorts, scout exercises, athletic teams, and kindred activities permit little time for those forms of sex activity that might really be dangerous.

Of vast importance during this period and before is the development of self-control. We cannot understand how a subsequent marriage is going to be successful if either partner is unable to control his or her temper or selfish inclinations. Parents are doing the consorts of their children a grave injustice when they permit children to grow up in such a way as to cause them always to consider their own welfare first. This may seem to some as if it were a subject that had nothing whatever to do with the subject of sex, but actually it has everything to do with it. The child that must have his own way, that must have everything that he wants, that has never been taught to give up, that doesn't know how to work, is likely to make a mess of marriage.

The question as to how much direct sex instruction should be given during this period is a rather knotty one. Sex during this period is probably less to the fore than at any time since babyhood, provided the curiosity of the preschool child has been properly satisfied as discussed in the preceding section. If the child knows in a general way about these matters, he will let it go at that until the problems of adolescence begin to assert themselves. Matters pertaining to sex in its simpler forms should be frankly discussed by the family in the presence of the child. Questions are answered, and basic principles underlying proper conduct are deeply implanted, and that is about all that is necessary. The subject is far less exciting in the open than when it is concealed.

The boy of this age is intensely idealistic. He has his heroes—men of action and high accomplishment. He dreams of hazardous stunts and well-nigh impossible achievements. All too often he is attracted as a moth to the flame by the supposedly brave exploits of the gangster and the gunman. In many cases this is because his own good parents and relatives are so unromantic as to bore him to death. Fathers need more to appreciate the intense desire that their sons have to be able to brag about their dads. The father should attend to his most important business—that of being a "real guy" in the eyes of his children.

Girls are being encouraged to be teachers, stenographers, concert pianists, prima donnas, lawyers, doctors, nurses. As a matter of fact, most of them—fortunately—will become housewives and mothers. Why cannot these objectives be held up also as ideals? Then, when they have a home of their own, they will find in the monotonous routine a purpose toward their ideal. In case, however, they have been taught that they are to have some glamorous career and then find themselves washing dishes for a family, they are nearly sure to despise their task. There are those who suppose that a career as a mother is a narrow experience as compared with that of typing letters for a concern that sells lumber or vacuum cleaners. Some suppose that a mother needs less education than a teacher who does nothing but teach a single subject in a high school. The mother must be a nurse, a physician, a teacher, a legal adviser, a cook, a dietitian, a financial genius, a diplomat, an authority on child psychology, and a hundred other things—at least, she should be. Why cannot this be made a career toward which girls can be pointed with pride?

Psychologists tell us that the child is half educated before he even starts to school. His mother has taught him—very often badly—the mother tongue, his habits, his manners, his attitude toward life, his self-control, his reliability, his respect for truth and right, his religion, his patriotism—and yet the task of a mother is considered too lowly to serve as an ideal! A wife, who has the responsibility of five children, once lamented that she envied a woman of her age who had attained a degree of success in bacteriology. She should be reminded that the other woman grew bacteria in culture tubes, while she was growing men and women in a home. All of this is very important in sex education. Indeed, it is the very heart of the whole thing. The girl who has been brought up to regard her womanhood as a career, the boy who is thoroughly instilled with the principles and practice of manliness, will probably not make great mistakes in their sex lives.

The pre-adolescent age is a period which is immensely important in the orientation of the boy or girl. Orientation is possible at this time for the reason that the strong sex impulses have as yet not taken definite direction because of their relatively immature state of development. A little later they will be so strong that they may take the bit in the mouth and run away. Happy is the adolescent who has been set in such a direction that he or she can permit his or her sex to run away for the good reason that it is running in the direction of the greatest advantage. Those driving men and glorious women who make the world go round are the ones, in large measure, who got their correct bearings in the pre-adolescent period and were able to drive full speed ahead into the business of being someone and of doing important things. Sex is a powerful *driving* force. In which direction, Oh parent, have you set that force driving in your child?

The Period of Adolescence

While a great many sex problems have their origin before the age of puberty and adolescence, the problems which arise at these times are much more urgent and difficult than those of the earlier years. This is the period of anxiety for parents.

This is the time when young people really need help and understanding. It is a time when powerful and utterly new forces are arising in them. New impulses are driving them they know not where. Elated with the new sensation of being comparatively grown up, and intoxicated with the previously unknown freedom which is usually granted them, they go plunging from one extreme to another. While there is some doubt about the matter of their maturity they must do everything possible *to prove that they are grown up,* and so the boys learn to smoke and to swear great and supposedly manly oaths. They affect deep knowledge of women and girls and tell of their conquests with this and that and the other one. They rarely, if ever, drive a car under seventy miles an hour, if one is to believe everything that he hears. It is, of course, obvious to those who understand something of the psychology of the period that they are overcompensating for their all too evident inexperience—whistling to prove that they are unafraid.

The girl usually passes through a "boy-struck" period. She giggles and makes herself conspicuous. Unless carefully controlled or endowed with unusual reserve, she is likely to go in for excessively high heels, extremes in dress, and large use of cosmetics. During this period of unrest she is sadly in need of intelligent and *sympathetic* guidance. Such guidance, however, is likely to be extremely distasteful to her. It will be impossible for parents who have neglected the matter of sex education until this time to pick up the reins of control and go serenely forward. Only those children who have been gradually led up to a realization of the forces at work within themselves will be in a position to appreciate the advice that wise parents can give. How may a mother who has told her daughter that babies slid down rainbows now hope to get control of the situation? Long before the time of adolescence the children have learned that their parents *are* sources of accurate information on the subject, or that they *are not* sources of accurate information. They may be expected to behave accordingly.

In continuation of sex education into the period of adolescence the parent or teacher must know that generalities are no longer sufficient. It is not enough to tell them to behave themselves and be good children. A concrete and detailed instruction in vital matters in which they may be concerned now becomes a necessity. By this we do not mean that every episode in sex life must be carefully diagrammed, but rather that the problems which the boys and girls are likely to meet should be discussed with them in a perfectly natural manner. It will, indeed, be well if the instruction is so natural and so unassumed that the boy or girl is hardly conscious that he has been instructed. Young people of this age should be included in the family conversation about many matters related to the subject of sex. The value of a good example on the part of the parents cannot be overstressed.

Let us assume here that adolescent boys and girls have had their minds thoroughly satisfied concerning the positive and beautiful phases of the subject. They are then ready to have some of the negative phases mentioned. This part of the education must not be made so graphic that it shocks or alarms excessively, but these young people should know about the possibilities of conception out of wedlock, and that under such circumstances the mother and child are sure to suffer severely from the social stigma which such a birth imposes. They should know something of venereal disease, which is perfectly capable of ruining them, their loved ones, and their careers. They should know of the depreciation of character which invariably follows the cheap promiscuity which seems so enticing under certain circumstances. These are not pleasant matters to explain, but children of this age should be treated somewhat as men and women, though they are still boys and girls. Life is coming to be real at this period; it is getting to be rather earnest. Young people will appreciate the confidence that is shown when such matters are frankly discussed, and they will really be grateful, though they may seem not to be so. It is important, of course, that discussion between young and old should be as casual as possible. The parent must not be dictatorial and he or she must be able to speak without embarrassment.

In case the young people have had no proper instruction in matters pertaining to sex during their earlier years; if they have no dignified vocabulary in terms of which these matters may be discussed; if they see in sex only the possibility of sensuous gratification, it will be difficult indeed—or well-nigh impossible—to correct the omission. Still, one can do no less than try. It is unfortunate if one must begin with the negative aspects of the subject, but even so such instruction may be necessary.

It is perfectly possible for boys and girls of the age under discussion to be parents of children. Such being the case, the careful parent can do no less than explain to his children something of the details of the sexual act. Only those who are willfully blind will pretend that it is possible or desirable to keep young people of the age ignorant of so vital a function. If there were any assurance that they might get such information in a relatively truthful form, there would be less need to insist upon parental instruction, but there is absolutely no such assurance. It is doubtful if there is so much misinformation on any other known subject. It is not so much that parents are ignorant, but rather that they "know so much that ain't so." They should be made to understand that sexual relations are of the utmost consequence to the welfare of the individual, the family, and the race, but that they are only for those who are sufficiently mature to bear and rear children, and are married so that they can do so. Unless this can be done in a way that convinces the young people themselves, it had as well not be done at all. Merely to admonish them in abstract terms is of little or no value. The sexual act must not be made an utterly delectable act utterly divorced from all sense of responsibility.

Provided the biology teacher of the high school has an appreciation of the possibilities of his subject, we strongly suggest that at least one course in this subject be taken in high school. Young people are usually safe when they are on familiar ground. It is possible in a biology class to discuss fundamental matters of sex in the most casual manner and in this way to lay an impersonal foundation for a sound understanding of the subject. When home influences and parental instruction then supplement scientific instruction, little concern need be entertained concerning the welfare of youths and maids who have normal poise and self-control.

Of much importance to the youth of this age is an appreciation of the fundamental reasons for the existence of a stable family life. Without the carefully integrated family the human infant or child is placed at a serious disadvantage and may not be able to overcome the handicap. While it is perfectly possible for persons to live in a satisfactory manner without wedlock, it is evident that marriage is fundamentally necessary, and in spite of the fact that many marriages go on the rocks, it is rather certain that men and women are normally better satisfied and happier in that relation than out of it. Marriage should then be held before young people as a probable goal, and careful thought and planning may well be given to the matter. All too frequently boys and girls break out into a scarlet rash as soon as marriage is mentioned. Giggling and protesting, they disclaim any such intentions. As a matter of fact, this behavior is a discredit not so much to these boys and girls as to their parents, for it shows clearly they have not frankly discussed such subjects with their offspring.

The sanctity of marriage may well be taught and illustrated at any age of development, but it is important that it be increasingly emphasized as the child approaches the age when he or she may be expected to enter into such a contract. Unfortunately there are a great many people who cannot understand the reasons why marriage should be more than a mere civil contract. The reason why marriage is more than a civil contract is to be found in the fact that children will probably result from such a union. Conventional marriage is the foundation on which is built the home, and the home is the basis of every one of the other social institutions—the school, the church, the government, industry, and social relations. Without the home it is hard to see how we could get along in any sort of acceptable manner. A community of good homes invariably has good schools, influential churches, thrifty, industrious, intelligent, educated people, and an acceptable government. A community of bad homes is hopelessly in the mire. These are facts that can be made plain to young people, who will consciously or unconsciously adjust themselves accordingly. Happy marriages and healthy homes are not the products of accident, the writers of melodrama to the contrary. They are worked out by persons informed in matters pertaining to real human values.

We shall do well, before we criticize the young people of today, to consider the difficult position in which we place them. They develop sexually earlier than they should and would were it not for the omnipresent sex stimulation which they are constantly receiving. They see moving pictures of the most sophisticated sort; they pick up *risqué* books or hear such books discussed; they hear suggestive songs; they see all sorts of irregularities. At any early age they have been more or less intimately introduced to the urges and passions, but are not permitted to marry until they are well into their twenties, as a rule.

In contrast to this situation is that of our parents, of earlier generations who were not let out into society until they were sixteen or seventeen, and were solidly married, frequently, at the age of eighteen or nineteen. In the early months of the period of courtship they were so awkward and green that they could hardly get into serious mischief, and by the time they were well out of that period marriage was usually consummated. If we are going to bring children up in such a way as to avoid the awkward and green stage, we are under obligation to help them take care of the passions which are aroused but may not be gratified. The awkwardness of the adolescent boy or girl is a protective device of no mean consequence. It is likely that those children who come through this adolescent period slowly and naturally will be better adjusted than those who are hurried through by socially ambitious parents, or who are turned loose on the streets.

It is for this reason that athletics are so important for boys and girls of this age. Many suppose that athletics are for the purpose of developing the physique. They are of much more consequence when they develop character. As a matter of fact, strenuous athletics at this time in life may, and frequently do, actually injure the body when not properly controlled. Play and recreation, rather than highly competitive sports, are needed. The boy who plays tennis, basketball, baseball, or engages in any of the many other wholesome sports, is not in much danger of giving too much thought to the girls. Very often, indeed, he has a fine scorn for the members of the so-called weaker sex because they cannot equal him in the manly sports. He plays until he is tired enough, when he goes to bed, to go promptly to sleep. He has something to think about; he has training rules to keep; he learns to give and take.

Girls will usually be somewhat less interested in athletics, though there are many exceptions. The reaction of girls toward athletics is essentially like that of boys, but there are certain differences which should not be entirely forgotten. There are, for example, the limitations imposed by the regular recurrence of the menstrual period. We do not wish to make invalids of girls, but insist that some consideration be given this matter. This point will be discussed later. The pelvis of the girl is broader and more loosely jointed than that of the boy. This is a relation which is necessary, as the pelvis must be built in such a way as to sacrifice strength for the contingencies of future childbirth. Heavy or excessive muscular exercise, or the carrying of heavy weights can for this reason more seriously injure the girl than the boy. Furthermore, there is an adjustment of the blood supply that is of much consequence. Nature insists that the demands of the reproductive system shall come first. For this reason the blood supply of the pregnant or nursing woman is commandeered for the reproductive organs and the breasts. If a girl is allowed to develop herself too highly in athletic lines she is able, in not a few instances, to train her muscles so that they will make such a drain upon the blood supply as will cheat somewhat the reproductive organs. It is well known that rather poorly developed women often have beautiful babies, while it is also well known that women of the muscular type are often sterile or have puny, poorly nourished (from the breast) babies. An analogy is seen in the fact that beef (muscular) cattle give poor milk and little of it, while the bony Jersey and Guernsey cows give large amounts of rich milk. We strongly believe in athletics for girls, but insist that they should be somewhat less strenuous and competitive. Girls do much better with the types of games that are mostly individual endeavor; boys need the highly coöperative games. This is in line with their probable needs in later life, when men, as a rule, work with others, while a housewife for the most part does her work alone.

Every child of adolescent age should have a hobby. Parents should make the way easy for the development of any special interest that the child may have. Collections of all sorts are made by interested young people: butterflies, beetles, plants, stamps, match-box covers, marbles, buttons, and a thousand and one other things. What a vast amount of mischief can be avoided by such means! The exercises prescribed by the Scout Manual have been of incalculable value in keeping boys and girls in pursuits which permit them to come along without too much attention to the developing forces within them. Of two boys of our acquaintance, one spent his spare time loafing on street corners, while the other was constantly looking for new plants for his herbarium, which already numbered several hundred specimens. It is not hard to guess which was developing best.

The parent who calls the child in from play in order to give him his weekly instruction in sex is entirely out of step. Sex is life. It is just plain wholesome living and doing. Therefore the teaching of this subject must be casual and matter of fact, except under certain conditions, when it must be highly idealistic and romantic. The wise parent will know when to look the other way and likewise when to set up the sanctuary. The best that the adolescent can do is to grow and develop, naturally, normally. When the new-found powers begin to assert themselves, they must be met with frankness and understanding—a sacred trust—a hostage to the future.

The habit of masturbation is likely to be developed during this period. Depending on their moral attitude to this habit, a boy or girl may worry about it or feel degraded by it. Physically, however, masturbation is of little consequence. The charge, often made in the past, that masturbation causes all sorts of maladies is without foundation. If masturbation caused only a small part of the ailments of which it has been accused the human race would be in a bad way, indeed.

Boys are frequently alarmed by the occurrence of seminal emissions or discharges of prostatic and seminal secretions while asleep. Mothers finding the stained sheets are sometimes greatly alarmed. It means nothing except that the boy is developing properly and is probably not indulging in masturbation or sexual relations. It is sometimes said that sexual relations are necessary after a certain age is reached, else the organs of the male will atrophy from disuse. Nonsense! Nature is not so dumb as to permit such a misfortune to that system which she so highly cherishes. She has provided the reproductive organs with a safety valve in the form of these seminal emissions. They are perfectly normal, and are indeed an accurate indication of proper and safe development. In the same category are the voluptuous dreams which boys and occasionally girls may experience. Think nothing of them.

Before she is twelve years old the girl should have the phenomenon of menstruation explained to her. Otherwise she is likely to be frightened by it and may be ashamed to say anything about it if she is not accustomed to confide in her mother. Formerly it was the custom of careful mothers to put their daughters to bed for a day or two at each menstrual period and to interdict all activity and bathing during this time. The girl was taught that she was "sick" and that she might expect for the next thirty years to be an invalid once a month and then to pass through a "change of life" that would probably kill her. In all too many instances the girl and woman lived up to the program expected of her. She was taught to be an invalid. Recently we have seen the absurdity of such a method, and now it is customary to go nearly as badly to the opposite extreme. The girl is told to pay no attention to it except to protect her clothing from soilage and to go ahead and do *anything* that she might otherwise do. Some girls can get by with this program just as some got by with the other.

A much more sensible approach is that which takes into consideration the altered condition of the parts but does not emphasize the condition as being morbid. Menstruation is a normal process, but in many respects approaches the pathological. Bleeding, for example, is otherwise always associated with pathology of some grade, as also is pain. The uterus of the menstruating woman is congested, and there are marked changes in the distribution of the blood; the nervous system is often considerably more unstable at such a time, and there are other evidences of altered physiology. Moderate exercise is rarely harmful; exposure to fresh air at such a time will be of no consequence unless there is chilling; bathing in warm water will rarely have a bad effect. It must be borne in mind that chilling of the skin usually tends to increase internal congestion of some sort, and so judgment must be exercised. Certainly the girl should be taught that the menstrual function is essentially physiological and that it should be treated as being such except when there is reason to believe that it is definitely pathological.

Children frequently experience rather intense love affairs. The adolescent is, of course, considerably more inclined to such attacks of "puppy love." On the other hand, some young people become so self-conscious in matters pertaining to sex that they go to the opposite extreme. Either reaction is easily understood and may be regarded as normal. Boys who are so delighted with their developing manhood are likely to become rather contemptuous of girls who have not their virile qualities, and so they sometimes think girls are quite impossible. It is not unlikely, however, that at times they may admire mightily from a distance. Girls who are becoming more careful of many little fine points of life are sometimes inclined to regard boys as being hopelessly uncouth. These reactions are also quite natural and do not presage a continuance of such feelings. As a matter of fact, rather the opposite is true as a rule, inasmuch as overreactions are common. Concerning all of these manifestations we can only say that they are normal, and strictly the affair of the individual concerned. For the rest of us, "Hands Off." The boy or girl should be allowed to develop his or her own individuality provided he or she is not taking a route that leads to deviations from what is considered to be a normal reaction.

Adolescence is a period of much dreaming and idealization. Children at this period are frequently dubbed lazy because of their propensity for dreaming and also because nature is protecting their rapidly growing and developing bodies from injury that might be inflicted by too energetic parents wishing to capitalize on the apparent—but more apparent than real—strength. The spirit of the youngster must not be injured by telling him that he is shiftless and will come to nothing. High ideals and religious motives are characteristic also of this period and may be utilized in helping to hold the young people to trends of action that may be considered safe.

The Mating Period

There comes a time in the life of every normal youth and maid when he or she is vastly interested in members of the opposite sex. The urge to mate, first in a process of courting and later in a permanent marriage, becomes the dominant factor in the determination of conduct. Older and younger persons may marvel why otherwise sensible persons should appear so foolish, but the young people themselves are intent on having their fling and their fun while they may.

In this country, particularly, the way of the lover is made easy. Young people may choose their own mates almost without help from their elders. Free choice is the inalienable right of every young person. No one is so unpopular as the stern parent who frowns on the dashing young dare-devil who for the moment sends his daughter into a state of ecstasy. In many other countries the young people have little or nothing to say about the matter and must mate according to the wishes or convenience of the parents. We are indeed glad to have this New World freedom, but it does impose a need for responsibility upon the part of the young people themselves. It is for this reason that the young people must be taught the facts of life as they are related to this subject.

Young people should be taught before the mating period is too urgently upon them that it is important indeed to look their companions over pretty carefully before allowing themselves to get too deeply involved. This is what is meant by "falling in love intelligently." We commonly speak of "falling in love" as if it were a sheer accident against which there was no protecting one's self. It is said that "love is blind," but surely this is a time for having the eyes wide open.

How may we hope to teach young people to use more discretion in the vital matter of marriage selection? Who is a suitable mate, anyway? How may one know whether the particular person is going to wear well or not? Obviously these questions are capable of being answered only in the most general of terms. Certainly the following points are extremely important:

1. The prospective mate should come from a family that is free of serious hereditary defects. Inasmuch as this is not a textbook of eugenics we shall not attempt to describe them. Furthermore, the family should be one of intelligence, industry, thrift, and such social standing as will be compatible with the status of the person making the choice.

2. The matter of the health of the individual is very important. The marrying of an invalid is a mistake that is rarely corrected. Physical attractiveness is of some importance, but exceptional beauty need not be required or particularly desired.

3. Similarity of interests and cultural background should by all means be considered. A vivacious wife and a phlegmatic husband are hardly likely to be happy. Likewise a boob, a boor, a clown, or a gigolo will be badly miscast among "in-laws" of the opposite type. Character, industry, thrift, honor, sobriety, and kindred qualities are by no means to be disregarded.

4. Education should be considered. By education we mean the ability to know what should be done in a given set of circumstances and when and how to do it. We have little respect for mere "book-learning" or diplomas in the present connection. Acceptable manners are a part of education, as are cooking, sewing, and the ability to earn funds and use them wisely.

5. It is well to know how the given individual treats the members of his or her family, and how he or she is regarded by the other members of his or her own and the opposite sex.

6. Each party should understand the attitude of the other toward children, toward sex, and toward sexual morality. When such matters are understood it would be very foolish to disregard such information in making the final decision to marry or not to marry.

7. Misgiving is sometimes expressed when the prospective husband is much larger than his mate. It is feared that she may have difficulty in giving birth to his children. This is much less serious than was formerly the case, for the good reason that obstetrical science is now far more proficient. Cæsarean section offers a solution in case trouble should arise. In general, it is better for the couple to be near the same size, but a match need not be called off because of difference of this nature. The small wife of a large man should in all cases see her physician as soon as she finds herself pregnant. If the child appears to be growing too large for safe delivery the physician has several resources which he may use.

8. An accurate inventory of cash on hand, assets, liabilities, the ability to maintain or take care of a home, and a frank understanding of the financial status is essential. By this we do not mean that we would condemn marriage to a person who is financially poor, but we are merely insisting that the situation be understood and soberly considered.

9. It will be much better if the individual has long been known and if the courtship has been long enough and under diverse conditions enough that the wearing qualities have been tested reasonably well before the marriage is actually consummated.

10. In general it will be much better if both of the mates are of the same race and social level. In some instances differences in religion, and even in politics, may cause trouble.

11. Concerning the matter of love for the individual there must be no doubt. One must be willing to make any sacrifice for the loved one, and to prefer him or her above all others. Anything short of a mutual unselfish devotion will almost surely break down in the stress and strain of married life.

It is not expected that many young people will have the discretion soberly to count the debits and credits of the suitor after the love affair has developed, but children who have had such ideals held up to them from an early age will be somewhat less likely to err in so vital a matter when they are older. Young people who understand and appreciate something of the nature of the problems of married life will be much more likely to use judgment. It is too much to expect that children who have had no instruction in sex and character will listen to their elders when they are in the heat of a fervid love affair.

Strangely enough, most parents, when they try to exert an influence upon the choice of mates which their children are making, produce an effect which is just the opposite of that which was desired. An undesirable young man brings daughter home from a function of some sort. The next morning she is questioned, and there is a scene. She is frequently told that he is worthless, good-for-nothing, and altogether impossible. She defends him, of course, and the thing is done because we come quickly to love those whom we defend. There is nothing which will so certainly drive a couple into matrimony as will the idea that the poor dear one is being mistreated and persecuted. It is human nature that we should desire that which we are told we cannot have. An uncouth young man, or a silly girl, can much more easily and certainly be eliminated by inviting him or her into the home and allowing the daughter or son to see him or her in comparison with persons of known value and merit. Many an unhappy marriage has been contracted because the young people have revolted against what they considered an infringement of their sacred right to choose.

Naturally the parent feels that he has some rights in the matter—as indeed he should have, if he has sense to be worthy of the opportunity—and as indeed he does have, if he has made the most of his opportunities in the training of the child. Does not a parent have the right to have some say as to who shall be the other parent of his grandchildren, in whom he will be tremendously interested? Does he not have some rights in saying who shall share the property which he will leave to his child? Does he not have the right to protect his child from what he believes is a disastrous marriage? The answer is that he does have some rights, but that he will have to use all the diplomacy and tact in his possession to get those rights. This is no place for the bungling despot of the home to "lay down the law" or "set his foot down." This is the prerogative of him who has spent two decades or more in preparing a son or daughter for the most important decision that he or she will ever make.

The superior experience of parents *should* make them capable of real aid to the young people, but in a great many cases the judgment of the young is much better. The mother who insists that her son or daughter shall consider social standing above everything else, and the father who demands a fat bank roll, think that they are looking after the welfare of son or daughter, but are really setting up obstacles which will be cleared with difficulty if at all. Loveless, sordid marriages made with an eye on the bank book will rarely be made by the young people themselves, and may be regarded as a legal form of prostitution. On the other hand, young people are rather prone to the "love-at-first-sight" sort of infatuation which may lead them into hasty, ill-considered marriages which rarely turn out well.

A difficult matter in modern courtship is that concerning the payment of expenses. Formerly it was possible for a couple to spend evening after evening in the most delightful companionship without the expenditure of a cent. There were no shows to attend, no gasoline to buy, no sodas, no expensive presents, no boxes of candy, no flowers. Now the matter of expense is one of considerable consequence. As likely as not the girl is earning as much or nearly as much as the man, but the old relic of chivalry demands that the man shall pay the bill and that he shall be ever so generous. Many girls are slipping a coin— or a bill—to the boy-friend sometimes, or are asking him not to spend more than is absolutely necessary, but there are others of the "give-me" type who are bleeding their consorts to the limit and are looking for boys with fat allowances and beautiful cars.

It is most unfortunate that there are expenses to be considered. Sometimes girls have been led to believe that they are under obligation to repay in ways that are destructive to morals and character. So long as the girl was entertaining in her own home, and furnishing lemonade or home-made fudge, she might bid her suitor begone when he made improper proposals; when, however, she has accepted a theater ticket, a soda, and an automobile ride and finds herself miles away from home in her friend's car, the situation is considerably more complicated, and it is not a matter of astonishment that an inexperienced girl who wishes to continue the theater parties, sodas, and rides will sometimes solve the problem in the wrong way. There is also a strong temptation for a sexually aggressive young man to take advantage of the situation. He reasons that he should have something in compensation for the outlay he has made. Being uninstructed in sex ideals, as are most boys, the form of the compensation desired is easily guessed.

Certain organizations in the large cities are giving parties and entertainments which will have the effect of throwing young people together with the express purpose of making it possible for courtship to progress as naturally as possible. Coeducational colleges serve a most useful purpose in this connection. Various church organizations and societies serve the same end. Rooming houses and girls' dormitories usually have some sort of parlor where a degree of privacy may be had. Private homes should give some thought to the matter of providing a place where the daughter may be the hostess and therefore in control of the situation. A midnight lunch from the family ice box will be deeply appreciated by the young chap who has none too much money to spend. It will also put him under a wholesome obligation to be a gentleman, whereas under a different set of circumstances the girl might feel obliged to repay him for favors received.

The matter of privacy is one of some consequence. In this country a young couple expects as their right a degree of privacy which is nearly equal to that which they will enjoy after they are actually married. Whether this is right or wrong, there is apparently little or nothing that can be done about it. To deny it would be to drive them to places where they could get privacy under much less favorable circumstances, or to appear to persecute them, which would have the effect of making them tend to wish to abuse whatever opportunities for privacy they might have. The use of a living room from which other members of the family are not entirely and rigidly excluded would seem to be a proper medium.

Interesting is the fact that the city mother used to worry when she had reason to believe that her daughter was alone with her friend on country roads. All sorts of terrible possibilities arose to worry her, though she felt no such qualms when the couple were together in the city. The country mother, on the other hand, thought nothing of her daughter driving alone with a young man in the country, but was afraid for them to go to the city unless someone went with them. Each mother rather intuitively understood that the young people were most in danger when they were in unfamiliar surroundings. Now that the distinction between city and country has mostly been wiped out, this reaction of mothers is less familiar, but it is still a fact that the young people are most likely to get into trouble when they are treading unfamiliar territory. This is the reason why they should be instructed thoroughly—but not morbidly—in matters pertaining to sex. Just as a democracy must educate the citizens who are the electorate, so must we educate our young people in these matters if we are safely to allow them the privacy that is customary in this country.

Some have supposed that they can control the relation of the two sexes by the use of chaperons. It is true that they can control the more obvious forms of indecency, but that is all. A chaperon thinks that she is saving the virtue of a girl when she compels a couple to use some restraint in their dancing positions. If the possible results were not so serious the idea would be humorous. The couple that wishes to dance in an indecent manner will not be restrained by a chaperon who all too often has been a prim dowager who hasn't the slightest idea what the whole thing is about. We need chaperons, and lots of them, but the chaperons should be *built into the character of the young people themselves;* otherwise they are simply figureheads who believe that there is no mischief simply because they have seen none. The conventional chaperon, of course, serves a useful purpose when she prevents couples who are improper from suggesting such activity to those who otherwise would have had no thought of it.

We must remember that our young people are already tremendously stimulated. We give them dancing lessons early so that they will quickly pass through the awkward age; we show them stimulating and *risqué* motion pictures; we have on our tables books that are written to sell and consequently made as "sexy" as possible; we scoff at conventions and laws which do not happen to suit our tastes; we wink at vice, graft, and illicit liaisons. After stimulating our young people in such manner, we set up economic and cultural standards which will not permit them to marry until they are much older than was the evident biological intention of Nature. According to Nature's standards a couple is ready to marry when fifteen or sixteen years old, but the requirements of conventional society set the time much later. Under such circumstances we marvel that there is no more immorality than there is.

Love between the two sexes is a pure and fine emotion, but those who cast their pearls before swine will soon lose them. For an individual to simulate the expressions of deep affection when such feelings are really not held is to invite an inevitable deterioration of character which will eventually rob that individual of the power of fine and noble emotions of this sort. A girl will soon find herself marked as one who has been pawed over; a boy will soon lose his respect for clean and sweet womanhood. Marriage for the sordid purposes of fortune and social position is an unclean thing which soon soils its nest. He who cheapens so precious an emotion as love will rue it if he has any of the finer sensibilities. He who sincerely and deeply loves another and who has earned the right to legitimate favors is entitled to them, but this presupposes that he would wish to bestow his affection only upon the favored one and has a legal right to do so.

Marriage is of such consequence that it should be carefully considered. The couple expecting to make such a contract should thoroughly discuss every phase of the subject before doing so. All reliable sources of information should be sought, and notes should be compared. Each should frankly tell the other what he or she expects.

There is nothing finer and more beautiful, nothing more useful, nothing more pure than those prenuptial agreements and arrangements which insure that the couple are really ready to marry and to assume the sacred obligations which marriage entails.

THE HONEYMOON

The honeymoon is the period between the marriage ceremony and the time when the young people shall have become more or less settled into the routine of a married couple. It is frequently used to designate a trip that is taken for the purpose of getting away from prying eyes. It is a period of adjustment to the new regimen and may be wisely or unwisely spent. Not a few marriages are utterly wrecked during this time, and a great many others are so strained as to weaken or damage the prospect of future happiness and usefulness. It is a time of high emotional tension and needs to be rather soberly considered. The obvious purpose of the honeymoon is to grant to the newly married lovers an unusual degree of privacy while they are experimenting with the new status in which they find themselves.

It is unfortunate that there have grown up so many ugly customs about so beautiful a thing as a wedding. Pranks without number are played upon the couple; many of these pranks are in exceedingly bad taste, and not a few are positively indecent, or dangerous.

Wealthy families are inclined to make much of a wedding. There are parties, showers, receptions, and elaborate ceremonies, and finally a long and tiresome honeymoon is planned. A trip to Europe or a tour around the world seems like an ideal wedding present, but is entirely too long and tiresome. On such a trip the lovers are thrown entirely too much into each other's company and may utterly exhaust themselves and their interest in each other. The fatigue of travel and of sight-seeing, added to the strain of adjustment and the enervating effects of excessive sexual exercise, is entirely too much. It would be better if the trip were short and the demands made upon physical and emotional resources were light. A cabin in the woods, or a room at a summer or a winter resort, according to season, is likely to be much better. It is easy also for the pair to lose themselves in a large city, where hotels afford any degree of seclusion that may be desired, and the myriad diversions of the city furnish opportunity for any degree of activity that may be needed.

Families in moderate circumstances often exceed their means in attempting to give their young people a big and elaborate wedding and trip. The worry as to whether the funds will hold out, and the consciousness that the rocket-like celebration is going to end with a thud, make a bad start. Better no honeymoon at all than one that cannot be afforded.

The most important relations of the period, however, are not those which are commonly called the honeymoon. They are those which take place in the very first days and nights of married life. The happiness and even the health of the couple may be seriously crippled by the bungling caresses of one who is not ready for real marriage or is utterly lacking in understanding of the processes involved.

Biologic marriage and conventional marriage have entirely different purposes, but the two are supplementary to each other and are best consummated at approximately the same time. In case the biologic marriage has lagged and one or another of the pair is not ready for the actual union, the process of courtship should continue until the mate—usually the bride—is really ready for sexual relations. Theoretically, legal marriage gives each the right to the body of the other, and many men have been crass enough to insist on those rights as soon as the privacy of the bedroom has been reached. Embarrassed, shocked, frightened, and even sometimes subjected to physical pain, the bride is essentially forced by one who has but a short time before promised to love and cherish her. Under such circumstances she is set against the whole process and, indeed, may never learn to take a normal attitude toward a relation which should be exquisitely pleasurable to both partners. In a short time the husband, being disappointed in the fact that his wife is no longer a lover, may become disgusted and seek mistresses who can take an interest in such things. Modesty is fine and splendid, but a ruined marriage is too big a price to pay for *mock* modesty.

Every prospective bridegroom should understand that, unless he has positive and first-hand assurance to the contrary, the bride may probably wish to delay the climax of the ceremony which has just been performed. Brides without previous sexual experience may be reluctant indeed, in spite of the fact that they are intensely in love with their new husbands. In such case there is nothing for the *gentleman* to do but bide his time and divert himself in the gallant and romantic manner which has so far won her approval that she has been willing to take his name, and share her life with him. The rights which the law gives him are as worthless as dust until they have been ratified by her approval. "Women first" is the code of the gentleman. If this fact could be impressed on the consciousness of bridegrooms most of them would be only too glad to wait until the loved one is ready to invite his amorous advances. Young people, when newly married, are in a highly idealistic and romantic state and are more liberal and unselfish probably than at any other time in their lives. But the young man, being intensely stimulated himself and never having been told that the feeling of the bride may be different, supposes that she as well as he is eager to bring about the consummation of their marriage. If she is so, very well! There is not the least reason for formality in cases where courting has progressed to such a stage. When, however, the bride is reluctant, courtship must be continued, and courtship only.

All or most of these difficulties can be avoided by a frank prenuptial understanding. The couple who are so excessively modest that they cannot discuss this subject had better grow up a little, learn something about themselves, and really get in love before going ahead with a wedding. If the girl seems reluctant, her fiancé can make her happy and reassured if he will promise her that he will consider her wishes in these matters as well after marriage as before. She, in turn, should assure him that she understands the purpose and nature of marriage, and that she will do her best to become interested in that which is so vital to happiness and unity.

In times past there is reason to believe that such an understanding has often not been attained, and that a green, inexperienced, awkward youth and a shy, embarrassed, undeveloped girl were commonly thrown together in utter ignorance of all the arts of conjugal life. Such, indeed, was considered to be the ideal condition, and mothers were prone to boast that their daughters knew absolutely nothing about such matters. It is no wonder that so many marriages went on the rocks. Probably the only reason that so many escaped is that the daughters were rarely so dumb as fond mamma supposed. Young people are much better prepared in this respect for marriage nowadays. There are opportunities to learn; there is a vocabulary in which they may speak to their prospective mates; there are books, pamphlets, and lectures from which they may learn much; and in most instances there is the practice of those intimacies which are the proper prelude to marriage.

Sheer clothing, athletic uniforms, and brief bathing suits have accustomed both sexes to the general appearance of the body of the other sex. It is to be hoped that this has helped greatly to prevent excessive embarrassment in the act of disrobing, and that it also will tend to temper somewhat the excitement of one or both. To one who stands in great reverence of the significance of the marriage relation it seems that a couple intensely in love and entering into a relation of such significance and beauty might find an exquisite delight in coming frankly and gladly together devoid of every covering and artifice. This is no time for silly giggling and undressing in the closet. It is a time for truth, dignity, and that fine sense of self-respect that is proud to proclaim to all the world that this man and this woman are grown up and are taking their places in the long line of those who have lived and loved.

The Young Married Couple

Much has been said about the advisability of the wife working after marriage. Until the couple can get a start there can certainly be no objection to the wife's holding her former job or getting another one. It will mean extra hours of work and less leisure now that she has the care of a home or an apartment, but it is all for the good of the cause. It would be a poor wife, indeed, who would not put her shoulder to the family wheel and help to make it turn.

Unfortunately, however, there is more to the matter than just that. It will be hard later for her to give up the outside job and devote herself exclusively to home-making with its comparatively intangible rewards. We need not be surprised that she is loath to give up the independence that comes with a check at the end of the week. There are so many things that are needed and can be had only if the wife as well as the husband earns.

So it is customary to put off, and put off, and put off the real purpose and culmination of marriage—children. If two have trouble making ends meet with two salaries—as two commonly do—how shall three or four or five live on one salary? And so by sex repression, which often eats into the hearts of both, by the use of more or less distasteful contraceptive methods, or sometimes by resort to criminal abortion, the couple more or less successfully cheats Mother Nature of her due. From month to month, with fear and hope combined, the coming of the menses is awaited as if its failure would be a worldwide catastrophe. Years pass, and the couple are still in need of both pay checks. Educated tastes have been developed and seemingly must be pampered; children are forgotten, or are pushed farther and farther into the future. Usually they say that "some day" they want children but hardly see how they can manage it just yet. "Some day" they are going to have beautiful blue-eyed boys and golden-haired girls, but when "some day" comes Nature has often become tired of being turned away, and the Gate of Life is closed.   The error that young people are so likely to make is to believe that parties, shows, elegant furniture, and sport roadsters can bring more happiness than children. Once they have had the children they would know that nothing can bring the soul-satisfying rapture that a baby brings, but, of course, they haven't had such experience, and quite naturally cannot fully appreciate it. Such marriages are easily broken. With no children, with little property investment as a rule, with both having an income, the slightest friction is likely to cause a serious split.

If the wife works there should be a definite understanding concerning the time when she shall be promoted to the much more important work of real home-making. Marriages when both parties are poor but in good health and willing to work are frequently the very best of marriages. Stories told of the hard times that grandfather and grandmother had in the old days are familiar family lore, and will be a century hence. We frequently see the young wife working to help her husband complete his education, and it makes a most inspiring picture. Likewise, the wife may continue her education after marriage. These are the people who know what an education is. They will get along.

For those couples who cannot for some reason bear children there are infinite possibilities in the adoption of orphans. With care the adopted child that has come from a good family has an even chance with the blood descendant of the same age and physical opportunity. It cannot be shown that adopted children turn out worse than others. They may on the average do better, when they have been carefully selected. A careful physical and mental examination should be made of all children who are being considered for adoption. Couples without children may also satisfy their parental instincts and do a great service by taking up some phase of work which has to do with the welfare of children and young people. It is the only way to stay young and keep sweet. "Suffer little children to come unto Me and forbid them not, for of such is the Kingdom of Heaven" is no idle dogma. It is the essence of life.

Marriage is not a lark. There is no more serious business in all the world than that of building a home and rearing children. Prospective husbands and wives had better grow up before undertaking the honorable responsibilities that come to those who assume the social and biological status known as marriage. When happily consummated and honestly lived it is tremendously effective in bringing into being the happiest and most satisfying of all human relationships.

An ideal family is like nothing so much as a beautiful flower. There is present in each a male or father element and a female or mother element. Beautiful in design, arrangement, color, and fragrance, the parts of the flower act together as a unit for the production and preservation of seeds—children —until they have attained such a degree of maturity that they may be safely entrusted to the dangers of the outside environment. By such means the perpetuity of the species is insured so long as the flower shall continue to exercise its primary function—the production of seeds—the rearing of children.

Sex in Middle and Advanced Life

Most men and women experience a considerable shock as they approach and pass the age of forty. They have learned to look upon "fat and forty" as being the zero hour of romance. As young people they have supposed that one so old has lost every good reason for living. To be a solid burgher or thrifty housewife of forty has been supposed to be the end of everything, and now to find one's self at the halfway place in life or a little beyond seems incredible. Actually, however, a large percentage of people are happier after this age than before.   Particularly is this true of those who have lived and loved wisely. The individual who can adjust his life and thinking to the fact that he is no longer a gay and irresponsible young thing will find many compensations for the fact that he can no longer swim across the lake or beat the young fellows at tennis. The woman who can relax a bit at this time and smile indulgently at the mad struggle for beauty and youth has before her many happy days of comparative quiet and serenity.

It is difficult for younger people to see in this period anything but a tiresome and monotonous existence, and there are many who find themselves at forty or above in an openly rebellious attitude. They want one more fling at "life" and may do foolish things in the effort to get it. The man who has been circumspect and careful about all such matters may get sympathetic for himself and think he has missed a great deal. Somewhat bored with the faithful but unromantic wife, he is prone to yearn for a younger and more vivacious companion. If some degree of affluence has rewarded his labors, he is in a position to indulge himself—and be an easy mark for gold-diggers who really hold him in contempt. Occasionally a woman of forty retains her youth better than her husband and may be tempted to "step out" a bit with a snappy "gigolo" or a neighbor whose "wife doesn't understand him." She yearns for a lover instead of a tired workhorse who prefers his house slippers and shirt sleeves to a "tux" and a ballroom. It is not unlikely that this period offers more urgent temptations than does any other. Certain it is that the opportunities for making a fool of one's self during this time are unexcelled.

It is not uncommon to hear men say that when they are no longer interested in a pretty face or figure they will be ready to die—life will no longer be worth living. The loss of virility in men is looked on as a calamity of the highest degree. Such an attitude reveals an utter lack of understanding of the real meaning of life.

Loss of virility is Nature's way of insuring against "exhaustion products"; it is her way of making sure that fathers will probably live until the work of rearing the child is accomplished; it is her protection for the weakened and wasted organs of the body which in the wear and tear of life have likely become injured to such an extent that ardent wooing and frequent sexual embraces are exhausting. What a fool is the man who seeks rejuvenation by some sort of gland operation or transplantation! Even if gland transplantations were successful, which they are not, little good could come from such meddling. It is like putting a powerful new motor into a rickety old chassis in the expectation of roaring along at eighty m.p.h. Of course something breaks—usually an artery in the brain—and there is real trouble. "New wine in old bottles" has been a dangerous combination for so long that it looks as if the fact might be better appreciated.

The elderly widower gets himself a young wife. How can a young woman be really in love with a man thirty or forty years her senior? For that matter, how can a man of that age who understands things be truly in love with a young woman? Ten years more will find him an old man while she will be just starting. Clashes between the wife and his children—as old as she perhaps—are inevitable. The suspicion that she loves his money rather than him; the fear that she may be stepping out with younger men; the painful effort to entertain her as a young wife deserves to be entertained; the fear that children may be borne at a period in life when children would be a burden; and a dozen other fears real and imaginary, take away every iota of the tranquillity that should be the heritage of him who has lived long. Much wiser indeed is he who chooses a companion who is near his own age.

Respect for gray hairs is a duty of the young. It is even more the duty of those who have the gray hairs. The young people are right when they tell grandma to "be her age." By this we do not mean that men and women of middle age should don the funereal black that used to be the custom, and that they should fold their hands and get ready to die. Quite the contrary! Dyeing the hair, having face-lifting operations, refusing to wear the glasses that they need, nervously driving themselves to act as if they were mere girls, these wretched men and women fool no one and wear themselves out trying to make the stream of life start over at the source. If it could be done there would be some excuse for the effort, but of course they always lose. Almost any young girl can be pretty or even beautiful, but it takes a "heap o' livin' " to make a beautiful old face. The lines of age are simply the character lines that have been developed through years of habitual smiling; or frowning; and constitute real beauty—or ugliness. The beauty of youth is skin deep, but the beauty of age really goes to the bone.

The Hygiene of the Reproductive System

A fine watch does best when it is meddled with least. The same is true of any complicated mechanism and in particular of the generative apparatus. A policy of "hands off" is hard to beat in this connection. There are, to be sure, elemental points in the care of the organs which should be understood by everyone, but further than this the layman should not go. There has been so much ignorance and misinformation concerning the sexual apparatus that the layman may hardly trust anything that he has learned from the usual source. When there is reason to believe that something is really wrong, the family physician or a specialist whom he may designate should be consulted at once. It surely is needless to say that the physician should be furnished with a full and frank history of the ailment and its possible causes. Furthermore, he must be permitted to make such examinations and to ask such questions of the parents as he may think necessary. Some of his questions will seem impertinent but it is exactly such questions as may bring out the basic difficulty.

CLEANLINESS

The first principle to be considered in the hygiene of the reproductive system is cleanliness. By this we do not mean to imply that lack of cleanliness will often jeopardize the physical health of the individual. Actually there is more danger that meddlesome methods of attaining cleanliness will cause disease than that lack of cleanliness will cause it. This is particularly true in the case of the female. But there is more to this matter of hygiene than mere maintenance of health. The reproductive organs must be clean if they are to be held in high regard; they must be free of odor; they must be wholesome; they must not offend. They are so exceedingly important to the welfare of the race, the self-respect of the individual, and the happiness of family, and yet they are so likely to be regarded as being vulgar by those who do not understand that there must not be any doubt about their basic wholesomeness.

Odor is undoubtedly of first consideration. The fact that we wear clothing complicates the matter for the good reason that the clothing does not permit the free ventilation that will carry away odors before they become concentrated and will permit the rapid evaporation of perspiration. Clothing should be as light and as well ventilated as comfort will permit. Great improvement in underwear has been made in recent years. Undergarments should be changed as often as one's finances will permit and should of course never be worn after they are definitely soiled. Night clothing should entirely replace the underwear that has been worn through the day. This will give opportunity for airing and drying of the various garments which would be most likely to offend.

Frequent washing of the external genitalia is of course extremely important. It is the *external* organs that need washing and not the internal. Much harm has undoubtedly been done by the use of antiseptic or even cleansing douches as many women use them. In the first place they are not necessary from the standpoint of preventing odors for the good reason that the odors of the vagina proper are practically never concentrated enough to cause trouble if the external organs are clean. The normal vagina nearly always contains great numbers of germs which are known collectively as "Doderlein's bacilli." These germs are not only harmless, but actually beneficial, because they prevent the growth of other germs which can really cause trouble. Incidentally these germs are closely related to, or by some are considered to be identified with, the germs that are deliberately put into acidophilus milk which is much used for restoring healthy conditions in the bowels. There is not a bit of doubt that the presence of these acid producing organisms is of positive value in the vagina. If they are frequently washed away with cleansing douches or inhibited with antiseptics, abnormal conditions may develop in the vagina, and real trouble may ensue. Furthermore, strong antiseptics frequently irritate the mucous membrane and make it more susceptible to invasion by other bacteria. Not a few of the commonly used douches are definitely irritating or even poisonous when used in too concentrated form or when used frequently. This is particularly true of bichloride of mercury and lysol.

Sometimes, particularly in the male, it is impossible to hold down odors merely by washing the external genitalia. In some individuals the foreskin is so tight about the end of the penis that it cannot be retracted and the groove beneath it cleaned of the white secretion—known as smegma—which accumulates there. This secretion is of an oily nature and easily becomes rancid, producing exceedingly bad odors and also irritation of the mucous membrane. At the time of birth every male child should be carefully examined to determine whether or not he is in need of circumcision which consists in removing the foreskin. When done in the early days of life the operation is a trivial one. Later it is somewhat more serious, but never dangerous when performed by a competent surgeon. Even those individuals who are not in need of circumcision should retract the foreskin and clean the groove beneath it carefully at least once a day. A child in need of circumcision is often made nervous by the irritation of the rancid secretions and will be constantly twisting, squirming, and pulling at himself. He may also develop the habit of masturbation as a result of the irritation which induces him to handle his penis. We do not advocate that all boys and men should be circumcised, but are emphatic in recommending such treatment when there is difficulty in keeping the parts clean otherwise. Girls are also occasionally in need of circumcision, or what is essentially the same thing.

Occasionally discharges of various sorts from the genital organs will greatly complicate the habit of cleanliness. In *every* case in either sex the cause of any discharge should be ascertained if possible. The family physician or a reliable specialist should be consulted, *always*. *Never* should patent medicines or home remedies be used as a substitute for careful examination and treatment by a physician. *Never* must the patient go to an advertising physician or to one who is known to be, or suspected of being a quack. In case the discharge can be cured and the cause removed the problem is solved. When the condition cannot be corrected, the greatest of care will be needed to prevent offensive odors and a disgusting local condition.

MENSTRUATION

The peculiar demands of menstruation call for attention in a discussion of hygiene. There is first to be considered the necessity of caring for the actual physiological needs. During this period the pelvic organs of the female are considerably congested, and for this reason are more subject to infection and circulatory disturbances. It is for this reason that excessively long hours of standing on the feet, dancing, strenuous athletics, and similar activities are not advisable for many women. Likewise sexual excitement will intensify the effect, and may cause trouble. Bathing was formerly interdicted, but is now permitted in most cases if the water is warm. There is, of course, additional need of cleanliness at such a time, and local bathing is always perfectly safe. There are many women and girls who can even swim in cold water while menstruating, but such chilling of the skin is likely to drive the blood inward and increase the internal congestion or cause severe cramping.

In case the menstrual periods should cease in a girl or woman who is probably not pregnant, careful physical examination should be made to determine the cause. In earlier times this cessation was supposed to cause tuberculosis. Now we understand that in most such cases tuberculosis is already present and the checking of this drain is a means by which Nature seeks to conserve the patient's strength. Patients with anemia of any sort or those with nervous disturbances are also likely to cease menstruating until they are restored to their normal condition. Of great importance is the mental attitude of the woman toward her menstrual periods, and toward the "change of life," at which time the periods gradually cease from natural causes. In times past girls were literally taught to make invalids of themselves, and women were led to believe that "the change" was something greatly to be dreaded and a time of danger. We understand now that menstruation is a perfectly normal process, and that the menopause need cause little apprehension if it is approached with understanding and poise. The fact that women are now so much less embarrassed in visiting a physician about such matters has opened a way of escape from many of the dangers and discomforts. The frank consideration of all subjects relative to sex and the far more natural attitude toward them has in large measure taken them out of the limbo to which they were formerly assigned.

With so much advertising of absorbent pads and other aids to feminine hygiene it is hardly necessary to describe in detail the means by which women may avoid the soiling of their clothing with the menstrual discharges. As stated elsewhere, young girls should have these matters explained before they are twelve years of age, or by the time they are ten or eleven if they are somewhat precocious in their development. It is important that the girl be taught so that she will not be frightened by the first appearance but will come to her mother for aid and advice. This is, of course, an excellent opportunity for the mother to explain something of the nature and purpose of the genital organs and to impress the girl with the value of the process of which the menstrual cycle is a part.

In recent years there has been much discussion of the use of a vaginal tampon as a means of controlling menstrual bleeding. Medical opinion is now pretty well agreed that the method is safe provided the tampons are of proper size and are removed as may be needed. When—as in virgins—the opening in the hymen is small, there is difficulty in inserting and particularly in removing the tampon. The objection to this method of feminine hygiene is for the most part a traditional objection to putting anything into the virgin vagina.

DISEASES OF THE GENITAL ORGANS

There are various serious diseases of the genital organs which need to be understood so that they may be detected at the earliest possible moment. We shall not describe the venereal diseases in this place, as they will be discussed in a later chapter. Various other chronic inflammations and injuries resulting from childbirth or injury usually manifest themselves by symptoms or pain of some sort. Of greatest importance are the various forms of cancer which may be found. Unfortunately cancers are not painful in their earlier stages. To be sure, they are terribly painful later, and this fact may mislead persons who are really in danger and will not believe that they are so because they are not in pain.

At the present time about one woman in seven above the age of forty years is dying of cancer of one kind or another. About one third of these cancers are of the womb, usually the mouth of the womb. We shall not attempt to give such a description as will enable the layman to make an unerring diagnosis of cancer of the womb, but merely call attention to the fact that any sort of unnatural bleeding from the privates should be investigated thoroughly. Excessive bleeding, bleeding after the change of life, continuous bleeding, or the passing of *clotted* blood, constitute "unnatural" bleeding. These signs do not mean that a given person surely has cancer, but they do mean that there is *something* wrong, and that a *thorough examination is needed*. The physician should be required to prove if at all possible that it is *not* cancer before the investigation is ended. Once the diagnosis of cancer is made, treatment in the hands of a reliable surgeon or radiologist is the only hope. It is believed that unrepaired tears of the mouth of the womb may be the cause of cancer in many instances, since they cause long continued irritation.

Another third of all deaths from cancer among women is from cancer of the breast. These growths are always small before they are large, always localized before they are generalized, and always painless before they are painful. The growth usually manifests itself as a lump or nodule in the breast, or sometimes as a thick place in the skin reminding one of a piece of bacon rind. It is usually irregular in shape, attached to the skin and deeper tissues, and solitary in number in the earlier stages at least. As the breast is moved the nodules cause dimpling. If near the nipple, they commonly cause the nipple to be drawn in. The chances for recovery are good if the diagnosis is made early and the appropriate treatment begun at once. If surgical treatment is delayed, the operation is much more severe, and there is less chance of cure. Rarely cancer of the breast is seen in the male.

Cancer of the prostate and bladder are fairly common in the male. The earliest symptom is usually blood in the urine or difficulty in emptying the bladder. These symptoms should call for an immediate examination to determine the cause.

The reproductive system of the female is much more complicated than that of the male and is for this reason more subject to disease and injury. It furthermore is under far greater stress in the performance of its function of reproduction. For this reason care must be taken to avoid as many as possible of the dangers which beset the sexual life. In the first place, women—and men, too, for that matter—should not marry unless they are reasonably sure that they are free from disease and deformity. Women who have suffered from rickets as children should make sure that the pelvic opening is large enough to permit the passage of a child at the time of birth. In recent years it has been possible for such women to bear children by submitting to Cæsarean section, but even in such cases it is better if the obstetrician knows beforehand that the child cannot pass through the birth canal. Women who have reason to believe that they are suffering from active or recently arrested tuberculosis should refrain from childbearing both for their own sake and for the sake of the child.

We believe there is no legitimate excuse for an intelligent woman to go into maternity without informing herself thoroughly concerning the risks and the means of reducing those risks to the minimum. Certainly there is no excuse for delay after she finds herself actually pregnant. She should consult her family physician or the specialist of her choice as soon as she becomes aware of her condition. If the pregnancy is the first, there is additional reason for such professional care. Likewise the women beyond the age usual for childbearing and those who have reason to believe that they may have weak hearts and kidneys should take extra precaution. All pregnant women should have their blood type known. In case the wife is RH negative while her husband is RH positive there is particular reason to know and be prepared to cope with the situation. With modern care the condition is usually handled with success, without such care the results are often disastrous to the child.

SEXUAL INTERCOURSE IN PREGNANCY

Many couples wonder if sexual intercourse may be indulged in during the period of pregnancy. This will depend upon several factors. Certainly it should not if there is a feeling that the act is degrading during this time. Likewise it may only be practised when both mates desire it. There is good reason from the standpoint of the possibility of infection for refraining during the last few weeks of the pregnancy. In case the wife seems to have been injured by marital relations on previous occasions, or if she is one who is easily aborted, continence is the only safe rule. In those instances—and they are many—in which the wife desires the relation at this time and does not seem to be injured by it there is no real objection. The fear that the child may be injured is quite without foundation except in those women who are easily aborted.

SEX GLANDS

SEX GLANDS (See also, *Internal Secreting or Endocrine Glands*) The glands of sex serve a double function: they provide the necessary materials for reproduction of the human being, the male sex cell uniting with the female sex cell; they also provide material which goes directly from the glands into the blood and which determines the nature of the growth of the body. If the amount of the material secreted by the gland into the blood is insufficient, definite changes will take place in the body inclining towards the female side if the male sex tissue is insufficient and to the masculine side in the woman if the female sex tissue is insufficient.

A deficiency of the male sex material may result from absence or destruction of the gland or from failure to function in case the pituitary gland does not produce the trophic hormone that stimulates the male sex gland. Again there may be disturbance of the function of the cells within the gland without actual destruction of the tissue.

A deficiency of male glandular material varies in its effects according to the age at which it occurred. If the material is completely absent, the condition called eunuchism is developed; this usually refers to a complete loss. When the loss of sexual gland function takes place before the time of maturation into an adolescent, a deficiency is shown in growth. The skin is delicate; the hair that ordinarily covers the surface of the body of the male is absent; there also may be exaggerated length of the arms and legs with broad hips and a tendency towards the development of a "pot belly;" sometimes also the breasts of the male will enlarge.

SEX GLAND DEFICIENCY—If a deficiency of sex gland hormones takes place after adolescence, the changes include a retardation of the growth of the beard and thinning of the skin with lessened pigmentation and perhaps also a diminution or complete absence of hair under the arms and around the sex organs. Interestingly there is also a failure to grow hairs on the ear which is rather typical of men past twenty-five or thirty years of age.

After men have matured and have reached the age of forty-five or fifty, they do not usually suffer the changes that come on in women about the same time and which are known as the climacteric. The specialists believe that this is due to the fact that the sexual function of men declines gradually rather than abruptly as occurs with women. The changes that occur in men are not visible in any way in the structure of the body since this has been well established by the age of forty-five, but are more definitely related to the functions of the body and to symptoms that are manifest often in the nervous system.

When there is an absence of sex gland material as is determined by some of the signs that have been described, administration of the artificially prepared material is now possible due to the development of the glandular material called testosterone. The amount of the material to be given and the duration of the time over which it is to be given depends, of course, on the condition of the patient, whom the doctor watches carefully. Actually there may be the growth of pimples and in the case of women, a tendency towards a masculine appearance from too much sex gland material. There are also effects on the handling of salt and water by the body. It has been established that excesses of testosterone, particularly in young boys, may result in difficulty in the development of sperm cells necessary for reproduction.

EXCESSIVE MALE SEX GLAND ACTION—Excessive production of male sex hormones is observed in men particularly when there are tumors of the male sex glands. Such tumors have been observed by physicians in many cases. Occasionally excessive growth of tissue of the anterior pituitary gland or in other portions of the brain may stimulate the sex glands excessively so that large amounts of male sex hormone are thrown into the circulation. The manifestations of excessive secretion vary with the time when the condition occurs. If it comes on before the young boy has reached puberty, the excessive sex gland material may cause puberty to come on much sooner than normally. Associated with this precocious pseudo-puberty is a too early development of all of the male sex characteristics including excessive growth of the sex organs, the development of a large amount of hair around the sex organs and under the arms, and even in little boys, the development of a beard and a mustache, a deep voice and similar conditions. Physicians have observed that excessive amounts of male sex gland material will cause increased secretion of the oil glands in the skin and associated acne is not uncommon. There may often also be changes in the growth of the skeleton. In this instance the trunk, the arms and legs are found to be short due to too early closure of the points from which the bones grow. Associated also with these developments may be excessive and definitely increased muscular development and strength; the so-called "infant Hercules."

If the excessive secretion of glandular material comes on after the body has passed puberty, the condition manifests itself by accentuation of the masculine character. Obviously the skeleton has already developed so that there cannot be effects on the skeleton.

The only known treatment for excessive activity is removal of the tumor which is responsible. Removal of portions of the tumor or of all of the tumor would naturally result in lessening the amount of sex gland material.

This can be measured by chemical study so that the return to normal can be definitely known. If, however, the tumor material should return and grow again, the excess of glandular secretion can be determined through examination of the urine. In this way the physician can trace the progress of the tumor growth.

Fortunately tumors of the male sex gland are relatively rare. Doctors believe that these tumors occur more often when there has been failure of the male sex gland to descend into the sac which it normally does before ten or eleven years of age, if not sooner. Experience has shown that the best thing to do whenever there is any tumor of this area is to have it removed by surgery as soon as possible. If the tumor, is not a malignant tumor, it is in any event a threat. If, however, it is a malignant tumor, the growth quite certainly threatens life itself. In fact, so definitely is that threat known that it has become customary to use the X ray to irradiate the area from which the tumor has been removed to make certain that all excessive action has been stopped.

If the male sex gland is retained and fails to descend into the sac, its function may be destroyed by the heat to which it is subjected in the body.

Failure of sexual gland function causes psychosexual changes in the males including loss of initiative and drive. Some psychiatrists feel this effect is wholly mental and results from a feeling of inferiority because the person knows of his deficiency.

Sexual precocity associated with excess of testosterone or androsterone has also been noted with adrenal and pituitary gland tumors.

OVARIES—FEMALE SEX GLANDS—The ovary, which is the female sex gland, has, like the male sex gland, the function of preparing an egg cell called the ovum. This is involved in reproduction. Following the development of this egg cell, the ovary prepares hormones or glandular materials which go into the blood and which are significant in the functioning of a woman's body. The periodic functions of women are largely regulated by these hormones from the ovary. The ovary, in turn, is regulated by hormones which come from the pituitary gland and which are necessary in order for ovulation to occur. Following ovulation the ovary develops a substance called the *corpus luteum* which provides a hormone called progesterone. Progesterone is responsible for the preparation of the uterus to receive the egg cell. When the egg cell fails to be fertilized, the uterus gets rid of the material by the usual flow.

The follicle which prepares the ovum or egg cell also is important in the formation of estrogen which is known as the female sex hormone. Although the function of the ovary was recognized as far back as 1673, only within recent years has this understanding of the glandular materials developed by the ovary come to light.

When a girl matures, the flow occurs which is usually seen between the ages of twelve and sixteen. This is a rhythmical or periodic function, taking place generally about every twenty-eight days although many cases are known in which the flow occurs at shorter or longer periods. Usually ovulation discontinues at the time of the menopause which generally takes place between forty-five and fifty-five years of age, the average being forty-eight. Estimates indicate that at the time when the girl matures there are approximately 300,000 possible egg cells ready for development. Only a few of these mature and eventually come to the surface.

After an ovum has been developed each month the follicle ruptures and the ovum travels by way of the Fallopian tubes into the uterus. If a male sex cell reaches the ovum and fertilizes it, the ovum remains in the uterus and pregnancy occurs.

In the absence of the female sex hormones, changes occur in the body of a woman which reflect the lack of these chemical regulators of the body.

OVARIAN DEFICIENCY—If the ovary is not adequate, or if it is absent following surgical removal, an insufficient secretion of the female sex hormones occurs. Absence of such hormones is associated with a disappearance of the usual menstrual flow. Development of the body is complete and the characteristics of women which are peculiar to the sex disappear.

As with a deficiency of the male sex hormone, absence of ovarian secretion results in overgrowth of the long bones which fail to close their points of growth during adolescence. An insufficiency of ovarian secretion may lead to failure of the sexual organs to develop so that they appear infantile in type. Associated is a lack of development of the breast and a lack of the usual growth of hair under the arms and around the sex organs.

If there is an adequate amount of female sex hormone up to the time of puberty and a failure to secrete thereafter, the symptoms are different, because the child will have achieved rather full growth by the time it comes to adolescence.

Fortunately substitutes for the usual hormones have been found. These can be prescribed by the doctor in amounts as needed and thus cause a return to normal conditions.

As with the male sex hormone, the function of the ovary is dependent on hormones that come from the pituitary or master gland in the brain. Failure of the pituitary gland to send its hormones will result in failure of the ovary to develop normally. With this comes lack of menstruation, lack of development of the breasts and delay in appearance of the other secondary female characteristics.

FAILING OVARIAN FUNCTION—If the ovary is not functioning following the time when the girl reaches adolescence, as may occur when there is a necessity for surgical removal or when cysts form in the ovary and destroy the ovarian tissue, a number of significant conditions may appear. One of the most important is development of irregularity of the usual rhythmic flow, sometimes culminating in complete absence of the flow. With this there is a tendency to put on too much weight, to grow extra hair and to develop a pasty skin.

Occasionally the menopause comes on in a woman long before she is forty-eight years of age. This is definitely abnormal. Such an occurrence should lead to an immediate medical examination because it may be associated with social and psychological difficulties. The doctor who is called to study such a patient can bring relief in many instances by prescribing the necessary hormones according to the condition in each patient.

The menopause may occur quite suddenly. When it does, a number of serious symptoms may develop including excessive flow and what are commonly called "hot flashes" with drenching sweats, the development of a ravenous appetite and a rapid gain in weight. There are also sometimes changes in the bones and joints, giving rise to the condition known as menopausal arthritis. Obviously such symptoms are serious, affecting the entire life of the women concerned. They should be an indication for a complete and careful study of the case and for the administration of such hormones as might be considered by the physician to be desirable.

For the arthritis of the menopause the use of Cortone or ACTH has already been shown to be helpful in bringing about relief.

The physician always remembers that the glands are an interlocking chain and the source for disturbance may be not only the sex gland itself, but quite as often the pituitary gland or occasionally the thyroid gland. In any event, the psychologic aspects must be studied. It is impossible for anyone to treat himself successfully for disorders of glandular functions such as I have described.

EXCESSIVE OVARIAN ACTION—Excessive secretion of glandular materials from the ovary is manifested most often by disturbances of the usual rhythmical functions of women. The disturbance may be reflected in abnormal bleeding, frequent bleeding, excessive bleeding, or similar symptoms. Whenever there is irregularity in the duration or frequency of flow, a careful examination should be made to find out the cause.

Of course bleeding is a serious symptom whenever it occurs from any portion of the body. Any bleeding before the child has matured or after the cessation of the regular flow is an indication which demands immediate study. In over half of such cases the necessity for determining the presence of any serious growth is obvious.

Excessive action of the ovary before the time of maturation into adolescence is manifested by bleeding, associated with excessive development of the breasts and premature establishment of growth of hair under the arms and on the sex organs. Rapid growth of the skeleton and occasionally an interest in the opposite sex which is far above the normal may occur. All this is called precocious puberty.

Any time the rhythmical flow is established before the age of ten, an investigation should be made. As in the case of men, the presence of tumors can cause excessive activity of any glandular organ including the female sex glands.

As was previously mentioned, the mechanism for the process of reproduction is in women quite complicated. It begins with the coming of glandular materials from the pituitary gland which, in turn, stimulate the ovary to produce its egg cell regularly every twenty-eight days. Following the production of this cell, the ovary produces another hormone. This, in turn, is associated with the activity of the uterus. Hence any excessive activity of any portion of the glandular chain will bring about definite changes in the body of the woman concerned. The conditions are now known to be reflected in changes in the temperature of the woman and also in such changes as the pigmentation of the skin, the growth of hair on various portions of the body, irregular bleeding and many other symptoms. The one which concerns women most is, of course, bleeding. In the treatment of such bleeding a variety of hormones are used, depending on the nature of the condition, the time when it occurs, and the facts that are determined by the doctor following his examination.

SEX HORMONE MEDICATION
(See also discussion under *Estrogens, Menopause, Ovary*) A study was made of the effects of male and female sex hormones, androgens and estrogens, on eleven elderly women who ranged from 64 to 89 years old. A control group was given inert medication in the same form. The women had been careless about cleanliness and dress, but after they received the hormones they showed new interest in their personal hygiene and appearance. They said they felt better and had more vitality. And their sociability and helpfulness in domestic matters also increased. The changes became apparent two or three months after treatment was begun. Psychological tests indicated an improvement in the women's memory and learning ability also.

A French doctor has reported complete control of symptoms of the menopause—including hot flashes, emotional states, and anxiety—by administration of hormones such as estrogens, androgens, and progesterones according to the nature of the symptoms. He treats the changes due to aging by injecting under the skin a mixture of hormones that includes testosterone, estrogens, progesterones, and desoxycorticosterone (male and female sex hormones produced by the ovary after pregnancy and by the adrenal cortex). The physician reports that in many instances the skin lost its dryness, the body contour became more youthful, the fingernails became less brittle, the hair regained its luster, physical activity increased, and the emotional and intellectual tone of the patient was improved. The treatment was accompanied by psychotherapy.

SHAKING PALSY (See also discussion under *Paralysis Agitans*) Parkinson's disease or the shaking palsy was formerly considered a progressive disorder in which there was not much to be done. Now new approaches to Parkinson's disease involve a number of drugs which control the tremors such as pagetane, artane and many other derivatives from belladonna. In addition a new operative procedure involves tying off the blood supply to the portion of the brain responsible for the tremors and also the injection of alcohol into the area concerned.

New drugs for the shaking palsy include kemadrin and parasidol. Both seem to have some increased efficiency in certain cases beyond that of artane.

SHINGLES An important fact about the occurrence of shingles, or herpes zoster, is the appearance of the blisters in groups along the course of one or more of the nerves of sensation in the skin of the body. The condition is thus quite definitely a nervous disease as well as a skin disease. Shingles usually are found in people whose nervous resistance has been lowered by overwork, disease, or some long-continued toxic action on the human body. The blisters are usually preceded by pain of a neuralgic character in the region of the body that is affected and the disappearance of the blisters is not infrequently followed by burning, tingling, or other irritation.

Sometimes one crop of blisters will persist for a week or ten days, then dry up, form crusts, and disappear. Shortly thereafter a new crop of blisters will appear at the same place or near by. The blisters vary in size from a pinhead to that of a small pea. The walls are thick but they will break eventually. Then a fine fluid appears and dries. If, however, there has been secondary infection of the blisters, they will be filled with a white puslike material.

Young people usually get over the shingles in short order but when they appear in old people they are painful and are quite frequently followed by repeated attacks of nerve pain in the region affected.

In most cases the shingles appear on the sides of the chest, the back, or above the eye. They may appear in the groin and actually, of course, on any portion of the surface of the body.

There are all sorts of superstitions about shingles, one of which is that when shingles occur on both sides of the body and meet in the center the condition will be fatal. This, of course, is ridiculous.

In persistent cases of shingles the specialist in diseases of the skin is sometimes able to prevent recurrences by the use of the X ray, ultraviolet ray, and by various other measures applied directly to the area concerned. A real advance in the control of shingles has been the use of ACTH or Cortisone. In some cases antihistamines have helped.

SHINGLES—See SKIN, article THE SKIN.

SHINGLES—chicken pox induces: See CHILDHOOD DISEASES, article INFECTIOUS DISEASES OF CHILDHOOD.

SHINGLES—lesions may require ointments: See CHILDHOOD DISEASES, article INFECTIOUS DISEASES OF CHILDHOOD.

SHINGLES—old age: See article OLD AGE.

SHOCK The condition called shock has been in the past one of the most difficult emergencies that confronts a physician. Loss of blood is one of the most serious effects of a wound. Many physicians are convinced that the cause of shock is in most instances loss of blood. Therefore the modern treatment of shock places emphasis on maintaining the blood supply through the use of blood plasma. The first change that occurs in shock is dilation of the blood vessels on the surface of the body. In connection with the dilation of these blood vessels, perspiration occurs and the skin is relatively warm. The blood pressure becomes low and the pulse feeble and slow.

The first step in aiding the person in shock is to place him with the head low because a loss of blood from the brain may result in a failure of that tissue to function. The patient in shock must be kept comfortably warm. Pain is relieved by sedative drugs because it is known that pain may be a contributing factor to the intensity of shock.

Following initial shock from a wound or an injury there develops a condition called secondary shock due to the damage of the tissues. This may come on an hour or more after an injury. People with secondary shock are pale, weak, or exhausted. They may complain of thirst if they are conscious; the perspiration is cold and clammy; the pulse is rapid and thready; the breathing rapid and shallow; the blood pressure low; and the superficial blood vessels are collapsed. This type of shock is seen particularly after severe burns or as a late manifestation following a surgical operation. Fortunately the condition is preventable to a large extent, so that in modern surgery continuous transfusion of blood or of plasma may be a feature of the operative procedure and thus greatly lessen the incidence of shock.

SHOCK—electric, first aid: See article FIRST AID.

SHOCK—resulting from burns, treatment of: See article FIRST AID.

SHOCK—treatment for mental patients: See MENTAL, article NERVOUS AND MENTAL DISORDERS.

SHOULDER The shoulder is a joint in which several bones, ligaments, and muscles are involved. This joint has the greatest range of motion of any joint in the body. For that very reason the shoulder is injured most easily. If the shoulder joint gets stiff and painful, you may as well quit work, for any further effort will merely make it worse. Scientific authorities believe that the shoulder evolved from a walking joint like that possessed by animals which walk on four legs and changed to a weight-carrying joint. Therefore the shoulder has lost much of its stability, strength, and durability.

The shoulder joint may, like any other joint in the body, become infected or injured in various ways. One of the most frequent injuries is a torn tendon, which gives rise to what is called a stiff, painful shoulder. Such a tendon may tear due to dislocation of the shoulder or to a fall or to an unusual strain such as occurs when one is trying to tie a rope or pull a chain hoist. A middle-aged woman slipped on an oiled floor and in trying to save her balance threw her arm up so high that she tore a tendon in the shoulder.

Fractures of any of the bones involved in the shoulder joint demand surgical attention. Dislocations also demand setting of the bones in the proper position and frequently bandaging, often the use of a cast.

There are also bursas in the region of the shoulder joint which may become inflamed and thus produce inability to move the joint properly.

Whenever there is serious pain in the shoulder joint after a sprain, a severe infection, or the tearing of a ligament, it is desirable that there be no excessive motion. The position of greatest comfort is to have the arm carried in a sling, which permits the arm to be supported and to be held rather close to the side. Often this treatment in itself is sufficient to prevent any further difficulties.

In other forms of injury to the joint it is desirable that the arm be held in a position away from the body or in the abduction position. In order to secure this position it may be necessary to put a splint and a plaster cast on the body.

Heat, massage, and early active exercise, which will utilize not only the shoulder joint but the other joints in that vicinity, as soon as possible after the splint and the plaster cast have been removed are important in preventing loss of function.

A rather common disability is a recurrent dislocation of the shoulder joint. Apparently this is controllable only by surgical operation, with subsequent use of a plaster cast and still later suitable exercise of the joint.

SHOULDERS, ROUND—See article POSTURE.

SILICONE OINTMENT (See also *Cosmetics,* discussion under *Child Care, Eczema, Skin*) Mother's cosmetics may occasionally be helpful to baby. Among the new cosmetics are silicone-containing ointments and lotions which are used for inflammations of the skin of the hands caused by soap and water or detergents and water. The condition of the skin is commonly called housewife's eczema and also dishpan hands. The silicone preparations are also used for chapping of the lips, hands and face. Recent trials have shown that they are also useful in diaper rash and also for the irritation and roughening of the skin around the mouth of the baby which has been called saliva eczema. This is due to drooling, licking, thumb sucking and lip biting. The silicone preparations provide an invisible film that interferes with irritation from harsh substances or harsh water; by eliminating continued irritation, they aid the body in healing itself.

SINUSES The sinuses are cavities in the bones of the head which connect with the inside of the nose by means of small openings. The sinus in the cheekbone is called the antrum, the one above the eyes is the frontal sinus, and deeper behind the nose is the ethmoid sinus.

Infectious germs gain access to the sinuses and infect the membranes which line their walls. If the opening of the sinus into the nose becomes blocked, the presence of infectious material causes headache and pain, and the absorption of infectious material leads to fever. An ordinary cold will clear up in three to five days, but if the sinuses become infected, the symptoms will last for weeks and weeks. Eventually such conditions become chronic, and there is an exacerbation which is like the original infection.

When a patient with an infection of the sinuses comes to the doctor, the doctor usually cleans the nose, shrinks the membranes by applying adrenalin or epinephrine, and then studies the openings from the sinuses into the nose to see whether or not infectious material is coming out. The sinuses are also studied by use of the X ray and by transillumination. Any blocking of the sinuses is shown by a shadow. It is also possible, when the physician believes there are growths like polyps or tumors in the sinuses, to inject an opaque substance into the sinuses and then to make an X-ray picture.

The presence of infection may be controlled with drugs given by mouth, materials applied directly to the nose by washing out the sinuses, and sometimes by surgical procedures. Modern developments in drug treatment, including the sulfonamides and penicillin, are known to be especially valuable in some of the infections that attack the sinuses.

Some of the recent studies on infections of the sinuses have shown that nutritional deficiencies are sometimes related to persistent infections of the sinuses. This applies particularly to deficiencies of vitamin A, since this vitamin is associated with the proper development of mucous membranes. Some have insisted that an excess of starch in the diet is responsible for sinus infections, and others say that calcium is an important factor. All of this merely means that the nutrition of the patient needs to be properly controlled in order that he may receive all of the essential substances.

People with infections of the sinuses should avoid swimming, diving, and strenuous outdoor exercises. Sometimes they find relief where the climate is hot and dry.

SINUSES—See EAR, article THE EAR, TONGUE, NOSE, AND THROAT.

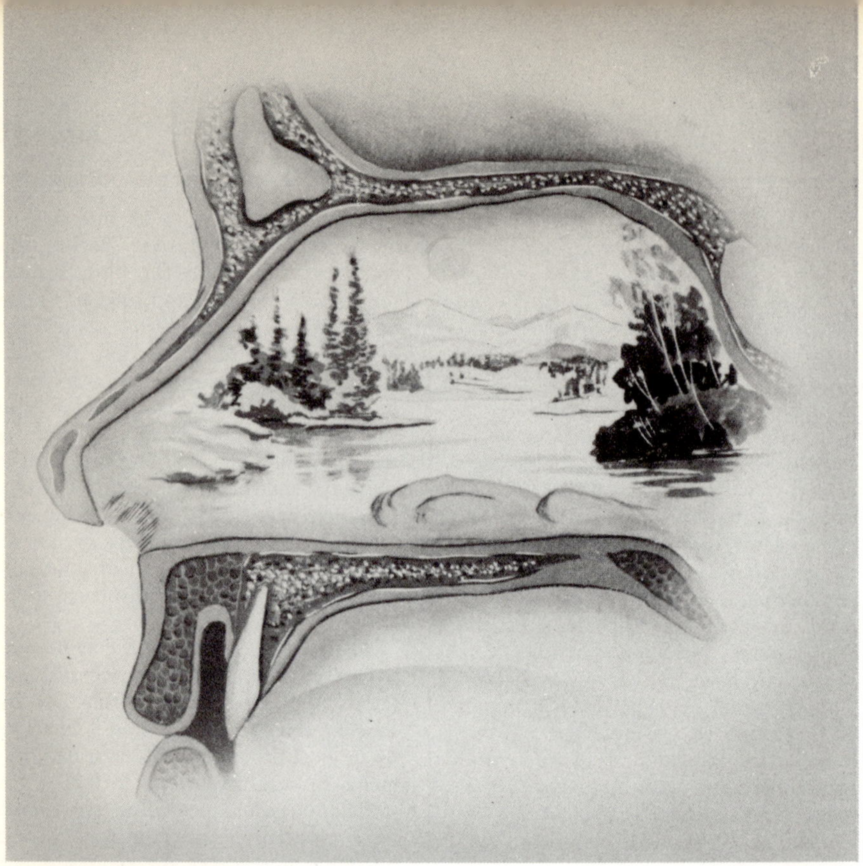

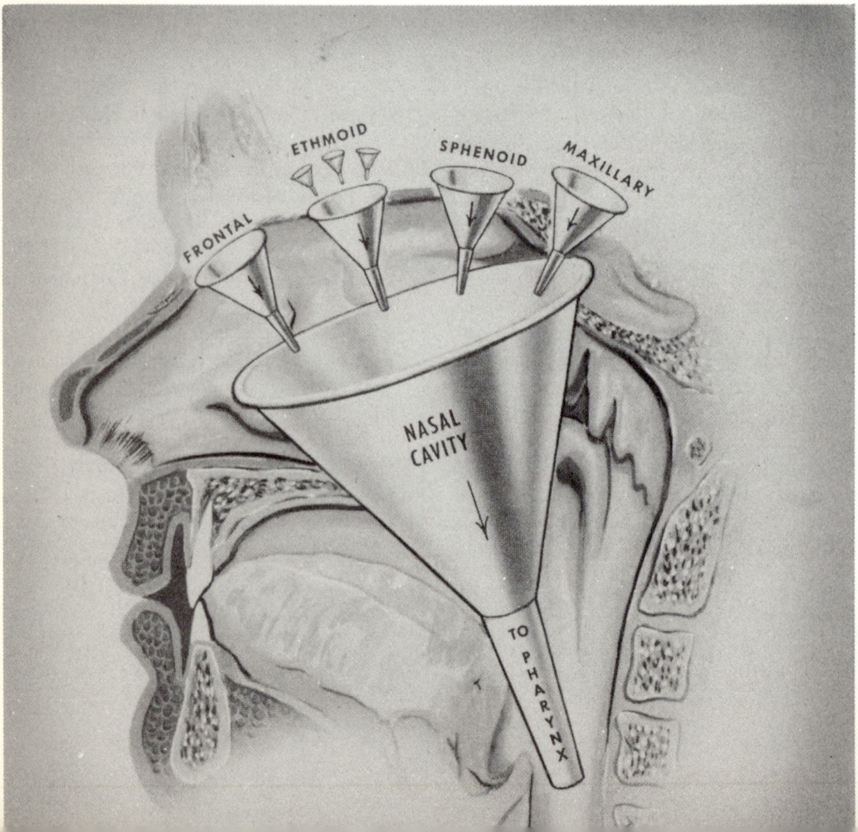
ETHMOID
SPHENOID
MAXILLARY
FRONTAL
NASAL CAVITY
TO PHARYNX

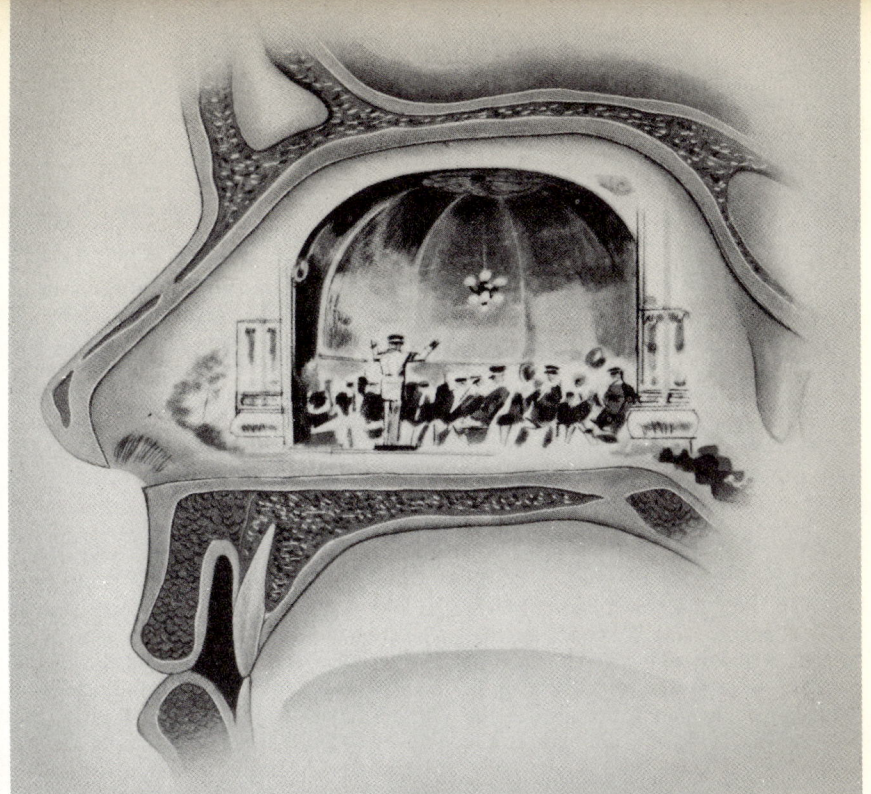

THE FUNCTION OF THE SINUSES

The sinuses, which surround the nose including the frontal sinuses above, the maxillary sinuses on each side, and the ethmoid sinus in back of the nose, help in various ways the physiology of the body. The mucous membrane that lines the sinuses is much thinner than that of the nasal cavity. In this mucous membrane are cells called goblet cells which pour out a substance called mucus. This mucus is ordinarily eliminated from the sinuses by the movement of the tiny hairs that line its walls.

If the openings of the sinuses are not blocked by inflammation or swelling, drainage of mucus goes on constantly and with it foreign material such as germs passes into the nasal cavity and the throat.

The functions of the sinuses shown symbolically in these three drawings are 1) the provision of moisture and warmth to air that is taken into the body; 2) drainage of material from these open areas in the skull cavity which help to lessen the weight of the skull and maintain balance on the neck; and 3) the resonance that is given by the sinuses to the voice exactly as a resonant chamber may be used to heighten and broaden the tone of the voice for radio amplification.   Winthrop-Stearns, Inc.

SINUSES—disease: See EAR, article THE EAR, TONGUE, NOSE, AND THROAT.

SINUSES—infections: See INFECTIOUS DISEASE, article THE PREVENTION AND TREATMENT OF INFECTIOUS DISEASE.

SINUSES—migraine: See article FIRST AID.

SINUSITIS—nasal allergy differentiated from: See article ALLERGY.

SINUSITIS—pollen injections make hay fever patient less likely to develop: See article ALLERGY.

SKIN The skin is living tissue, not just an envelope on the outside of the body. The skin of a grown person weighs about 6 pounds and if spread out flat on the ground would cover an area of about 16 to 20 square feet. The skin on the palms of the hands, the soles of the feet, the shoulders, and the back of the neck is the thickest skin of the body, varying from .02 of an inch to .16 of an inch in thickness.

Externally the skin is full of furrows which are formed by the attachment of the skin to the structures underneath and by the movement of the skin. These furrows are constant for each person. Between the furrows are ridges which are dotted with numerous depressions that are openings of the pores which release sweat through the skin.

Doctors view the skin as being made of three layers—an outer layer, which is called the cuticle; the next layer, which is the true skin; and finally, the lowest layer where the blood vessels, lymph vessels, and similar structures necessary for the health and life of the skin are located. Here also are some of the glands and the beginnings of the hair follicles. The blood vessels are extremely important to the skin because

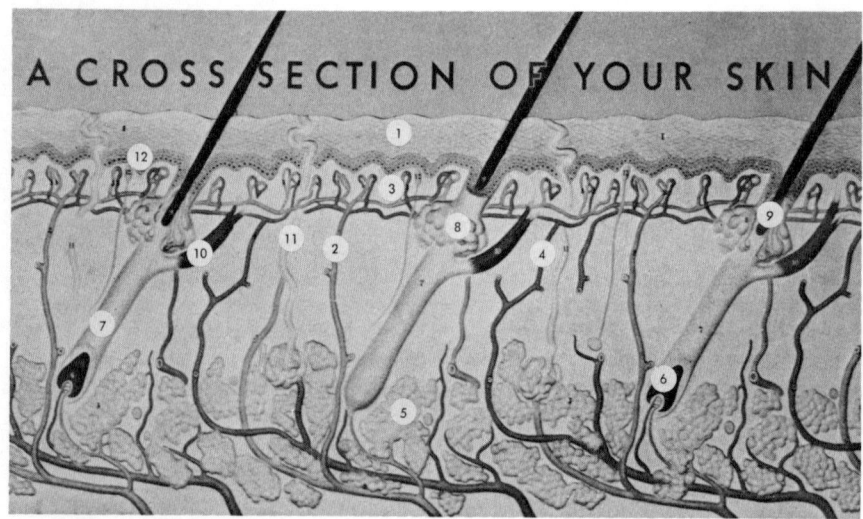

A cross-section of skin showing (1) outer layer, (2) arteries, (3) capillaries, (4) veins, (5) fat tissue, (6) hair root, (7) hair shaft, (8) oil gland, (9) hair, (10) hair muscle, (11) sweat gland, and (12) touch nerve.

Cleveland Health Museum

the skin receives one third of all of the blood that circulates in order to nourish it.

The skin is constantly rejuvenating itself until old age comes on. The outermost layers are detached as the lower layers produce new cells. Billions of new cells are made every day and billions of dead horny cells are shed by the body. There are thirty layers of cells constantly being added to from below and shed from above.

One of the functions of the skin is the evaporation of heat from the body so as to maintain a constant temperature. The amount of heat radiated depends on the climate in which one lives. The skin keeps the body from drying up through evaporation of fluid. Other glands in the skin secrete an oil or grease which maintains the skin in a flexible condition. On the palms of the hand there are more than 5000 sweat glands for each square inch of surface.

The skin is an organ of the body just as are the liver, the heart, and the lungs. When the flow of blood to the skin is hindered for any reason, the skin hardens, thickens, and loses its normal appearance. In old age when the circulation to the skin is lessened, the skin loses its youthful appearance. Wrinkles form and the color of the skin also changes.

The color of the skin is dependent to some extent on the effects of sunlight. In most people the pigment or color of the skin depends on inheritance and, finally, on the amount of blood that circulates through the skin.

Many people believe that it is possible to feed the skin or cause it to fill out by the use of oils, creams, pastes, ointments, or similar preparations which are rubbed on or into the skin. There is no way to feed the skin by anything put on the surface. Fatty substances and ointments placed on the skin are not absorbed but if they are rubbed hard enough they may be pushed into the glands, from which they are taken up by the blood. Thus some substances rubbed on the skin are picked up by the blood.

With a reasonable amount of cleanliness the skin gets along quite well. The skin of a baby requires more attention than that of an adult since it becomes more easily irritated by rubbing between the folds of the skin or by the constant contact with secretions of the body. If the skin is kept clean, it will seldom become irritated except through rubbing or from exposure to irritating substances.

Any inflammation of the skin is called dermatitis. Ninety-five per cent of people who come to doctors with disturbances of the skin have simple inflammations that are due to some external cause such as an irritating chemical or an infection.

The amount of attention given to the skin depends on the kind of skin it is.

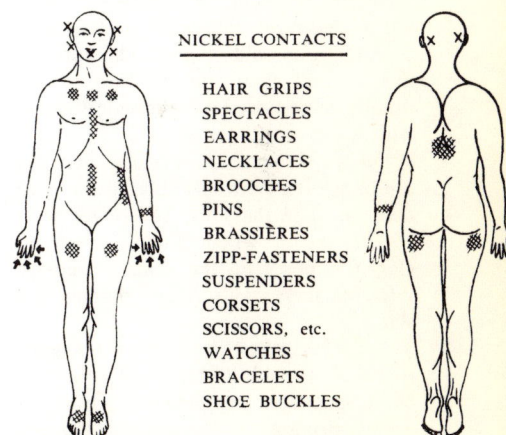

NICKEL CONTACTS

HAIR GRIPS
SPECTACLES
EARRINGS
NECKLACES
BROOCHES
PINS
BRASSIÈRES
ZIPP-FASTENERS
SUSPENDERS
CORSETS
SCISSORS, etc.
WATCHES
BRACELETS
SHOE BUCKLES

Schematic drawing to illustrate sites of primary eruption on individuals who are sensitive to the nickel in metal found on pieces of wearing apparel.

An oily skin may require more cleaning and a different type of cleaning than a skin that tends to be dry. The skin of a baby is often benefited by being oiled, since the oil serves as a protection. People with oily skins need to bathe more frequently than those with dry skins. People with dry skins may require added oil.

The face is usually adapted by years of exposure to sunlight, fresh air, and the elements to get along satisfactorily merely with simple cleansing. This means washing two or three times a day either with water alone or with soap and water. The face may be washed more frequently, however, if it needs it. Generally it is satisfactory to wash the face frequently with plain water during the day and then to give it a thorough washing with warm water and soap before going to bed at night.

Men who shave frequently put plenty of soap and water on the face during the shaving process. Women often like to steam the skin by covering it with hot towels and thereafter softening it by rubbing in cold creams. The application of any cream to the face should usually be preceded by thorough washing with warm water and soap.

For a skin that is especially dry, the use of a toilet powder aids in preventing damage. The daily use of creams with powder on top will incline, however, to clog the pores of the skin. Secondary infection then may seriously damage the skin.

Nowadays there is a great tendency to expose the skin to tanning by the sun. Most specialists are convinced that excessive exposure to the sun will damage the texture of the skin and, in older people, perhaps set up processes which, in the long run, are quite harmful.

In many of the deficiency diseases, such as pellagra, changes in the skin are prominent. We know that the vitamins have a definite relationship to the skin. There are six conditions affecting the skin which are also definitely related to vitamin deficiencies. Practically all the vitamins have been offered at one time or another for specific effects for ordinary acne with pimples and blackheads. Actually, however, the use of the vitamins for the control of pimples and blackheads has not been proved to be especially beneficial. In some instances improved activity of the bowels brought about by the taking of yeast or the vitamin B complex has been found to be of some help to the skin. This, however, is not a specific vitamin action.

A deficiency of vitamin B_2 (called riboflavin) has been definitely related to the appearance of blisters and cracking at the corner of the mouth. If it can be shown in such a case that there is a deficiency of riboflavin in the diet or if it can be shown that the riboflavin is not absorbed, the use of the riboflavin may be helpful. There are, however, many cases of blistering and cracking at the corner of the mouth in which the giving of extra riboflavin does not bring about a cure.

It has been well established that a deficiency of vitamin C will produce scurvy with hemorrhages in the gums and in the skin. The claim has been made that excessively large doses of vitamin D will help patients with psoriasis. However, careful testing of great numbers of patients indicates that there are many in whom this form of treatment has not been helpful. A well-established deficiency of vitamin A will be associated with a dryness of the skin and hair. However, the taking of excessive doses of vitamin A does not seem to benefit most people who complain of excessive dryness of the skin and hair.

This all adds up to the explanation that the human body is a highly complex mechanism and that many different factors may be involved in the conditions described, so that the mere addition of one vitamin or of several vitamins may not bring about improvement.

Many people feel that all of their skin troubles are due to something that they ate. There is hardly a skin disease that has not at one time or another been treated by a diet of one kind or another. In the majority of instances, however, attempts to control a skin disease by diet alone are not satisfactory. An examination of the books on nutrition shows that there is no single diet that is specific for any single inflammation of the skin. This does not mean that dieting is without value; it means rather that many diseases of the skin that are said to be due to foods are not related to food at all. The skin diseases that with certainty are related to diet are those like urticaria and forms of eczema, which represent a sensitivity of the body to certain proteins.

All sorts of diets have been tried for pimples and blackheads including diets without meat, diets without sugar, and diets without fats. At present most specialists agree that a low fat diet is useful because there is an overactivity of the glands in the skin that secrete oils. Such a diet is said to be helpful, but, again, there are many of these cases in which the adoption of a low fat diet is not necessarily associated with a cure. Here again the constitution of the body and particularly its glandular mechanism is such that the condition cannot be controlled by diet alone. One fact is certain: the skin, like every other tissue of the body, needs to be nourished by proper amounts of all of the essential substances. A well-balanced diet is helpful in every disease.

THE SKIN IN WINTER—In winter the cold slows down the circulation of blood in the skin and as a result there is a lessened amount of secretion of oil from the skin. This failure to keep the skin well lubricated results in dryness, irritation, and cracking. Incidentally, the extreme dry heat of most modern apartments and homes merely intensifies the exposure of the skin to dry heat.

Next most serious are the sudden changes of temperature that are inevitable when you leave your home or your office to go outdoors and submit yourself to cold and wind. People who have skin diseases such as psoriasis, eczema, inflammations of the skin, and chilblains discover frequently that the skin gets much worse during the winter. People who work a great deal with the hands are more likely to have cracked and chapped skin and to become secondarily infected. The modern habit of girls of going out in cold weather without stockings has been reported to bring about inflammations and difficulties with the skin in winter.

Fortunately there are available today a great variety of treatments for chapping of the skin and for the lack of a sufficient amount of lubrication. Any of the widely advertised hand lotions will be useful if properly used during the winter months.

Certainly the ears, the cheeks, and the nose should be protected against frostbite. The wearing of babushkas or scarfs is a great help in this direction. When the hands are washed in winter, they should be thoroughly dried and treated with a suitable hand lotion or with a powder.

One must be sure that clothing is warm but not so tight as to restrict the circulation of the blood. This is an added factor of danger to the skin in winter.

CORTISONE IN SKIN DISEASES—One hundred and thirty-four patients of various ages suffering from inflammation of the skin, including twenty-nine who had inflammation resulting from contact with poison ivy, were treated at the University of Cincinnati with various forms of cortisone. Chronic cases of psoriasis, pemphigus, and lupus erythematosus were among the inflammations treated there. Cortisone was found effective in many of these cases. Results were as satisfactory when the drug was taken orally as when it was injected. Indeed, dose for dose, hydrocortisone tablets (taken orally) proved to be more effective than either hydrocortisone acetate or cortisone acetate (injected).

SKIN—See SKIN, article THE SKIN.
SKIN—abnormal functioning: See SKIN, article THE SKIN.
SKIN—adolescence: See SKIN, article THE SKIN.
SKIN—adrenal glands: See SKIN, article THE SKIN.
SKIN—aging: See SKIN, article THE SKIN.
SKIN—allergy: See article ALLERGY; SKIN, article THE SKIN.
SKIN—antiseptics: See SKIN, article THE SKIN.
SKIN—bathing: See SKIN, article THE SKIN.
SKIN—blue discoloration: See article OCCUPATION AND HEALTH.
SKIN—body odor: See SKIN, article THE SKIN.
SKIN—boils: See SKIN, article THE SKIN.
SKIN—burning, how to relieve: See INFECTIOUS DISEASE, article THE PREVENTION AND TREATMENT OF INFECTIOUS DISEASE.
SKIN—cancer: See article CANCER; SKIN, article THE SKIN.
SKIN—capillaries: See SKIN, article THE SKIN.
SKIN—carbuncles: See SKIN, article THE SKIN.
SKIN—care: See SKIN, article THE SKIN.
SKIN—chafing: See SKIN, article THE SKIN.
SKIN—change during stress: See article STRESS AND DISEASE.
SKIN—chapped: See SKIN, article THE SKIN.
SKIN—childhood: See SKIN, article THE SKIN.

SKIN—cold cream: See SKIN, article THE SKIN.
SKIN—color: See SKIN, article THE SKIN.
SKIN—constipation causes eruptions: See article DIGESTION AND DIGESTIVE DISEASES.
SKIN—dermatitis from external irritants: See SKIN, article THE SKIN.
SKIN—dressings, wet: See SKIN, article THE SKIN.
SKIN—drug rashes: See SKIN, article THE SKIN.
SKIN—dryness: See SKIN, article THE SKIN.
SKIN—eczema: See SKIN, article THE SKIN.
SKIN—emotional disorders: See SKIN, article THE SKIN.
SKIN—endocrine glands: See SKIN, article THE SKIN.
SKIN—eruptions caused by infectious diseases: See INFECTIOUS DISEASE, article THE PREVENTION AND TREATMENT OF INFECTIOUS DISEASE.
SKIN—erysipelas inflammation: See article TRANSMISSIBLE DISEASES.
SKIN—excessive functioning: See SKIN, article THE SKIN.
SKIN—feeding: See SKIN, article THE SKIN.
SKIN—folliculitis: See SKIN, article THE SKIN.
SKIN—frostbite: See SKIN, article THE SKIN.
SKIN—functions: See SKIN, article THE SKIN.
SKIN—growths: See SKIN, article THE SKIN.
SKIN—heat rash: See SKIN, article THE SKIN.
SKIN—herpes simplex: See SKIN, article THE SKIN.
SKIN—herpes zoster: See SKIN, article THE SKIN.
SKIN—hydroquinone affects pigmentation: See article OCCUPATION AND HEALTH.
SKIN—hypersensitivity: See SKIN, ar-

ticle The Skin.
Skin—impetigo: See Skin, article The Skin.
Skin—infancy: See Skin, article The Skin.
Skin—infections: See Skin, article The Skin.
Skin—inflammations: See Skin, article The Skin.
Skin—inner layer: See Skin, article The Skin.
Skin—intestinal function: See Skin, article The Skin.
Skin—itching: See Skin, article The Skin.
Skin—itching, how to relieve: See Infectious Disease, article The Prevention and Treatment of Infectious Disease.
Skin—lotions: See Skin, article The Skin.
Skin—massage: See Skin, article The Skin.
Skin—nervous tension: See Skin, article The Skin.
Skin—nutrition: See Skin, article The Skin.
Skin—occupational diseases: See article Occupation and Health.
Skin—oil glands: See Skin, article The Skin.
Skin—oiliness: See Skin, article The Skin.
Skin—outer: See Skin, article The Skin.
Skin—ovaries: See Skin, article The Skin.
Skin—parasites: See Skin, article The Skin.
Skin—parathyroid: See Skin, article The Skin.
Skin—peeling in scarlet fever: See Childhood Diseases, article Infectious Diseases of Childhood.
Skin—perspiration: See Skin, article The Skin.
Skin—pigmentation: See article Occupation and Health; Skin, article The Skin.

Skin—pituitary gland: See Skin, article The Skin.
Skin—pores: See Skin, article The Skin.
Skin—powders: See Skin, article The Skin.
Skin—pregnancy stretches: See Skin, article The Skin.
Skin—prickly heat: See Skin, article The Skin.
Skin—protection: See Skin, article The Skin.
Skin—pus-producing infections: See Skin, article The Skin.
Skin—rashes: See Childhood Diseases, article Infectious Diseases of Childhood; Skin, article The Skin.
Skin—regenerative power: See Skin, article The Skin.
Skin—ringworm: See Skin, article The Skin.
Skin—scales: See Childhood Diseases, article Infectious Diseases of Childhood.
Skin—scarlet fever: See Childhood Diseases, article Infectious Diseases of Childhood.
Skin—scar tissue: See Skin, article The Skin.
Skin—sebaceous glands: See Skin, article The Skin.
Skin—seborrhea: See Skin, article The Skin.
Skin—shingles: See Skin, article The Skin.
Skin—soap: See Skin, article The Skin.
Skin—spirochetes: See Skin, article The Skin.
Skin—steaming: See Skin, article The Skin.
Skin—structure: See Skin, article The Skin.
Skin—sugar stored in: See article Diabetes.
Skin—sun baths: See Skin, article The Skin.
Skin—sunburn: See Skin, article The Skin.

SKIN—sweat glands: See BIRTH, article CARE OF MOTHERS BEFORE AND AFTER CHILDBIRTH; SKIN, article THE SKIN.
SKIN—sweating: See SKIN, article THE SKIN.
SKIN—syphilis: See SKIN, article THE SKIN.
SKIN—testes: See SKIN, article THE SKIN.
SKIN—tests do not harm children: See article ALLERGY.
SKIN—tests to determine allergy: See article ALLERGY; SKIN, article THE SKIN.
SKIN—tests to determine tuberculosis: See RESPIRATORY DISEASES, article THE RESPIRATORY DISEASES.
SKIN—texture: See SKIN, article THE SKIN.
SKIN—third layer: See SKIN, article THE SKIN.
SKIN—thyroid gland: See SKIN, article THE SKIN.
SKIN—tuberculosis test: See RESPIRATORY DISEASES, article THE RESPIRATORY DISEASES.
SKIN—virus infections: See SKIN, article THE SKIN.
SKIN—vitamin A: See SKIN, article THE SKIN.
SKIN—vitamin B complex: See SKIN, article THE SKIN.
SKIN—vitamin C: See SKIN, article THE SKIN.
SKIN—vitamin D: See SKIN, article THE SKIN.
SKIN—vitamin E: See SKIN, article THE SKIN.
SKIN—wet dressings: See SKIN, article THE SKIN.
SKIN—wrinkling: See SKIN, article THE SKIN.
SKIN—yellow: See article OCCUPATION AND HEALTH; and entry JAUNDICE.

The Skin

BY

HOWARD T. BEHRMAN, M.D.

Chief of Clinic in Dermatology and Syphilology, Mount Sinai Hospital, New York. Assistant Attending Dermatologist, University Hospital, New York University and Bellevue Medical Center, New York.

MANY PEOPLE think of the skin as a sort of envelope into which the rest of the body has been stuffed. This is far from true, as the skin is essentially one of the most important parts of the body and performs many functions which are necessary for both life and health. This complex and sensitive organ shows many different variations, depending upon age, sex, climate, and race; and, in addition, it shows considerable changes in different parts of the same person. For example, in some parts of the body such as the lips and the eyelids, the skin is soft, smooth, and exquisitely sensitive. On the hands and feet, as well as over the surfaces of the joints, the skin is tough and dry and sometimes even on the rough side. The skin is a useful part of the body. In its far-flung stretches, there are millions of minute factories at work producing oil, sweat, hair, and nails. So too, there are numerous waste-disposal stations where busy little cells and groups of cells are at work getting rid of waste products, bringing blood to the surface of the skin so that the temperature will be regulated, helping absorb or neutralize various substances from the surface, and trying to protect the skin from the ravages of various bacteria, chemicals, and all sorts of external irritants. In many ways the skin is a mirror of what is going on inside the body and will often show changes along its surface which indicate the presence of some internal illness. These illnesses vary from the minor ones, such as a sore throat beginning with a fever blister, all the way to the covering of the entire body by the ugly spots of smallpox. The skin plays a part of great importance as far as the human being is concerned, and the following paragraphs will show how these activities are specifically regulated.

Structure of the Skin

The skin consists of two main divisions, an outer layer called the epidermis, or outer skin, and an inner layer called the corium or true skin. The corium is a sort of meshwork support for all the important little organs, blood vessels, and nerves which supply and nourish the skin. Underneath the skin itself is a third layer called the subcutaneous tissue, which also contains additional fat and fibrous supporting structures.

THE OUTER LAYER OF THE SKIN (EPIDERMIS)

The epidermis, or cuticle, is made up also of several layers. The main layers are the corneous or horny outer layer, and the mucous or deepest layer of the epidermis. The corneous or horny layer is the very top covering of the skin, and it is composed of practically lifeless cells which are being constantly shed from the surface as new cells from below move up and take their place. Its chief function is the protection of the skin. The deep or mucous layer is the most important layer of the epidermis because it is the living one and the one which produces new cells. It is composed of several layers of cells which are many-sided and joined to each other by tiny bridges of cell substance under which flow minute canals. As the cells in the deep mucous layer grow, and push those above them toward the surface, the top cells become flatter, dryer, and more shriveled in appearance. When they finally reach the surface, they are dried, horny, and wrinkled and are constantly shed from the surface as new cells from below take their place. The other two layers of the epidermis are called the clear layer and the granular layer. Their functions are relatively minor in importance.

The pigment cells, which are responsible for the color of the skin, are also produced in the mucous layer of the epidermis. These cells may vary from merely a few in number, or none at all, as in the albino, to the concentration of many cells heavily laden with pigment as in the darkly colored races. Pigment cells may also be found in the inner layer or corium of the skin. This is especially true in the colored races, in whom the pigment cells are more highly developed and the corium itself is deeply pigmented.

THE INNER LAYER OF THE SKIN (CORIUM)

The inner or connective tissue layer of the skin is its most important part. It is composed of parallel fibers forming a meshwork support for the blood vessels, nerves, oil and sweat glands, and hair which travel through it. As seen under the microscope, the line between the outer and inner layers of the skin is not a straight one because of the presence of little nipple-like prominences in the corium called papillae. These little structures dovetail into depressions on the under surface of the epidermis, thus serving to fasten the two layers together securely and increasing their flexibility. The papillae in general have two main functions, depending upon their origin. One type of papilla carries blood vessels and is responsible for the nutrition of the skin and all its minute parts. The other type of papilla carries various specialized types of nerves and is responsible for the feelings of touch, pressure, pain, and any of the many other sensations that originate in the skin. Even the sensation of tickling has a special type of nerve ending which notifies its owner that he should laugh. Estimates indicate that there are approximately five thousand of these specialized papillae to the square inch of skin surface. In addition to the papillae, the true skin is composed primarily of bundles of stringy fibers arranged in the form of an intricate mesh and forming sort of a crisscross network. This network runs directly into the third layer or subcutaneous tissue, and in many places is composed of a great deal of fat as it gets farther down in the skin. These layers form a comfortable cushion on which the skin rests and protects the delicate glands, vessels, and nerves from injury. In addition, it also gives the rounded appearance to the body which adds so much to beauty, provided it is not too rounded. Scattered through these layers are also found many little elastic fibers, which act like a layer of rubber bands in the skin. These fibers are primarily responsible for the elasticity of the skin, and if these fibers are numerous and healthy, the skin is likely to be smooth and have a good tone. If they are few in number, or shriveled because of age, the skin becomes saggy and wrinkled. Because of these fibers, the skin can accommodate itself to a moderate degree of stretching, such as occurs during exercise, and still return to its original smooth condition. However, there are limits to which the skin can be stretched, and this is demonstrated during certain states such as pregnancy, when the elastic fibers often stretch to the breaking point, and subsequently return almost to normal, leaving the white lines often seen on the abdomen of women who have had children. It is also common these days to see these white lines in the skin of women who have undergone periods of rapid reducing. The skin which had been stretched to the extreme, as in the very obese, cannot accommodate itself rapidly enough to the contraction of the fatty layer and hangs in apronlike folds. A similar process is in operation as we get older and the skin loses its elasticity, so that normal lines deepen and wrinkles become more apparent and noticeable.

Advancing age is inevitably associated with a certain degree of wrinkling of the skin. The only way really to escape wrinkles would be never to move a muscle in the face. Even such pleasant functions as eating and drinking require the use of facial muscles, and the inevitable appearance of lines and wrinkles in the face. This brief survey of the anatomical reasons for wrinkling and aging of the skin will not suffice to deter women from spending millions of dollars a year in attempts to lessen or minimize the ravages of time.

SWEAT GLANDS

The sweat glands are corkscrew-shaped tubes beginning in the true skin and spiraling up to the cutaneous surface. Their openings in the skin surface are called pores, and literally millions of them are scattered over the surface of the skin, especially on the palms and soles. The larger sweat glands are found in the armpits and are primarily responsible for various types of body odor. The secretion of sweat is one of the most important functions performed by the skin.

SEBACEOUS OR OIL GLANDS

The sebaceous or oil glands are composed of a number of baggy pouches grouped together, along the sides of the hair shafts. They produce an oily, semifluid material of a whitish or yellow color, which is excreted directly along the upper part of the hair follicle onto the skin surface. This semisolid, greasy secretion lubricates the hairs and the skin surface, protecting it in part from all external agents and keeping it in a constant well-oiled state. As we grow older the oil glands function less and less adequately; for this reason the skin becomes dried with advancing age. Several million glandular oil factories are scattered over the body surface; the largest of these are found in the free margins of the eyelids, where they are called Meibomian glands. Beneath the sebaceous gland is a small involuntary muscle which is also associated with the hair follicle. During periods of stress or fear this muscle squeezes the gland and at the same time is responsible for the erection of the hair. Thus your hair can actually stand on end, as all of us who have had "goose flesh" at some time or other are well aware.

SKIN TEXTURE

The normal texture of the skin is smooth and fine, because the scales covering it are minute, oiled, and covered with delicate hair. The skin may be coarse, like that on many noses, because of large sebaceous ducts. Often faces that are scarred are referred to as having large pores. This is incorrect, as the scars are actually little pits unrelated to the pore openings. On the skin, as best seen on the palms and soles, there are many fine ridges arranged in patterns which are characteristic for each person and are often used for identification (fingerprints). On these ridges the sweat pores open. Coarser, less regular lines are caused by motion and stretching of the skin with eventual folding of the skin along these lines. Still larger lines are caused partly by motion and partly by the attachment of the skin to the underlying tissue about the joints and under the breasts. Dimples are caused by the attachment of the skin to the muscles of expression, thus drawing in the skin at this point when they contract. It almost seems a shame to break down the bare anatomical reasons for a dimple, but there you have it!

COLOR OF THE SKIN

The color of the skin depends upon the amount of pigment in the lower layer of the epidermis and by the color of the neighboring blood and the size of the surface blood vessels. Through the skin of the average blonde (if there is such a woman as an *average* blonde), the red color shows diffusely as through ground glass, with just enough effect of the pigment to make the color creamy. Brunettes have even more pigment, and other races than the white race have still more, until in the black race the red color of the blood is largely concealed. In many instances the skin may be quite light at the time of birth and become progressively darker with age. As is well known, the babies of the colored race are born with a comparatively light skin, and the pigmentation becomes progressively darker during the first few months of life, until the final skin color has been attained. In a few instances, when experiments have been performed with skin grafts, it has been found that a white man's skin grafted to the skin of a Negro will rapidly become dark and vice-versa.

The color of the skin may be temporarily affected by flushing or blushing of the skin surface. This momentary change in color is due to the opening of the small blood vessels near the surface and a flooding of the skin itself with blood. This may occur as a result of exposure to excessive heat or as a result of some local inflammatory change. However, the skin is so readily influenced by the emotions that even a mild degree of embarrassment will result in temporary redness of the face. Now you know what the humorists meant when they said that "your skin is showing." The skin reacts so vigorously to an emotion that we can see an immediate redness of the skin as a result of embarrassment, "goose flesh" as a result of fear, excessive sweating of the palms and under the arms prior to an interview with the boss or that quarrel with your in-laws, and so on down the line. The unusual person can develop a poker face. These examples illustrate how the skin readily mirrors not only the health and functions of the body but also of the mind.

NUTRITION OF THE SKIN

The skin feeds on the blood which seeps into its layers from the small blood vessels in the corium or true skin. These blood vessels also bring all nutritional necessities to the glands, the hair follicles, and the papillae. In the papillae the smallest blood vessels, which are called capillaries, exude a serum which passes into the little canals of the epidermis and circulates between the cells. As it circulates it gives up its nutritive substances and picks up the waste products, and flows down again to the papillae where it finds its way back to the blood vessels or lymph vessels, and is carried away. From this description of the structure of the skin it is obvious that food for the skin does not come from its outer surface. The skin receives its nourishment from the blood stream and from the essential ingredients of the blood stream. There is actually no such thing as a skin food because, like every other part of the body, the skin feeds on what is brought to it by the blood stream. Yet millions of dollars are spent yearly for nourishing creams, skin foods, and the like, under the mistaken impression that these preparations feed the skin and are responsible for its health and beauty. It would be almost as unintelligent to attempt to increase knowledge by rubbing the head with some learned treatise as it is to attempt to feed the skin from the outside.

THE FUNCTIONS OF THE SKIN

The skin has many uses and important functions. In general, these include the protection of the rest of the body from injury, to minimize the absorption of dangerous substances, to act as an organ of sensation and touch, to excrete waste products, and to regulate heat. Besides this, some of its nerve organs are connected with sexual gratification and other physiological stimuli.

The chief function of the skin is protection. A dry skin is a good insulator against all but high-voltage electrical currents. Insulation against body cold is aided by the contraction of the tiny muscles of the hair follicles, which lift the skin to form "goose flesh" and at the same time close off the surface pores and blood vessels, thus preventing the loss of the body's heat.

The prevention of evaporation of the body fluids is also of great importance. This provision against drying out made it possible, millions of years ago, for living beings to emerge from the sea and risk the drying effect of air, a bitter enemy of life.

Not less important than the loss of fluids from within is the prevention of the entrance of water and other harmful substances from without. The normal skin is almost entirely waterproof, but when its surface has been injured, water is readily absorbed. Usually, however, only small quantities of water filter through, and when this happens the cells of the outer layer "drink" it up and swell in the process. Have you ever weighed yourself before and after a long tub bath? The change in weight is due to the extra fluid absorbed by the cells in the top layer of the skin.

The skin can protect itself during long-continued slight exposure to mild acids but not to prolonged contact with a strong acid. Against alkalies the protection is only fair, for the alkalies soften the horn cells and, together with other chemicals of a fat-removing nature, they can reduce the resistance of the skin and favor penetration.

Radiation of heat is one of the chief functions of the skin, protecting it against the harmful effects of fever. In hot weather or during a fever the surface blood vessels become opened or dilated, thereby increasing the amount of blood exposed to the cooling air, and at the same time increasing the production of sweat which helps in the evaporation of heat. The production of sweat is also one of the important functions of the skin. Its value as an eliminant of waste products from within the body is slight, for only volatile bodies are eliminated in the perspiration. The odor of the sweat is the chief source of body odor, now popularized as "B.O.," about which so much is said by the advertising profession. The odor is due partly to these volatile substances from within and partly to the fatty acids in the skin. While sometimes unpleasant, giving the unfortunate possessor much mental distress, cases are also on record of a pleasant, violet-like odor of the sweat, but don't count on it! Recently there has been a great fanfare concerning the use of chlorophyll to lessen body odors. This harmless product does seem to cut down some mild odors but will not really lessen the obnoxious odor of large amounts of garlic and similar dietary indiscretions.

Under ordinary circumstances, absorption through the outer skin is slight even for greasy substances. By friction, fats may be forced into the hair follicles and absorbed, carrying other substances with them. The quantity of such absorbed substances is so small that while it may be valuable when strong medicines are applied to the skin, for the purpose of "skin food," it is too slight to be of consequence and must be redigested by the internal organs before the skin can use it. The popular idea that oils applied to the surface can feed the skin is a fallacy. Oils or creams thus applied only serve a useful purpose by keeping the skin supple, preventing scaling and cracking, and maintaining the resistance of abnormally dry skins, even though small portions of these creams or their ingredients may be absorbed.

The nerves of the skin protect the body against harm by warning us of the dangers of excessive heat or cold or sharpness. They also help us to become acquainted with the world about us, and provide one of our sources of pleasure in the feel of marble, fine woods, smooth skin, velvet, and the like.

By pigment formation the skin can protect the body successfully against exposure to ordinary sunlight and ultraviolet rays. The skin cannot protect itself from overexposure to X-rays and the rays of radium, and its efforts, though often manifested by pigmentation, are of no avail because these rays penetrate the pigmented skin as easily as they do the non-pigmented. And when it comes to the atomic bomb, the skin has no protective defenses whatsoever. If compensatory changes of evolution continue, we can conceive of centuries of exposure to atomic radiations resulting in a thick, bombproof skin if the human race has not been wiped out by some type of chain reaction.

Besides these more or less obvious functions of the skin, it has also the ability to clear its surface of germs within a short time. The mechanism of this action is not completely understood. Against some bacteria the skin is powerless; it cannot rid itself of them. Even against these germs the normal skin is an important first line of defense. Further, if germs do gain entrance to the skin, whether from without or through the blood stream, the normal skin can produce chemical substances which may inhibit their growth or wholly destroy them. Of course, some agents of infection are too strong to be controlled in this way, and the resistance of the skin is futile. These efforts of the skin to protect itself and the whole organism against infection often take the form of an inflammatory reaction in the skin. This skin reaction is the basis for many of the tests used to develop or determine resistance or immunity to tetanus, tuberculosis, diphtheria, scarlet fever, or other infectious diseases. Various skin tests have also been devised to detect allergic causes in asthma, hay fever, hives, and eczema. They are all of more or less value in diagnosis. Thus the skin has become a useful bureau of information, ready to report on the state of affairs in relation to protection against these diseases or on the presence of unusual sensitivities to organisms, chemicals, drugs, and the like, whenever requested to do so by the physician. Here again, we can understand why it is often referred to as the mirror of the body. In addition to its ability to protect against infection, the skin produces the vitamin (vitamin D) that protects against and cures rickets. This explains in part the beneficial effects of sun baths and ultraviolet light baths, particularly for infants.

Of course, there are still many functions connected with the skin about whose purpose we can only speculate. For example, we know that the secretion of the oil glands or sebum is of primary value in keeping the skin normally lubricated and also to supply a small amount of lubrication for the hairs. And yet recent work has shown that some of the secretions from these oil glands may become concentrated in certain abnormal conditions of the scalp and may actually result in the loss of hair, so that too much of some secretions may do harm rather than good. Another function of the oily secretion is to prevent the absorption of any toxic or poisonous material through the surface of the skin. Accordingly, if we wish to treat a certain area of skin with some drug or medication in a grease, it is important to wash the area thoroughly to remove its normal oily secretion and thus to get penetration of the specific drug contained in the externally applied grease.

Finally, one of the most unusual and important functions of the skin is to renew itself after it has been injured. The human being cannot quite compare with the lobster which can regrow a claw after it has lost one, but the skin certainly does show remarkable powers of regeneration. Very frequently extremely extensive areas of the skin will have been lost or injured, as in an accident or a severe burn. In many instances, these areas will completely regrow without leaving a trace of the original injury. However, if the injury has been extensive and deep, the normal skin will not regrow but the area will be replaced with a different type of tissue called scar tissue. Sometimes it is necessary to help the regrowth of this tissue by performing grafts with skin taken from other parts of the body. Modern science has made great strides in this direction and even now there are many ways in which ugly and disfiguring scars can be made almost insignificant in appearance.

Nutrition

From a general point of view, proper diet is fundamental as far as the health of the skin is concerned. Faddist regimes and so-called health diets are not essential as far as the skin is concerned. A well-balanced diet, with proper attention to balanced meals and adequate vitamin and mineral intake is of fundamental importance. As shown in the chapter on diet, certain foods are required for health.

Special diets should be avoided unless you are allergic to some particular component of a diet. There are also certain diseases in which special diets are indicated, and the skin has its share of such disorders. In the last few years there has been much research concerning the fact that the skin is often the first indicator of a serious deficiency in the diet, and much has been written concerning the rôle of vitamins in the skin health.

In the following brief survey the vitamins are considered primarily from the point of view of their internal administration related to the skin and not from external application.

VITAMIN A

When vitamin A is missing from the diet, the effect on the entire system is pronounced. Some of these effects of vitamin A deficiency are lowered resistance to infection, poor appetite, disturbed digestion, eye disease called xerophthalmia, and loss of hair. The condition of the skin is also changed in deficient states. Generally, it becomes dry, rough, and darker than normal. Small spots, resembling goose flesh, appear on the arms and thighs, and gradually spread to involve the leg, abdomen, buttocks, and neck. Sometimes these tiny lumps resemble acne. Confirmation of the diagnosis of A deficiency may be obtained by various technical means, such as the biomicroscopic examination of the eyes under slit lamp illumination. Estimation of the vitamin A level in the blood is also helpful in diagnosis. The minimum daily requirements of vitamin A are approximately 4,000 U.S.P. units. The treatment dose ranges from 10,000 to 300,000 units daily. Large amounts of vitamin A should not be taken over long periods of time without medical supervision because an excess of this vitamin may give rise to toxic manifestations. Surprisingly enough, one of these symptoms may be loss of hair.

VITAMIN B COMPLEX

Slight deficiences of this vitamin lead to a decreased appetite, fatigue, and burning sensations of the hands and feet.

Vitamin B_2 or riboflavin is well distributed in our diet, and so deficiency states are not too common. A deficiency of it leads to itching and burning of the eyes, dimness of the vision, and a sensitivity to light. The skin shows characteristic changes as a result of a deficiency of riboflavin. These changes include scaling and redness of the lips, cracks at the angles of the mouth, and an oily scale on the nose and ears. These changes about the eye and mouth have been called "sharklike" in appearance. The tongue is usually bright and red and shiny. Recent studies have shown that the vitamin may be helpful in the treatment of psoriasis. The minimum daily requirement is 2 milligrams.

Vitamin P-P, or niacin or nicotinic acid, is still another member of the B complex. A deficiency of it leads to the disease known as pellagra. In medical parlance, this disease is known to produce the three D's—dermatitis (skin rash), diarrhea (intestinal upsets), and dementia (mental changes). The victim is usually nervous, restless, and easily fatigued, and complains of vague aches and pains. The skin changes are present on the exposed parts of the body (hands and face) and vaguely suggest sunburn. The minimum daily requirement is approximately 25 milligrams.

Vitamin B_6 or pyridoxine is considered necessary to the body because of its rôle in aiding in the use of certain essential fats in the food. This may be the reason for the lessened secretion of fat from the skin when pyridoxine is given to persons with oily and greasy faces. It may even help clear up the excessive oiliness and blackhead formation of a sufferer from acne or "pimples." Nothing is known of the minimal daily requirements of this vitamin. Therapeutically, as high as 50 to 100 milligrams daily have been used.

Pantothenic acid, another part of the B complex, is of interest in view of its alleged effects on hair. Also, a deficiency of it may be a factor in the development of gray hair. This effect may occur indirectly through its effects on the glands, as its exclusion from animal diet leads to the destruction of several of the glands of internal secretion. Workers in the field have not been able to demonstrate an exact relationship between the results in animals and in human beings. Accordingly, its value in the treatment of color changes of the hair is still questionable, as is discussed subsequently under the heading of gray hair. The daily requirements are not known, although 1,000 milligrams are tolerated therapeutically.

Inositol, a little known factor of the B complex, is a substance of extreme interest to scientists engaged in the study of hair growth. Experimental investigation has shown that inositol will cure baldness in mice. This dramatic change can sometimes be produced within as short a period as three days. This definite growth response has been checked by workers in different laboratories. The relationship of inositol to human baldness is still in the investigative stage, although it has so far proved of little value. Effects produced in laboratory animals cannot be applied directly to human beings. Perhaps the future will unveil this substance or some allied drug as the direct stimulant of hair growth.

Biotin, or vitamin H, is a term employed in the past to designate a number of different substances, but it is now considered a member of the B complex. Biotin concentrates prevent a scaly rash in chicks, but its importance to the human still remains to be clarified. It has recently been studied with reference to its preventive effects in minimizing the development of cancer.

Para-aminobenzoic acid, still another B-complex factor, has also received widespread publicity as a cure for gray hair. This publicity followed the announcement that this vitamin restored the black color to the hair of rats which had become gray on a diet deficient in the substance. This is another of those unfortunate examples of the ease with which a gullible public may be misled by results obtained in animals. Well-controlled studies on human beings have failed to substantiate the claims advanced for this substance. No drugs have been discovered, as yet, which will restore gray hairs to their natural color.

Choline is the last member of the vitamin B complex of any importance at the date of the present writing. It is related to growth, the metabolism of food, and the prevention of fatty livers in animals. It is still in the investigative stage.

VITAMIN C

Lack of this vitamin is the cause of scurvy. The value of foods containing it, as being anti-scorbutic, was recognized long before the vitamin principle was known. Whalers and other ships bound on long voyages kept supplies of lime juice and lemons and potatoes aboard as preventives of scurvy. The British sailor was called a "limey" for this reason. This disease manifests itself by bleeding gums, hemorrhage into various joints, swelling, and bloody diarrhea. The skin changes are of particular interest because they are easily seen and enable the doctor to make an early diagnosis. The changes consist of red spots around the hair follicles and openings of the sweat pores. This is most common on the legs and thighs or wherever pressure exposes the extreme weakness and fragility of the small blood vessels. Irritability, lack of stamina, and retardation of growth may be due to insufficient amounts of this substance, and there also results a susceptibility to infectious diseases. The minimal daily requirement is 600 U.S.P. units.

VITAMIN D

Vitamin D is abundant in the liver of fishes, chiefly the codfish. The discovery of this vitamin disclosed the secret of rickets. This disease is characterized by enlargement of the wrists, knees, and ankles, bowed legs, and other bony changes. It is closely tied with the absorption and use of the minerals, calcium and phosphorus. Accordingly, it is of importance in the growth and development of normal teeth. A very interesting fact here is that ultraviolet rays can produce the same effect on the bodily health and growth as vitamin D; and, as a matter of fact, children suffering from rickets improve miraculously under the ultraviolet-ray therapy, provided other necessary minerals and substances are present in the body. The minimal daily requirement is 400 to 1,200 U.S.P. units.

VITAMIN E

The wide distribution of vitamin E in natural foods has led to the belief that human deficiency of this vitamin is not likely. However, it has been found to play a rôle of importance as far as repair of the skin is concerned, and it is believed of increasing importance in the treatment of certain skin diseases where the corium or true skin is involved. It has also been found of some value in the healing of ulcers of the skin and certain long-standing disorders of the fibrous or connective tissue. The normal requirements of this vitamin are unknown. It is usually prescribed in the form of mixed tocopherols.

This brief discussion of the vitamins is merely intended to show that they are of importance as far as the health of the skin is concerned. It must always be remembered that vitamins are essential to health as accessory food factors and that they are not the *only* important factors from a dietary standpoint, despite the tremendous advertising campaigns which might lead us to believe otherwise. To maintain proper health of the body and the skin, proteins, carbohydrates, and fats and a number of mineral salts are also necessary. Some of the minerals of particular importance as far as the skin is concerned are calcium, phosphorus, iron, sulfur, and other substances.

INTESTINAL FUNCTION

The health of the skin is definitely influenced by the functions of the intestinal tract. Failure to eliminate waste through the bowels and absorption of toxic substance from the bowels injures the proper sanitation and nutrition of the skin. For many years great stress has been laid upon the importance of inner cleanliness to skin health. Although this is true in great measure, it must be realized that the term "constipation" is a much overworked and little understood word. A slight degree of constipation is preferable to looseness, although healthy evacuation is more important. The irritative effect of cathartics on the bowels may favor the absorption of the so-called toxic agents they are intended to eliminate. Obviously, the routine administration of laxatives is to be deplored as it leads to looseness of the stools with consequent lack of muscular effect and tone, with resultant aggravation of the very condition which it is desired to cure. Today it is known that there is little absorption of poisonous toxins if the bowel contents are solid, but that unhealthy absorption of such contents may occur when they are rendered on the soft or even loose side, and that in this state bacterial decomposition is even greater. As far as the skin is concerned, the proper functioning of the intestines is important, and this should be regulated by diet and medical guidance, rather than by the constant use of cathartics. People who take mineral oil for constipation must recognize that mineral oil depletes the body's source of vitamin A, a vitamin, as we have already learned, of considerable importance as far as the skin is concerned. Where it is essential that the mineral oil be continued, the intake of vitamin A should be considerably increased.

The Endocrine Glands

The last decade has witnessed great strides in the direction of knowledge of the glandular secretions and their functions as far as the skin is concerned. These glands supply substances known as hormones which have profound effects on the skin and the structures within the skin.

THYROID

If hypothyroidism develops early in life, the individual remains small; the hair becomes dry, thin, and brittle. If an adult develops hypothyroidism, the condition is usually known as myxedema. The skin develops a peculiar swollen appearance, especially over the forehead, cheeks, nose, and lips. The skin is sallow or yellowish in color and dry, coarse, and cold to the touch. The nails are thin and brittle, and sweating is much diminished. The hair tends to fall out or is short, thin, and dry. It is often entirely absent on the chin, under the arms, and around the sex organs. The outer third of the eyebrows is frequently missing.

Overactivity of the gland leads to hyperthyroidism or excessive secretion of thyroxine. This produces an increased metabolism, loss of weight (body fuel is burned up too rapidly), and a rapid pulse. In addition, excessive sweating, shortness of breath, and nervous symptoms are usually present. The latter include trembling of the hands and fingers, restlessness, fidgety motions, mental irritability, and troubled sleep. The eyes occasionally protrude and the heart may become enlarged. The skin becomes hot and flushed. The hair is usually thin and silky. The nails are frequently lined and ridged. Treatment consists of the proper use of iodine, and surgical removal. Milder cases respond to sedation and drug therapy, especially to new drugs of the thiouracil group.

PARATHYROID

These glands are small bean-shaped masses located in pairs above and below the thyroid. A deficiency of the secretion from these glands gives rise to a condition known as tetany. In this disease the nerves become irritable. The nails are ridged and brittle and the teeth show defects of the enamel. The skin may develop a peculiar hardness known as scleroderma. In animals the hair frequently falls out, and this occasionally occurs in humans.

ADRENAL

The cortex, or outer part of the adrenal glands, has a direct relationship to the skin and to hair growth. A deficiency of the secretion of the cortex produces a condition known as Addison's disease. In this disease the victim shows extreme fatigue following a slight exertion. A peculiar pigmentation often develops which first attracts the patient's friends. The degree of color ranges from a bright yellow to a bronze-brown or tan, so white persons are often mistaken for mulattoes. The pigmentation may be difficult to distinguish from "sun tan," for, in both, the color is deeper on exposed parts. The patient gradually loses weight, the blood pressure drops, and diarrhea occurs. If treatment is not instituted, death may result. Primarily, it is in conditions due to hyperfunction (overactivity) of the adrenal cortex that we see effects on the hair structures. Overactivity of this gland gives rise to a peculiar chain of symptoms. In affected people there is an increase in hair over the entire body. This hair growth may be very heavy. The eyebrows are usually bushy and thick. The skin becomes thick and the sweat glands large. It is the overfunction of this gland in children which produces the so-called "infant Hercules." These children are much taller than their age, of broad stature, great muscular development, and especially well-developed sex organs. A boy of five may require daily shaving and have the hairy chest and mature sexual organs of an adult. A girl of five may have well-developed breasts, hair around the genital region, and may even menstruate. An adult woman may show the secondary sex characteristics of a man (growth of a beard, deep voice, and flat chest). The new wonder drug, cortisone, is produced by the adrenal cortex. It has been found helpful in the treatment of certain skin diseases. It must be taken with great caution because of certain side effects. As far as the skin is concerned, these side effects include the development of acne and the growth of facial hair.

PITUITARY

In those people who suffer from an oversecretion of the anterior pituitary growth factor, in addition to their tremendous increase in size, the skin becomes dry and yellowish in color. The entire body usually shows an increased growth of hair. In individuals who show an oversecretion of the pituitary sex hormone, a peculiar group of symptoms may develop. These symptoms also appear when ACTH (one of the pituitary hormones) or cortisone is administered in the treatment of disease. These symptoms include a rapidly progressing weight increase of the face, neck, and abdomen (buffalo type). In addition, these individuals develop high blood pressure and peculiar purplish lines on the abdomen. An extreme degree of hairiness is present. In conditions due to an undersecretion of this pituitary sex hormone, the individuals are known as Fröhlich types. Pickwick's "fat boy" is an example of this disorder. The victims are fat around the face, breasts, abdomen, and hips. The skin is delicate, soft, and cool. Dryness, falling hair, and nail changes are rare. The genitals remain undeveloped and infantile. Even when maturity is reached, the men have a distinctly feminine appearance and manner. The face remains hairless, fat deposits occur about the hips, and the voice remains high-pitched.

The posterior lobe of the pituitary has various effects on the blood pressure, lungs, intestines, and kidneys, but it bears no known relationship to skin changes or hair growth.

MALE SEX GLANDS

The testes are the primary sex glands of man. They produce secretions which are responsible for the male appearance and development. They also produce the sperm cells, which are responsible for the propagation of the race following fertilization of the eggs produced by the female organs of reproduction. The secretion produced by the testes include the androgens or male sex hormones. These hormones are extremely potent, and a study of their behavior effects in animals is amusing; female canaries given male hormones sing like males, and hens crow; the social order of chickens can be manipulated, because birds receiving the hormone become very domineering and quarrelsome. A deficiency of this hormone in humans leads to retention of a high-pitched voice, reduction of hair growth, particularly around the sex organs and the chin, a slim figure, and poorly developed sex organs. The extreme form of this deficiency is evident in castrated individuals or eunuchs. It is extremely interesting to note that these people rarely if ever lose the hair from their head. Whether this fact is due to a deficiency of androgen or to other secretions contained in the testes, or through remote effects on other organs, is discussed in detail under the heading of hair growth. An excessive amount of male hormones is also considered to play a causative role in the development of acne or "pimples," and this fact must be considered when treating resistant or severe cases of this disease.

FEMALE SEX ORGANS

The ovaries are two in number and are located on each side of the lower abdomen. The ovaries usually produce one egg each month. Fertilization of the egg leads to pregnancy. The ovarian hormones are responsible for the characteristics of the female and influence the development of the breasts, uterus, and accessory female organs of reproduction. At the time of puberty these secretions lead to slight alterations in the voice, the enlargement of the breasts, and the acquisition of feminine characteristics. They also influence the development of hair under the arms and around the genitals. The average woman goes through several periods of glandular change. The first of these occurs at puberty, then at sexual maturity, and finally following the menopause or change of life. During the first cycle, an irregularity of the secretions may lead to acne of the face, chest, and back, and an increased hair growth on the face. The hair may also be affected at the time of the menopause when there is frequently an increased fall of hair from the scalp and a thinning of the individual hairs. Due to lessened activity of the oil glands, dryness of the skin may also accompany the menopause. Pregnancy may also be followed by a diffuse loss of hair, which is usually due to a temporary lack of hormones almost in the nature of a "miniature menopause." With proper treatment, this hair loss may be restored. Pregnancy may also be accompanied by an increased growth of facial hair. Certain tumors of the ovary and the adrenal cortex are frequently accompanied by masculine changes in the affected women, as shown by an increased growth of hair over the entire body but especially on the face, under the arms, and around the genitals. This is due to an excessive production of male hormones similar chemically to cortisone and ACTH, and the same changes may also be produced by these drugs.

Allergy (Hypersensitivity)

Many skin conditions are produced or aggravated by a peculiar idiosyncrasy to a food, a drug, or some external application. Many people show an unusual susceptibility in their reactions to various foods and develop annoying rashes on their skins if they eat these foods. The most common offenders are eggs, strawberries, fish, chocolate, and related substances. In the majority of cases these foods produce a skin reaction known as "hives" or urticaria, which shows itself as itchy, raised "bumps" frequently shifting to involve different parts of the body. This is not always the case, as there are various other forms of skin reactions to foods and drugs. Sometimes it is possible to determine the offending agent by performing so-called skin or allergy tests. The suspected agent is either injected into the skin or scratched into the surface of the skin, and the sensitivity of the individual is determined by the development of an irritative patch of skin around the tested site. These tests are not infallible, and in many instances the allergic manifestation can only be brought out by swallowing the food or actually taking the drug, rather than by the performance of skin tests. The doctor must always be on the lookout for these drug eruptions as there are many old and new drugs which are capable of producing such reactions. In the early days of penicillin therapy this wonder drug was considered completely harmless, but as time went on numerous people were found to be sensitive to penicillin in various forms. Many of the newer drugs which are constantly being discovered are heralded in the beginning as completely harmless and incapable of doing damage. As their usage continues for long periods of time, many side effects and complications are observed to develop, and the skin is often the first to show these complications.

NERVOUS TENSION AND EMOTIONAL DISORDERS

Many eruptions on the skin are related to nervous tension, emotional upsets, and the like. We have all become familiar with the term "psychosomatic" and recognize the fact that it means the interplay of body functions with emotional or psychic factors. At present many diseases are called psychosomatic or "nervous" which are not entitled to the use of this term. Before dismissing a skin complaint as being due to nerves or emotions, it is advisable to obtain the opinion of your doctor first. The great strides that are being made in medicine are still due to the early recognition of disease rather than dismissing it on the basis of some emotional upset. Nevertheless, relaxation and rest are helpful in the treatment of many disorders of the skin, and understanding and insight into your own emotional background is also of great benefit. We have advanced too far in the treatment of ulcers, heart disease, and similar illnesses from the standpoint of their origin along the lines of emotional difficulties ever to dismiss the subject lightly in the matter of long-standing and resistant skin conditions. Our modern daily life provides many factors of tension and strain. The nerves especially suffer from the tension under which we live, and the skin is indirectly affected by it. Where skin disturbances are associated with an accompanying emotional disturbance, the physician can be of great help in assisting the patient to express his fears and worries, and to bring them out in the open for a frank discussion and understanding of their nature. It is amazing how much benefit can be observed in some chronic skin conditions following a reassuring discussion and a helpful adjustment in a life situation.

The Care of the Normal Skin

It is of importance to understand how to take care of the skin and how to apply external preparations to keep it healthy and free from disease. The measures discussed in the following paragraphs are those accepted as adequate for maintaining a healthy skin.

BATHING

Local care is, of course, of great importance to the skin. Besides the removal of grease and dirt, bathing, particularly if the bath is ended with a cold shower, has a beneficial effect on the circulation. This is accentuated by the rubbing necessary to drying, especially because of the feeling of vigor consequent on the cold shower. Frequency of bathing is an individual problem. Some find frequent bathing enervating, while on others it has the opposite effect. Some people cannot get a good reaction to cold baths and therefore should not take them. Often such persons react better to a mild application of cool water and can train themselves to the cold shower by gradual increase in the duration and decrease in the temperature of the bath. People with dry skins should not bathe frequently because constant washing removes their own meager supply of oil and merely degreases and defats a skin which desperately requires all of its own available oil supply.

The use of soap in the bath is to be regulated according to the kind of bath and the kind of skin that is being bathed, and according to the season of the year. In the summertime we perspire so profusely that soap can be used more freely by most of us. In fact, we usually start to produce more sweat and oil immediately following the bath, and there is no danger of depriving the skin of the oil necessary to its welfare. In winter, however, the skin secretes less sweat and oil, the cold air is dry, and so is the warm, overdried air of our steam-heated dwellings. Frequent bathing only serves to aggravate the dryness of the skin. The skin resents it by becoming flaky and itchy, especially after a bath. This can be corrected by limiting the use of soap during the winter months to the armpits and groin and to the parts that get the dirtiest, the hands and feet.

Some women and a few men find that their abnormally dry skins will not tolerate soap on the face at any season. The skin becomes scaly and itches and, if the irritation is carried farther, becomes red in patches, the condition known as chapping. For such people cold cream is a justifiable substitute for soap. More refreshing, however, is oatmeal water, made by boiling oatmeal for five minutes in a bag made of several layers of gauze. A handful of oatmeal should suffice in a gallon of water. It removes dirt better than plain water, taking the place of soap to a considerable degree, and can be used on some irritable skins with impunity. The introduction of sulfonated oils as soap substitutes for cleansing the skin has given us another method, valuable for those whose skins are sensitive to soap. The best of these oils are acid in reaction, as is the surface of the normal skin, and they cleanse without forming suds and without drying the skin. Those with greasy skins, however, must recognize that these methods are not for them; but that their skins are best cared for by vigorous washing with hot water and soap, followed by a cold shower.

For long periods of immersion in water, as in the use of a tub bath containing some medication intended to soothe the skin, the water temperature is best kept lukewarm. Ordinarily, both hot and cold baths are stimulating, and the greatest effect of this kind is obtained from a hot bath followed by a cold shower, which stimulates the circulation, preventing chilling and increasing resistance against infection. Rubbing the skin with the hands or the washcloth while in the water and vigorous rubbing while drying assist in obtaining this effect. The duration of the bath should be short, unless a soothing effect is desired. We are all aware of the relaxing and soothing effects of a warm bath at night. On the other hand, a short cold shower in the morning is stimulating and helps wake one up in preparation for a day of activity. Sweat baths, among which the Turkish bath is the most popular, are not essential and are, in fact, enervating. If benefit can be derived from them, they should be taken with the approval of the physician. The same rule applies to medicated baths, mud baths, and sulphur baths, for under some circumstances they may prove to be too much of a strain and should, therefore, not be taken indiscriminately. Certain types of skin conditions are made worse by excessive sweating, and this type of bathing is absolutely contraindicated in the presence of these disorders.

Open-air bathing is one of the most popular of the sports of today and of past ages, and deservedly so. At the beginning of the season care should be used to avoid too long exposure to the sun, and the same warning applies to those who go to the southern beaches during the winter. The skin, long protected from light, cannot stand much of it at first. Severe sunburn damages rather than benefits and should be avoided. This applies particularly to people with blue eyes and light complexions, inasmuch as constant exposure of such skins to strong sunlight may eventually lead to extreme dryness, warty growths, and even cancer of the skin.

SOAP

The surroundings of our present-day life, with constant exposure to the smoke and dirt of the cities, make frequent washing and the use of a good soap a necessity rather than a luxury.

As the result of the application of modern scientific research, there have been tremendous advances and changes in the formulation of soaps. A good soap must cleanse the skin thoroughly without irritation and without removing all of the skin oils. It should not be harsh nor excessively alkaline. It should preferably produce a thick creamy lather in both soft and hard water, without leaving an insoluble scum in the water. The manufacturing chemist has set his sights on the production of such a preparation, and there are several excellent soaps on the market. When fats are boiled with a solution of an alkali, they are split into glycerin and fatty acids and the latter unite with the alkali to form soap. The glycerin is a valuable by-product. Potassium hydrate forms soft soap, of which the green soap used in the hospital is the familiar example. Sodium hydrate forms hard soaps such as ordinary laundry or toilet soap. The solution of these in water is viscid, that is, it has the power of holding together, illustrated by the formation of bubbles, which are globules of air separated from the rest of the air by a film of soap. This viscid character of soapsuds enables it to emulsify the grease on the skin, carrying with it the dirt, and they both then dissolve in the water and are carried away.

In the making of soap there is always a part of the alkali not combined with the fatty acids, and this is the "free alkali" so often mentioned in connection with toilet soap. It makes the soap strong, loosening the dirt and grease so that it can better be removed. For rough work considerable free alkali is needed; but for the average skins it is desirable that the free alkali should be reduced to the minimum. Strong soap removes more fat from the skin than is good for its health and leaves it red and irritated, an easy victim to skin eruptions and infection. In good toilet soap the free alkali should not exceed ¼ of 1 per cent. For dry and delicate skins superfatted soap is made by removing as much as possible of the free alkali and adding wool fat. This does not become rancid and leaves a film upon the skin to replace that removed in washing. These superfatted soaps are only a little less efficient as cleansers than the regular soaps and are particularly recommended for infants and for older persons with dry skins.

Green soap is strong; that is, it contains a considerable amount of free alkali. The surgeon prefers it because of this fact, in order to get his hands and arms as free from germs as possible. Not uncommonly, however, he suffers from its irritating quality. Pure green soap is not green but yellow. At present most hospitals have discontinued green soap because of its harsh reactions on the skin after long periods of use. Some of the newer antiseptics, such as hexachlorophene, are even more germicidal in action, and may be incorporated in a mild soap mixture, thereby minimizing the dangers of skin irritation.

Hard water soaps are often only ordinary soaps with an excess of coconut oil. This oil enables them to form suds more readily with water containing too much calcium. Coconut oil is an ingredient of most soaps and is not harmful as long as the amount is small; but in excess it may be irritating to delicate skins.

There are now available various types of water softener. When these substances are added to hard water, they prevent the combination of calcium and soap, thus softening the water and enabling it to form soapsuds more readily. The solution of such a salt in hard water prevents the deposit on the skin of a scum which holds and protects bacteria. Thus the water softener aids in ridding the surface of the skin of infectious agents. Sodium hexametaphosphate is one of the best softening agents.

Soap is not only cleansing in its action, but actually kills most of the ordinary germs. Unfortunately, two, the typhoid bacillus and that cause of most of the boils and other skin infections, the ubiquitous staphylococcus, are able to resist it. It seems better to maintain the normal germ-killing efficiency of the skin by proper care rather than to attempt direct action upon the bacteria with antiseptics combined in soap.

The best soaps usually contain approximately 20 to 30 per cent of water. The best type of soap is a comparatively neutral form containing no mcre than ¼ to 1 per cent of free alkali. Transparent soaps contain more water, 25 to 35 per cent. Floating soaps also contain large amounts of water, although their brilliancy is due to the air stirred into them during their manufacture. Superfatted soaps are milder and less irritating due to the fact that the alkali has been neutralized by the addition of lanolin. A good soap need not be expensive, as the well-known brands put out by the leading manufacturers are usually priced within a reasonable range. For the average skin they are adequate. The highly perfumed soaps made up in expensive packages and given misleading names are not superior to the average inexpensive toilet soap. As a matter of fact, they are frequently less effective from the standpoint of cleansing and minimal irritation. Choose a soap adapted to your need and made by a leading manufacturer, and it should be adequate for the average skin.

POWDERS

Dusting powders and face powders are soothing, cooling, and drying, as well as protective and decorative. Each tiny particle of powder acts to increase the available surface for the evaporation of insensible perspiration, thus cooling and drying the skin. It also protects against the irritation of cold air or sunshine and the rubbing of clothing. The requirements for a good powder are that it be fine and non-irritating. Talcum is the best known and most widely used powder. It is of light weight, very fine texture, and adheres well to the skin.

Zinc stearate is heavier and also a good adherent. The starches, potato, wheat, or corn, are useful but absorb moisture and swell, making them less desirable where moisture is present in any quantity. Boric acid in small amounts is often added to dusting powders for its action in deterring the growth of germs. Stout people and babies are the chief beneficiaries of dusting powders. Without them, they are apt to suffer from irritation in the folds of the skin (armpits, groin, buttocks), known as intertrigo. In applying powder to the infant, great care should be taken to have it in one of the patent containers made to prevent the possibility of the baby getting the open end of the container into its mouth, for severe consequences have been caused by the baby's shaking an antiseptic powder (boric acid) into its mouth and inhaling it. For this reason I prefer a bland type of baby powder with a minimum of added antiseptic ingredients. Where the skin folds are irritated (as in the diaper region), a powder of a more adherent nature with water-repellent powers, due to its content of cod liver oil (Desitin powder), is often of value.

Since powders are widely used on account of the smooth and cooling feeling which they give to the skin, they must be correctly formulated in order to exert this cooling effect. Although a good powder could be made from talc alone, it would not have good absorbing properties, and for that reason various metallic salts are usually added. In addition, when powders are used as aids to the complexion, they must have additional chemicals added in order to cover defects of the skin and to lessen the shine of the oil secretion. Unfortunately, the trend in recent years has been to mask completely the shine due to the secretions of the sweat and sebaceous glands, and the resultant powder gives a smooth, mask-like appearance to the face. Aside from the appearance, the use of these heavy powders (cake make-up, foundations) results in the undesirable side effect of blocking the skin secretions for a period of time. The constant use of heavy foundations and cake make-up, without adequate cleansing of the skin, often results in the appearance of blackheads and other minor complexion difficulties, much to the distress of the wearer. If a woman must use a foundation, she should apply it infrequently and cleanse her skin thoroughly following its use.

LOTIONS

Most lotions are actually water solutions containing powder. The usual preparation often requires thorough shaking prior to its use. The lotion is then spread on the skin and allowed to dry. The evaporation of the fluid leads to a cooling off of the skin, and the residual coat of powder which it leaves on the skin continues its action and so soothes both normal and inflamed skin. The well-known calamine lotion is just such a mixture. Part of its effectiveness is due to the fact that it is extremely bland and cannot irritate or aggravate an already inflamed skin. If most home remedies applied to the skin were of a similar bland and harmless nature, the doctor would see fewer cases of aggravated and irritated skin disorders.

COLD CREAM

The oil in the skin is an important ingredient. It keeps the horny layer of the skin soft, flexible, and watertight and forms a thin protective film on its surface. When oil is deficient the skin becomes rough, dry, and scaly, often inflamed, and much more liable to infection. The owner of such a skin is notified of this condition by a feeling of stiffness or even itching or pain. In common words, the skin is chapped. This happens most often in the winter, when cold dry winds are prevalent. To counteract it, oil may be supplied to the skin in the form of cold cream, supplementing nature. Creams are oils that contain water. When applied to the skin, the water evaporates and the cream absorbs water from the skin. If there is inflammation present, this results in a cooling of the skin, whence the name, cold cream. To avoid the overly frequent removal of oil by ordinary washing with soap and water, cold cream is rubbed on the skin and wiped off, removing much of the dirt with it. This does not compare, of course, with the cleansing attained by the use of soap, but is fairly efficient. Cleanliness may be next to godliness, but is not an unmixed blessing for those with dry skins. It can be overdone, or, rather, it can be done in the wrong way. In those with greasy skins, however, cream is harmful if it takes the place of hot water and soap cleansing. Cream adds to the grease already too plentiful in the skin, and in cases of blackheads and acne increases the tendency to form pus pimples.

Many different fats are available for anointing the skin; but cold cream, ointment of rose water, a perfumed emulsion of fat and water, is deservedly the most popular. There are many formulas for it; but all have about the same effect upon the skin. Light, soft creams are called cleansing creams and are sometimes advertised as "skin foods," which of course is a misnomer and a false claim, for the skin is fed only through the stomach, as the rest of the body is fed. Other preparations advertised as greaseless cold creams and recommended as cleansing creams are not creams at all but soaps made with sodium carbonate. Of course, they cleanse better than real cold cream, but they also defeat the purpose of creams, for they take oil out of the skin instead of adding to it. Some cold creams become rancid in time. This can be delayed by adding a small amount of boric acid, 5 or 10 per cent, to the cream. Many of the commercial cold creams are now made with petrolatum (mineral oil) in place of animal fats. Petrolatum is not a fat, but a derivative of petroleum which has many of the properties of fats but does not become rancid.

Creams are best used at bedtime following thorough washing of the skin with soap and water. From the point of view of their true value, the chief use of creams is to cleanse and protect the skin as well as to supply a small amount of oil and fat when the skin is on the dry side. In recent years there has been a great deal of discussion concerning the value of hormones in creams as an aid in minimizing the aging process. Up to the present time there has been no specific proof that hormones in creams will halt or lessen the process of wrinkle formation and maintain or produce a constant state of rejuvenation. If you are actually deficient in sex hormones, they should be administered in adequate dosage by your physician. It is very difficult for the average person to read between the lines of a skillful advertisement proclaiming an easy method for obtaining glamour and facial beauty. Experts in the field can do no more than advise caution and intelligence in reading highly publicized reports concerning a new easy road to perpetual youth and a beautiful complexion.

ANTISEPTICS

For application to small wounds, tincture of iodine is probably the most widely known antiseptic. It should be painted on, one coat only. More than this does not add to the good effect and increases the danger of irritation. The bottle must be kept tightly stoppered, preferably with a rubber stopper, for if the tincture is exposed to the air it evaporates and becomes so strong that even one application may cause a severe reaction. After iodine has been applied, no preparation of mercury should be used on the same area for several days for fear of an unpleasant skin irritation. The stain of iodine can be removed by alcohol, and it is usually advisable to follow an iodine application with an alcohol application.

Boric acid in saturated solution is a deservedly popular household remedy. Though it does not kill germs, it limits their growth and is soothing rather than irritating to inflamed skin. It should be made by filling a clean (boiled or scalded) fruit jar or large bottle one fourth full of the boric acid crystals, then adding boiled water to fill the jar. When this has cooled, it is a saturated solution, and what is needed can be poured off. By keeping crystals at the bottom, water above, a saturated solution is always ready for use. These bottles must be carefully labeled and kept in a safe place out of the reach of a child, as the solution is poisonous if swallowed. For infections, the boric acid solution should be heated and applied on a large dressing covered to retain heat as long as possible. For most acute skin irritations, however, it is best applied cool on a thin compress, allowing for evaporation. The compress should be kept thoroughly saturated if it is to be effective.

The solution of hydrogen peroxide is a useful household remedy. It does not kill germs, except those that cannot grow in the presence of oxygen. These occur in the mouth and other cavities of the body. More often, peroxide is used for cleansing wounds. It attacks and destroys pus and blood, and at the same time gets into small crevices where it forms oxygen gas and loosens dirt so that it can be wiped or washed away. It should not be applied too frequently as it may delay the healing of a wound. Care must be taken not to put peroxide into a cavity from which it cannot easily escape, for under these circumstances the gas may form under pressure and cause great pain and actual damage to the tissues.

Carbolic acid, often used in the household, is a dangerous chemical. It does not dissolve well in water, and when the attempt is made to make such a solution, concentrated carbolic acid often comes into contact with the skin and burns it. It should be used only under the direction of the doctor.

Within the past few years many new drugs and chemicals have been discovered. These agents have the common effect of killing or at least inhibiting many of the organisms which are present on the surface of the skin. A partial list of their names would have to include the sulfa drugs, penicillin, bacitracin, streptomycin, terramycin, aureomycin, chloromycetin, and many others. Although these drugs are effective from the standpoint of sterilizing the surface of the skin, they should be taken only under the supervision of a physician because of their capability of producing undesirable toxic or allergic reactions. Also their use in a skin cream for a minor infection may result in the development of an allergy to the drug, thereby preventing its use at some later date, for a more serious internal infection.

WET DRESSINGS

Wet dressings are helpful in the treatment of minor skin disorders, and some of them have already been described under the heading of antiseptics. Sometimes the application of a wet solution to an inflamed area of skin will accomplish a remarkable degree of healing and soothing action within a short period of time. In most instances it is important to apply the wet dressing every few hours for at least twenty to thirty minutes. Wet dressings are one of the most effective ways of removing crusts and dried secretions from the surface of the skin and in maintaining some drainage from infected areas. They serve as very effective local applications of heat, and may also be used to prevent rapid changes in the temperature of the skin surface. They are very useful in the treatment of skin eruptions with extensive blister formation, in that they tend to open these blistered sites and bring the effective medication in the wet dressing to the irritated area. The most widely used and effective wet dressings are a weak salt solution, Burow's solution (usually used in solutions containing ten to twenty times as much water); potassium permanganate solution in a weak form (approximately 1 part of potassium permanganate to 5,000 parts of water), a 2 to 5 per cent boric acid solution, and a magnesium sulfate or Epsom salt solution containing approximately ½ to 1 tablespoon of the salt to a quart of water. There are two main types of wet dressing, and it must be realized that their effects are considerably different. The open type of wet dressing, in which the solution is merely soaked in several layers of cotton or gauze and applied to the skin, is used when cooling is desired and maceration of the underlying skin is not advisable (poison ivy, burns). The so-called closed type of wet dressing, in which the layers of gauze or cotton are covered with oiled silk or cellophane, is used where local heat and maceration of the top layer of the skin are desired (boils, carbuncles). It is important that the dressing be kept sopping wet by constantly changing the entire thickness of gauze or cotton, or applying a completely new and fresh application. The hands and feet can also be treated by merely soaking the affected part in a basin containing the solution.

MASSAGE

Massage, including rubbing and kneading, is a well-established means of maintaining circulation in those prevented by disease from exercising, and of restoring circulation to parts of the body in which it is deficient. The face, however, seldom lacks exercise. Our days are full of facial exercise. At mealtimes we chew our food thoroughly (let us hope), and between meals we talk and allow the play of our emotions to find expression on the face. The rubbing in of cold cream is not necessary, for it exerts all its benefit on being applied gently. Massage is refreshing, however, and if followed by a good washing, as it always should be, does no harm in most cases. In any active inflammatory condition of the skin massage is harmful. In acne it is of doubtful benefit, and the grease that always accompanies its application is harmful. In any real infection, such as boils, it is dangerous, particularly on the face.

STEAMING

Steaming the face or other involved parts of the skin (back, chest) is a valuable measure in greasy skins containing blackheads. It causes increased perspiration and acts more vigorously than washing with hot water. It should not be carried to the point of causing the face to get very red and should always be followed by a cold application to restore tone to the vessels. Like the hot bath, if used too frequently, it may cause drying or even chapping of the skin.

SUN BATHS AND ARTIFICIAL SUBSTITUTES

The use of arc lights and quartz mercury vapor lamps in the home is being popularized. There is no doubt of the beneficial action of these rays and of the sun's rays under proper conditions and control. Light baths of any type should be given cautiously, allowing the skin to become accustomed to the light and to respond with pigmentation, instead of being burned. People with blue eyes and fair skins should exercise particular care to protect the skin from the harmful effects of light. The overly frequent exposure of the normal skin to ultraviolet rays for the purpose of a temporary cosmetic effect is not without the possibility of ultimate harm to the skin. There are some abnormalities and diseases of the skin, as well as some internal conditions, in which light is actually harmful.

On the water or snow the reflected rays may greatly increase the degree of the skin's exposure to ultraviolet irradiation. Hats are no protection against these rays, which contain the ultraviolet rays that are most active in producing irritation. Particularly at high altitudes, their penetration is great, and the effect of sunlight much greater than its visual intensity indicates. At low altitudes these rays are largely absorbed by the atmosphere, and comparatively few of them reach us. People who are strongly sensitive to the sun may now protect themselves by the use of creams and lotions containing physical or chemical sun screens. One of the best chemical sun screens is para-aminobenzoic acid and its derivatives, and it has been incorporated in several preparations now commercially available.

Care of the Skin at Various Periods of Life
INFANCY

The skin of an infant requires gentle treatment. Soap should be of the mildest superfatted kind, and even this should be employed only when absolutely necessary. It is preferable to clean an infant's skin with a bland oil containing small amounts of one of the newer and less irritating surface antiseptics such as hexachlorophene. After the bath a bland powder should be used, care being taken that the baby cannot get the opportunity to shake the powder into its mouth and lungs. The folds of the body should receive more powder than the rest of the skin. The clothing should be soft, carefully rinsed after washing, and not too heavy. Many infants are kept too warm and suffer from heat rash, which may, as a result of scratching, become infected and eventuate in more serious skin disease. Infants frequently develop chafing of the skin in the diaper region due to prolonged contact with urine and feces. This area may be protected by the application of soothing creams of a slightly water-repellent nature due to their cod liver oil content (Desitin ointment).

CHILDHOOD

The same rules apply as in infancy, except that the young child and the older small boy or tomboy girl require for their hands (and too often for other parts of the body) more soap and water. The mother should not, however, let her love of cleanliness carry her too far with the scrubbing process, for it is better that the child be a little less than perfectly clean rather than hampered in its exercise. Precautions against overcleanliness can be safely left to the defensive power of the child in most cases. Both boys and girls, if they have blond skin that freckles, should be urged to wear hats in the sun and to protect the skin before going outdoors. Modern sunburn protection includes the use of preparations containing para-aminobenzoic acid and derivatives, as well as salol, menthyl and benzyl salicylates, and other agents. The average sunburn is effectively soothed by applications of cold, weak boric acid solutions and a mild lotion such as calamine containing 1 per cent of phenol. The fair-skinned youngster should be taught in childhood that severe sunburn is dangerous and should be taught how to protect the skin from the sun's rays.

ADOLESCENCE

The chief change seen in the skin at puberty is the greasiness which appears in so many skins at this time, often accompanied by blackheads and pimples. The measures to be described later under the heading of acne must be instituted at once, and include frequent washing with hot water and soap and the insistence on good habits of hygiene.

MIDDLE LIFE

This is the active, strenuous time, when health is most often neglected for the sake of work or even sometimes for the sake of play. Loss of sleep, irregular meals, worry, all have their effect upon the health of the skin, as well as on the rest of the body. Worry, hurry, and impatience hasten the onset of age, which is often announced too early by the condition of the skin. The use of cold cream upon the female skin becomes more generally justifiable because of lessening oil production and decreasing glandular activity.

AGE

Age brings lessened nutrition to all parts, including the skin, and the latter loses both elasticity and oil to become wrinkled and rough. The skin loses its resistance and tolerance to the sun and various chemicals such as soap. Oil should be applied artificially, soap used sparingly, and the skin protected as much as possible. If hormones are necessary, they should be used only under the guidance of a physician.

Inflammations of the Skin
ECZEMA

Years ago almost any skin disease involving a patch of red, scaling, itching, and weeping skin was attributed to eczema; no one really knew what produced the symptoms. Accordingly, at some stage in development more than half of all skin diseases were called "eczema."

Eczema is a common inflammation of the skin. Its symptoms are: redness, itching, small blisters, and the discharge from the skin of a fluid that stiffens linen and tends to dry into scales and crusts. Incidentally, eczema is *not* catching.

This sounds specific enough—but, unfortunately, many other skin diseases have exactly the same symptoms. Actually, a skin disease is called eczema when it has all the features just mentioned, and is apparently caused by some unknown agent, either inside or outside the body.

For example, a man visited his physician and complained of an eruption of this type on the outside of his thigh. Without modern scientific investigation, it was classified as eczema of an unknown origin. Later, when the eruption had spread to the hands, face, and neck, the patient became seriously worried. Again he consulted a physician, this time a specialist in diseases of the skin. The second doctor made a detailed investigation. It revealed that the patient always carried a box of matches of foreign manufacture in his trouser pocket. The box rested against his thigh at the spot where the trouble began. The doctor found that the sulphur and phosphorus mixture on the striking side of the box and also on the match heads had an irritating effect on this particular patient's skin.

This man's reaction to these chemicals was so violent that he would have become a hospital case, with an entire body rash, had the cause not been discovered and the matches removed from his pocket.

Another instance, also an actual case, concerned a woman who asked her physician about an itching, red rash on her hands and forearms, a type of irritation that many chemicals and substances produce. This woman did not normally come in contact with strong chemicals, soaps, or other irritants. She was the sort of woman who used her hands for holding cocktails, waving people out of her way, and playing Mah-Jongg (before the days of Canasta). After questioning, the doctor discovered that a friend had given her a beautiful set of Mah-Jongg tiles, made in Japan. It was finally discovered that these Japanese tiles were covered with a lacquer made from a distant relation of poison ivy! The Japanese Mah-Jongg sets sold well, and, as a result, many women developed skin rashes from playing with the "poison ivy" tiles.

Neither the woman nor the man mentioned here had eczema. If the cause of their skin eruptions had not been discovered or determined, it would have been diagnosed as eczema, for want of a better explanation.

There is a lesson to be learned from these illustrations. It is of the greatest importance for patients to provide their doctors with all details of their daily lives when consulting them about skin condition.

There are other examples of specific skin diseases.

Among these are those fellow Americans who would develop a rash on Sunday nights, after a relaxing, restful day spent with pipe, slippers, and the Sunday papers. This rash improved during the week and flared up again on Sunday night.

"Aha, my friend," exclaims Sherlock Holmes the dermatologist, "you're rather fond of the rotogravure sections."

"Yes—so what?" replies our fellow American.

Well, you've guessed it! The rotogravure sections of the Sunday papers were the clue to the mystery of the Sunday-night rash. The ink from which they were printed frequently contained a red dye, which is an irritant to some people's skin. The irritation took several hours to develop—if it did not, it might have been a Sunday-afternoon rash. The rotogravure sections have disappeared from the Sunday papers, although an occasional person may be found sensitive to ordinary newsprint.

From the foregoing examples, there are irritants that affect certain people and not others. Likewise, there are certain substances that affect only certain parts of the body. For example, the scalp, face, and neck may react to a hair dye, a cold wave lotion, or to a perfume; the forehead to hat bands, especially those recently cleaned; the ears and nose to plastic or metal eyeglass frames; and the eyelids and neck to nail polish. The latter may sound strange—but the damage is done by contact with the fingernails.

Underwear shorts may affect the thighs or abdomen. Plastic watch straps may inflame the wrists. Even, forgive me, nylon stockings might affect the legs!

I can hear the American housewife say: "Just give me the nylons; I'll take my chances."

And, she is right. Ill effects from wearing nylons are infrequent. Yet the few women who are susceptible can develop an annoying and itching eruption from wearing these stockings.

There are innumerable other instances where diagnoses could not be made until after long and detailed investigations. A baffling case was that of an attractive young woman on whose lips a severe itching and burning broke out. Many tests were made, with lipsticks, cosmetics, foods, and other substances. Yet these and other precedures produced no effect. At long last the cause of the irritation was tracked down—her fiancé's mustache wax!

We seem to be concerned not with what eczema is, but with what it is not. This is necessary. The importance of the cases described is that there are some diseases classified as eczema that are due to specific agents. These agents can only be discovered by means of painstaking examinations.

The number of cases classified as eczema has been shrinking steadily. It will continue to do so as our methods and means for ferreting out hitherto unknown causes improve.

For our purposes, eczema can now be defined more exactly. It is a skin eruption in which there are certain complex internal factors more important than the local existing cause. In other words, though there may be a local existing cause, such as a matchbox, Mah-Jongg tile, or mustache wax—the removal of this cause, while essential, may not affect the cure. What is more, a skin irritation due to some such simple cause may develop into an eczema. Even though you track down and remove the primary cause, the irritation process goes on as eczema.

Again heredity comes into the picture. Some people are apt to develop eczema because of family tendencies. Blondes and redheads usually have sensitive skins that are irritated by sun, wind, and other agents. Other people are susceptible to eczema because of an infection in the teeth, tonsils, or sinuses. People with dry or oily skins may be predisposed to skin eruptions. People with dry skins are easily irritated by soap and, in general, lack sufficient resistance to skin infections. There are people whose sweat glands do not function well. Consequently, they don't perspire enough to remove irritants from the skin or cool the body.

Poor nutrition may also cause eczema. Lack of vitamins may lower skin resistance to the disease. Lack of vitamin A can cause a type of eczema complicated by pus formation. Lack of vitamin B can cause scaling of the nose and lips. Deficiency of various elements of the vitamin B family can cause a peculiar eruption on the arms and legs.

Various internal parts of the body influence the skin in the development of eczema. Among these are poorly functioning glands, such as the thyroid and others; and upset stomachs, livers, and kidneys. Often a good doctor tracks down some unsuspected disease elsewhere in the body following an eczema clue.

These conditions, and others, can predispose a man or woman to eczema. In other words, they are indirect causes. There are also causes directly responsible for it. Some people are hypersensitive, or allergic, to drugs or proprietary remedies which may do others good. If the hypersensitive individual takes these drugs, it may easily produce a skin disorder, or predispose him to it.

If you have a skin eruption, it may be possible that a supposedly harmless laxative, tonic, or blood purifier in your medicine chest is either the cause or part of the cause of your trouble. Perhaps you get a rash in the spring or fall of the year. You probably attribute it either to the weather or astrology. It's more likely to be caused by the insect spray or moth destroyer you use during these seasons.

Of course, there are many more factors which bear on this disease than can be briefly mentioned. Nerves also enter the picture. A period of emotional tension can produce inflammation of the skin. Does this sound far-fetched? If so, reflect on what happens when you are embarrassed—your face gets red. What happens when you're nervous or excited?—you break out in little pimples, known as "goose flesh." So—you see—mere thoughts and emotions do produce definite skin changes. When these thoughts and emotions take firm hold, they can also play an important rôle in the production of skin eruptions.

The patient, on being convinced that he has eczema, next wants to know the answer to the question that doctors hear many times a day, "All right, what can you do for me?"

The answer is—a great deal. One of the first jobs is to determine the cause and to eliminate it.

Another decision the doctor must make is whether the condition is acute or chronic. If it is acute, the itching must be relieved and the inflammation reduced as soon as possible. Normally, the patient will be given wet dressings and soothing lotions at this stage. The doctor will urge him to avoid such irritants as soap and water. If there are any predisposing factors—such as the matchbox, Mah-Jongg tiles, hair dyes, or hat bands—and also specific worries or digestive troubles—these must be eliminated or modified. Proper diet is important; so is proper intestinal functioning.

In chronic or long-standing eczema, the skin becomes thick and leathery. The irreverent medical student calls it "pigskin" or "elephant's hide." When this stage is reached, the cure becomes a long and difficult task. It is important for the doctor to study the patient minutely, to eliminate all potential irritants. Each person presents an individual problem. The doctor must decide what investigation and laboratory tests to make and he must analyze and interpret the results. Careful attention should be given to the patient's diet. The rate at which the patient's body absorbs sugar from his food must be checked. Functioning of the glands should be tested, and a search made for specific infections.

In addition to his chronic eczema, if the patient has some mild skin eruption elsewhere, such as "athlete's foot," this should be treated at the same time. If not treated, it may aggravate the eczema.

A word of warning—if a local remedy is prescribed—the greatest care must be exercised in applying it. To apply it skillfully is often as important as to choose the right remedy. It is also essential to carefully follow instructions. Strong remedies require careful judgment, and you may be sure your physician has assessed your requirements.

In some cases of obstinate eruptions X-ray treatment, administered by an expert, may produce a cure when other methods have failed.

Eczema, then, occupies a unique position in the field of dermatology. It is not only the wastebasket for all unexplained eruptions with characteristic symptoms, but it is also the keystone of skin diseases. The specialist in this subject deals with the commonest and most distressing skin disorder. If he knows how to treat this disease, you may be certain that he is able to treat most skin disorders.

DRUG RASHES

Within the past few years rashes on the skin due to drugs taken for some reason or other have become one of the most important causes of skin disease. Every doctor who prescribes a drug is well aware of the many problems which arise both on the skin and elsewhere on the body, as a result of the same drugs which may do so much good internally. Although the physician may be well aware of the pitfalls and disadvantages of these drugs, the patient usually is not. This is especially unfortunate in view of the fact that many drugs may be bought in the neighborhood drugstore without the necessity of a prescription. Accordingly, the occasional person may be taking some proprietary remedy which is doing him more harm than good. As far as the skin is concerned, while many of the drugs embodied in these various remedies are harmless, many others produce skin eruptions varying from an occasional attack of hives to an extremely serious rash involving almost the entire body. At the present time it is probable that the two most important causes of drug eruptions are the sulfa drugs and penicillin. Even a drug as simple as the salicylates (most popular member of which is aspirin) may be the cause of a troublesome itch or recurrent eruption, often baffling to both the patient and to his doctor.

This brief paragraph cannot be regarded as adequate in view of the vast importance of the rôle played in chronic eruptions of the skin by one or several drugs. It may, however, serve to impress upon the reader that he must seek the services of a physician for advice concerning any chronic skin disorder and, of even greater importance, as to the necessity of continuing some highly vaunted home remedy or drug mixture. Many people, on being asked whether they take a drug, state that they do not. On further questioning, it develops that the remedy they have been taking over a period of years for constipation or for their liver, or whenever they have a headache, is just the drug that is producing the trouble with their skin. Even that so-called "harmless" hang-over remedy may be the cause of their troublesome rash, and that special cure of Grandma's may not only irritate the skin, but affect various other parts of the body even including the blood cells and certain vital structures. Don't take any of those home remedies unless you know exactly what is in them and the mixture has been approved by your physician.

DERMATITIS FROM EXTERNAL IRRITANTS

The common example of this type of rash is the inflammation caused by poison ivy, poison oak, or sumac. The plants, chemicals, fabrics, and other substances that may cause this form of dermatitis are as numerous as those causing eczema, and in fact the two are closely related, so that it is at times impossible to say definitely where one leaves off and the other begins. Children should be taught to recognize the appearance of poison ivy so that they may avoid it in their excursions to study nature. It has glossy foliage, arranged three leaflets on a stem. In the fall among the first to change color, the leaves turn a beautiful red, and are often collected for this reason by uninformed enthusiasts. A good working adage is: "Leaves of three, let it be!"

If contact with the plant has been unavoidable, the next procedure should be to wash thoroughly with soapsuds and hot water, followed by rinsing with strong grain alcohol. If the dermatitis has hardly begun, this may lessen the severity of the attack; but when it has become well established, this treatment comes too late and will irritate the skin and result in a more severe skin reaction. It should be employed preferably within a two-hour period following exposure to the plants.

Among house plants the primrose is a common cause of dermatitis. Tincture of iodine that has been allowed to become strong by evaporation, or the too enthusiastic application of the fresh preparation, often is responsible for it. One coat of a fresh preparation is all that is necessary, and more will not have any better effect but may have a bad one. In bygone days the mustard plaster also was a common cause, but today it is scarcely used. However, there are many new household cleansers, chemicals, and cosmetics which may result in skin irritation.

Severe cases of dermatitis may be caused by contact with certain chemicals. The conditions are just about the same as those caused by poison ivy. Paraphenylenediamine and mercury are among the most important of these chemicals, as they are contained in many hair dyes and toilet preparations. New York City has an amendment to the Sanitary Code prohibiting the sale and distribution of preparations containing these chemicals, except with certain precautions.

Paraphenylenediamine is a coal-tar derivative and a strong poison. It is commonly used in hair dyes and has recently become a source of common exposure due to the sudden popularity of home hair dyes. The scalp may react shortly after the hair is dyed, with severe itching, followed by swelling and blistering of the scalp and surrounding skin. On the other hand, the reaction to a hair dye may not appear for several days, depending on whether the reaction is due to irritation alone or to an allergy to the dye.

Mercury is another chemical often used in liniments, ointments, and lotions. Most freckle removers contain mercury. While it is a valuable agent for many purposes, it is sometimes an acute irritant, and it should not be used except when specifically prescribed by a physician.

Another frequent source of inflammation of the face and neck is traced to dye used on furs, a dye similar to that in hair dyes. The inflammation is usually severe, prolonged, and recurrent. Another form of dermatitis on the forehead is caused by the action of sweat on the dye and other chemicals contained in cheap sweatbands in hats. Mouth washes, lipsticks, and toothpaste may cause a dermatitis around the mouth, face, and neck. Many cosmetics and cosmetic applicators (rubber sponges) may also be the cause of unpleasant and uncomfortable facial rashes.

For these forms of dermatitis the treatment consists in the detection and removal of the source of irritation, whatever that may be. The doctor must really do some detective work in order to ferret out the cause of some of the more obscure skin eruptions. After the cause has been eliminated, soothing remedies are all the treatment that may be required.

CHAPPING

Chapping is one of the simplest forms of inflammation of the skin. It is seen commonly in the wintertime, on the tender skin of children and on the hands of housewives who do not protect their skin from constant contact with soap, detergents, and other household chemicals. The combination of a cold, dry, wintry climate and a dried-out, steam-heated room conspire with hot water and soap to remove the oil from the skin, causing red, dry, scaly areas. Ordinarily such areas, when spared the irritation of soap and lubricated with some oil, will promptly return to normal. This same combination of overdried and steam-heated rooms together with the winter season not only dries out the skin but the mucous membranes of the nose and throat. Do you have a very dry and rough skin during the winter together with frequent colds and sore throats? If so, get hold of a monkey wrench and fix the radiators so that no one can heat your rooms to that blood-drying level where your skin, nose, and throat literally pant for a little atmospheric moisture. Or at least keep a pan filled with water on the floor so that the hot air can pick up some of the fluid. The Eskimos hardly ever catch cold, and their skins are in excellent condition—and all this without steam-heated igloos.

Some people have a distinct tendency toward chapping. Usually their oil and sweat glands do not function adequately. Accordingly, it is important for them to wash as infrequently as possible, and to minimize their contact with harsh, strong soaps. They are far better off using bland oils, either mineral or vegetable in nature, for cleansing purposes, and lubricating their skins whenever possible with a soothing cold cream. Some of the new lotions and emulsions containing ingredients whose purpose it is to increase the oil content of the surfaces of the skin are also very helpful.

CHAFING

This occurs commonly in babies and obese adults. It is caused by the rubbing together of parts moistened by sweat, offering an excellent opportunity for infection to take place. The parts should be kept scrupulously clean and well powdered. If this does not suffice, a flat bag made of gauze may be filled with talcum powder and suspended between the opposing surfaces to prevent rubbing. Of value also are various lotions and pastes which absorb some of the excessive secretions and excretions from these sites (i.e., Lassar's, Desitin). In women with heavy thighs, chafing between the legs may be minimized by wearing a light, porous pantie specially designed to lessen friction in this region. If these simple measures are not successful, it is advisable to consult a physician because some form of infection may have been superimposed on the simple chafe.

SUNBURN

Sunburn is an inflammatory reaction of the skin to the rays of light, not to heat rays. It occurs on snow fields as well as in the hottest climates. The redness does not appear at once, but several hours after exposure to light. If given an opportunity, most skins can produce enough pigment to protect themselves against any ordinary exposure to the sun; but when they receive a large dose of light without any preparatory hardening, they react with an acute inflammation. Some skins do not produce pigment in all parts but only in small scattered patches—the well-known freckle. And the albino has a skin that apparently cannot produce pigment at all; sunburn in the albino can be a very serious malady.

People vary in their reaction to the sun's rays. Blondes, as is well known, are apt to grow very red, to burn instead of tan. Brunettes frequently do not redden at all but merely take on a tan color, due to increased pigmentation in the skin. If the exposure to the sun is prolonged or if the redness (erythema) has lasted for some time, the skin becomes dry, harsh, and what is called "dead." The top layers scale or peel off. Very sensitive skins, or those exposed to intense sunlight, may become severely inflamed. There is much swelling, blistering, oozing, and disfiguring. The eyelids, mouth, and nose swell greatly. Some persons react so severely to sunburn that after a short exposure which is only sufficient to cause a slight burn in the average person, they are generally upset and nauseated. Stronger exposures lead to more violent reactions with fever, chills, and severe surface burns.

Brunettes as a rule do not suffer from these reactions nearly so acutely as do blondes. The normally high percentage of pigmentation in brunette skins is what protects them. Pigmentation is the skin's chief protection from the sun's rays. The pigment-containing cells are called chromatophores, literally meaning "color-loving cells." Blondes have fewer chromatophores than brunettes. The colored races, naturally, have the greatest number of chromatophores, and therefore have greater resistance to the sun's rays.

Prevention against sunburn is worth many pounds of cure to those who react. Large, wide-brimmed hats should be worn. Parasols and the large type of beach umbrella are of great help, especially at the seashore, where the strongest rays are felt. Applications of oils, lotions, and creams keep the rays from penetrating the skin to some extent. Para-aminobenzoic acid in various liquid or solid forms is a very efficient protection against sunburn, as is red veterinary petrolatum (a very effective but messy preparation). Salol (5 to 10 per cent) in a vanishing cream base is also pleasant and efficient. Other new drugs are effective and not unpleasant for application, but when trying a new sunburn cream, use it carefully for the first few times. It may not protect sufficiently, or the very chemical designed to protect your skin may do just the reverse if you are allergic to it.

When the first signs of sunburn appear, a cold cream should be applied. If there is swelling, a wet dressing of a slightly astringent and cooling solution, such as 5 per cent of Burow's solution, boric acid, or witch hazel, should be applied, followed by a powdery liquid such as calamine lotion. These reduce the heat, cool the skin, and help absorb the water in the skin.

The action of cold creams is excellent. They cool, soothe, and protect the skin, and counteract the drying effect of the sun. They do not make hair grow on the face, as some people would have us believe. (If cold cream did that, it would do as much for the scalp, and every bald-headed man in the country would be frantically massaging his scalp with his wife's newest and most expensive cold cream.)

Exposure to strong sunlight occasionally results in a very severe burn, usually of a first- or second-degree character, but never third degree. The so-called first-degree burns are really comparatively mild and produce only a redness of the skin. Second-degree burns occur simultaneously with the first-degree type, and in addition to redness, there are many blisters scattered over the burned area. The second-degree burns do not destroy the complete thickness of the skin, so that the remaining tissue can spontaneously regenerate the burned areas. It is only in third-degree burns, which practically never occur from sunburn, which cause complete destruction of the entire skin, and are far and away the most serious in that the burned victim is seriously ill and requires various types of plastic operation in order to correct the permanent damage to the tissues. First- and second-degree burns occur not only from some sun exposure, but primarily as a direct effect of exposure to heat. This heat may be due to exposure to fire, hot liquids, steam, and flash burns. Although we worry to a certain extent about the dangers of atomic bombs, the real medical problem of exposure to the atomic bomb is not the atomic radiation but the direct effect of heat.

Although the principal measures involved in the treatment of burns are primarily medical problems, their main features are the relief of pain, the prevention of shock and infection, and the actual treatment of the burned areas. With sunburn, the ordinary first-aid measures are adequate, such as the use of a simple mineral oil ointment containing a mild cooling agent such as menthol in a very weak concentration, in order to help relieve the pain. If not available, the application of a heavy paste made of water and sodium bicarbonate is also a useful first-aid measure. The more severe burns resulting from the direct effect of heat rather than sunburn should only be treated by a physician. While waiting, however, the victim may be made more comfortable by the application of a cool wet dressing, minimizing contact with the hands so that infection is not apt to occur. These extensive second- and third-degree burns are best covered with a clean, freshly ironed towel or sterile dressing moistened with a weak bicarbonate of soda solution until the doctor arrives. The newest method of treatment includes the surgical removal of all blisters and dead tissue, preferably in a sterile operating room. Subsequently, the burned area is washed with an antiseptic soap and sterile water, but in a very mild fashion, in order not to remove any of the still living tissue. The soap is then removed by rinsing with a sterile salt solution. There are many variations in the treatment of severe burns, depending upon the training of the physician. At the present time the most popular methods include the use of pressure dressings over a simple mineral oil application to the wound itself. Although many authorities feel that the ointment should contain some antiseptic or antibiotic, it would seem as though the best results have been secured by using the antibiotic internally, rather than locally. Another strange thing that has been found out is that it is preferable to leave the dressings in place for several days rather than to change them frequently. The reason for this is that there is less chance of infection developing, and the tissues seem to heal better when they are not disturbed.

Certain people are extremely sensitive to sunlight and should never expose themselves unnecessarily. Still others, particularly those suffering from a skin disease known as lupus erythematosus, should avoid sunlight as they would a plague. One strong exposure might initiate a fatal flare-up of the disease. People with a tendency toward skin cancer must also avoid the sun.

FROSTBITE

The skin may become irritated as a result of exposure to extreme cold. Usually it is most evident on prominent parts, such as the cheekbones, tip of the nose, ears, and chin. This is frostbite or chilblain, and it usually begins with a painful whiteness of the frozen part. Subsequently, the skin becomes cold, dark red, and painful. It may then lose all sensation. If the exposure is prolonged, the extremities may turn a black color, and in extreme cases the skin becomes gangrenous or dead.

The recent war has resulted in a considerable knowledge concerning the treatment of frostbite. These measures were learned, unfortunately, by the observation of aviators whose hands were frozen at high altitudes, and also from poor "G.I. Joe," who developed trench foot due to exposure of the feet to cold and wet for days at a time. Formerly we were all aware of the age-old custom of massaging the skin with snow, but this has long since been thrown out. In fact, massage of these almost brittle areas of the skin may actually lead to gangrene. The present methods of treatment of frostbite include gradual increase in the skin temperature by putting the patient first in a cool room and allowing the frozen part to thaw out slowly. It is of the utmost importance that the frozen tissue be thawed out slowly, because any rapid increase in the skin temperature will result in death of the skin cells and gangrene of the tissue. Gradually the frostbitten victim is warmed up with hot stimulating drinks, and if the freezing is extensive, transfusions of blood or plasma are usually necessary. Very little is done with the skin itself, other than keeping it extremely clean. The trend has been to give all the necessary antiseptics and antibiotics internally rather than locally, and this procedure has resulted in fewer cases of lost fingers and toes.

Excessive and Abnormal Functioning of the Skin or of Its Oil and Sweat Glands

EXCESSIVE SWEATING

Excessive sweating may prove annoying, and the pads worn in the armpits and the various chemical applications to this area are not fully satisfactory remedies. Many chemicals act as deodorants when externally applied, and some are also anti-perspirants. The most effective anti-perspirant preparations are the aluminum salts, although some people may be allergic to these chemicals and they must be tried out with caution. As a deodorant, plain bicarbonate of soda as a dusting powder is effective. In recent years some of the newer internally acting drugs such as banthine have been successfully used for the control of excessive sweating, but only under medical supervision because of their effects on other parts of the body.

BODY ODOR

Body odor is usually synonymous with the odor of the sweat. Certain perfumers advise the use of perfume suited to the body odor of the client, but that sounds rather unpleasant. Foul-odored sweat is a great affliction, fortunately not common. Some of the newer soaps and deodorants are effective in the control of unpleasant body odors. Many of these preparations contain hexachlorophene and other effective antiseptics. Chlorophyll enjoys great popularity, not entirely deserved.

PRICKLY HEAT

Heat rash (prickly heat) is an acute inflammatory disorder due, obviously, to an inability of the skin to adapt itself to an increase in temperature. It occurs more often in infants than in older persons, and is most prevalent during periods of heat and humidity.

The eruption consists of tiny elevations ranging in size from a pinpoint to a pinhead and usually containing a clear fluid. Actually, these tiny elevations are present over the pore openings and are due to the fact that the sweat secretions have been blocked by a surface inflammation of the skin. The surrounding skin is usually of a pinkish shade. The prickles may remain separate, but not infrequently they join with one another and form large patches of irritation, as in eczema. If these areas are not properly treated, secondary infection may result with pus formation and rapid spread.

Prickly heat is best prevented by the avoidance of too heavy clothing and frequent use of bath and dusting powder. Do not dress babies and children too warmly during the summer months. Bathe them frequently, and make certain that they drink enough water and other fluids. After the eruption is present, it will frequently yield promptly to cooling measures such as weak, cold applications followed by the use of a bland dusting powder or calamine lotion. The skin should not be cleansed with soap, which is very apt to irritate the condition. For the purposes of cleansing, mineral or vegetable oils may be employed in alternation with the local applications of powder and soothing lotions. If these simple local procedures fail to improve the condition, a physician should be consulted, as such eruptions afford an excellent invasion center for infections of the skin.

EXCESSIVE OILING

Excessive oiliness of the skin is one of the commonest causes of large pores and a generally poor complexion. It is most common around the age of puberty or adolescence, and this may be considered due to the increased activity of the sex glands during this period of life. The oiliness of the skin occurs about equally in both sexes, although it is presumed to be due to the secretion of male, rather than female, sex hormones. It is usually referred to medically as seborrhéa, and is characterized by the presence of an excessive amount of oily secretion on the face and the scalp, and occasionally elsewhere on the body. This greasy secretion appears as oily droplets oozing through the pores of the skin and often on the scalp. The result is a greasy layer of oil droplets which can be wiped off the surfaces of the skin with a handkerchief at frequent intervals. In time the pore openings become blocked with oily secretion which can be squeezed out in the form of little wormlike bodies. In addition, these oily droplets serve as sort of a catch-basket for all the dirt floating in the air, and so the surface of these oil droplets or the secretion in the pores themselves is often of a blackish color and is referred to as "blackhead." The black color is not actually dependent on dirt, as certain chemical changes are responsible for the blackish color. The scalp is always affected, and the free oily material results in a glistening and shining appearance of the scalp. In women with long hair the secretion may be so extreme as to mat the locks together in a sort of glue-like paste. Although in former years this was believed to be responsible in great measure for early baldness, the relative importance of oil secretions in producing baldness is still an unsolved problem.

Although the glands of internal secretion are primarily responsible for the excessive greasiness and oiliness of the skin, other predisposing causes include any internal change which lowers the vitality and general nutrition. Seborrhea may appear following any one of a number of infections and is often associated with constipation, lack of fresh air and exercise, and poor diet. When seborrhea has persisted for a long time, it may be responsible for the formation of crusts and scales on the scalp and around the ears and nose. This may even go on to a more severe form of the disorder, often referred to as seborrheic dermatitis.

In the average case of seborrhea frequent washing with soap and water and the use of a mild astringent may be all that is required. However, in the usual instance it is important to take care of both the external and internal factors if an effective cure is desired. Ordinary common-sense hygienic measures are indicated. Sunlight, nutritious food, and plenty of fresh air and exercise are important. An adequate intake of vitamins, especially of members of the B-complex family, is especially indicated. The latter vitamins contain substances which have been shown to lessen the greasiness and scaling of the skin both in animals and human beings. Vitamin B_{12} has been reputed of particular benefit in this disorder. For the direct treatment of the skin, frequent use of soap and water on the face and frequent shampooing of the scalp are highly recommended. Bland soaps or soap substitutes such as sulfonated oils are of value in many instances, especially if the skin is sensitive and easily irritated. One thing that is definitely contraindicated is the use of massage by the beautician and barber, both of the face and scalp. Massage of the face is not only valueless in this condition, but will often increase the local irritation and accentuate the blocking and oil secretion of the skin. In addition to frequent washing of the skin, the use of a mild astringent at frequent intervals is effective.

Where the condition is more of a rash, rather than merely excessive oil secretion, various drugs have been employed and recommended, and these include sulfur, resorcin, salicylic acid, and similar agents. They are usually made up in the form of pomades of various types, although lotions are better adapted to some skins. Repeated application and patient care of the face and scalp are necessary to secure complete relief in the case of a disease as essentially chronic as seborrhea. These conditions require the services of a physician, as the local and internal measures require close watch and frequent change.

EXCESSIVE DRYNESS

This condition is the exact opposite of seborrhea, in that there is an inadequacy of the secretions of the oil glands. As a result, the skin is not satisfactorily lubricated, and this may occur as a natural phenomenon or as a result of constant bathing of the skin, or as a result of immersing the body in strongly alkaline solutions in the course of various occupations. Dryness of the skin frequently occurs in the wintertime in cold climates, and is often aggravated by the lack of humidity in heated rooms. It is often associated with other disturbances of the skin, and is not infrequently a forerunner of eczema. In extreme instances the skin is not only dry but becomes cracked, chapped, and split. Dryness of the skin is more typical of the older age groups, but it must be realized that various internal factors may also produce this state. For example, when the thyroid gland does not function adequately, the skin often becomes extremely dry and scaly.

If the dryness is merely due to various external causes, the condition can usually be simply remedied by the use of oils such as lanolin, almond oil, mineral oil, and other agents. The skin should be bathed as infrequently as possible, and soaps confined primarily to the skin under the arms and in the groin. Even the face should be cleaned with oils rather than soaps, and a protective layer of cold cream should be left on the skin overnight. Other effective solutions for the face include glycerin in rose water and the occasional local application of the white of an egg rubbed gently into the skin. If the condition does not respond to simple applications of creams and oily lotions, a search for some internally causative factor, such as a hormone deficiency, may often be rewarding.

ITCHING

The skin is the source of many peculiar sensations, including smarting, burning, prickling, tingling, creeping, and crawling. However, one of the most common sensations in the skin is itching. As a result of this sensation, we are provoked into rubbing and scratching the affected area in an attempt to relieve the undesirable sensation or to change it almost preferably to one of pain. When the itching is severe, self-control can seldom be mustered even by persons of unusually strong will power. These unhappy efforts of the sufferer to relieve himself result in the formation of bumps and infection as a result of the entrance of bacteria through self-inflicted wounds. Often the irritation is far more acute at night than during the day, and sleep becomes a thing of the past.

The causes of itching are many. In some instances it may be as simple as contact with a new soap, shaving lotion, hair tonic, or the like. In other instances it may be due to infection with some germ or parasite. Occasionally it may be a symptom of a severe underlying disease such as diabetes. Obviously, then, the only intelligent approach to the treatment of itching is to find out what has caused the symptom. To a trained observer, this may prove to be a simple problem, although, on the other hand, it may require an extremely careful medical and laboratory investigation.

The occurrence of itching is divided about equally among men and women, and, while no age level is exempt, there is a tendency for it to be more frequent after forty. Adults with dry skins often develop itching during the winter, especially if they bathe frequently and use more than their share of soap. It may also make its appearance during the menopause and result in itching of either one portion of the body or the entire body surface.

If the itching is due to a specific cause, removal of the offending substance will result in prompt and speedy relief. This relief will be increased by the use of cold wet dressings and soothing lotions. Within recent years new antihistaminic drugs have been found extremely effective in controlling sensations of itching, whatever their cause. Of course, these drugs should be taken only under the supervision of a physician. Unfortunately, the tendency at present is to employ them as a cure-all for all known skin diseases, but, as might be expected, they will not perform miracles. Not infrequently dietary measures are also of value in itchy states, and the elimination of tea, coffee, and alcohol may be of considerable benefit.

Itching of the skin may also be due to an associated nervous disorder, and the treatment of a difficult emotional situation may sometimes result in relief from that extremely uncomfortable and maddening itch. Where an itching condition has persisted for any period of time, do not attempt to treat the condition yourself but consult your physician.

Infections of the Skin

Bacterial Infections

Impetigo is the commonest of all skin infections and one of the easiest to cure. It is most frequently seen in children and is caused by pus germs, the streptococcus and staphylococcus. In the newborn baby, it can be serious because the baby has no immunity to the infection and it is fatal in approximately

25 per cent of all cases. For this reason children are not permitted to visit the maternity floor of the hospital. The disease is highly communicable and spreads rapidly from child to child. It can usually be recognized by the appearance of honey-colored crusts which look as though they were stuck on the skin. Impetigo prefers to attack children, and the face is the favorite site. The scalp is not uncommonly involved, especially in children with head lice.

The treatment of impetigo is based primarily on the use of antiseptics and general cleansing with soap and water. If the crusts do not come off easily, the application of a wet dressing or a soap poultice will serve to take them off in short order. Following removal of the crusts, the application of any one of several antiseptic ointments, such as those containing ammoniated mercury, or some of the newer antibiotic agents is extremely effective. Where the condition is widespread and serious, it may be necessary to employ some of the newer antibiotics, such as penicillin or terramycin, by mouth or by injection.

Folliculitis is similar in nature to impetigo, but the infection is in the hair follicle rather than on the surface of the skin. In other words, the infecting germs, either the staphylococcus or streptococcus, penetrate the deeper parts of the skin, usually through the mouth of the hair follicle or pore opening. Within a short time the skin surrounding the hair follicle becomes inflamed, sensitive, and tender and discharges pus. As with impetigo, the infection spreads rapidly from one hair follicle to another, most commonly on the beard or in the scalp. The infection sometimes is transmitted from unclean instruments or unsanitary procedures in the barber shop, and is more common in people with diseases such as diabetes. Even if true diabetes is not present, persons whose blood sugar or skin sugar content is high show a particular tendency toward the development of pus infections of the skin such as folliculitis, boils, and carbuncles. Recurrent attacks of these conditions are often successfully treated by a low sugar and starch diet in combination with proper hygiene and antiseptic agents.

Boils. When the same pus-forming bacteria that produce impetigo and folliculitis dig farther in and attack the deeper parts of the follicles and the oil glands, a deep, round, inflamed mass develops. The result is a boil.

Boils are common enough to be considered slightly amusing by everyone except their victims. They are painful, hard, red lumps like marbles surrounding each hair follicle. Some tend to soften and form a soft, pus-discharging core. That is, the center around the follicle discharges the pus and the rim remains hard and bright red. When the center has softened sufficiently, it may be removed. A pus-discharging ulcer is then left, which empties itself and heals, often leaving a scar.

Boils are quite frequently the accompaniment of constitutional disorders. Almost invariably they indicate a run-down condition, if not a serious disease.

Diabetes is often accompanied by boils. Frequent boils should send the patient to a physician for a general examination and treatment.

When the rim or wall of a boil is soft—because of a poor general resistance —the infection is not well confined and tends to spread and invade the blood. Abscesses may develop in other parts of the body, such as around the kidneys, and general blood infections may result. Sometimes these infections are fatal. Boils with firm borders are, therefore, more easily cured and less dangerous.

In certain occupations in which the skin is likely to be injured or exposed to dirt, tar, petroleum, or other chemicals, there is a constant danger of contracting boils. Bromides and iodides taken internally may produce boils and folliculitis. Both boils and folliculitis may affect any part of the face and neck. Folliculitis, of course, is more likely to occur on the bearded parts of the face. It is more chronic and obstinate, but boils are more painful.

A boil on the upper lip or in the nose is especially to be watched. It is extremely dangerous and may cause death. This is because the blood circulation of the upper lip is extensive, and also is upward to the brain. Poisons draining from the lip, therefore, may cause meningitis and abscesses of the brain.

Carbuncles. There is a widespread confusion of ideas about boils and carbuncles. A great many people rather naturally think they are the same thing. They are distinctly different, but the difference is more in degree than in kind.

A carbuncle is larger, deeper, more destructive, and vastly more serious than a boil. It is an infection by a pus-forming germ, like the boil; but it is always accompanied by the symptoms of a severe and acute illness.

A carbuncle is a hard, rounded, inflammatory mass, extending down through the corium into the subcutaneous tissues. It goes deeper than the boil, which seldom extends below the upper part of the corium. A boil affects only one hair follicle. A carbuncle affects several, through which pus is discharged from the inflamed center.

With carbuncles may be fever, chills, loss of weight, and general discomfort. In addition, there may be symptoms of a metabolic disease, such as diabetes. Because of this, a main feature of the treatment of carbuncles is the employment of every measure that will build up the body and help it to fight the disease.

The Treatment of Pus-Producing Infections
(Folliculitis, Boils, Carbuncles)

In the treatment of folliculitis, boils, and carbuncles, the doctor finds out if any constitutional disease is present and corrects it. Even if no such disease is discovered, it is advisable to clean out the bowels, remove sweets and indigestible foods from the diet, and take any measures necessary to bring the system's powers of resistance up to par. Plenty of fresh air and sunlight and a great deal of water, outside and inside, are highly desirable. Irritation, dirt, and harmful chemicals should be avoided, of course.

The physician may decide to rely on immunization in order to stimulate the defensive forces of the body. Either the so-called stock vaccines, or a vaccine made from germs in the pus given off by the patient may be used. It is necessary to regulate the dosage carefully, or there will be severe reactions. In recent years the sulfa drugs, penicillin, aureomycin, and other potent remedies of modern science have been remarkably effective in curing episodes of these diseases. They are usually not effective in the chronic and recurrent types, although small doses carefully supervised over a period of time may prove effective.

There are two main fallacies about the treatment of folliculitis and boils. One is that the face must not be shaved, and the other is that boils must always be cut. Actually, the face should be shaved daily. The reason for keeping hair off the face is that infection is minimized and the local applications can penetrate more readily. Boils usually need not be cut. Cutting breaks down the rim, or defensive wall that the body builds around the infection, and this opens up the blood and lymph vessels and so permits the spread of the infection. It is rarely necessary to cut boils, as a matter of fact; but when it is done, the most thorough asepsis and antisepsis must be enforced.

The main aim of treatment, indeed, should be the enforcement of cleanliness and personal hygiene and the administration of measures that will reduce and remove the infection. The boils and the skin around them should be washed several times a day with soap and water. Following the washings, alcohol and water or antiseptic solutions should be lightly dabbed on and then antiseptic dressings applied. Avoid irritating and infecting the skin around the boils.

When the boils are tense and tender, a wet dressing of a 5 per cent Burow's solution or a 5 per cent sodium propionate solution—not a compress—relieves the pain and encourages the softening and evacuation of pus. It is a mistake to put heavy bandages, oilskin, or gutta-percha over the gauze to form a compress. The dense texture of these materials causes a retention of the heat and the pus discharge, and nurtures the growth of the germs. In early cases wet applications are aided by X-ray treatments. Ultraviolet rays also are useful in improving some local infections. Of even greater value are a whole score of new drugs, including the sulfa drugs, penicillin, bacitracin, aureomycin, and terramycin. These drugs may be used either locally or internally, depending on the severity of the infection.

The same sort of treatment is employed for carbuncles, but here surgery may be necessary if wet dressings, the antibiotics, and X-ray therapy are not effective.

As may readily be imagined, these pus infections are not trivial. The best way to treat them is not to have them. And the best way to achieve that happy state is to keep the general constitution up to its highest tone, and to make a habit of strict cleanliness and an intelligent, balanced diet.

Spirochetes—Syphilis

Syphilis is no longer considered as a disease to be discussed in whispers by both younger and older generations. This is an era in which prudery has little, if any, place. We are more concerned in measures and effects that will improve the public health and which must be known by those who wish to protect themselves. We must understand the early and beginning symptoms of a disease such as syphilis, so that any suspicious symptom may be promptly investigated. At present the ease and speed of eradication of the disease depend chiefly on the early diagnosis of the condition. A disease such as syphilis does not merely affect one part of the body, but can spread to affect almost any organ or tissue in the system. Furthermore, if the initial symptoms are disregarded, the germs which cause the disease quietly dig into the internal organs and produce serious damage which cannot be remedied if it has been persistent for many years. In this chapter the purpose for describing and discussing this disease is not so that it can be treated at home. The average person is no better equipped to take care of syphilis than is the quack who preys on frightened and uninformed youngsters without a real knowledge of the proper treatment and fundamentals of medical care. If you develop any symptoms such as those mentioned under this disease, discuss them with your family physician and not with your friends or a so-called sex disease expert who may not even be a qualified physician.

The cause of syphilis is a tiny corkscrew-like germ which swims around in the fluid discharging from a syphilitic sore. It is an organism called a spirochete, and in fresh syphilitic sores the fluid literally swarms with these corkscrew-shaped organisms. This germ is rather delicate and is usually promptly destroyed outside of the body. For this reason, syphilis is usually transmitted only by direct contact with a person who is infected with the disease. Although syphilis may also be acquired and transmitted in other ways, these transmissions are quite uncommon and the disease is truthfully called a venereal disease. The germ usually requires the presence of an open wound or slightly irritated mucous membrane such as the mouth, rectum, or outer male and female genital organs, to enter the body. Although syphilis may be transmitted through the sputum, after kissing, this method of transmission is slight in comparison to sexual intercourse as the primary means of infecting another person with syphilis.

Syphilis is usually divided by the physician into three stages. During the first stage the infection usually appears as a small sore on the genital organs. This sore usually appears within two weeks following sexual intercourse. Any sore which develops on the genital region at this period of time should be examined by your physician. He can usually perform a test known as a dark field examination, which will promptly disclose the presence of spirochetes if the sore is due to syphilis. If it is not, you are better off being told that such is the case, rather than waiting to see what happens. At this stage the germ has only started to get into the blood stream and so the Wassermann test does not become positive until a later date. If this primary stage is disregarded, the sore usually heals in a few weeks and the glands in the groin, which are swollen at the time of this primary sore or chancre, usually go down. The germ is now being transported around the body, and the unfortunate victim is passing into the second stage. If the second stage is mild, the infected person may not know that he has syphilis for many years, when it will either be disclosed by the performance of a routine blood test, or by symptoms of a serious nature.

In the secondary stage of syphilis, which appears within six weeks or so, the chief symptoms are an extensive rash, a peculiar loss of hair, and often what seems to be an ordinary cold or sore throat accompanied by slight fever and achy or "grippy" symptoms. One of the unfortunate features of the disease is that the secondary stage may be mild, and the patient may feel that he merely has a slight cold. The rash may be mild enough to be overlooked, and he may be completely unaware of the fact that his entire system is going through a mighty battle in order to build up resistance against the germs which have spread to every part of the body by way of the blood stream. Another unfortunate feature of the disease is that lack of awareness of this stage means that the victim can easily transmit it. During this secondary period the saliva and all other body secretions are loaded with the organisms, and it is very easily transmitted. To get back to the rash, it may be stated that it looks like measles and is usually present on the body rather than on the face. The hair fall is of a peculiar type in that it usually consists of either a diffuse thinning of the entire scalp, or of the appearance of small bald patches. These bald patches are so characteristic, in that they look mangy or moth-eaten, that it is described in medical textbooks as the typical moth-eaten appearance of the scalp in secondary syphilis. During this stage the blood shows a strongly positive Wassermann test and the diagnosis can readily be established.

After several weeks or months the secondary stage passes, and the symptoms gradually disappear. If laboratory tests have not been performed on the blood and spinal fluid, the disease may pass unnoticed until the person passes into the final or tertiary stage of syphilis. This stage may not appear for many years and it is due to the destruction of various internal tissues and organs by the spirochete which eats away insidiously at these tissues over the years. This stage persists until the end of the patient's life and may even remain undiscovered if the symptoms are not sufficiently pronounced to bring the patient to the doctor. In the ignorant and uninformed this occasionally is the case. The average person with the tertiary stage of syphilis has usually had such mild primary and secondary stages that he was never aware of the presence of the disease. At some stage in his life either a routine blood test or a general examination brings to light the presence of the disease. The symptoms of the tertiary stage may consist of extensive sores on the skin, or changes involving any portion of the body, including the eyes, ears, nerves, blood vessels and heart, the liver, and the brain. These changes are usually so extensive and severe as to shorten the life span.

The symptoms described present the picture of a serious and unpleasant disease. The disease will only be eradicated in time by early diagnosis and prompt examination following any suspicious exposure. Don't let fear keep you away from the physician! He is sworn to secrecy and will protect your privacy as well as your health. Fortunately, public health authorities have made tremendous strides in wiping out the sources of infection among prostitutes and other groups which are responsible for the constant transmission of the disease. Only with lessened secrecy and more intelligent knowledge and information concerning the disease, will it eventually disappear. Modern treatment methods are such that the disease can be completely cured and its transmission prevented if an early diagnosis is made. Even the late and severe stages of the disease can be dramatically helped by prompt and adequate therapeutic measures. The old methods of treatment with arsenic, bismuth, and other heavy metals have to a great measure been displaced by the newer drugs, especially penicillin. Whereas formerly it was necessary to treat patients over a period of years, the disease is now practically completely eradicated in weeks with massive doses of penicillin, as well as some of the other drugs. The advances of science will eventually force the disappearance of this dread disease, but this will only come about with intelligent understanding and co-operation on the part of the general public.

Virus Infections

Fever Blisters (Herpes Simplex)

Small groups of blisters break out on the face when we catch cold or get too much sun. They usually appear around the mouth or nose as tender and tense small blisters which rapidly become crusted and sore. Herpes are due to a virus and are actually an infection, difficult to transmit. Some people seem to be peculiarly susceptible to them and get herpes regularly whenever they get a cold or sore throat. Others get herpes whenever they are exposed to too much sun or wind. The blisters seem to have a favorite site for recurrence so that some people always develop them around the mouth, yet others only get them around the nose or elsewhere on the body. They also occur in association with certain severe infections or high fevers, for example, pneumonia. They also occur at the time of menstruation, but this may often be due to some drug taken for the relief of menstrual cramps.

Herpes usually dry up and disappear within one week to ten days. The healing process may be accelerated by the use of drying lotions and powders. In the initial stage spirits of camphor or tincture of benzoin may make the tender area less sensitive and hasten the drying of the blisters. Of value also is plain zinc oxide ointment containing a fraction of a per cent of menthol. When herpes simplex recur constantly in the same spot, this may be prevented by a few X-ray treatments to the affected area. Other people who develop recurrent fever blisters may be immunized against them more or less permanently by four to eight smallpox vaccinations at intervals of two weeks. It seems as though the smallpox vaccination immunizes against the herpes virus as well as against the smallpox virus.

SHINGLES (HERPES ZOSTER)

Shingles is also a virus infection like herpes simplex, but is more severe in its effects. The name *zoster* is derived from the Greek and means girdle. It got that name because the virus infects part of a nerve and the eruption appears all along the course of the nerve, thereby girdling or encircling the body. Only one side of the body is involved, and so the rash appears as a group of blisters traveling from back to front along one side of the body. Because the nerve is infected, this eruption causes severe neuralgia and the pain may be very distressing. In fact, the pain often lasts long after the rash is gone, and the poor sufferer complains far more because of the neuralgia than because of the rash.

If shingles is treated early with antibiotics such as aureomycin or terramycin, the infection may disappear quickly. In other instances, if the pain is not great, the whole process may be treated satisfactorily with drying powders, lotions, and salves. The neuralgia may be so severe that drugs like codeine and others may be necessary. The occasional severe attack may even require blocking or destruction of the sensitive and irritated nerve. Fortunately, dangerous complications of shingles are rare, and the disease hardly ever recurs.

Parasites

Vegetable Parasites (Ringworm)

This old name of ringworm was given to the disease because of a misconception of the cause of the ring shape of the patches on the skin. It is a complete misnomer, because the disease, in most of its manifestations, is not in the shape of rings. Of course, worms have no part in producing the disease. It is due to many different cousins of the common molds which attack bread left in an open moist place. This has been known for many years by the medical profession. Only lately have the doctors realized how important and widespread these infections are.

On the feet this disease is carried between the toes of a large percentage of those who consider themselves perfectly healthy. The wonder is not that it breaks out in other parts now and then; but that this happens so seldom. So far as is now known, it is spread chiefly by walking on moist, infected floors of bathrooms, gymnasiums, and golf clubs, and in evidence of this fact is the more modern name "athlete's foot."

The treatment of these infections is often difficult and taxes the ingenuity of the physician. The hair and nail infections are most difficult of all forms to treat, and the latter is one of the important sources for the spread of the infection. Fortunately, many new remedies are now available both for control and treatment of the ringworm. The majority of these effective agents are derived from non-irritating, fatty acids first discovered in human sweat. These acids may be incorporated in liquids, powders, and ointments. Cleanliness of the feet and frequent powdering, particularly care to keep the clefts between the toes clean and dry, is of great importance in preventing infection. Women have less ringworm than the men, probably because of better care of their feet. There is little doubt that a great difference of susceptibility to these organisms exists, and those afflicted may not be lax in regard to cleanliness but only unfortunate in their susceptibility.

Treatment of most cases of ringworm should be kept up for a long time after cure has apparently been obtained. The organisms lurk among the skin cells and await an opportunity, perhaps in the form of simple moisture, to multiply rapidly and cause another outbreak.

Everyone has a pet remedy for his own case of ringworm, but the same remedy may wreak havoc on someone else's skin. If your athlete's foot or jockey itch does not get better from simple hygienic measures, don't use your friend's remedy but seek professional advice. Some of the newer drugs such as the undecylenates, propionates, salicylanilides, and many others may actually cure that "old faithful" ringworm of yours, so don't give up hope!

ANIMAL PARASITES

1. *Lice*—The three forms of lice which feed on man obtain their nourishment from blood sucked from the hair follicles. In procuring this food they inject a poison into the skin, which causes intense itching. Among ordinary folks the best known of this disgusting family of parasites is the head louse, pediculus capitis. The children of the family too frequently bring home samples of the parasite in the hair. Its eggs, called nits, are tiny white pear-shaped bodies glued to the hair. The parent louse has a semitranslucent gray body and is not easily distinguished through the hair. Scratch marks and bloody crusts, sometimes pustules and matting of the hair are seen.

Thorough soaking of the hair and scalp with a mixture of equal parts of kerosene and sweet oil is an old method of eradicating the lice. A cap is formed of cloths soaked in the mixture and left upon the head overnight. The next morning a thorough shampoo is given, and after this hot vinegar applied to loosen the nits, which then are removed with a fine comb. Modern methods of cure are much more effective. They include the use of DDT, HCH, and similar chemicals in the form of ointments or lotions applied for comparatively short periods of time. When large groups of children are infected, powder sprays of DDT have been very effective. They kill the parasites with speed and efficiency.

The body louse lives in the clothing and only moves to the skin at mealtime. It attaches its eggs to the fibers of the underwear. To obtain blood it marches over to the skin. This explains why the bloody crusts and itchy pimples which are typical signs of this disease are found most plentiful on parts like the waist and shoulders, where the clothing rests closely upon the skin. The derelict and the hobo, as well as those who neglect cleanliness of body and clothing, harbor body lice though it must be recognized that some people are much more attractive to the louse than are others. Body lice carry typhus, a dangerous disease fortunately rare in the United States, but a great problem when our troops entered Italy during the last war. A mild form of typhus is associated with rats, possibly carried by their fleas.

"Crabs" are caused by the pubic or "crab" louse, and this nasty parasite is found clinging to the pubic hairs with its head down close to the skin. At times the parasite travels to the armpits, the chests of hairy men, or even to the eyebrows and eyelashes. Although formerly a great nuisance and difficult to eradicate, the parasites are now destroyed with ease due to the use of DDT and similar chemicals in a form suitable for application to the pubic region. What a transition from the weeks of constant observation and the shamefaced isolation endured by the victims of "crabs" in former years!

2. *The Itch* (*Scabies*)—The itch mite, a member of the spider family, is

small. The male mite is smaller than the female. Living on the surface of the skin, his only purpose in life seems to be the propagation of his kind because the female often destroys him after impregnation. She then burrows into and along the upper part of the skin, depositing her eggs as she goes, producing a small canal about one fourth of an inch long. As the eggs hatch the canal loses its roof and appears as a dark, wavy silk thread, seen most easily between the fingers. Itching is more severe at night, because the female itch mite is a night worker.

The diagnosis of scabies is often difficult. A doctor should always be consulted. Much damage can be done by unsupervised home treatment of this disease and the other conditions frequently confused with it, whereas proper medical treatment employing benzyl benzoate, DDT, and sulfur may promptly eradicate the mites.

3. *Insect Bites*—Many insects use man as their source of food supply. Mosquitoes, flies, bedbugs, and fleas are some of the many insects which disturb our travels and trips to the country. They all produce somewhat similar reactions in the skin, depending upon the individual. Some people are completely immune to their bites, but the usual reaction consists of a tiny red spot at the site of the bite, followed by itching and a small, whitish swelling or bump. There are even reports of people so sensitive to these bites that fever, chills, and severe constitutional reactions may result from them.

The first problem is one of prevention and this may be accomplished by extermination of the particular pest. DDT sprays and various new insect repellents are effective with precautions taken to avoid overexposure to these chemicals by the humans rather than the insects. Thorough housecleaning and removal of dust and rubbish may also be necessary.

Treatment consists merely of soothing lotions and tinctures. Calamine lotion with 1 per cent phenol is still a useful remedy. The more severe reactions respond well to the antihistaminic drugs.

SKIN GROWTHS

CORNS

Corns are caused by pressure, as everyone knows, usually that of improperly shaped shoes. The world is slowly becoming more sensible in its dress, but tight-fitting shoes are still much in favor, and corns still flourish. The only effectual treatment is protection from pressure. Removing the central horny plug with a knife, or softening with a salicylic acid preparation, followed by soaking in hot water and scraping out the plug is good treatment, but is of no lasting benefit unless the pressure is removed. Sometimes a soft felt pad may take the pressure off the callus or corn and cause it to disappear. Anything that does not yield to such treatment over a period of a few weeks is probably a wart and requires treatment for that condition.

WARTS

Because they are at first tiny, flat, skin-colored elevations that are inconspicuous, warts are often neglected until they have had an opportunity to show their ability to grow and spread. The original wart may remain single and stationary for a time, but a month or so later a new wart may appear near this spot. This property is called autoinoculability; that is, we can infect ourselves again and again. In this way whole crops of warts are raised, like dandelions, where they are least desired. It is plain, therefore, that warts should not be picked with the teeth or fingernails or pared with the pocketknife. The virus that causes warts belongs to the interesting group of "filtrable viruses," whose ability to pass through the finest porcelain filter has given them the name.

Ordinarily warts are painless; but sometimes on the fingers, and commonly on the soles of the feet, they are tender, causing exquisite pain during walking, dancing, or as a support for someone else's feet.

Ever since prehistoric time warts have been treated successfully by suggestion. Tom Sawyer's method and many others like it which are still used by boys all over the world are survivors of the ancient practice of the witch or voodoo doctor. The modern child is often too sophisticated, even at an early age, to have any faith in such practices, and other methods must be used. The only objection to the faith cures is their encouragement of false beliefs and gullibility, which is even worse than warts. Warts respond to treatment with various chemicals, X-rays or radium, and the "electric needle." Some of the newer "wart" remedies include extremely potent chemicals such as tri-chloracetic acid and mixtures of podophyllin. Because warts are sometimes difficult to cure even with the most modern methods, the treatment is best left to the physician. A popular home treatment is the use of nitric acid. This is mentioned only to be condemned, for it often results in unsightly scars or even keloids.

Seborrheic warts are the brown to black-topped elevations that occur on the trunk, less often on the face or scalp, of people in middle life or later. They are of no consequence except for the fact that they are sometimes hard to distinguish from senile keratoses, which are important lesions in that they may be the forerunners of skin cancer.

SEBACEOUS CYSTS (WENS)

Sebaceous cysts or "wens" usually occur on the face, back, or scalp. However, they may appear on any part of the body surface in which there are oil glands. They are a result of a blocking of the mouth of the oil gland or hair follicle with an accumulation of oily or cheesy material under the skin. The skin around this cheesy secretion develops an actual cheese bag or pocket in order to contain this material. This bag or cyst continues to grow larger until it is a large lump in the surface of the skin. Sometimes a small black pore communicates with the interior of the cyst, and some of its cheesy contents can be squeezed out through this opening. Often several cysts of different sizes are scattered about this surface of the body. They should be removed because of the possibility of infection, and in a small percentage of cases of cancer.

These cysts may be cut out surgically, but they should not be opened unless a complete removal is planned. However, the resulting scar may be small if one of the newer techniques for removal is employed. By one of these methods, an electric needle is inserted into the cyst and its contents are actually "cooked." Subsequently the cooked cheesy material expels itself with the wall of the sac. Other methods include injection of the cyst with penicillin and other drugs and a gradual expression of its contents. When performed with painstaking care, this method may result in removal of the cyst with practically no scar formation.

MOLES

Moles are birthmarks, even though, as often happens, they do not appear until adult life. The ordinary skin-colored or brown mole, whether covered with hair or not, seldom becomes dangerous except when exposed to chronic irritation. When located so that the clothing rubs upon them, or so that they are frequently cut in shaving or possibly irritated in some other way, they should be removed thoroughly by the physician. Any mole that starts to grow rapidly, bleed easily, or show any type of unusual change, should be examined promptly by a physician and as promptly removed if the doctor considers it necessary.

Blue moles, much less common than the brown kind, but not rare, are in a class by themselves. They may last throughout life without change. Consult your physician about them if there is any question as to change in the mole.

KELOIDS (OVERGROWN SCARS)

Keloids are benign tumors (tumors that practically never become malignant) which grow in scars. At times there is no history of a preceding scar; but it may have been so slight that it was not noticed. Some people have the peculiar tendency to form keloids in their scars, or these tumors may occur in some of their scars and not in others. They should not be cut out because of their ability to return promptly, thereby resulting in a larger tumor than before the operation, unless treated at the same time with radium or X-rays which have a very beneficial effect on them. The careful application of solid carbon dioxide ("dry ice") by the physician has also been found of value in the treatment of keloids.

XANTHOMA (YELLOW SPOTS)

Xanthoma is the name given to the yellow tumors caused by the deposits of fat in the skin. Some of us seem to have an inability to dispose of fats in the normal way, and the skin serves as an exit station. The only form of this disease seen frequently involves the skin around the eyelids, most often the inner part of the lower lid, in the form of small yellowish elevations. They can be removed by the physician with the production of very slight scarring. They may return if the internal condition that causes them is still operative, though seldom sufficiently so to cause other symptoms.

VASCULAR BIRTHMARKS

Vascular birthmarks may be flat "port-wine marks," slightly elevated, flat-topped "strawberry marks," or egglike swellings composed of groups of veins in a grapelike mass. The large swellings are easily compressed, but return immediately to their original shape, and tend to become bluish and still larger when the baby cries. Often the skin over such a mark is the site of one of the flat kinds already mentioned. All these growths should be treated during infancy, when the skin is able to renew itself most readily and the resulting scars are smaller. Furthermore, although some of these bloody tumors may disappear, many of them grow larger rather than smaller.

The vascular tumors respond well to proper methods of treatment. The flat or port-wine stain may be improved by abrasive scraping with an electric drill. The strawberry mark can be removed by the electric needle, "dry ice," or by injection with a strong solution (sclerosing solution). The deep or cavernous type of bloody tumor may be removed by the two latter methods or by means of contact X-ray therapy or radium applications.

KERATOSES

Keratoses are of two kinds. The soft or seborrheic variety are brownish, velvety plaques which appear during middle age. They are of no significance and can easily be removed from the skin. They are commonly seen on the face and back.

The hard or senile keratosis is more serious in nature. It is a rough, scaly spot often found on the face and backs of the hands. People who are exposed to a great deal of sun and wind over a period of years often develop these spots. Farmers and sailors are particularly apt to develop these spots because of their constant exposure to the elements. These small scaly or warty growths must be removed because they may turn into cancers of the skin. Removal may be accomplished by cutting or burning them off. The only important fact is to make certain the removal is a complete one. People who develop senile keratoses should protect themselves from the sun and wind, following the removal of these growths.

CANCER OF THE SKIN

Cancer of the skin offers the doctor one peculiar advantage over cancer in other parts of the body in that it can be seen at its beginning and treated early. Inability to do this is the chief reason why cancer elsewhere cannot be cured as readily. Any unusual growth on or in the skin should be shown to the physician at once, without taking the great risk of home treatment or delaying treatment until ulceration occurs. The idea that cancer always causes pain is another very harmful one, for skin cancer seldom causes pain until it is in the last stage, when it is too late to save the patient's life. Home treatment is worse than simple delay, for it is like trying to put out a fire by pouring on gasoline. If anything will insure the change from a harmless to a malignant growth, or encourage one that is already malignant, the usually irritating home treatment will do so.

Scaly spots, warts, or growths on the lips and the hands should have attention early, for cancer occurring on these parts is apt to be more malignant than upon the face. The great strides made in the treatment of malignancy are due to the early recognition and removal of suspicious growths. Any "mole," "wart," or similar spot on the skin should be examined by your doctor promptly if it becomes sensitive, enlarges in size, bleeds readily, forms a crust, or ulcerates. Make certain that the wart or lump on your skin is harmless by having it examined rather than by waiting for trouble!

Miscellaneous Skin Conditions
ACNE VULGARIS

Acne vulgaris is a disease of the oil glands of the skin. At puberty, along with other changes in the body, these glands develop and frequently take on excessive activity, causing the skin to become greasy and plugs to form in the pores. These plugs of grease undergo a chemical change and show as black points on the skin, commonly called blackheads, and by the doctors, comedones. These plugs cause some irritation, as do all foreign bodies in the skin (wood, glass), and nature tries to eliminate them by the formation of pus. When the pustule breaks, the comedo is forced out with the pus. Unfortunately, if the pus remains too long in the deeper lesions before being freed, the pressure and dissolving action of the pus destroys the tissue about it. This loss must be replaced by scar tissue, leaving a permanent disfigurement. If scarring does not follow the pustule, the process may be repeated many times in the same follicle. Acne tends to clear up as the patient grows older, but the risk of scarring is too great and the distress of the young person at the disfigurement too acute to justify neglect of treatment. Don't neglect the early treatment of acne if you wish to have your child develop as few holes or pits in the skin as possible. And remember, at this impressionable age the seeds of an inferiority complex are easily sown. The physician, opening the pustules with a tiny knife, is not causing scars, as many think. He is preventing them by releasing the pus before it has time to destroy tissue.

Since acne occurs usually in greasy skins, acne is benefited by the free use of hot water and soap. Children affected with the disease should not be accused of causing it by reluctance to use these measures. No amount of scrubbing can cure a real case of acne. Neither is acne a sign of sexual irregularity, as some ignorant persons insinuate. The unfortunates afflicted with the disease are embarrassed enough because of their facial blemishes without the added cruelty of such insinuations.

In mild cases pustules may be few and comedones many, forming small yellowish elevations with a yellow, brown, or black point in the center. When the horny layer of the skin forms completely over the surface, the end of the fatty plug cannot become dirty but remains as a white pearl-like body called milium, or whitehead. These remain without much increase in size until removed and do not recur as promptly as the blackheads.

Acne is not always confined to the face, but also involves the chest, upper back, and outer sides of the arms. In persons of low resistance it becomes a disfiguring, distressing, and indeed serious disease. Cold cream or other greasy applications should not be used, for the skin already has too much fat. Massage is apt to do harm because of the cream employed. Patent medicines called "blood purifiers" are apt to make acne worse, because many of them contain iodides. The acne patient does not need this type of "blood purifier."

Removal of blackheads is beneficial, as can easily be understood when the method of formation of pus pimples is considered. It should be done with care, however, not to injure the skin by too much force. Many nervous patients increase their disfigurement by too enthusiastic attempts to remove blackheads by squeezing without preliminary loosening. The face should first be washed thoroughly with hot water and soap, hot towels applied for about ten minutes and then the skin sponged with alcohol. If necessary a needle, sterilized by flaming, or a blackhead remover, a small instrument with a hole about 1/16 of an inch in diameter in one end, may be used to help remove the blackheads. After the blackheads have thus been removed, the application of hot towels should be repeated, followed by a short application of cold water and drying with a towel. This second application of heat lessens the inflammatory reaction to the pressure. Deep pustules, the kind that are most apt to cause scars, should be opened by the physician.

Care of the health is important in all children, but particularly in those who have acne. Fresh air, good food, proper exercise, and plenty of sleep are essential to good health. Strict dieting seldom cures acne and may do harm if not properly supervised. Many youngsters with this disease need restraint, however, in the matter of eating and drinking, and should be particularly warned against the bad effect of sweet carbonated drinks, nuts, greasy foods, excessive condiments, chocolate candy and ice cream. Irregularity in the eating and sleeping schedule is also harmful. Constipation should be avoided by the generous use of vegetables and fruits and by the formation of regular habits of bowel evacuation.

This somewhat lengthy discourse on acne is not intended to convey the idea that acne can be cured by home treatment. Only the mildest cases can be handled without the help of the physician. Under medical supervision, the proper use of some of the newer drugs (both internally and externally) may result in rapid improvement of the condition.

Cleanliness is essential. Soap and water are fundamental, and the face should be vigorously washed several times daily. A good astringent should be rubbed into the skin after each washing. At night salves containing chemicals such as sulfur and resorcin are left on overnight to soften the blackheads and peel off the top layer of affected skin. In addition, your doctor applies various chemicals such as a carbon-dioxide slush and various peeling pastes to accelerate the cure. Ultraviolet light performs a similar aid in treatment. Although X-ray was formerly used in the treatment of many cases of acne, it is seldom used now except in the resistant and stubborn cases of acne. However, modern science has found out that certain hormones and chemicals such as the antibotics may be helpful in the treatment of acne. Even the pits and scars produced by the disease can be removed by the newer techniques of facial planing and drilling. Don't neglect your child's skin, because acne is a disease that can and should be controlled from its onset.

ROSACEA

Rosacea, or acne rosacea, is the disease that reddens the nose and cheeks, and in extreme cases causes enlargement of the end of the nose, popularly called "whiskey nose" or "grog blossom." This title is not justified, for many sufferers from this disease are strict abstainers from alcoholic drinks. The trouble is caused by a nervous reflex flushing of the sensitive blood vessels of these areas on the face as a response to internal changes or abnormal local conditions in the mouth or nose. Anything which tends to cause flushing or heating of the face should be avoided. The patient can do much to restrain its development by the avoidance of hot foods or drinks, spicy or peppery foods, and particularly alcoholic beverages. Alcohol irritates the stomach and sets up the reflex already mentioned, at the same time that it acts directly to dilate the peripheral blood vessels. After frequent dilatations, the vessels become paralyzed and remain as disfiguring red or bluish lines. The consequent slowing of the circulation is probably the chief reason for the enlargement of the end of the nose. This can be improved by treatment with proper diet and astringent, local measures including powdered carbon-dioxide "slush."

For direct treatment of the skin, the main thing is merely washing the face frequently. But it should be washed with soap and cold water, or rubbed with ice. This is a marvelous tonic; it peps up the muscles and blood vessels and keeps them small and contracted. It is difficult to resist the temptation to break into eulogy of water. No cosmetic ever devised can compare with plain cold water as a tonic, cleanser, and beautifier combined. The only drawback to water is its cheapness. If it could be obtained only in tiny, ornate flasks at ten dollars an ounce, it would sweep a vast amount of perfumed trash off the toilet table!

There are, however, certain preparations which help cold water in fighting rosacea. They are all astringent in nature. Rose water and boric acid solutions and emulsions containing sulphur are especially valuable. The best sulphur lotions, such as lotio alba, tend to prevent grease formation, and as they evaporate cool the skin, contract the blood vessels, and leave the sulphur powder on the skin.

Where there is irritation in addition to the redness, the skin should be soothed with wet dressings of boric acid (2 per cent), or zinc oxide lotions, such as calamine lotion, before the sulphur is employed. In using these preparations, some of the mixture should be poured into a saucer and applied with a piece of clean flannel cloth. The best time to apply any such preparation is at night, so that it can remain on the face until morning, when it should be washed off with cold water and soap. After this, a fine powder or a thin, invisible lotion may be dabbed on.

Vinegar, witch hazel, and weak alum in solutions of less than 5 per cent are good, mild astringents. Too strong a reaction of the skin is harmful; but drugs such as resorcin, ichthyol, and camphor are sometimes used successfully.

There is a general delusion that massage of the face is necessary in treating rosacea. Barbers are apt to prescribe it, as well as operators in beauty parlors. The fact is that massage of a diseased face is injurious. It irritates an inflamed skin and spreads infection. When the skin is unhealthy, it is very easy for it to contract infection from the masseur's fingers.

Electrolysis can do much to reduce telangiectasias—the enlarged blood vessels which show as purplish streaks. The operation is the same as that for the destruction of the follicles in hypertrichosis, or superfluous hair. The electric needle is inserted along the course of the vessel and the current allowed to flow until the vessel is destroyed. The application of the electric cautery will also destroy the unsightly vessels, if done skillfully. After such treatment, cold applications and astringents are applied.

These same methods of treatment are employed for cases where the nose is tremendously enlarged or has a hanging growth; but the quickest and best method is removal of this growth by surgical operation. The growth is cut away surgically; if the bleeding is profuse, it is easily stopped by pressure and ice. Operations by this technic usually produce excellent results. X-ray or caustics prevent the regrowth of tissue after the operation, and caustics are used to destroy the follicles which have produced the excess growth.

Rosacea is no longer a difficult problem. With proper diet and internal measures, plus effective external applications, the victim may again regain a normal complexion. It requires self-control and patience on his part, and both proper diagnosis and therapy on the part of his physician.

HIVES

Hives or urticaria affect many people. You may get it the first time you eat strawberries or peaches. Or you may spend an uncomfortable night after that delicious lobster. Or that last injection of penicillin which cured your boil shows up again one week later in the form of little swellings or wheals all over your body. The hive itself is a small whitish or pinkish bump which can appear anywhere on the body. It means that you are allergic to something or other, and if you are lucky you can quickly blame the strawberries, the lobster, or the penicillin. Alas, not all hive sufferers can find the cause of their symptoms so quickly, and a long, tedious search may be necessary if the hives keep on appearing over a prolonged period of time.

Usually the wheal is what is called evanescent. It comes and goes. It may last only for a second, or it may remain twenty-four hours. It sometimes appears so suddenly that it can actually be seen swelling. The wheals vary in size from that of a pea to a patch big enough to cover the whole face. Usually round or oval, they are sometimes irregular or ring-shaped, or they may develop like a map or become scalloped in shape.

There is usually itching, and sometimes burning or tingling or creeping sensations in the skin. Frequently the itching is intense. Another condition occurring with the hives is dermographism. This phenomenon consists in the appearance upon irritation of elevated white spots bounded by pink borders, which take the outline of the irritation that causes them. The irritation may be only slight pressure, or it may be pinching or scratching. In medical schools it is demonstrated to the students by stroking the patient's skin, or writing on it with a finger. The elevations appear whenever the finger touches the skin.

The wheal is produced by practically anything which affects the blood vessels of the skin. It is supposed to be due to a combined action of the nervous system acting on the blood vessels. The blood vessels are first closed in the central zone which results in the white area of the wheal. Those on the border are open to make the pink area.

Although hives may be produced by almost any kind of external or internal irritation, the more serious types are associated with constitutional and emotional disorders. Even when external causes are apparently the only ones, there is almost surely some disturbance or defect in the vasomotor system—the mechanism which controls the blood vessels and their nerves.

The internal disorders which produce hives fall into special groups. There are those due to allergy or to a sensitivity to proteins; those due to the taking of such drugs as quinine, aspirin, cathartics, or any other drug for which the individual has an idiosyncrasy; disturbances of the metabolism; disturbances of the blood; and nervous disorders. Still another group is due to intestinal disorders. Another group is due to the reaction from eating certain foods. Children especially suffer from this type of hives.

An attack of hives is usually of short duration. Twenty-four hours at most should cover the appearance and disappearance of the wheal. There are, however, short attacks which recur for several weeks. Other cases last for a long time. The itching is intense in the prolonged cases.

The great point is to discover the cause. In acute cases a simple diet is usually ordered and a thorough cleansing of the bowels. Large amounts of water should be imbibed—alkaline water is especially good—and a brief diet consisting mainly of skimmed milk, wheat-free cereal, lamb, and toast is advisable.

Chronic cases require a general examination and the care of a physician. Tests should be performed to determine sensitivity to various foods, pollens, and other possible causes of allergic reactions. Laboratory tests may be necessary, before the constitutional cause can be determined.

Certain drugs are of benefit in treating the hives. These include the new and potent antihistamine drugs, which work wonders in recent and acute attacks of hives. These so-called anti-allergic drugs are less effective in the chronic types.

Adrenalin, one of the most powerful of all drugs, is also valuable in acute cases. It has the special effect of causing the blood vessels to contract, thus diminishing the formation of the wheal. Frequently adrenalin causes the immediate disappearance of the wheals and itching. Ephedrine is also given. But all these drugs are to be taken only on a physician's orders. They may injure the eyes, heart, or nervous system, and may cause peculiar eruptions.

PSORIASIS

Psoriasis is a strange and capricious skin condition, characterized by the appearance of bright red, coin-shaped patches on the skin, especially on the knees and elbows. These bright red patches are often covered with delicate silvery-white scales. When these scales are scraped off the skin, a bright red surface with tiny bleeding spots is characteristic of the disease. Although this disease is not serious in that it does not affect the general health, it can be very annoying in that its constant appearance and reappearance, with spread to involve many different parts of the body, can be a source of great unhappiness. No one knows why this disease occurs. Strangely enough, the condition doesn't seem to bear any relationship whatsoever to various forms of internal or external illness and often affects people who are otherwise in the best of health. It is not infectious or communicable. In a small number of cases the condition may be associated with some form of arthritis.

One of the features of psoriasis has been that patients with the condition usually improve following exposure to sunshine. An old adage used to be that psoriasis does well with grease and water, soap and sunshine. This would mean, of course, the use of some drug in an ointment, following removal of the crusts by soap and water. The average patient with the condition requires a little more than the preceding if he really wants to know how to take care of the condition. Unfortunately, the permanent relief of a severe case of psoriasis cannot be promised as there is no remedy which will produce a permanent cure of the disease. However, the sufferers from this disease often find that common sense and the help of a physician who has had special experience in the treatment of this condition can get him through the severe episodes more rapidly and will often lessen the violence of a flare-up in the condition. The local measures which have been found to be of the greatest value include preparations containing tar, ammoniated mercury, salicylic acid, and chrysarobin. These are strong drugs and capable of doing a considerable amount of damage unless closely supervised by the physician. This is particularly so because the concentrations of the drugs to be employed are usually high if they are to be effective. Continued diligent treatment will often bring about the disappearance of large patches of the disease. Specialists in diseases of the skin have also found that, in certain instances, the use of various drugs taken by mouth will be helpful in improving or controlling the condition. Again, intelligent co-operation between the patient and his doctor is of great value. At the present stage of our medical knowledge, the patient with psoriasis must learn how to live with the disease rather than constantly to fight it. This knowledge can be gained from a combination of expert medical therapy and guidance, plus an intelligent approach to the problem.

Locally, wet dressings and tub baths containing starch or oatmeal may be comforting. The wet applications are more comfortable when cold. On the skin itself lotions or powders containing camphor, phenol, or menthol often afford considerable relief. The antihistaminic drugs (Benadryl, Pyribenzamine) in a cream or lotion form are also effective in relieving itching, but must be carefully watched as they may produce local irritation. In severe cases both cortisone and ACTH have been found to be useful, preferably for a short period of treatment.

LUPUS ERYTHEMATOSUS

This condition is an example of one of the skin diseases which can affect both the skin and the internal organs. The internal form is far more serious and may even occur in the absence of a rash on the skin. However, in the usual case it is associated with a reddish eruption involving the nose and the cheeks in what has been described as a "butterfly pattern." This form occurs most frequently in younger women and is related to overexposure to sunshine. In other words, there is a probability that a strong sunburn in a person who has had a preceding infection, or is predisposed to this disease, may be the aggravating or precipitating factor which touches off the whole process. The subsequent occurrence of changes in the heart, kidneys, and other internal organs would indicate the serious and often fatal nature of the condition. Although the disease has been treated with some success with cortisone and ACTH, these drugs usually serve merely to arrest or lessen the condition rather than result in a complete cure.

The external form is of a somewhat different type in that the victims are not necessarily sick. It also bears some relationship to preceding excessive exposure to sunshine, and is most often present on the nose and cheeks as a red butterfly-type of rash. In addition to the red rash on the face, the scalp is often involved and the skin may show patches of crusts, scars, and bald areas in the scalp. This disease is a serious one, and no attempt should be made to treat it at home. It requires the services of a skilled physician and the use of various internally acting drugs, such as bismuth, gold, arsenic, and others which may be potentially dangerous when taken without constant supervision.

CONTINUED IN VOLUME 8

ILLUSTRATED

MEDICAL

AND

HEALTH

ENCYCLOPEDIA

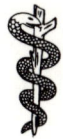

VOLUME 8
SKIN (continued) — ZYME

A Modern Medical and Health Library for the Family
. . . Includes all the Articles From "THE MODERN
HOME MEDICAL ADVISOR" and "THE POPULAR
MEDICAL ENCYCLOPEDIA" Plus Additional
Articles, Photographs and Charts.

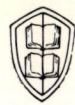

ILLUSTRATED
MEDICAL
AND
HEALTH
ENCYCLOPEDIA

EDITED BY
MORRIS FISHBEIN, M.D.

EDITOR, MEDICAL PROGRESS; EDITOR, MODERN HOME MEDICAL
ADVISER; MEDICAL EDITOR, BRITANNICA BOOK OF THE YEAR;
CONTRIBUTING-EDITOR, POST GRADUATE MEDICINE; AND
FOR 25 YEARS EDITOR OF THE JOURNAL OF
THE AMERICAN MEDICAL ASSOCIATION

WITH THE COLLABORATION OF LEADING
SPECIALISTS IN MEDICINE AND SURGERY

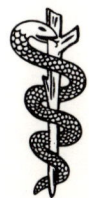

H. S. STUTTMAN CO., *Publishers*
NEW YORK, N. Y.

Copyright © 1957, 1959, 1963, 1966 by Doubleday & Company, Inc.
All Rights Reserved

ILLUSTRATED MEDICAL AND HEALTH ENCYCLOPEDIA contains new entries and illustrations plus material from THE MODERN HOME MEDICAL ADVISOR. (Copyright © 1935, 1939, 1940, 1941, 1942, 1948, 1951, 1953, 1956, by Doubleday and Company, Inc.) and THE POPULAR MEDICAL ENCYCLOPEDIA, revised and enlarged edition, (Copyright © 1946, 1950, 1953, 1956) by Doubleday and Company, Inc.

PRINTED IN THE UNITED STATES OF AMERICA
BY ROTARY GRAPHIC PRESS INC., NEW YORK 16, N. Y.
33P—11-67—15R

PEMPHIGUS

This is an extremely serious disease involving the skin. Its cause is unknown, although recent research would seem to indicate that it may be in part an infection and in part some disturbance in the general metabolism. It usually begins around the nose or mouth as a series of blisters or crusts, which get better or worse and never seem to heal completely. In time practically the entire body becomes covered with small and large blisters. These blisters may join together to form large areas of raw weeping skin. The unfortunate victim literally leaks his life fluid through these open surfaces of the skin. In the majority of instances the disease is fatal within a period of six months to several years. Within the past few years, the occasional patient may be helped considerably with cortisone and ACTH, although the results may merely be a prolongation of life, rather than an actual cure.

SCLERODERMA

This disease is also a serious skin problem. The sufferer develops the condition gradually after having complained of previous circulatory changes in the skin. The hands and feet are cold and bluish in the beginning and eventually become hard, tight, and ulcerate easily. In time both arms and legs may become stony hard and firm to the touch, and the process may even involve the entire body. Not much is known about its cause except that the fibrous tissue and small blood vessels in the true skin have been severely damaged by an unknown toxin. Treatment is not too satisfactory, although some patients have been helped by warm climates, measures designed to improve the circulation of the skin surface, and some of the newer drugs such as sodium paba, cortisone, and ACTH. None of these measures have proved constantly satisfactory or curative.

Disorders of Pigmentation

Freckles and Tanning

These changes in the skin are brought about by exposure to sunlight. The natural reaction of the skin to light and some other forms of irritation is the formation of pigment, tanning. Some skins, notably those lacking in pigment, are not able to produce pigment as readily as the darker ones and often produce it only in spots. Freckles, therefore, are the indication of a weakness of the skin in this important function. Such skins should not be needlessly exposed to light, for they cannot protect themselves or the owner from its sometimes harmful effects, which do not appear at once, but may come to notice much later as senile freckles, liable to change to rough, scaly spots and end in cancer of the skin. These are larger and fewer than the ordinary freckles of youth and are more persistent. Such a skin should be protected as much as is possible from direct sunlight; though, of course, this is locking the barn long after the horse has been stolen, for such a skin should have been protected since early childhood. After the damage has occurred, its progress may be delayed somewhat by the daily application of a good cold cream. Treatment of senile freckles is usually not necessary unless they are disfiguring or show some tendency to become rough and horny. They should then be eradicated. The freckles of youth are best treated by preventive measures, as already stated. The mild applications suggested for chloasma may be tried if the freckles are disfiguring; but time and protection from light are the most successful measures.

Chloasma

Chloasma is the unequal browning of the skin of the face that occurs in women more often than in men and, like all increases of pigment, in dark-complexioned persons oftener than in blondes. Its popular name is "liver spots"; but the liver cannot be held responsible. (Apparently a hormone from the pituitary called the MSH or melanocyte stimulating hormone is responsible.—Ed.) The treatment often unsatisfactory, consists in trying to remove the surface layers of the skin by means of an inflammatory reaction produced by irritants. These, when strong enough to be effective, are hard to control and often cause too great an inflammation with most unpleasant consequences to the patient. Peroxide solution, made active by the addition, at the time of using, of about 20 per cent of ammonia water, may be beneficial to some; this is questionable, however, and care should be used to stop the application before too great an irritation has been produced. All such remedies act by causing scaling, and this is seldom deep enough to affect the pigment without causing an unpleasant inflammatory reaction. In some instances careful electrosurgical removal of the pigmented patch may be successful. (A new ointment called Benoquin has been reported useful.—Ed.)

VITILIGO

This disease is almost the opposite of freckling. White spots suddenly appear on the skin, usually around the face or on the backs of the hands. In time they get larger in size, and new white areas appear elsewhere on the body surface. These white spots are due to a loss of the pigment cells in the affected areas, but no one knows why they occur. They may be due to deficiencies in the glands of internal secretion, metabolic alterations, or various unknown factors. They sometimes appear at the same time as alopecia areata, and may be due to similar emotional problems.

The spots become more conspicuous if the surrounding skin gets sunburned —so stay out of the sun. The whitish areas may be effectively concealed by Covermark. A new Egyptian chemical, derived from an herb, has been found of value in some instances. (This product is now marketed under the name of Oxsoralen. It must be prescribed by a physician.—Ed.)

BERLOCK DERMATITIS

This relatively common disorder appears as flat, dark brown spots, usually in a necklace or droplike appearance. It is more common in women and is due to the action of sunlight on skin previously covered with a sun oil, lotion, or perfume containing an essential perfume oil (bergamot). The usual sites are the sides of the neck, face, arms, and armpits, but any part of the body may be involved. The eruption is often produced by dripping or running down of the fluid on the skin, and this gives it the droplike appearance. It is due to light sensitivity, and the brown spots can appear with redness, inflammation, and even blistering. Treatment should consist at first of soothing creams and later of bleaching lotions. Cosmetics or other substances containing the essential causative oils must be avoided if recurrences are to be prevented.

SLEEP Sancho Panza, who accompanied Don Quixote on his travels, is famous for one of his most simple sayings: "God bless the man who first invented sleep." Most people know that sleep is necessary for health. People differ in sleep requirements. One investigator deprived himself for 115 hours, but all of the evidence shows that the longer a person goes without sleep the less he is able to carry on any kind of important activity and the less reliable to accept any kind of responsibility.

Fortunately sleep is rest, no matter whether it is taken in large or small doses. If one has difficulty in getting enough sleep at night, a nap of even just a few minutes is helpful. The difficulty with naps is that they tend to become prolonged. A number of people have invented technics for controlling the length of a nap. One New York captain of industry always took his nap with a bunch of keys in his hand. When his sleep became sufficiently sound, relaxation of the hand resulted in dropping the keys; the keys would jangle, and he would wake up.

An important journalist takes his nap immediately after lunch each day in a barbershop. He has become accustomed to fall asleep the moment he gets into the chair for his shave, and he awakens when the shave is completed.

A number of people insist that they cannot sleep at night if they sleep at all during the day. However, the physiologists say there is no essential or inherent inappropriateness in reversing the time of sleep. Night watchmen, newspaper workers, railroad men, factory men on night shifts, and a great many others became accustomed during the period of accelerated war industry to sleeping in the day and working at night. Just as soon as daytime sleep became sufficiently established as a habit, they obtained adequate rest from their sleep during this period.

Some people find it especially difficult to sleep while traveling. For a long time there was a superstition that one sleeps better with the head toward the north. Others insist that they sleep better with the head toward the east. It should not make the slightest difference whether you sleep with your head toward the north, south, east, or west, provided you do not have in your mind the continual question of whether the position in which you lie is the most healthful one. In most European countries passengers always ride sidewise in sleeping cars, and in many of our modern American sleeping cars the sidewise position has been adopted.

Much of the ability to sleep while riding in trains depends on the ventilation, which has been continuously improved, on the comfort of the mattress, the number of pillows, and a good many other small factors which do or do not duplicate the sleeping conditions at home. One may become a nuisance to the porter by insisting on a duplication of home habits of sleep as much as possible when traveling, but, nuisance or not, it is well to attempt such duplication if sleep is to be sound and comfortable.

How Long Can You Go without Sleep?—The first experimental study of the ability of human beings to get along without sleep was made by two investigators in 1896. They kept three young men awake for from 88 to 90 hours and reported that there was no significant change except a decrease in reaction time, slower motor performance, failures to memorize, and a slight loss of ability to perceive.

Since that time studies have been made on other people who have gone without sleep for periods like 65 hours. Not long ago some experts at the University of Chicago tested thirty-five students who were willing to try the experiment. They found that sleepiness comes in waves, with the greatest difficulty from three to six in the morning. When sleepiness occurs, there is increased difficulty in writing, reading, and studying. The eyes feel and become tired. Sometimes one begins to see double. The effect on the emotions is to make the individual resentful and irritable.

Dr. Kleitman, who made these studies, concluded that the effects of loss of sleep are to produce a general disturbance of the body and that greatly increased amounts of effort are demanded for any performance when there is loss of sleep for periods longer than 24 hours.

Investigators at the University of Georgia have studied the effects of loss of sleep for 100 consecutive hours, utilizing a number of volunteers. They found, too, that sleepiness comes in waves and that people who have been going without sleep feel quite wide-awake sometime after breakfast and early in the evening.

After 48 hours without sleep it is difficult to read. Eventually one finds it difficult to maintain balance and may stagger. Some people suffer severe headaches. Many people see flashes of light. Some who go without sleep have the feeling of a band pressing on the head. The longer one goes without sleep the less becomes the ability to be certain as to one's location or destination when walking.

The irritability of one man who tried to do without sleep became so great that he reported that he felt like fighting all the time. A girl who took part in the experiment began hearing voices which sounded far away. Another girl constantly counted the people to see if everybody was there and found one missing all the time; this person was herself.

Especially interesting also was the report as to how long it takes to recover after one goes 100 hours without sleep. Some made up their sleep with about half the sleep that they had lost. One man reported that he did not feel recovered until he had had extra sleep for two weeks. The smallest and least athletic man recovered in 57 per cent of the time lost, but the most powerful made recovery in 86 per cent of the lost time. The women came through the experiment as well as or better than the men. The smaller and lighter individual suffered the least; the stronger and more athletic men suffered the most.

Everyone likes to have a good night's sleep.

Inadequate feeding, colic, hunger, thirst, temperature of the room, lights, and noise are likely to interfere with a baby's sleep. If these obstacles are eliminated, it will be found that babies like to sleep. Many authorities hold that babies cannot get too much sleep. Yet even among babies there are variations.

Doctors agree that methods of putting children to sleep artificially by means of monotonous sensations are not desirable. This includes rocking of babies in cradles or in the arms, and singing of monotonous lullabies. The latter method is in the nature of hypnotism.

Investigators have found that young children will get enough sleep almost regardless of direction by their parents. Over a long period of time each child finds the normal amount of sleep that he needs, provided of course he is a healthful child.

Authorities are convinced that it does not make much difference what hour a child goes to bed, except that he must get enough sleep. One expert feels that children are put to bed early in the evening not for their own benefit but for the parents to be able to arrange their evening as freely as possible. Thus the baby is put to bed early more to get him out of the way than to give him enough sleep.

Another expert insists that children

ought to go to bed later in the winter so they will not wake up in the dark. These views may be revolutionary, but there seems to be a certain amount of truth behind them.

There is a great deal of agitation about the problem of a daytime nap for older children. This is another factor that cannot be regulated by any sort of an absolute law.

Some experts recommend one to two hours a day in bed for children from the ages of six to thirteen. Afternoon naps should be encouraged until they seem to delay the onset of sleep in the evening.

Anything that causes a child to remain awake after going to bed is undesirable. It is a bad habit to put a child to bed and then to have him play, read, look at pictures, or do anything else that keeps him from associating going to bed with going to sleep. This may set up habits which persist in later life and which may bring about insomnia in the adult.

Experts who have studied sleep in children claim that heavy evening meals have a disturbing effect on children as have mental work and exciting games in the evening, certain types of motion pictures, and serious emotional states.

The question as to how long an adult ought to sleep has never been satisfactorily answered, and probably never will be, because of the differences in human beings.

It is hard to study the matter because many people get enough sleep and complain that they do not rest; others do not get enough sleep and say nothing about it. Some people sleep too long. Experts say that oversleeping is just as bad as overeating.

The mental aspects of sleep have been insufficiently studied. Some people have a good night's sleep and still wake up moody and mean. Others will sleep only five or six hours and awaken in the best of spirits, quite refreshed.

There has been some study of the optimum time for going to bed. One expert says that an hour before midnight is worth two after midnight.

Another expert says that there are two types of sleepers. One is tired in the evening, quickly falls asleep, soon reaches the greatest depth of sleep, and wakes up refreshed and well rested. The other is alert in the evening, does not fall asleep easily, reaches the greatest depth of sleep during the early hours of the morning, and wakes up feeling tired.

Some people have two phases of sleep. They awaken from a first phase but are not quite rested. After lying awake for a brief time they fall asleep again and awaken shortly quite refreshed.

Any effort that upsets the routine of daily life may bring about a restless night. The eating of foods to which people are sensitive or which they find difficult to digest may result in restless sleep. Authorities have found that an empty stomach is irritable and that any light snack taken around bedtime tends to enhance restful sleep. Yet some people are restless if they eat or drink anything at all before going to bed.

City dwellers take great pains in purchasing sleeping equipment. It is possible not only to get mattresses which are especially designed for good sleep, but also eyeshades to keep out the light, ear stops to keep out noise, and many special kinds of pillows.

A large portion of mankind sleeps on bedsprings on the ground, sometimes only on mats, sometimes on the bare floor or soil.

These people seem, once they have established the habit, to sleep as well as those who use a hard mattress, a soft mattress, a spring mattress, or a solid mattress.

Specialists in orthopedic surgery say certain forms of mattress prevent spinal curves by placing stress on the bones of the spine.

The argument has been made that a sag in the middle of the bed is bad for good sleep. A cat sleeps curled up, the Japanese sleep on the ground and do not make it conform to the curves of their bodies, and sailors who sleep in sagging hammocks sleep quite soundly.

The sagging of a mattress and bedsprings may discourage frequent changes in position of the sleeper once he has become used to that particular mattress and spring. Most of these matters seem to be questions of individual likes and dislikes.

This is true also of bedcovers. Some people sleep better on cool nights with a full covering of quilts and blankets. Others sleep better when they use no covers. There are some people who cannot sleep well unless they wear gowns or pajamas; others insist the only way they can sleep well is "in the raw."

A few sleepers insist the only way to sleep comfortably is with the face and stomach down. Others never feel well unless they are lying on their backs.

Before there was suitable indoor heating, it was customary to use a bed warmer. Some people prefer an ice-cold bed. They say they fall asleep quicker as they must lie still in order to warm up the part of the bed with which they are in contact.

As early as 1834 an expert found that a person changes his sleeping positions frequently during the night. With the development of the motion picture and suitable timing devices, studies have been made which establish definitely the fact that no normal person sleeps "like a log," but that all of us change our positions frequently during sleeping hours.

If we remain too long in one position, there is likely to be a feeling of discomfort and stiffness which disturbs sleep. This happens particularly with people who are exceedingly tired when they go to bed or with people who have taken enough alcoholic liquor to make them semiconscious.

It is desirable to have the air in the room sufficiently cool because too much warmth and humidity interfere with sleep. It is well to have the air mildly in motion, but a draft will interfere with sleep.

A question of more importance is whether everyone should sleep alone or whether the bed should be shared by two people. Apparently some people sleep better double and others single. This indicates that habits are of the utmost importance in relationship to sound sleep.

Some people insist that exercise before going to bed makes them rest better. Some practice breathing exercises before an open window, others practice complete relaxation. These factors again indicate that there is no absolute rule for every person and that the establishment of a good routine is of the utmost importance.

The psychology of falling asleep has brought on a number of formulas like the counting of sheep. Other rituals suggested include the repetition of prayers, the naming of large numbers of animals or objects in certain classifications (i.e., everything made of wood, every animal that walks on four feet), or any other routine and monotonous task.

One psychologist suggests that all one has to do is to paint a large imaginary figure 3 on an imaginary wall by means of an imaginary brush and a can of imaginary white paint. He says that anybody who has painted three of these 3s will shortly find it impossible to stay awake. You can easily imagine why.

Practically all that has been really learned about the hygiene of sleep is that the adaptation of the body to a regular rhythm of sleeping and wakefulness in the 24-hour cycle of day and night is an individual affair; that it depends on the mind to a large extent for its establishment and maintenance; and that the development of regular habits with respect to the activities of the waking hours, as well as those of sleep, is most significant in falling asleep promptly and in sleeping restfully.

Sleep, as a factor in the development of the child, was given special consideration in a recent survey of the growth and development of the child, made under the auspices of the White House Conference on Child Health and Protection.

Even though numerous physiologists throughout the world have studied the phenomena of sleep, it has not been possible to determine satisfactorily just why we go to sleep, why we remain asleep, or why we awaken. There are numerous theories, however, all of which have a fair amount of reason behind them.

Most of these theories are based on the idea that fatigue gradually develops in the body due to action of the nerves and muscles and that as a result chemical changes occur which lead to the development of sleep. During sleep the reverse process goes on and when fatigue is overcome the body awakens.

However, it must be pointed out that the hours of waking and of sleeping are usually rhythmical and associated in periodicity with the movements of the planet on which we live.

There is usually a drop in the blood pressure during sleep. The sleep becomes more intense during the first hour and then gradually lessens. Young children tend to sleep more quietly than older children, but there are also differences in the sexes, the time of the year, and other factors.

In one series of scientific investigations it was found that there was a slight tendency to sleep less at night among children who had taken a long nap during the day, but at the same time that children who took no nap at all or who took only a nap for a few minutes had a definite reduction in the total number of hours of sleep in the 24 hours; that is to say, sleeping at night does not compensate for the loss of the nap during the day.

Up to four years of age a nap taken in the daytime rarely interferes with sleep at night. However, after four years of age children as a rule should not be allowed to sleep more than one and a half hours during the day because this will tend to interfere with going to sleep at night.

The authorities believe that children up to the seventh or eighth year should sleep 12 hours daily and at the sixteenth year 9 hours.

If good sleeping habits are established early in life, they tend to persist. It is recognized, however, that there is considerable individual variation in requirements of sleep and that there is not yet sufficient scientific knowledge to make absolute rules.

Newborn babies sleep most of the time except as the demands of nature serve to stimulate and awaken them. The desire for food, pain in the digestive tract, sudden noises or flashes of light, or sudden changes in the temperature of the body will awaken the baby.

If, therefore, the child is kept warm, is placed in the crib in such a manner as to avoid muscular activity, if the stomach is kept free from discomfort by proper feeding, if the clothing is not too tight and the room not too warm, the child will probably sleep well. However, children can be taught to disregard slight noises, slight changes in lighting, the position of the bed, and similar external factors to which it is possible to become accustomed.

The one interference that is serious is irregularity in the hour of going to sleep. The child is therefore best put to bed at a regular hour and if left alone will probably go to sleep by himself.

Psychologists recommend that the attitude of children toward sleep should always be pleasant. They should not be punished just at bedtime.

There must be no possible suggestion that will induce fear connected with the dark or with being left alone. Adults should not discuss before children their own difficulties in sleeping. Too much excitement just before bedtime is likely to make sleep difficult.

For this reason it is extremely unfortunate that many modern radio programs planned for children are exciting mystery stories or detective stories full of warfare, shooting, explosions, and murders rather than the type of material that will lead to a rested mind.

Authorities suggest that the infant, from birth on, be accustomed to sleep in a room by himself. But he should not be so secluded as to have artificial conditions develop which are not likely to be followed later in life; by this is meant complete absence of all noise or the daily activities of life.

SLEEP OF THE CHILD—People spend approximately a third of their time in sleeping, which naturally results in sleep being one of the most important and interesting subjects for human discussion. A research was devoted to the sleep habits of preschool children. In this study 29 boys and 29 girls were included and the investigators made a most meticulous record of their daily lives including eating, speaking, eliminating, learning, which are quite normal in human conduct, and also thumb and finger sucking, nail biting, nose picking, handling of the sex organs, patterns of sleep, the duration of sleep, restlessness and similar characteristics. Specific inquiries were made as to anxiety, fears, and dreams. This was not the first research done on the subject of sleep, since it has interested the medical profession for many years.

Children two or three years old sleep about twelve and a half hours out of twenty-four and those three to five years old sleep from eleven to twelve hours. However, as great variations were found as to the amount of sleep required by different boys and girls as can be found among adults. Some parents have rigid standards about hours of sleep and even try to force children to sleep by threatening not to love them any more. Some parents give children candy to get them to sleep. Obviously these are also abnormal reactions.

Among the children studied, some had their own rooms and slept alone, some slept in a room with a nurse, some slept with another child in the room, frequently a baby, and one child slept in a room with his mother, who happened to be a divorcee. Frequently the presence of another person in the room makes a great deal of difference in falling asleep and in the duration of sleep. Children vary greatly in the length of time required to fall asleep. Some fall asleep immediately and others take anywhere from a few minutes to half an hour to fall asleep. One child slept usually ten hours but took two hours to fall asleep. Many children are restless during sleep, moving around in the bed, removing the covers, getting up, crying, and in some instances almost invariably going to the bed of the mother. Early attitudes toward parents are observed in that some boys consistently went to the mother's bed while one girl consistently went to her father's bed during periods of restlessness. One boy went to a doll's bed or a nurse's bed when his sister did not let him sleep in her bed.

Parents develop all sorts of patterns toward getting the child to go to sleep. Some play with the child, others tell stories, and some cuddle and rock the child to sleep. Some children reported that they were being spanked and being locked in their rooms and told to go to sleep. The majority of children sleep face down or on their backs. Children who suck their thumbs are usually those who sleep face down. Most school children, even including those who sucked their thumbs, sleep on their side. Among the children who were restless at night, one third were also bed-wetters. Out of the whole study comes the conclusion that most parents are too rigid about children's sleep and will do much better by less strictness. Many a sleep problem was developed by parents putting too much attention on the number of hours of sleep that had to be obtained daily at all costs. When the means selected by parents to force children to sleep are wrong, the child tends to develop methods of deceiving the parents and that may give him a sense of guilt. When a child develops an elaborate ritual about going to sleep, the pattern is usually developed to overcome a sense of anxiety.

SLEEP PRODUCERS—Among the greatest blessings of mankind are those drugs and preparations which either completely remove consciousness from the human being or temporarily inhibit it so that the human being becomes insensible to pain or to outside stimuli. The ancient Arabs and Egyptians were familiar with the drugs that would produce sleep or temporary unconsciousness. Only with the coming of modern centuries, however, have we been able to develop a great variety of such drugs and preparations, so that they vary in their strength from those which act for a few moments only and which produce slight degrees of insensibility to those which may produce complete unconsciousness for long periods of time.

All such drugs are poisons if taken in large quantities. They should, therefore, be used with the utmost caution, preferably never except under the advice of a physician. In many places druggists are not permitted to sell such preparations to anyone without a doctor's prescription. If they have been prescribed by the doctor for use according to his directions, they should always be kept safely so as to avoid any possibility of error in their use.

BROMIDES—Among the older sleep producers are the bromides, which are now available in many forms. They are used chiefly to quiet the spasms and convulsions associated with epilepsy, but the dose and intervals of taking them must always be regulated by the doctor. Bromides used to be the chief ingredients of patent medicines sold for epilepsy. Today most patent medicines sold for epilepsy contain some derivative of barbituric acid. These vary in their strength or toxicity and poisoning character.

NOT TO BE KEPT IN FAMILY MEDICINE CHEST!—The narcotic preparations should never be used by anyone without a doctor's prescription. Any drug that has to be administered with a hypodermic syringe should not be kept in the average family medicine chest. There are some persons with diabetes who have been taught by the doctors to inject themselves with insulin. Even these people should always keep their syringe outfits separate from the family medicine chest.

CHILDREN'S SLEEP—Using the encephalograph (an instrument for recording brain waives), investigators have identified five depths of sleep: (1) the stage of dropping off, when the person is neither asleep nor awake; (2) light sleep; (3) a deeper stage, in which the person is still easily disturbed; (4) sound sleep, when the person is not easily disturbed; and (5) very deep sleep. Children's sleep is sound within an hour, gets progressivly lighter until the sixth hour, deepens again and reaches sound sleep during the eighth and ninth hours. The investigators conclude that if a child is hard to waken in the morning, he has not completed his sleep cycle and has not had as much sleep as he needs. It was noted that out of 250 children, 184 awoke of their own accord, 53 awoke easily on being called, and 13 were hard to waken. Most of a group of eleven-year-olds slept ten to eleven hours, but some who had difficulty falling asleep actually slept only seven hours.

SLEEP—children's requirements: See INFANCY, article CARE AND FEEDING OF THE CHILD.

SLEEP—drugs to produce: See MEDICINE CHEST, article THE FAMILY MEDICINE CHEST.

SLEEPLESSNESS See *Insomnia.*

SLIPPED DISKS (See also discussion under *Nervous Diseases and Spine*) When intervertebral disks, cartilage cushions that lie between the bones of the spine, slip out partially, they may cause trouble. Pinching of a disk may be associated with severe neck pains that radiate down the shoulders, or severe nervous troubles that result from compression of the nerve roots in the spinal cord. The condition can usually be diagnosed by the taking of X rays, accompanied sometimes by the injection of substances that make the tissues more visible in X rays. If the condition is allowed to persist too long before surgery is performed, it may not be completely corrected because the disks have calcified or because the changes in the tissues of the nervous system have become permanent and cannot be reversed. A London surgeon has given a report on five hundred patients followed up for periods of one to twelve years. He finds that when patients are treated promptly, only a small proportion of them require surgical removal of disks. When surgery was used in proper cases, 92 per cent of the patients were later found to be either free from symptoms or greatly improved; only a fraction of 1 per cent of the patients stated that the disability was as bad after the operation as before.

SLOW LEARNERS (See also discussion under *Child Care, Intelligence, Speech*) Psychoanalysts have been trying to find out why a seemingly normal child fails to learn. They now say that if a child is to learn during the early months of life, he must feel unconditionally loved and must have a desire to do what his mother wants him to do. He imitates his mother and attempts to feel and act as she does. If an infant does not have a loved person to emulate, or if his parents have overprotected him and restricted his independence, he won't develop normally. If he has an infantile person as an object for imitation, he will remain infantile. Infantile personalities sometimes conceal their condition by parroting words and phrases, to give an impression of maturity, without having any real idea of their meaning. They display dependence and fear, and are easily frustrated.

SMALLPOX Most of the civilized countries of the world now control smallpox by isolation, quarantine, and vaccination. In the United States we still have more smallpox than any other civilized country in the world except British India. In thirteen of our states, with a population of more than 42,000,000, vaccination is compulsory. In these thirteen states there are each year about 230 cases of smallpox or 1 case for every 200,000 people. In fourteen states every town is permitted to decide for itself whether or not its citizens ought to be vaccinated against smallpox. In these fourteen states the population reaches more than 38,000,000 people, and in these states there are more than

1300 cases of smallpox every year, or 7 cases of smallpox for every 200,000 people. Now there are still twenty-two other states, including the District of Columbia, in which vaccination is not compulsory in any form. In these states there are 44,000,000 people who have more than 6000 cases of smallpox every year. They have 28 cases for every 200,000 people.

Smallpox is a foul disease. Once it was so frequent that the rare person in any community was the one without scars on his face from this disease. Now it is rare to see a person with scars of smallpox. They are a manifestation of ignorance or stupidity either on the part of the person concerned or on the part of those responsible for him.

In the typical case of smallpox chills, high temperature, vomiting, aches, and pains begin ten to fourteen days after exposure. The characteristic eruption appears about fourteen days after exposure. It consists of blisters which become filled with pus. In some cases the infection is so severe that hemorrhages occur.

How pitiful that there should still be instances in which this condition is permitted to occur to a child who is unable to protect himself. Practically every school in the United States that is conducted along scientific lines now requires that a child bring with him on his first day of school a certificate that he has had a recent and satisfactory vaccination against smallpox. Vaccination against smallpox is as safe a procedure as is known to medicine. Complications are rare when the vaccination is properly performed. The protection is so certain that neglect of this scientific procedure represents the height of foolhardiness.

While this procedure brings about immunity in the vast majority of cases, there are a few instances in which repeated vaccination may be necessary to build up immunity. This means not only that a person should be vaccinated at certain definite periods of life but also that he should be revaccinated whenever there is the possibility of being brought into contact with smallpox. The fact that smallpox is now so rare has made many people neglectful or evasive of vaccination.

The recent experiences in Great Britain, where there were outbreaks of smallpox both in civil communities and

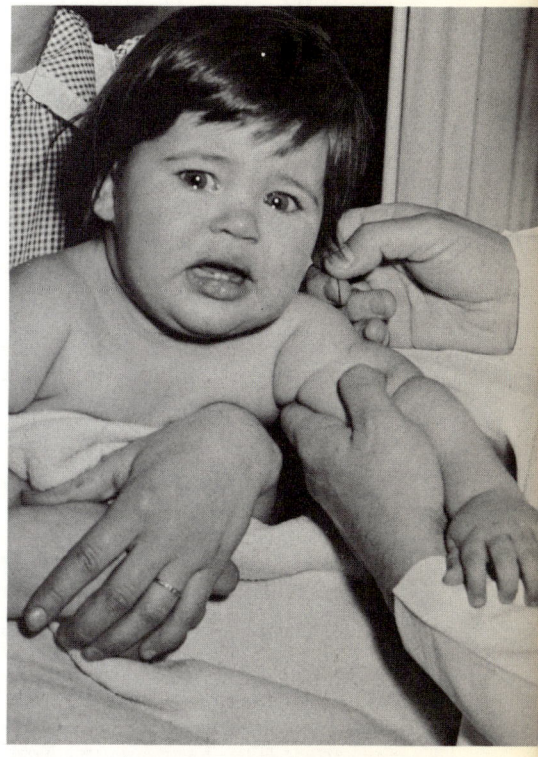

Child being vaccinated against smallpox. Since immunity to smallpox is not permanent, vaccinations should be repeated. *Hygeia*

SMALLPOX　　　　　　　　　　　　　　　　　　　　　　　　　　SMELL

in troops, indicate the desirability of keeping the danger constantly in mind. Indeed one British physician says that the situation there in relation to smallpox is like the situation that existed in foreign affairs among the democratic nations in 1933 when the prophets kept on saying that there was danger ahead and that we ought to be preparing whereas the stupid and the conscientious objectors kept on insisting on "peace in our time."

SMALLPOX—albuminuria may result: See KIDNEY, article THE KIDNEY: ITS DISEASES AND DISTURBANCES.

SMALLPOX—blamable: See article DIABETES.

SMALLPOX—chicken pox mistaken for: See CHILDHOOD DISEASES, article INFECTIOUS DISEASES OF CHILDHOOD.

SMALLPOX—confused with measles: See CHILDHOOD DISEASES, article INFECTIOUS DISEASES OF CHILDHOOD.

SMALLPOX—control: See INFECTIOUS DISEASE, article THE PREVENTION AND TREATMENT OF INFECTIOUS DISEASE.

SMALLPOX—incidence: See INFECTIOUS DISEASE, article THE PREVENTION AND TREATMENT OF INFECTIOUS DISEASE.

SMALLPOX—incubation period: See INFECTIOUS DISEASE, article THE PREVENTION AND TREATMENT OF INFECTIOUS DISEASE.

SMALLPOX—inflammation of colon: See article DIGESTION AND DIGESTIVE DISEASES.

SMALLPOX—pneumonia frequently follows: See RESPIRATORY DISEASES, article THE RESPIRATORY DISEASES.

SMALLPOX—tongue inflammation: See EAR, article THE EAR, TONGUE, NOSE, AND THROAT.

SMALLPOX—vaccination: See article ALLERGY.

SMALLPOX—vaccination immunizes against herpes virus: See SKIN, article THE SKIN.

SMELL Odors are sometimes pleasant and sometimes disagreeable. Usually the sense of pleasure is associated with some previous experience; likewise the sense of displeasure. The smell of roses is more pleasant than that of asafetida. One man who smelled camphor immediately associated it with the door of the wardrobe and was then reminded that he had been placed in a closet in which were clothes that had been treated with camphor as a moth preventive over thirty years previously. A girl who smelled cedarwood oil associated it with a summer evening on the Norwegian coast and with the cigar box in which her mother had kept the family funds. A woman who smelled cedarwood oil thought about spring cleaning and the use of the mop. A Scotchman who smelled asafetida thought of a streetcar in Edinburgh and it was discovered that these cars were formerly lighted by acetylene gas which gave off a similar odor.

The odors of the human body vary with different races, although some people insist that the odor is wholly a matter of cleanliness. An ethnologist has said that Indians smell of acetylene, Australians of phosphorus; the Chinese are said to have a musty odor and the Negro an odor slightly suggesting ammonia.

Once doctors thought that certain diseases had a definite smell associated with them, particularly diphtheria and diabetes. It is now recognized that the odor of diphtheria is the odor of infection in the throat which has injured the tissues. The odor of diabetes is the sweet acetone odor associated with acidosis.

In some people the sense of smell is greatly deficient; in others it is exceedingly sensitive. Usually the sense of sight dominates by far the sense of smell, so that even when the sense of smell is wholly lost, life is not greatly affected except by such pleasures as come from perfumes.

In testing sensitivity to smell, certain well-defined odors are used. An extremely sensitive person can detect camphor in a solution of 1:400,000; musk in a solution of 1:30,000,000; and vanilla in a concentration of 1:10,000,000. Apparently the strongest odor is that of the substance called mercaptan. This can be detected when 1/23,000,000th of a milligram is present in a quart of water.

SMELL—sense of: See EAR, article THE EAR, TONGUE, NOSE, AND THROAT.

SMILES (See also discussion under *Child Care and Laughter*) The newborn baby smiles more often on one side only. Gesell who observed children born in the seventh or eighth month, speaks of "unilateral grimaces; the brow corrugates, sometimes only half a brow, for bilateral integration is not yet firmly achieved, the lips purse in a rabbit-like manner; they mince; they draw into a smile." This early smiling lasts rarely longer than one second, and that is also why it is so often overlooked. Evidently, it is an expression of comfort from the beginning, for it happens most often after a meal or when uneasiness turns into ease. Children born blind smile as well as those who can see. With increasing amusement, the smile turns to laughing and finally to loud laughter. Clearly, it is not learned by imitation of a seen model; the innate motor coordination is an instinct.

SMOKING AND LUNG CANCER (See also *Cancer, Detection of Cancer, Lung Cancer, Mortality in Cancer, Research in Cancer*) Statisticians found evidence of increasing numbers of deaths from cancer of the lung in various portions of the world and were inclined definitely to relate these to the increase in the smoking of cigarettes. Many scientists argued that the considerable increase was not due to cigarettte smoke but to some other factor that might cause irritation of the lung. The suggestion was made that polluted air over our big cities is much more to blame for the increase of cancer of the lung than is tobacco smoking. Proof from the British Cancer Research Council established that irritants in polluted air are capable of producing cancers on the skin of mice that belong to a strain in which cancer is prevalent. Answers are not yet available as to why persons who never smoke develop cancer of the lung, why more cases of cancer of the lung develop in air polluted cities than in rural areas or why there is less cancer of the larynx and mouth than of the lung since smoke reaches the larynx and mouth also. A study made by the British Empire Cancer Campaign demonstrated that the incidence of cancer of the lung tends to increase with the density of the population. These investigators believe that the effects of tobacco smoking and pollution of the air supplement each other. For this reason tobacco smoking should be more dangerous for a town dweller than for a country dweller and many newly developed statistics indicate that this is the case.

Several statisticians, notably, Berkson of the Mayo Clinic and Brownlee of the University of Chicago Committee on Statistics have attacked the analysis of figures related to cancer of the lung and smoking. Brownlee considers these to be quite misleading. He emphasizes that the claims of causation are ludicrous and that the most that can be expected is proof of some association. It is generally agreed by statisticians that the restrospective study, where attempts were made to provide a matched set of controls were unsatisfactory. Brownlee indicates that almost any conceivable death ratio among smokers and non-smokers can result from the prospective studies. The sampling in the prospective studies appears to have been uncontrolled and subject to the whims of the sampler, he says. Furthermore, he pointed out that the general question generated violent emotions and that these modified greatly the scientific inquiry.

SNEEZING A sneeze is elicited by irritation of the mucous membrane of the nose. The impulses responsible for a sneeze are set up by the irritation of the nerve endings of the trigeminal nerves and probably also by the stimulation of the nerves that are concerned with detecting odors. A sneeze usually begins, as does a cough, with the taking of a deep breath and the violent expulsion of the air. The deeper the breath taken the longer and louder will be the sneeze.

Experts, using flash photography, have studied the effects of the sneeze on contamination of the surrounding air. When you sneeze, most of the droplets that are expelled come from the mouth but there is also a large discharge of material from the nose. The material carried from the nose is carried forward horizontally by the blast from the mouth. The size of the droplets varies greatly. When the mouth is open, the droplets are larger; when the sneezing is done with the mouth closed or partially closed, the droplets are smaller.

A British bacteriologist exposed some culture plates before a healthy sneezer at a distance of three feet from the nose. Then the germs deposited on the culture plate were counted after they had grown. The investigators counted 19,000 different colonies, which would mean that a least 19,000 different droplets must have been projected at least three feet.

The droplets with the germs that they carry will hang in the air for some time. After a man sneezed in a dry, dust-free room, some plates were put out twenty minutes later. Some 493 germ colonies grew on these plates.

Since it is known that coughs and sneezes spread diseases, various means have been sought to control such contamination. The wearing of a gauze mask helps but the mask becomes messy after there have been many sneezes through it. A large handkerchief would prevent the escape of droplets almost entirely but the bits of flimsy linen used by most women permit droplets to escape around it. Masks of cellulose acetate which are used sometimes now in surgeries apparently trap everything but they are often warm and uncomfortable. The placing of a hand to the mouth and nose will deflect the spray but it contaminates the hand, after which everything in the neighborhood of the hand may become contaminated. One Britisher suggested that the best way to sneeze is from a short distance directly into a coal fire or a grate fire.

During the great influenza epidemic of 1918 the wearing of gauze masks was popular. It was then found that a thin gauze mask is an inefficient filter. A six-layer gauze mask will filter away 97 per cent of the germs. Laundering tends to destroy the ability of the mask as a filter of germs.

SNEEZING—antihistamines relieve: See article ALLERGY.

SNEEZING—infectious disease carried: See INFECTIOUS DISEASE, article THE PREVENTION AND TREATMENT OF INFECTIOUS DISEASE.

SNEEZING—summer colds: See RESPIRATORY DISEASES, article THE RESPIRATORY DISEASES.

SNORING Somehow the habit of snoring in sleep is usually greeted with a good deal of ridicule and embarrassment. Whenever the question arises in any home, the father and mother will affirm positively that each of them individually never snores, yet each is likely to affirm with equal glee that the other snores to the high heavens.

Old people are likely to say—with a good deal of irritation over the accusation—that they not only do not snore but never did snore. Now practically everyone under certain circumstances may snore, because the conditions that cause snoring may occur at one time or another in every person.

The actual noises made by the snorer are due to intermittent passage of air at places in the nose and throat where there may be partial obstruction to the passage. What are the conditions that may bring about such obstruction?

First, there may occur during sleep a partial relaxation of the muscles holding the vocal cords, so that they fall more or less closely together and thus interfere with the passage of air.

Second, when a person in deep sleep or one who is unconscious lies on his back, the tongue may fall back and partially close the opening through which the air passes.

Third, when a person lies on his back, the muscles controlling the soft palate may fail to hold it, so that it falls against the hard palate and obstructs the passage of air up through the nose.

Fourth, because of irritation or inflammation mucus may collect in the nose or in the passages behind the nose.

Fifth, the muscles associated with the throat and nose may be abnormally tense and thus create interference to the passing of air.

Sixth, if the nose is blocked and the lips are held rather close to the air, a whistling sound occurs as the air passes out.

Many people can produce snoring sounds during their waking hours by trying any or all of the muscle arrangements that have been mentioned. This, however, is not an especially desirable performance because snoring sounds are seldom pleasant.

It is interesting to realize that snoring seldom disturbs the soundness of the sleep of the snorer himself. Even though he is sensitive to noise while asleep, his own noises do not wake him up.

The most that we can do to prevent snoring is to make sure there are no obstructions in the nose and throat. Then snoring is less liable to occur if the person goes to sleep and stays asleep on either the side or the abdomen instead of on the back.

SODIUM BICARBONATE The common name for this drug is baking soda. Its chief uses are to overcome excess acidity of the juices of the stomach and excess acidity of the body generally. In cases of acidosis large doses of baking soda are usually given by mouth. The drug is also used occasionally as a mild alkaline wash. Baking soda baths are sometimes used to overcome itching.

SODIUM BICARBONATE—burning skin: See INFECTIOUS DISEASE, article THE PREVENTION AND TREATMENT OF INFECTIOUS DISEASE.

SODIUM BICARBONATE—deodorant: See SKIN, article THE SKIN.

SODIUM BICARBONATE—heartburn: See BIRTH, article CARE OF MOTHERS BEFORE AND AFTER CHILDBIRTH.

SODIUM BICARBONATE—itching skin: See INFECTIOUS DISEASE, article THE PREVENTION AND TREATMENT OF INFECTIOUS DISEASE.

SODIUM BICARBONATE—lemonade made more alkaline by: See RESPIRATORY DISEASES, article THE RESPIRATORY DISEASES.

SODIUM BICARBONATE—medicine chest: See MEDICINE CHEST, article THE FAMILY MEDICINE CHEST.

Sodium Bicarbonate—mouth wash: See Ear, article The Ear, Tongue, Nose, and Throat.
Sodium Bicarbonate—sunburn: See Skin, article The Skin.
Sodium Bicarbonate—treatment of burns: See article First Aid.

SOMNAMBULISM This term comes from two Greek words meaning sleep and walk. Therefore any person who habitually walks in his sleep is known as a somnambulist. There are many different causes for this condition. In practically every instance, however, the condition is due to stimulation of the brain by thoughts that are carried over from the waking period into the sleeping state. Proper mental hygiene and attention to the stimuli which may disturb sleep are helpful in the control of this condition.

SPARKS AND FLASHES (See also, *Eye*) Many persons complain of seeing sparks or flashes of light. These are sometimes due to disturbances of the circulation of the blood of the eye. In cases in which one of the lining membranes of the eye may be inflamed the sensation of dazzling flashes of light of various colors may be very pronounced.

Some people complain particularly of constant showers of golden dust or of large numbers of black specks floating in front of the eyes or of stationary spots of large sizes. In many instances these are due to difficulties of color vision or of vision generally. Sometimes the wearing of blue-colored glasses, which cut off the red rays, will relieve the person concerned of his symptoms.

No doubt the best advice that can possibly be given to people generally is to tell them to see a competent specialist in diseases of the eyes at least once each year and not to take lightly any disturbance of vision. The eye, once damaged, does not recover with ease; neither does any other highly specialized organ of the body. Disturbances seen early are treated to better advantage than if there is considerable delay.

SPASMS A spasm is any sudden contraction of a muscle that occurs without any desire or wish on the part of the person affected. Almost anybody can at one time or another have a muscle spasm. Sudden chilling of the body after swimming may bring about spasm of the muscles. Whenever the circulation of the blood in any part of the body is greatly diminished, sudden involuntary contractions of the muscles may occur. Of this type is the muscle spasm of the calf of the leg that is called intermittent claudication. This may be so severe as to bring about pain and inability to walk. If the person will rest for a few minutes or more, he finds that he is able to walk again. The spasm of the muscle relaxes and the circulation improves.

Difficulties in the nervous system, as for instance the death of a nerve cell in the interior portion of the spinal cord, may result in paralysis of the muscles with spasm of the opposing muscles.

Spasms are not to be confused with what are called tics. Tics occur as a result of habit. Among the most common of all spasms are those that affect the face. This is particularly due to the fact that the muscles of the face are easily movable. They are affected easily by many different emotions or activities. Spasms of the face may be sudden and pass so quickly that they go unnoticed. Sometimes they affect only the little muscles around the eye. Sometimes when the eye becomes especially tired the eyelids will develop a spasm or twitching which is known as blepharospasm.

The habit spasms of children are not to be confused with chorea, or St. Vitus' dance, which is a rheumatic disorder. The movements of habit spasms differ from those of chorea by being quicker and always being repeated in the same way. The movements of chorea are irregular and variable.

Whenever a spasm of the muscle occurs, it needs investigation with a view to removing the cause. If the cause is in a condition affecting the nerves, medical or surgical treatment may be required. In some instances the only way to stop a spasm is to inject various substances around the nerves of the area involved.

Sometimes the spasms in children occur in association with distress, such as fear of punishment. These children do well with encouragement and pleasantness. Constant faultfinding makes them worse.

SPASMS—rabies: See article TRANSMISSIBLE DISEASES.

SPEECH About the most exciting time in an average family is the moment when the new baby begins to talk. In the first few months of life babies make sounds which have little significance to those who hear them but which must be a source of satisfaction to the baby; otherwise the baby would not spend so much time working at it.

The first sounds that a baby makes are variations of the sounds of *a* and *u*. Then the consonants *m, p,* and *b* are added to these vowels. These are the sounds that can be made with the lips closed. After the baby is three months old he will combine these sounds so that *umm, da, ma* and *goo* are formed. When he puts two *da's* together, the father is flattered. When he puts two *vah's* together, the mother insists that the baby wants water. Soon the baby begins to see that there is value in the sounds he makes. People bring things. Then the baby imitates adult sounds and thus learns to speak. As soon as possible the baby makes noises that sound like words and people begin praising and encouraging him. This causes the baby to try to imitate himself and he becomes proud of his ability. This encouragement also helps him to speak.

A baby can probably understand a number of words before he can say any of them. A bright baby will speak his first word about the time he is eight or nine months old. Almost any baby can be expected to say something about the time he reaches the tenth or twelfth month. Some babies know one or two words by the time they are a year old. The ability to combine words in phrases and sentences comes usually between the time the child is one and a half to two years old. The vocabulary grows almost daily. By the time the child is seven years old, he is probably familiar with about 3000 words. However, the number of words that a child can use varies with his intelligence. In general smart children talk earlier and dull children talk later than the average. The development of speech is one of the methods that experts use for measuring intelligence.

Speech is the chief characteristic by which we distinguish men from animals. Twenty-five or thirty years ago the country was well covered with elocution teachers. Many little boys and girls were taught to recite poetry with gestures. Nowadays less attention is paid to such recitation and much more attention is paid to simple talking for purposes of living.

Children learn speech largely through imitation. Many a child is ruined as to his speech habits by the bad speaking habits of his older brothers and sisters, his mother and father, and his playmates. When children enter kindergarten, the teachers classify them according to their ability to express themselves. Statistics show that about 10 per cent of people have speech defects. At least 1,500,000 children stutter and stammer. Many others just have bad speaking habits.

One writer has coined the phrase "lip laziness" to describe people who do not trouble to talk correctly. The ability to speak distinctly requires a certain amount of attention to the formation of sounds exactly as ability to swing a baseball bat or a golf club requires mental and physical co-ordination.

When young children are learning to speak, they may be made to realize the importance of speaking correctly by suitable rewards for correct speech. The words used by a small child are not nearly so important as the manner in which the words are spoken. Children who live in homes in which the parents speak distinctly and use correct words will, if they have ordinary intelligence, learn to use the same words in the same way.

Here are seven rules which parents should follow in developing habits of good speech in their children.

1. Do not correct the child's pronunciation or enunciation. Applaud that which is right. Do not stress that which is wrong.

2. Do not imitate the child's baby talk. When you say "dravy" for "gravy" and "wed" for "red," simply because the baby talks that way, you confirm him in his difficulty. But do not correct him too severely. If you keep on talking English, he will talk it as soon as he can.

3. Never talk down to babies and little children.

4. Do not nag, coax, or raise your

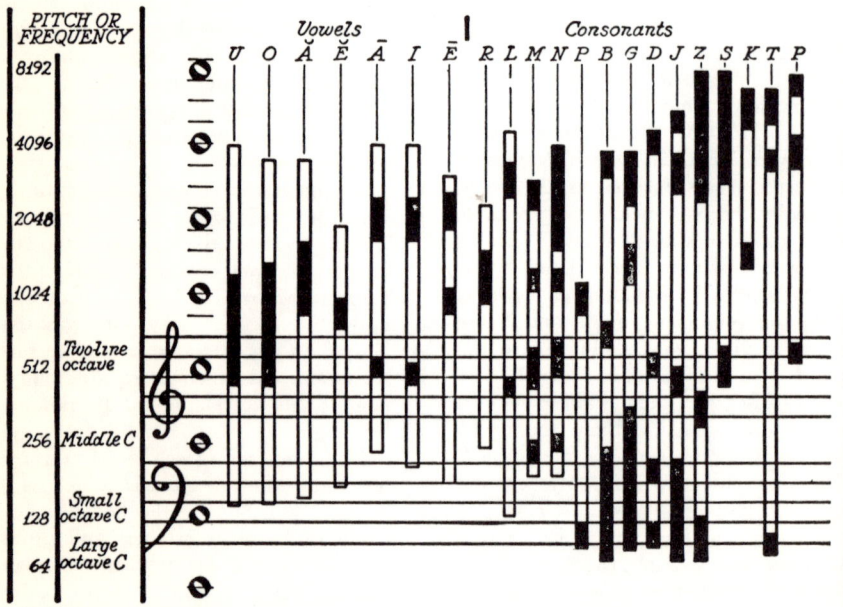

Musical scale indicating pitch or wave frequency of various sounds used in speaking.

voice in an effort to get the baby to talk. Speech will come naturally.

5. If the baby's uncle and aunt stammer, or if you stammer yourself, give the baby a chance to learn how to talk from someone else. Children will imitate.

6. Give the child a chance to talk, and listen to him when he talks. This will encourage him.

7. Tell the child to listen. Do not ignore him, but include him whenever possible in the conversation.

SPEECH AND MENTAL HEALTH—Language and speech are important indications of mental health. Patterns of association of words are used as diagnostic tests of personality disorders. The emotional climate in the home affects the child's personality adjustment and his language development. An ignorant or illiterate servant whose speech affords a poor model may injure the child's language and speech. A mother who encourages in her children excessive use of games or viewing of television, to keep them out of her way, is not merely depriving them of opportunities to practice language; she is depriving them of herself and of the real, vital, interpersonal experiences such as storytelling, picnics, tea parties, etc., that are the essence of family life.

SPIDER BITES The only venomous spider in the Western Hemisphere is the black widow. When a person is bitten by a spider the first step is to stop the absorption of the poison into the circulation. The wound can be disinfected with tincture of iodine or any other good antiseptic. If any considerable amount of poison has been taken into the body the area of the bite can be put under suction.

Following the bite of the black widow spider, one feels a sharp pain. Then come swelling and redness at the bitten spot, and the whole body reacts with dizziness and weakness, tremor of the legs, and even abdominal cramps. Small children may have difficulty in breathing and even stupor or convulsions. A serum or antitoxin has been developed but has to be secured in most cases from the health department or directly from the manufacturer.

SPINA BIFIDA In 1 out of every 1000 childbirths the infant comes into the world not quite properly grown together, at least as far as the lower portion of the spine is concerned. In most instances the difficulty is simply a failure of the coverings of the spinal cord to grow together. In some instances, however, one or more of the bones of the spine may be lacking. In such instances there may be a hernia or projection of the coverings of the spinal cord to the exterior. This makes a large sac or balloon filled with fluid. The condition is serious because it exposes a part of the nervous system directly to the exterior.

Occasionally a failure of the spinal tissues to grow together properly is associated with a collection of fluid inside the skull and enlargement of the bones of the skull occurs to make room for the fluid. This condition is called hydrocephalus, meaning water on the brain. Such people have tiny bodies and large heads.

If nothing is done for a child with spina bifida, there occurs such pressure and stretching of the nerves of the spinal cord that they do not function satisfactorily. If the condition is in the lower part of the spine and damage to that part of the spine occurs, the child will suffer with paralysis, including inability to control the motions of the bowels and bladder. There may be ulcers on the legs due to the fact that certain portions of the skin do not have a satisfactory nerve supply.

Certainly a child with this deformity should be taken to a doctor as soon as possible, so that the doctor may study the condition to see what is the most that can be done. In some instances a simple surgical operation to eliminate the protrusion of the coverings of the spinal cord and to repair the sac will yield a satisfactory result. This type of surgery is called reconstructive or plastic surgery. At least one half of the babies born with this deformity can be helped by surgery. Everything possible should be done to see that help is given to them early, since cure is much more likely when help is given early.

SPINAL CURVATURE The spine sometimes curves to one side or another. To this the scientific name of scoliosis is given. This may be a symptom or a sequel to many different diseases but often seems to be a condition of the spine itself. Occasionally it results from an insufficiency of the muscles and ligaments that hold the bones in place. Sometimes it occurs from the permanent adoption of a faulty posture. In still other instances the bones themselves are at fault and a breakdown in the structure of a bone allows other tissues to collapse.

In the early stages of twisting of the spine due to bad posture there will not be found any definite changes in the tissues of the spine. If, however, the condition is not corrected, such changes do occur, and when the tissues have changed, the condition is more or less permanent.

Naturally, with the twisting of the spine, changes in the position of the organs occur. The lung may be compressed more on one side than on another. Often there is an absence of important symptoms except for the appearance, so that a child with a twisted spine is first brought to the doctor because of the bad posture. Eventually pain will develop because of pressure of the ribs on the thighbone or pressure on various nerves. In such cases it is customary to examine the child and to make certain of the alignment of the spine. The child should be examined with the body fully exposed. The outline of the back is examined both with the child trying to stand erect and with relaxation in the habitual position. Sometimes a plumb line is used to find out just how straight the spine really is.

Every parent should watch carefully the postural development of a child, and everything possible should be done to avoid faulty attitudes. Sometimes gymnastic treatment and exercise will correct bad posture and encourage the strength of the muscles necessary to hold the spine in proper position. In serious cases an orthopedic surgeon gives help by the use of braces and supports, sometimes even by a plaster cast.

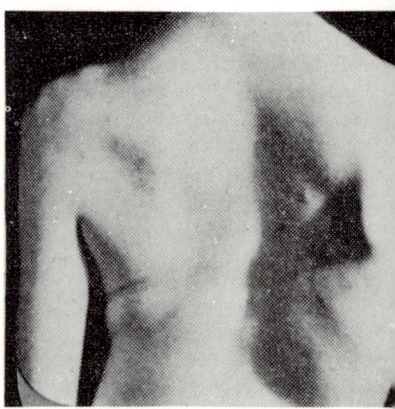

Curvature of the spinal column of unknown causation. Curvatures may result from faulty development of the spine or from diseases of the spinal column itself.

Postgraduate Medicine

However, it is considered to be unwise to use spinal supports until everything possible has been accomplished by suitable exercises and training.

SCOLIOSIS—poor posture may cause: See article POSTURE.

SPINAL FRACTURE A broken back used to be considered about as serious an injury as could occur to a human being. In those days the only way to be certain that anyone had a broken back was the presence of paralysis of certain portions of the body due to injury to the nervous system. Now, with the discovery of the X ray and with improvements in the use of the X ray, breaks in the bones of the spine are detected much more frequently.

Most injuries to the spine occur when people fall from a height, in traffic accidents, in being thrown from a horse, or in sudden pressures resulting from lifting or straining.

Fractures of the spine may occur in the upper portion of the spine called the neck or the cervical region, in the middle, or at the bottom. Most of the serious breaks occur in the neck region. A broken neck is much more serious than a break in the spine lower down. Sometimes a serious injury to the spinal cord will occur when the bones of the spine are twisted away from each other without actually breaking a portion of one of the bones.

The most serious results follow when there is a break directly into the spinal cord with hemorrhage into the spinal cord or tearing of the spinal cord itself.

Sometimes following an injury to the back there is loss of sensation below the level at which the injury occurred and loss of control of the ordinary actions of the bowel and the urinary bladder. The appearance of these symptoms is a clear indication of a serious condition demanding immediate medical attention.

The doctor will suggest first of all that anyone with an injury to the spine should be moved only when lying on a flat board and with the minimum amount of manipulation. If the injury is in the region of the neck, some technic should be found to hold the neck absolutely still. Usually an injury to the spine that is serious will bring on shock. This means again that the patient must lie with the head down and with sufficient warmth to maintain the circulation of the body.

As soon as the condition of the patient permits, the diagnosis of fractures of the spine should be verified by the use of the X ray in order to determine how much damage has occurred. Then a surgeon or orthopedic surgeon will get the bones in proper position and provide supports and braces to hold the tissues in proper position until there has been healing and as much recovery as possible.

During the period of recovery it may be necessary to aid the action of the bowels and the urinary bladder until the person is recovered.

When there has been injury to the spine or any other portion of the nervous system, a specialist in conditions affecting the nervous system will have to make a complete study to determine the extent of the damage that has been done and the possibilities for bringing about a full recovery through specialized treatment.

Curvature of the spine sometimes results from tuberculous infection of the bones so that they fall together. In the worst cases of curvature of the spine the difficulty may be due to disease. The earliest possible application of modern methods is necessary in such cases to prevent serious deformity.

SPINE The spinal cord is one of the most remarkable mechanisms of the human body. It is strong enough to support many hundreds of pounds; at the same time it is pliant and elastic. The muscles and tendons attached to the bones away from the spine help to move it in every direction.

Between each two of the bones of the spine there is a soft cushion which is known as the intervertebral disk. This serves like a ball bearing and a shock absorber. Shock between the bones of the spine that occurs when walking or sitting down is absorbed by this cushion. Its presence permits the bones of the spine to rotate more easily one on the other.

In the middle of this intervertebral disk is a soft material called nucleus pulposus. A sudden shock such as occurs when an airplane comes down or in a traffic accident, may cause the whole intervertebral disk to be pinched or pushed out of place. Occasionally it will break the nucleus pulposus and permit loss of fluid.

Only recently has the importance of this tissue come to be realized. Squeezing or dislocation of the intervertebral disk may produce constant and long-continued pain in the back. A new disease called "jeep disease" is simply an injury to the intervertebral disk which was common during World War II among drivers of jeeps and tanks and which occurred as they bounced over ditches and foxholes.

Exercises that involve sudden strains on the spine, such as football, soccer, baseball, and cricket, are sometimes productive of injury to the disk. Even organized gymnastics, or what the British call "organized jerks," may, if taken too precipitously or with too much force, injure the delicate tissues of the spine. These movements are especially dangerous for people with long legs and short arms who have a special problem of balance.

The presence of an injury to an inter-

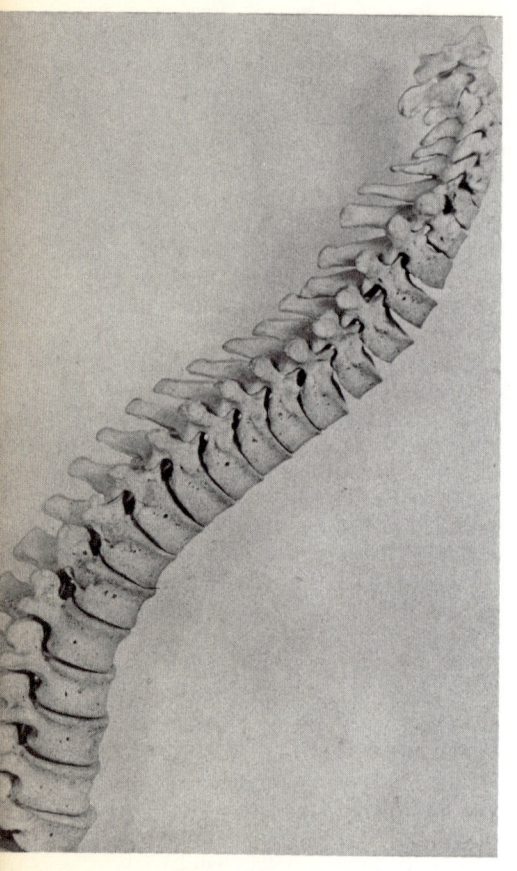

Model showing the position of the backbone when a person is bent forward with the head held erect. The spine is viewed from the right side. The bones of the spinal column increase in size downward. The cervical at the top is the smallest bone and the lumbar toward the bottom is the largest.
Cleveland Health Museum

vertebral disk cannot be detected simply by running the fingers up and down the spine or by asking questions. The doctor is aided in determining such injury by taking an X-ray picture, often first injecting into the area concerned a substance which makes the position of the bones and soft tissues of the spine quite clear. This type of study, combined with application of the knowledge that the doctor has of the structure of the spine, will give him the necessary information to determine whether or not the condition can be corrected by braces and supports or whether or not a surgical operation is required.

SPINE—pneumococcus: See INFECTIOUS DISEASE, article THE PREVENTION AND TREATMENT OF INFECTIOUS DISEASE.

SPINE—rheumatoid arthritis, X-ray treatment for: See article ARTHRITIS, RHEUMATISM, AND GOUT.

SPLEEN In the abdomen on the left side there is a large pulpy organ known as the spleen. From the earliest times the spleen has been associated with emotions of anger. From this came the phrase "to vent one's spleen."

Even today all of the functions of the human body are not clearly understood. Contraction of the spleen occurs with the forcing of blood out of the spleen into the circulation. This has given rise

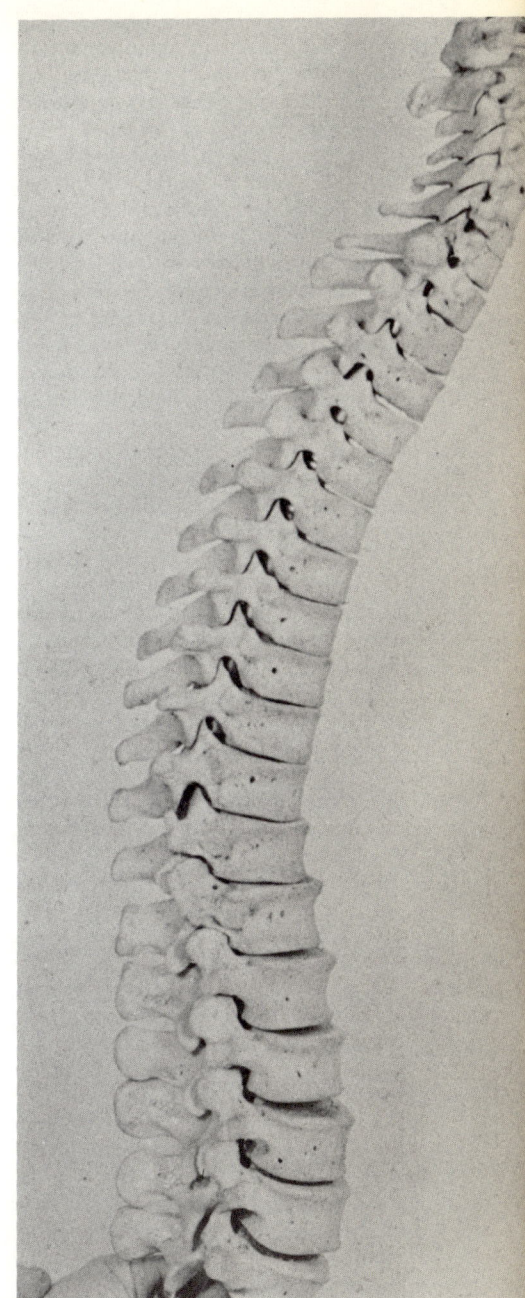

Model of the backbone in the erect position as seen from the right side. The spine is made up of 33 vertebrae, 24 of which are movable. The pattern of the spine permits flexibility in bending. When in the erect position, the spine forms a normal shallow S curvature.

to the concept that the function of the spleen is to maintain a proper amount of blood in the blood vessels, thus keeping up the blood pressure through controlling the volume of the blood.

For some time it has been thought that the spleen is concerned not only with the breaking down and disposal of worn-out blood cells but also with the production of new blood cells.

Some of the studies of the spleen have been made by a very interesting process. Using an animal for the experiment, the doctor puts a celluloid window in the wall of the body and watches directly the function of the organ. It is also possible to transplant an organ outside the abdominal cavity and thus observe its action. The spleen itself is insensitive to pain.

When an animal exercises severely, the spleen contracts due to the discharge of blood into the circulation. Also when an animal exercises severely, the kidney may be deprived of blood to the extent of being actually injured. Injury to the kidney has been known to accompany severe and excessive exercise. Thus the spleen is helpful in putting more blood into the circulation and preventing damage to the vital organs, like the kidney.

Some truth must lie in the idea that the spleen is associated with emotions. The famous physiologist, Dr. Joseph Barcroft, made some tests on a dog which had developed the habit of chasing any cat in the neighborhood. If this dog lay on a table and a duster was placed in front of its nose, the spleen remain unaltered. If that duster were removed and another which had been in a basket with a cat was held in front of the dog's nose, the spleen would contract, even though none of the muscles of the dog moved. The noise of a cat mewing in another room caused the spleen of the dog to contract.

These observations help to explain why a person gets pale when he gets angry and how he can get so mad that he will faint away.

SPLEEN—anti-platelet factor: See BLOOD, article THE BLOOD AND ITS DISEASES.

SPLEEN—enlarged: See article TRANSMISSIBLE DISEASES; BLOOD, article THE BLOOD AND ITS DISEASES; article CANCER.

SPLEEN—leukemia: See article CANCER.

SPLEEN—leukopenia: See BLOOD, article THE BLOOD AND ITS DISEASES.

SPLEEN—malaria: See article TRANSMISSIBLE DISEASES.

SPLEEN—spherocytosis cured by removal: See BLOOD, article THE BLOOD AND ITS DISEASES.

SPLEEN—subacute endocarditis: See HEART, article DISEASES OF THE HEART AND CIRCULATION.

SPLEEN—white blood cells manufactured by: See BLOOD, article THE BLOOD AND ITS DISEASES.

SPLENIC PUNCTURE—See BLOOD, article THE BLOOD AND ITS DISEASES.

SPLEEN REMOVAL, SURGERY AND

(See also discussion under *Spleen, Splenic Disease, Hematura, Hemorrhage, Purpura Hemorrhagica*) For years the spleen has been removed when necessary because of accident or disease and the body is apparently able to compensate through other organs for the removal of this tissue. The principal reason for this operation has been the occurrence of a condition called thrombocytopenia in which the blood platelets are tremendously reduced and the blood does not coagulate easily. Nowadays research has shown that the giving of adequate doses of ACTH or Cortisone in some manner changes the system, reinforcing the walls of the capillary blood vessels and thus making the operation for removal of the spleen one which is done only when other medical methods have failed in this disease.

SPLENIC DISEASE The spleen is one of the large organs of the body least understood by medical science. It lies in the abdomen on the left side under the ribs. It seems to be concerned in the formation of blood cells, perhaps also in their destruction. In certain diseases the spleen enlarges greatly. Like other tissues of the body, it may be subjected to injuries such as occur in motor accidents, gunshot wounds, or falls. The spleen is likely to become much enlarged in leukemia, in which there are a tremendous number of white blood cells in the circulation.

Among unusual conditions affecting this organ are the appearance of accessory spleens scattered through the abdomen. Sometimes the spleen becomes detached or the tissues which hold it in place become relaxed, so that the spleen will move from the position it ordinarily occupies. It then is called a floating or wandering spleen, a condition which occurs far more often in women than in men.

When the spleen is ruptured or broken, as occurs in a road accident, the bleeding is usually severe because of the extensive amount of blood going through this organ. A rupture of the spleen is followed by an intense hemorrhage into the abdomen.

The spleen is often found enlarged in malaria and in blood diseases of various kinds. It is particularly large in a condition called Banti's disease, when the tremendous enlargement of the spleen is associated with severe anemia.

In certain diseases surgical removal of the spleen is considered to be especially helpful, for instance in severe cases of purpura hemorrhagica, a condition in which the blood does not clot easily. The spleen may also be removed because of the presence of tumors. Removal of the spleen has not been considered especially desirable in Banti's disease.

The spleen is not necessary to life as is the liver.

SPITTING UP Babies in the first year or year and a half of life will occasionally spit up or regurgitate a little milk or milk and cereal soon after eating. This is usually simply a sign that the baby has eaten too much or too fast and should not be a cause for worry. As the baby grows older the spitting up will gradually decrease in frequency and eventually stop by the time he is two or two and a half. If the baby spits up regularly after every meal he may be eating more than he can handle, or may need a change in formula. In any case, you should consult your doctor if the spitting up continues over too long a time.

One common mistake that many young mothers make is confusing spitting up with true vomiting. If food is ejected from the stomach with great force after a feeding, the cause is usually a stomach upset or a gastric or intestinal disturbance. If the baby seems otherwise in good health try feeding him again after a few minutes. If the projectile vomiting is repeated, a physician should be consulted. One cause of frequent forcible vomiting is the chronic malfunctioning of the pyloric valve. This is a comparatively rare condition, however.

SPLENIUS The splenius is a flat muscle of the neck. One is found on either side of the back of the neck. They are used in rotating the head.

SPLINT A splint is any rigid appliance, usually a flat piece of wood or metal which is used in first-aid treatment of a broken bone. As a general rule you should never attempt to administer first-aid to someone with a broken bone further than trying to keep him comfortable until a physician can be brought to him. There may be times, however, when someone who has a badly broken leg or arm must be moved before a doctor can be called. In these cases the broken limb must be immobilized as much as possible to prevent pain to the sufferer and further injury to the broken bone. The best way to do this is with a splint.

Splints can be made from anything that can keep the injured part immobilized—anything from an umbrella to a heavy magazine to some tightly rolled newspaper. If a hard object is used it should be wrapped in towels or cloth of some kind to keep from bruising the arm or leg. The splint should be strapped with a belt, or tied to the injured part. Always be careful not to cinch the splint too tight as you may run the risk of stopping the circulation. It should cover the break and be long enough to immobilize the joint adjacent to the break. If the fractured bone has broken through the skin be sure to cover the break in the skin with a cloth or other bandage of some soft material to protect it from dirt.

SPLINTERS Splinters are dangerous because they may introduce germs and become the seat of potentially dangerous infections. In most cases of splinters removal is simple and there is no necessity for worry. The splinter can usually be squeezed out to a point when it can be removed by a tweezers. If the splinter cannot be reached with a tweezers a sterilized needle can be used to pluck out the splinter. After the splinter has been removed the wound should be squeezed gently until blood circulates in it. This cleans the wound from the inside. A disinfectant should then be applied.

Splinters that have been driven under a fingernail or toenail occasionally require medical attention if they are too deeply imbedded to be easily reached. The doctor will cut away whatever part of the nail must be removed in order to reach it. Never attempt to perform this operation yourself as a physician's skill and the aseptic techniques which are part of his routine are necessary to prevent infection.

One of the most serious of industrial accidents is the lodging of a metal sliver in the eye. Care of this condition most certainly comes in the province of the eye specialist. In recent years new techniques have been developed for the quick and safe removal of such splinters which in the past have caused many cases of blindness.

SPOILED FOOD (See also *Botulism* and *Food Poisoning*) Poor handling and faulty refrigeration are frequent causes of contaminated food and subsequent cases of food poisoning. Some foods tend to spoil more quickly than others. Sea food should always be kept under refrigeration as it will spoil almost immediately at room temperature. Meats and poultry, even after cooking should not be allowed to stand out in the open air. The danger with spoiled foods is that they may be spoiled not just by old age but by organisms which could prove extremely harmful to humans. There are a few basic rules of food storing and handling which, if followed, will protect you and your family from the possibility of unsettling illness.

1. Never refreeze a frozen food product which has thawed.
2. Keep all foods with an oily base in the refrigerator.
3. Wrap all leftovers in wax paper or

foil and keep under refrigeration.

SPONGE, ALCOHOL An alcohol sponge is a therapeutic measure used to reduce a fever without chilling the sufferer. It is also used as a bath to relax bedridden patients and to help prevent bedsores with people who must stay prone in the same position for a long time. The procedures for giving an alcohol sponge are similar to those used in giving a bed bath. The bedclothes should be protected with a bath blanket and the patient should be rubbed on his chest, arms, legs and back with a solution of ½ water and ½ rubbing alcohol.

If the doctor has recommended that an alcohol sponge be given specifically to lower temperature, then the same procedure is used with certain additions. An ice bag is placed at the patient's head and a hot water bottle wrapped in a towel so as not to burn, at his feet. A cloth which has been soaked in the solution and then wrung out is placed at the patient's abdomen. With another cloth rub the chest slowly and gently for several minutes, then dry thoroughly. Follow this procedure on the arms and legs, then turn the patient over and rub the back with the solution. Remove the hot water bottle, the ice bag and the wet cloth.

SPONDYLOLISTHESIS, or slipped vertebra, a condition in which an exaggerated lumbar curve is formed when the fifth vertebra is so disturbed as to slip forward toward the front of the body. This abnormality is caused by defective growth of bone in the neural arch. Because support is lacking, the condition causes backache, which disappears when the person rests. The pain reappears on exertion and is felt down the thigh and leg.

SPOROTRICHOSIS, an infection of the skin and mucous membranes, caused by a fungus, the Sporotrichum schenckii, which grows on plants and brush. Persons exposed to vegetation, such as gardeners or farmers, are most apt to become infected, usually by acquiring the fungus on the skin or a break in the skin. Sporotrichosis has also been found in horses, dogs, and cats.

SPOTS BEFORE THE EYES (See also, *Eye*) One of the most common Symptoms complained of by many people is a sense of spots floating before the eyes. Scientifically, these are called *muscae volitantes*. The specialist in diseases of the eye attaches little significance to these spots, unless such spots can be seen on special examination of the eye with the ophthalmoscope, the instrument with which the specialist looks into the eye. These floating spots have been attributed to irritations of the eye, to congestion of the tissues, to eyestrain, and various constitutional diseases. Generally speaking, they are not important. If the person concerned has the right kind of glasses and keeps himself in good physical condition the spots will disappear.

SPRAINS Among the most common injuries which affect human beings are sprains, particularly of the ankles and the wrists. A sudden movement or a fall will stretch or overstretch a ligament so that it tears. Fluid or blood then gets into a joint. Sometimes a sprain is so severe that a bone is broken. For this reason every serious sprain should be subjected to an X-ray picture. The opening of the football season and the coming of winter produce a sudden increase in the number of sprains, particularly of the ankles.

Ordinarily a simple sprain is treated by rest, elevation of the leg and ankle, and the application of an ice bag. The doctor can immobilize the joint with strapping—use adhesive—or even with a plaster cast. Modern treatment, however, calls for movement of the joint. Since this is likely to produce pain, the physician in some instances injects an anesthetic substance into the injured area and permits the patient to use the foot or the hand.

After a joint has been fixed in one position for a considerable length of time and particularly if there has been much inflammation and swelling, it is difficult to move the joint. In such cases movement is not attempted rapidly but slowly; massage is used to aid softening of the tissues and relaxation of the stiffness. Heat should not be applied to a sprained ankle until the danger of congestion and hemorrhage has been controlled. The value of heat is greatest in the final stages when repair has begun in order to encourage circulation and absorption of excess fluid.

SPRAINED ANKLE—See FOOT, article THE FOOT.

SPONTANEOUS DISAPPEARANCE OF CANCER

(See also discussion under *Detection of Cancer, Cancer, Mortality in Cancer, Research in Cancer, Stomach Cancer*) For many years investigators have been convinced that cancer cells sometimes have the effect of stimulating the defenses of the body to act against them in the same way that immunity can be developed to germs and viruses of various kinds. A recent review establishes that many cases of spontaneous regression of cancer have been authenticated and recorded. Several investigators refused to believe such evidence even after they had seen it. With the increase in our knowledge of cancer the belief that the cancer structure was an autonomous process which depended on the host only for the blood supply and that the cancer is essentially a behavior of a growing structure not susceptible to modification has been altered. In 1918 one investigator published a survey of 302 cases of temporary or permanent regression of cancer. The famous pathologist Ewing noted that under peculiar conditions involving changes in the blood supply and nature of growth, they could regress or disappear from the body. The regression of tumors cannot be wholly explained on the basis of an insufficient blood supply. Huggins and his associates, whose work has already been mentioned and who showed that cancer of the prostate regressed and tended to disappear after removal of the testicles and removal of the adrenal glands or the pituitary, indicate that cancer growths are dependent on chemical substances derived from various tissues of the body. Similarly, the gradual alteration of breast cancer by the administration of male and female sex hormones is now recognized. These experiments also indicate that the tumor depends upon chemical substances derived from the host.

The body is capable of defensive action against invading cancers as is shown by the development in the body of specific antibodies against the cancer. The appearance of such antibodies is leading to the development of specific blood tests which will detect the presence of cancer. The recognition of spontaneous regression of cancer leads to hope that specific methods can be found which will increase the rate of regression and stop the wild and unrestrained growth that we recognize as most significant in this devastating disease.

SPRUE

Among the tropical conditions which affected a good many of our soldiers in the war was one called sprue. In this condition diarrhea, loss of weight, and inflammation of the mouth are the chief symptoms. Often the condition is mistaken for food poisoning. The tongue becomes red and sore, the abdomen is suddenly swollen with gas, and there may be repeated cramps.

The word "sprue" comes from a Dutch word that is used to describe an inflammation of the mouth. The disease was known more than two thousand years ago. The exact cause of sprue is not now known but the generally accepted view is that sprue follows some nutritional deficiency. This impression is confirmed by the fact that proper feeding with certain materials brings about improvement. The symptoms of sprue are like those of pellagra and pernicious anemia, in both of which the addition of certain substances to the diet brings about improvement. Incidentally the existence of sprue is associated with the growth of a yeastlike fungus called the monilia, but the evidence that the monilia is the cause of the sprue is not generally accepted.

Because there are many types of infection in tropical areas associated with dysentery, inflammation, and even bleeding from the bowel, a correct diagnosis of sprue is most important. The doctor, therefore, must get a careful record of the diet and of the action of the bowel. The failure of appetite in these patients makes it more likely that they will have an inadequate diet. Often patients with sprue lose one third to one half their normal weight.

The material from the bowel in a case of sprue has a large excess of fat. Apparently the difficulty is the inability of the body to take up this material. Until recently sprue was treated with a great variety of special diets. Then it was found that liver treatment is just as effective in sprue as it is in pernicious anemia. When the treatment with liver is begun early, the results are brilliant. In far-advanced cases the damage to the tissues of the body has been so great that complete recovery is impossible. Because of the nature of the disease the feeding of liver alone never gets as good a result as injection of liver into the body by the veins or the blood. During the course of treatment the diet is also modified to cut down the fats and to provide extra protein and extra vitamins. Often these patients improve tremendously merely with a high-protein and high-vitamin diet.

Sprue—gastritis: See article Digestion and Digestive Diseases.

SQUINT See discussion of *Cross-Eyes* under *Eye*.

STAMMERING See *Stuttering and Stammering*.

STAPHYLOCOCCUS INFECTIONS—(See also, *Infections and Immunity*) Staphylococci used to be among the most feared of all the germs that attack mankind. In their various forms they could attack mucous membranes, the tissues of the heart, even the entire blood. Boils, carbuncles, and similar manifestations of staphylococcus infection were frequent. The germs would get into the centers of bones and cause the condition called osteomyelitis. Many a child was crippled for life by the inability of medicine to control this infection.

Occasionally staphylococci attack the bowel through entrance with food. Staphylococcus food poisoning results from the absorption of the toxin given off by the germ. The response is cramping pain, usually coming on two to four hours after the food is taken, with nausea, vomiting, and diarrhea. This lasts for a few hours, seldom more than a day. After twenty-four hours, the attack subsides, leaving the patient weak. The best treatment is to go right to bed and stop taking food for at least twenty-four hours. Paregoric is usually given to relieve the diarrhea and the cramping. Of course a doctor has to make sure that the condition is not appendicitis or some similar disturbance.

Penicillin is the drug that is most frequently recommended for treating staphylococcal infections. When the germs are resistant to penicillin some of the other antibiotic drugs may be used including the sulfonamides. Mixtures of several sulfonamides, such as streptomycin, aureomycin, or terramycin, are sometimes successfully used. The sulfonamides and the antibiotics are so effective in combatting staphylococci that the only additional treatment usually required is good nursing. Surgery helps by opening accumulations of pus and draining away infected material after which healing occurs promptly.

STERILITY The future of any nation depends on the continued growth of its population. When people do not have children, nations must seek elsewhere for their population. An example is the way in which Germany imported workers because her men were all engaged in war. Fortunately the desire to have children is a natural human desire. Unfortunately some people who want children, who are even anxious to have them, do not do so because physical conditions prevent.

People who have many children are called fertile. Sterility is the opposite of fertility and it means inability to have children. Either the woman or the man may be responsible. In many cases the responsibility is shared by both. Some people make up their minds early in their married life that they do not want children and take steps to prevent childbirth. Experts say that at least 10 per cent of marriages in Great Britain and in the United States are completely sterile. This means that there is nothing that can be done that will cause these people to have children.

Many people are not absolutely sterile but merely relatively sterile—that is to say, they are sterile under the conditions of the marriage but might not be sterile under some other conditions.

Once, when we knew far less about childbirth than we know now, it was taken for granted that failure to have children meant that the woman was responsible. Nowadays we realize that investigations of childless marriages involve exhaustive examination of both husband and wife before it may be determined which is responsible and to what extent.

From the point of view of the woman who is sterile, the doctor determines whether or not the ovaries produce and give off eggs capable of being fertilized. He must find out whether or not such eggs pass down through the tubes into the uterus in which the child develops before birth. He must know whether or not it is possible for the male cells to reach the female cell in the uterus. He must know whether or not the lining of the uterus is capable of forming tissues that are necessary for the development of the child.

From the point of view of the man, the doctor must find out whether or not the male sex glands produce the fertilizing element in sufficient amount and with sufficient strength or life to travel the necessary distance to reach the female cell.

If any of these prerequisites fall short of perfection, the result is a definite lessening of the possibility that a child may be conceived or developed.

The most recently accumulated figures show that the man is responsible wholly or in part for from 30 to 40 per cent of all cases in which a family does not have children. The first step in sterility studies should always be an investigation of the husband. In case a

STERILITY

complete absence of the fertilizing element is demonstrated, there is no further need to examine the wife. In many instances the number of male elements is small and the product is weak. Frequently several examinations are necessary because these qualifications differ from time to time.

When a man and woman marry and live an apparently normal sex life and still fail to have children, physical conditions are usually responsible for the failure. When such people consult the doctor to determine what is wrong, they must realize that conditions affecting the man are just as likely to be responsible as conditions affecting his wife. Since the child is formed by the union of a cell from the man with a cell from the woman, the study must include an actual investigation of the ability of the man and of the woman to provide the necessary cells.

Furthermore, there must be certainty that the cells of the father can travel the necessary route to join the cell from the mother in the organ in which the child is carried after conception. The physician must make certain that the cell from the mother developed by the ovary can travel successfully down the tube into the uterus. The male cells undergo greater risk of damage or destruction in their route to join the female cell than does the ovum of the mother in passing from the ovary to the uterus. The normal male can provide each time from 3,000,000 to 4,000,000 cells; yet only one of these is neccessary to fertilize the female cell. The destruction of the male cells or damage to them en route by secretions or other materials

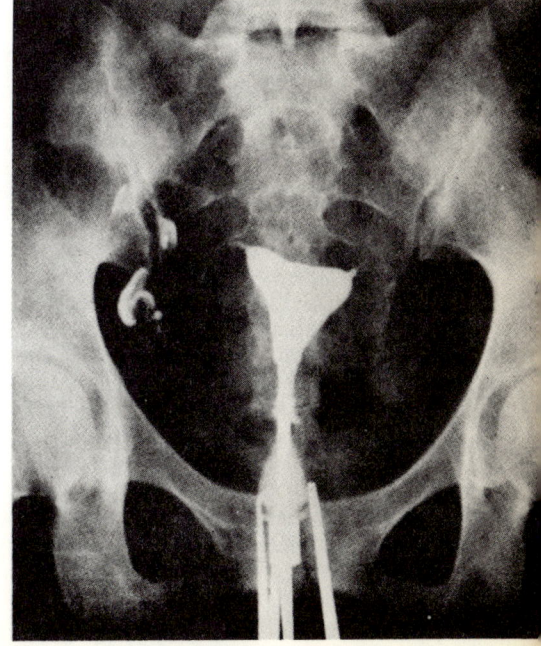

Some couples who are concerned about their inability to have children consult a physician. Since the cause of infertility may lie with either husband or wife or both, tests must be conducted on both. This X-ray shows the results of one of the tests done on the wife to determine the normalcy and patency of the uterus and tubes. A radiopaque solution is injected into these structures and passage of the substance can be watched by X-ray. A normal uterus (white, triangular area), one patent tube (on the left in the X-ray) and one blocked tube are demonstrated in this particular X-ray.

Postgraduate Medicine

on the path that they follow may be responsible for failure of the woman to conceive.

Obviously, if the number of male cells deposited is less than it should be, or if the cells are without the necessary vitality to travel their course, the chance of conception is greatly lessened.

Another factor of importance is the time when the female cell reaches the uterus in relationship to the time when the male cells start their journey. There are about two weeks between the periodical functions of the woman when impregnation of an ovum by a sperm cell is exceedingly unlikely.

The term "sterility" usually means that a woman has not given birth to a child after living with her husband for three years, during which time no efforts have been made to interfere with conception. This does not mean, however, that the woman cannot become pregnant. Some women become pregnant ten years after marriage, while others may never be able to become pregnant.

If the tubes which carry the egg cell from the ovary to the uterus are permanently blocked as the result of abnormal construction or disease, the woman cannot possibly become pregnant. There may have been infections early in life which injured the organs involved in this procedure. For instance, mumps is known to affect the organs involved in the production of the sex cells. Experiments with animals have indicated that diets seriously deficient in certain necessary vitamins may damage the reproductive function. Indeed, even serious mental or emotional disturbances may affect the physical relationships to such an extent as to make conception unlikely. If, therefore, any couple is disturbed about failure to have children, a complete physical examination of both the prospective father and mother is necessary in order to determine the responsibility for the failure. The examination may include a study of the cells developed by the father, the use of modern methods to determine whether or not the tubes of the mother are open, and finally a complete record of the sex life of the people concerned.

Unfortunately the tubes of the woman, once sealed by serious disease, are not likely to be capable of repair by surgical procedures, or by blowing of air through the tubes or other technics which physicians use.

Duke University investigators have found that the best treatment many childless couples who want children can have is assurance from a doctor that they are capable of having children. In a group of 150 couples in whom nothing physically wrong could be found, 80 of the wives became pregnant after they were examined and assured that they could have children. Studies are now being made to determine why the other 70 women did not become pregnant. Among other treatments given were use of antibiotic drugs to overcome moderate infections, and use of thyroid in cases where there was underactivity of this gland.

STERILITY—gonorrhea causes: See VENEREAL DISEASES, article THE VENEREAL DISEASES.

STERILITY—syphilis not the only cause: See VENEREAL DISEASES, article THE VENEREAL DISEASES.

STERILIZATION—after third Caesarian operation: See BIRTH, article CARE OF MOTHERS BEFORE AND AFTER CHILDBIRTH.

STERILIZATION—no deleterious effect: See BIRTH, article CARE OF MOTHERS BEFORE AND AFTER CHILDBIRTH.

STOMACH CANCER (See also discussion under *Cancer, Detection of Cancer, Research in Cancer*) Since the one hope in certain forms of internal forms of cancer such as cancer of the stomach is successful removal by operation, much attention has been given to improving surgery. The average mortality for patients with complete removal of the stomach was previously about 16%. This has been reduced in competent surgical clinics to about 8%. In one large clinic, of all patients who had such removal, because of cancer, an estimated 31.6% were still living five years after operation, 23.2% were living ten years after operation, 17.2% were living fifteen years after operation and 12.2% were living twenty years after operation. Almost all of the patients who had simple palliative operations had died when five years had elapsed. Therefore the outlook regarding cancer of the stomach is much less pessimistic than it was formerly. The crux of the matter is obviously to get more patients to the surgeon while the growth is still susceptible of complete removal and before spread has taken place to other organs of the body. In the attack on cancer of the stomach, the use of the fluoroscope for observation and of the gastroscope for looking directly at the changes in the stomach walls, the examination of cells taken from the stomach, and earlier and more frequent operations on all suspicious small ulcerating lesions are believed to be most significant in lowering still further the death rate from cancer of the stomach. For extra safety, some surgeons advocate what is called a second look operation particularly to be used when the first operation does not yield relief.

STOMACH, SURGERY OF (See also discussion under *Cancer, Esophagus, Indigestion, Stomach Ulcers*) The stomach was once considered the most vital of all the organs of the human body and was even considered to be the seat of the soul. Many years elapsed before surgeons began to make routine the operations on this organ. The operations proceeded from simple cutting away of the diseased portions to the removal of a portion of the stomach, then of a half of the stomach and now of all of the stomach. This procedure, called "total gastrectomy," is widely employed, particularly for treatment of cancer of the stomach. The mortality is steadily diminishing so that some clinics report as few as 10% of deaths. Most surgeons today seem to prefer what is called a "subtotal" gastric operation.

The treatment of ulcers of the stomach by vagotomy which is the cutting of the vagus nerve to the stomach is one of the innovations in medicine which has developed greatly in recent years. Surgeons however still debate the desirability of vagotomy over subtotal gastrectomy. The operations are frequently combined with various short circuiting operations such as gastroenterostomy, which involves connecting the intestine to the stomach or pyloroplasty which is a remaking of the valve at the lower end of the stomach.

In all types of surgery on the stomach and the intestines, the use of x-ray has been invaluable not only in making the diagnosis but also in tracing the healing and in watching the functions of the stomach and the intestines before and after operation. Modern surgeons would not think of attempting surgery of the stomach or the intestines without the aid that is provided by x-ray. As has already been mentioned, modern surgery now involves the removal of great amounts of tissue from the gastrointestinal tract so that the cutting away of several feet of the intestine which is some 32 feet long as a means of ridding the body of diseased tissue is not considered an extraordinary procedure.

STOMACH ULCERS The stresses and exigencies of war resulted every-

STOMACH ULCERS

where in an increase in the incidence of ulcers of the stomach and duodenum. The duodenum, the portion of the intestines which comes immediately after the stomach, was called that by the ancients because it was about twelve fingers long.

Ulcers of the duodenum have been described as the commonest disease of the upper part of the intestinal system and the condition is found four times as often in men as in women. Also ulcers are found ten times as often in the duodenum as they are in the stomach. Occurring usually in people who live under high tension, the condition has often been called "nervous indigestion."

Simply because we are not certain of any one cause of ulcers of the stomach or duodenum, we are likely to assign any one of a number of causes. Apparently they are more prevalent in certain families, but this can be related to the fact that a nervous constitution occurs also in certain families.

Undoubtedly there are physical causes as well as mental, but apparently the physical causes become operative under certain mental conditions. When there are stock-market crashes, when there are wars, when there are constant bickerings and arguments in the family, ulcers appear.

There has been a tendency to associate the presence of ulcers with an increased amount of acid in the stomach. The excess acid is responsible for the continuation of the symptoms. It has been customary to treat the condition largely with a view to combating the excess acidity. An ulcer of the stomach or of the intestines is like an ulcer elsewhere in the body: when it heals, there is a tendency to form a scar.

Because of the increased emphasis on psychological relationship in ulcers, modern treatment calls for mental rest and special attention to decreasing the worry or strain from which the patients suffer. Many men with ulcers improve when they take a vacation. It has been observed that when patients travel long distances to get some kind of treatment they sometimes arrive at their destination with the beginning of healing already in progress.

Apparently the continuation of the stress and strain will be reflected in the nervous system. The drugs used are antacids, antispasmodics like atropine, banthine, or prantal which block the nerve impulses, and sedatives. In severe uncontrollable cases surgical treatment prevents perforation and leads to more permanent results.

The big problem for the doctor is to correct the excess acidity by the provision of a proper diet and proper drugs. Diets have to be calculated for the individual patient, and they must take into account the necessity for vitamins and mineral salts in order to maintain general health as well as the treatment of the ulcer.

In the hygiene of the person with ulcers, authorities recommend discontinuation of smoking and of the use of alcohol and of excessive exercise. In occasional instances change of occupation and of residence seem to make the difference between health and continued disease.

DUODENAL ULCERS—See article DIGESTION AND DIGESTIVE DISEASES.

DUODENAL ULCERS—angina pectoris caused by: See HEART, article DISEASES OF THE HEART AND CIRCULATION.

DUODENAL ULCERS—cancer unlikely to follow: See article DIGESTION AND DIGESTIVE DISEASES.

DUODENAL ULCERS—reaction to stress: See article STRESS AND DISEASE.

GASTRIC ULCERS—See article DIGESTION AND DIGESTIVE DISEASES.

STOMACH ULCERS—See article DIGESTION AND DIGESTIVE DISEASES.

STOMACH ULCERS—ACTH contraindicated: See article ALLERGY.

STOMACH ULCERS—cancer may follow: See article DIGESTION AND DIGESTIVE DISEASES.

STOMACH ULCERS—cortisone contraindicated: See article ALLERGY.

STOMACH ULCERS—diet: See DIET, article ADVICE ON THE DIET.

STOMACH ULCERS—emotional disorders may cause: See MENTAL, article NERVOUS AND MENTAL DISORDERS.

STOMACH ULCERS—polycythemia: See BLOOD, article THE BLOOD AND ITS DISEASES.

STRABISMUS Another word for *Cross-Eyes*. See under *Eye*.

STRAWBERRY BIRTHMARKS (See also discussion under *Birthmarks* and *Skin*) Collections of dilated small blood vessels commonly called "strawberry birthmarks" tend to disappear as babies grow older. A Missouri physician observed 39 cases over a number of years. In 24 cases the marks had gone between 1 and 14 years of age; 14 of the remainder seemed to be regressing. Should such marks at any time show signs of growth, they are removed surgically or destroyed by other techniques such as freezing with carbon dioxide snow or electric coagulation.

STREPTOCOCCUS VIRIDANS (See also discussion under *Heart*) Various germs can cause endocarditis but the one most frequently responsible is called the streptococcus viridans.

Stress and Disease

BY

HAROLD G. WOLFF, M.D.

Professor of Medicine (Neurology), Cornell University Medical College, New York City.

Our language bears witness that men have been long aware that feelings and bodily changes are related. A few indicative phrases are:

> He got red in the face; he was pale with rage; it took one's breath away; he got into a cold sweat; it makes me sick; it turns my stomach; he had a lump in his throat; he got a weight off his chest; he trembled with fear; he shook with rage; he had cold feet.

Industry has not been blind to these facts. A thousand people sweat approximately 100 pounds of moisture in one hour under ordinary conditions, but under the emotionally charged conditions of a thrilling motion picture the moisture output rises to 150 pounds per thousand persons.

Bartlett's *Familiar Quotations* has in its index nine columns of phrases including the word "heart." Roget's *Thesaurus* has "heart" in the index more often than any other word. Indeed, "heart" has become a symbol of the human spirit, thus, "hard-hearted," "warm-hearted," "cold-hearted," "steel-hearted." We continually use words that indicate our knowledge that the body participates in reactions to experience. How pertinent these bodily changes are to health, and how these changes begin to disturb a man's effectiveness and jeopardize his life, will be seen in the following pages.

SKIN

The skin offers dramatic demonstrations of change during stress. For example, the minute vessels of a man's skin were tested as regards their ability to retain blood within them, called, for convenience, capillary tone. The left arm was forcefully struck, and immediately a red area appeared which began to swell, and the deterioration of the capillary tone was charted. The skin of the right arm behaved in the same way even though it was not struck. The left arm gradually returned to its former state; the right arm reached that state a little sooner. The experiment was repeated, but, instead of bringing the ferrule down onto the forearm, it was brought just short of the arm. Even though no injury was inflicted by this sham blow, the skin of the left arm behaved just as it had before. That of the right arm did not respond. Gradually the left returned to its former state. In other words, this person, through his skin, reacted not only to an actual blow but also to the symbol of a blow by putting into his tissues a certain amount of fluid, perhaps representing not only a reaction to tissue injury, but also a means to protect him from injury. The whole procedure was repeated, except that this time the subject was told what was going to happen; after the expected sham blow, no bodily change took place.

Another man with a complaint of hives was studied. A record was made of the ability of his capillaries to hold their contents. Instead of striking him with a ferrule, we discussed a situation involving his family which made him feel as though he were being hit. At the same time, his skin behaved as though he were actually struck, and he developed "hives." In a little while they disappeared. In this instance a bodily pattern serving to protect from injury was used in a way in which it was of no specific value.

A man's skin was tested for ability to react to stroking, and to the chemical poisons, histamine and pilocarpine. His skin was insensitive to all of these. He was then exposed to a discussion about his family troubles which made him feel as though he were "taking a beating." At the height of his reaction the very same mechanical and chemical stimuli that failed before to produce an effect produced a great effect, seen as hives. In other words, he became at this time vulnerable to a great many assaults, not only to the effects which came from the discussion of his family troubles, but also to other noxious influences. He was, at that moment, in a weakened or vulnerable state. With reassurance he soon returned to his original condition.

Stenographic records of remarks during such bodily changes were made. During a conversation in which a man was developing hives, we heard: "They did a lot of things to me and I couldn't do anything about it." "I was getting pushed around." "I had to sit and take it." "I was taking a beating." "They were cracking a whip over me." "My mother is constantly hammering on me." "He walked all over me." In other words, while his body is acting as though it were "taking a beating," he feels as though he were being exposed to such an assault. The organism deals with an assault in a given way and uses that pattern again and again, sometimes in reaction to noxious interpersonal relations where it can serve no useful or appropriate end.

Stomach

A man was offered food which interested him, and immediately the measured blood flow in the lining of his stomach increased. A record of the mechanical action of the stomach showed that it was churning and contracting. Also the digestive secretions had increased in amount, i.e., the stomach was preparing for the act of digestion even though the man was only look-

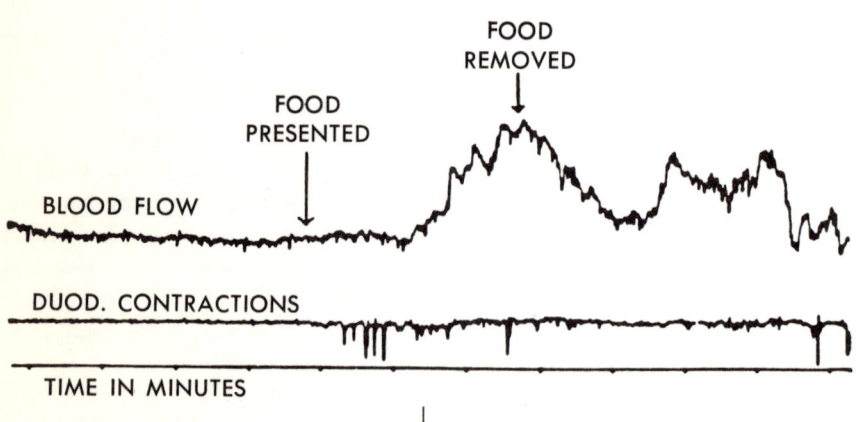

Changes in blood flow and motility associated with the sight and smell of appetizing food.

ing at food. When the food was removed, the blood flow and contractions gradually returned to their initial level. Other food was offered which did not appeal to him; his "appetite" was not stimulated and consequently there was no change noted in the function of his stomach.

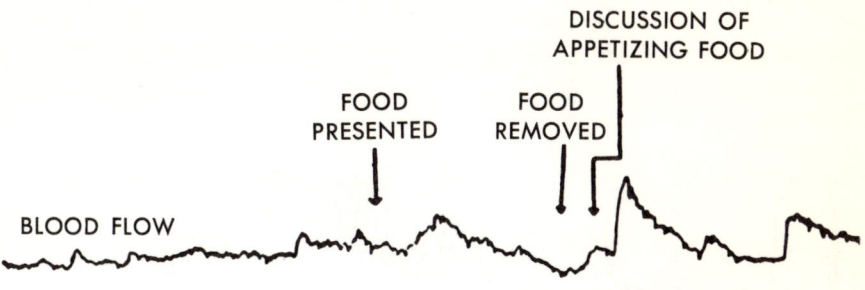
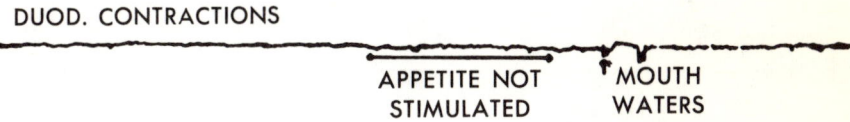

Changes in blood flow and motility associated with the discussion of appetizing food. Note the absence of changes with the sight and smell of un-appetizing food.

Next, the food was removed from view, and instead of introducing something he could see or smell, food that he liked was discussed. Immediately his stomach prepared for digestive activity. Words symbolic of food rather than food itself were the stimuli. A topic which was extremely poisonous to this patient was then presented. During an absence due to illness, his business partner had carried on some shady business deals which had brought him disrepute. As he discussed his partner's behavior he became exceedingly angry, and his stomach and upper gastro-intestinal tract acted as though they were preparing to digest.

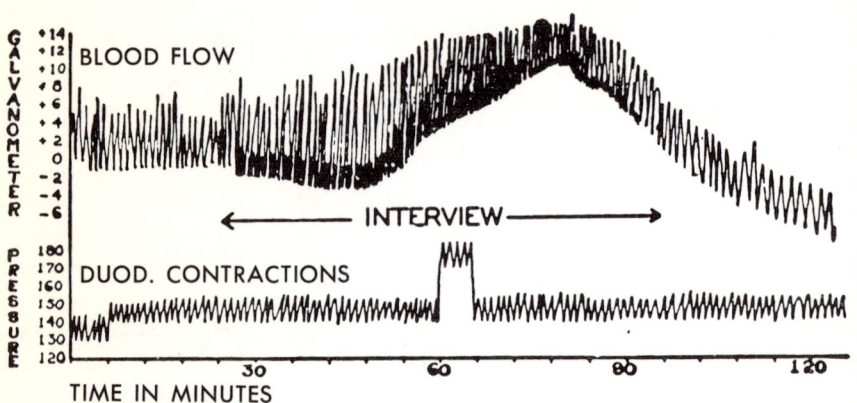

Gastroduodenal blood flow in man. Increase in duodenal blood flow accompanying anxiety, tension and resentment. (The pressure is calibrated in mm. of water.) The rise in the upper recording indicates an increase of blood flow in the walls of the duodenal portion of the intestine, during an interview which aroused feelings of anxiety, tension and resentment.

One of our subjects, "Tom," now about age sixty-five, experienced a serious accident when he was nine. He came home from school one day, thirsty and warm, and mistakenly drank scalding hot clam chowder. He thus blocked his gullet and could not swallow. In order to keep him alive surgeons created a hole in his abdomen leading to his stomach, and through this opening he has since fed himself twice a day for more than half a century. He is a good citizen, father, and worker. He is shy, taciturn, with strong feelings about "respectability" and his capacity to take his place in the community. He is now employed as a helper in the New York Hospital. He comes into the laboratory every day, and the blood flow in his stomach lining is measured—the more blood flow, the redder the lining; the less blood flow, the paler the lining. The secretion of gastric juices and the churning activity of his stomach are also ascertained. At the same time a note is made of his current fears, hopes, wishes, frustrations, and satisfactions.

On one occasion while "Tom" was in the laboratory a physician entered saying that a certain important protocol, the safekeeping of which was Tom's responsibility, was missing. Gradually he grew pale in face and stomach as his terror increased. The troubled doctor opened and closed drawers, muttering imprecations. He finally found the protocol and left. Tom said, "I was scared that I had lost my job." This statement has to be seen in symbolic terms. The man was in terror that he had lost his position not only as our fellow worker, but also that he had "lost face" as one who had been entrusted with responsibility. His stomach was pale, hypoactive, non-functioning. It was "out of condition," distended, and digestion was slowed. He complained of flatulence, food remained in the stomach a long time, he experienced gaseous eructations, and felt nauseated. Under comparable circumstances at other times, he vomited through the opening in his abdomen. This may serve as an example of an organ hypofunctioning under circumstances of stress.

In contrast, the following observation was made on Tom when, again resting on the observation table, he was told that an additional job of dusting and cleaning which he had undertaken was improperly done. As he was being told about his inadequacy Tom got red in the face, red in the stomach, the acid in his stomach increased in amount, his stomach began to churn, and when told that he was "fired" it became exceedingly red. His accuser then left, whereupon Tom muttered, "I'd like to wring his neck." Along with this expression of anger he felt abused and "put upon."

Such changes in the stomach may last for weeks. The acid secretion and the color of the stomach before, during, and after a period of crisis are exemplified in the following situation: Receiving a small salary, Tom was obliged to accept the contributions of a benefactor who meddled in his personal affairs. This threatened his independence and he repeatedly made efforts to throw off his benefactor. Finally, during a two-week period the meddling was particularly irksome, and his stomach exhibited a high acid secretion and a deep red color. A slight raise in salary enabled him to be rid of his benefactor, and his stomach returned to its former state.

Also studied was another man who had a similar abdominal aperture through which his stomach could be viewed. The lining of the stomach had a pink color when he was tranquil. But when a certain doctor was mentioned whom he hated because he believed he had failed to diagnose his illness, which he feared was to cost him his life, he became exceedingly angry. He sputtered and became profane, and his stomach mucosa became dark red. Thus as part of his reactions to the poisonous topic involving his hates and fears, impulses went down the vagus nerve which converted the mucous membrane of the stomach from a resting state to one of readiness for eating, and one, which if sustained, could lead to ulcer formation. It became necessary to cut this major nerve to the stomach, i.e., the vagus. After surgery, discussion of this same doctor was associated with every outward show of anger, but there was no change within his stomach.

Attitudes

Feelings are part of our reaction to events. They should not be spoken of as causing bodily changes. What one feels is not truly causative, but only another manifestation of one's reaction to experience. In other words, when something happens to you, you develop an attitude which has two components. First, what meaning has this experience for me? Secondly, what do I do about it? This attitude is, for the most part, unconscious. When a person rids himself of something by vomiting because it is disgusting or unattractive, he expresses a characteristic attitude. Recorded statements included: "I wish it hadn't happened." "I didn't want this." "Why did it have to happen?" "I wish things were the way they were before." "I wish I hadn't gotten into this." "I wish I hadn't listened to him."

Much has been said concerning the conscious versus the unconscious, but an appraisal of the *meaning of a situation for the individual person* is far more relevant. If it be conscious, it has a chance of being dealt with; if it be unconscious, it is less accessible and the person may suffer its effects for indefinitely long periods. Often matters are so dreadful and so overwhelming that they are dismissed from consciousness. But to repeat: important for consideration is, "What is the *meaning* of an experience or a stimulus or a threat or a statement?" and then, "What do I do about it?"

Bowel

Four people with abdominal apertures allowing views of the large bowel gave us much information about the connection between the bowel and life experiences. One man had a thumbscrew arrangement put on top of his head. He willingly volunteered, although he knew that he was going to be hurt. Painfully squeezing his head with the thumbscrews caused his bowel to get red and to contract. He felt angry and anxious, but placidly accepted the assault. The second man, despite the fact that he wished to participate and knew what was going to happen, became angry and showed it. Indeed, he would not permit the experiment to continue. Also, this second man had, in reaction to exactly the same stimulus under the same circumstances, precisely the opposite bodily reaction as did the first man. His bowel got pale, and contractile activity stopped. A general principle is thus exemplified: Here were two people exposed to the same assault, yet, because its meaning was different, they experienced opposite reactions. The assault engendered a distinctly individual attitude in each of the men, leading to different ways of meeting the threat and danger.

In a similar study it was observed that a person's bowel when he was in a state of relative tranquillity was pink in color. During a period featured by dejection or sadness, it became pale and relaxed. During a period with anger it contracted and became dark red, and a balloon inserted within the bowel showed it to be hypermotile. Also, about twenty minutes after eating, it became red and hypermotile even during a period of tranquillity. This is the so-called gastrocolic reflex and it is the basis of the urge to empty the bowel shortly after meals. It serves a good purpose, but it is not good for this condition to be maintained by anger. The same man was observed on another day after lunch, under ostensibly the same circumstances, but reacting to the lunch not at all as regards to change in color and blood supply of his mucosa, or the contractile state of his bowel. He was dejected because of an unfortunate and humiliating incident involving a neighbor which occurred just a few hours before. The subject under these circumstances would have no urge to evacuate the bowel and indeed might consider himself "constipated."

The Significance of the Topic

When a topic is introduced that sets off a given reaction during an interview, it does not mean that the subject matter is the key to the person's life difficulties and that if this particular problem be solved, all of his troubles would end. The topic under discussion is merely representative of many which are looked upon as threats and reacted to in a similar way. For example, we discussed with a sensitive man something about his sister-in-law. This man's bowel trouble, known as ulcerative colitis, began shortly after the death of his mother upon whom he was overdependent. He was devastated by her death. He duly assumed the position of head of the family with vigor, but without conviction or effectiveness. His younger brother married and brought into the home a woman who, by her attitude and behavior, threatened the patient's position as head of the family. Merely discussing this woman caused his bowel to contract and become dark red. His sister-in-law had become a threatening symbol. He reacted to many other threats in the same manner. The bowel acted as though it were trying to get rid of an irritant.

A sailor, with similarly exposed colon, believed that because of his religious affiliations he was not given a "good berth" on ship. Discussion of the problem caused his feelings to be roused, anger expressed, and his bowel to contract, become overactive, and dark red. He was easily diverted, however, and within a few minutes the bowel became paler and relaxed. Again, within a few minutes he felt much threatened and challenged by questions which he took to indicate that his integrity was in doubt, and again the bowel became dark red and contracted vigorously.

The overcontracted, hypermotile gastro-intestinal tract with a dark red mucous membrane becomes very fragile. When a person is relaxed and tranquil, a negative pressure of up to 200 mm. of mercury applied to the bowel surface may be withstood for six minutes without damage or bleeding. But when a person subject to ulcerative colitis becomes insecure and angry and the bowel is in an overactive, congested state, it takes very little—say 60 mm. of mercury pressure for 1½ minutes, or even the gut's own contractions—to cause the tissue to tear and bleed. Under these circumstances when bleeding

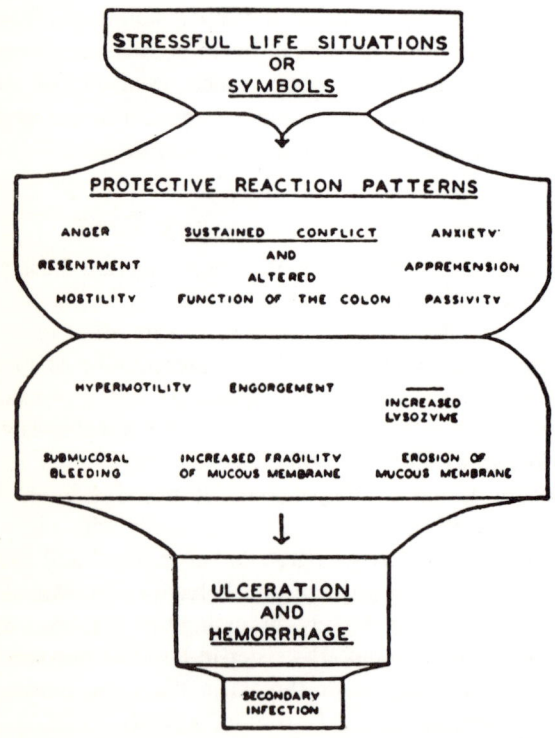

A schema suggesting the relationship of life situations, emotional reactions and bodily defects which lead to ulceration of the colon.

so readily occurs, many small erosions and ulcers may appear. In other words, this exposed portion of mucous membrane goes to pieces under circumstances that can have little to do with the nature of the colonic content or the feces. These damaged areas may become the sites of serious hemorrhage which occasionally cause death.

Thus a stressful life circumstance or a symbol thereof evokes protective reactions—in this particular instance, the desire to get rid of something by pushing it out of the gut, by vomiting, or diarrhea. The person feels angry, resentful, hostile, as well as anxious and apprehensive, although his outward behavior may be passive at the same time. Concurrently manifesting itself, although not causally related, is altered function of the colon with increased contractility, increased blood flow, engorgement, alteration of secretion with bleeding, tearing of the gut, erosions, ulcerations, hemorrhages, and perhaps secondary infection.

On the other hand, when a patient bleeding profusely from the bowels, with fever and weight loss, makes contact with another human being who helps alter his attitudes, re-establish his self-esteem, re-establish his faith and trust in himself and others, his body may also restore itself. In so doing, his temperature becomes normal, he gains in weight, and the body diarrhea, which is the inappropriate expression of the drive to get rid of something, stops.

Constipation and diarrhea are opposites in their functional significance. Diarrhea serves to rid the organism of some noxious agent it has inadvertently admitted by mouth or otherwise and is associated with increased redness, contraction, and heightened motility of the bowel, so that as quickly as possible the noxious agent may be emitted. Constipation is associated with a large, relaxed, pale bowel showing ineffective contractions of the terminal portions, with retention of ingested substances for longer than the usual periods. Contraction of the muscles around the outlet further impedes the ejection of the bowel contents.

What does such a person feel? What attitudes does he express at the time that these patterns are being enacted? The person with diarrhea or ulcerative colitis is likely to say: "If I can only get rid of it." "I want to get this over with." "I wanted to be done with it." "I want this to be finished." "I want it to be all over." Men facing a firing line have diarrhea. In contrast, the one with constipation, grimly determined to carry on even though faced with little hope of change, says: "This is a lousy job but it is the best I can get. I will have to keep on with this, but I know I'm not going to like it. It will never be any better. I don't want to do it, but I will go through with it. It's no good, but I won't quit."

The Interpretation of Bodily Changes

Is it purely by chance that one organ, part, or bodily system is used rather than another? No, because the choice in any person is predictable. One person under stress gets diarrhea again and again, another constipation, another vomiting, and still another a duodenal ulcer. Is this a state of general excitement only, so that with spread of excitation most any sort of change may occur? Were this so, then during great excitement there should be an indiscriminate show of protective patterns. But, on the contrary, there is evidence that in the general excitement that occurs during battle it is uncommon for a person to develop asthma, or bleeding from ulceration, colitis, or peptic ulcer. Further, there is no evidence of purely isolated responses representing the activity of only one part of the nervous system. Thus it does not help to view the reaction in terms of the function of a unique part of the nervous system or of any particular endocrine gland.

The person at times of stress is using protective or adaptive patterns which have in their literal application a highly useful purpose, i.e., to improve ventilation, to maintain nutrition, circulation, or to get rid of a poison. When dealing with a poison it is useful to vomit or have diarrhea. When dealing with one's sister-in-law it is of no use. In the latter instance it is inappropriate, and therefore may become an excessively prolonged pattern of action; appropriately used, it serves a good end, but when used awkwardly and, because of that, excessively, the person may be damaged.

That does not mean that these patterns in action do not serve a useful purpose. A good display of tears with frustration, for example, will often make one feel better. A pattern in action—running, jumping, crying out, weeping, vomiting—brings with it a degree of tranquillity even though no resolution has occurred. But the price is often high, and if the pattern continues in operation excessively or too long, tissues may be damaged. The person who shows such an uneconomic and inappropriate use of equipment is punished accordingly.

Airways

A man was examined as regards the color of his nasal mucous membranes by simply looking into his nostrils. Day after day the color of his mucous membranes went along in a steady way, as contrasted with that of another man. The latter's nasal mucous membranes were red one day and pale the next, red on one side and pale on the other. When a person is exposed to smelling salts, he suddenly gasps, and the mucous membrane of the nose gets dark red and swollen; water pours out, and he hardly can get any air through; he may not be able to speak; his chest seems held in a vise. It would appear that he is attempting to neutralize, wash away, and shut out a very unattractive feature of the environment. When exposed to rose pollen, a sensitive man developed symptoms of "hay fever," and his nose reacted as it did when exposed to smelling salts. He attempted, seemingly, to shut out, wash away, and neutralize the noxious agent to which he had been exposed. He exhibited a proper use of the nose.

But consider a woman with a long history of nose troubles, resulting in several operations. She couldn't get air freely, and her nose seemed to be stopped up much of the time, particularly at night and especially when her husband was in the room smoking. It was suggested by her physician in an interview that perhaps her troubles were related to her attitudes and her husband. She violently rejected the suggestion and burst into tears. The mucous membrane on the inside of her nose became dark red and there was much secretion and swelling. A little while later it appeared pale, boggy, and solidly occluded. This woman acted as though she were shutting out, neutralizing, and washing away some noxious agent. Illustration shows what took place in

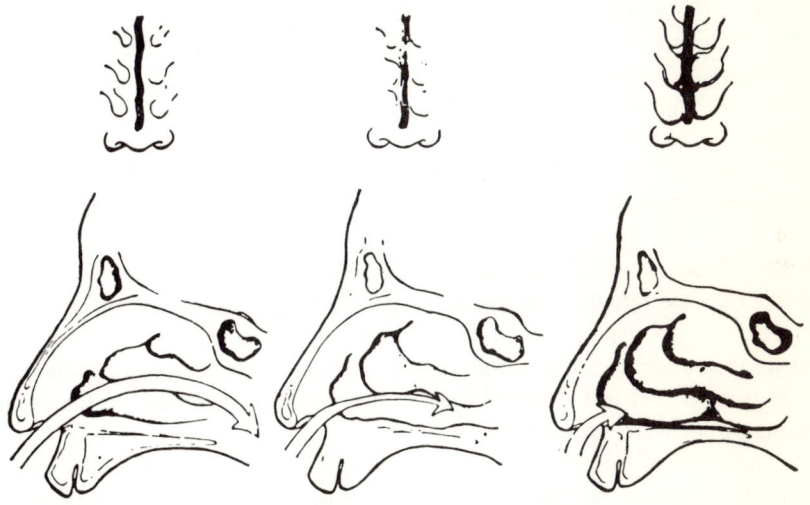

Diagrammatic representation of the turbinate bones and their mucous membrane coverings and their appearance in various stages of swelling. Obstruction to air passage is indicated schematically by arrows. Note that minor deviations in the septum (see vertical line in upper pictures) may become important when the turbinates are swollen.

her airways during the discussion. The membranes of this woman's airways became redder, more swollen, wetter, and the air passage was completely closed.

These changes may last minutes, or days, as exhibited by an ambitious young physician who was much concerned with his career and was obliged to work intimately with a professional partner in his hospital some years his senior, but junior in experience and wisdom. He resented working with this colleague and feared that his future was jeopardized by the inadequate performance of his associate. Their relationship deteriorated rapidly. During a two-week period, while his conflicts with this colleague were most severe, he exhibited red and swollen mucous membranes, with quantities of fluid pouring out and scarcely any space for the passage of air. He developed headache, which he called "sinus headache," and had red eyes, tender swollen flushed cheeks, and tender forehead. His nasal mucous membranes were exceedingly sensitive to touch. During an interview the mucous membranes swelled further, additional secretion poured out, and increased quantities of pus cells appeared in the secretion. It was possible to separate these men, and soon thereafter the patient became symptom free and his nasal mucous membranes became paler and much less swollen, with little secretion and no obstruction.

Summative effects are evident when one kind of noxious stimulus is added to another. A patient was brought into a room containing a constant amount of circulating pollen in the air. She had "hay fever" in the pollen season and was sensitive to this pollen, and as she sat in this room her mucous membranes began to redden and swell slightly. Then, in addition to the irritating pollen, a topic concerning her troubles and her quarrels with her father was introduced. Immediately her symptoms were greatly augmented and her airways became obstructed. She was then reassured by the words of her physician, and, despite the fact that she remained in the room laden with pollen, the membranes were restored even to their initial state, akin to that noted before she entered the pollen-laden room. In this instance, then, the more important noxious agent of the two seemed to be her relation to her father, rather than to the pollen, although both were operating.

An anatomical defect in the nose, present since birth, can under certain circumstances take on importance in middle life or later. For example, a deviated septum which has been present for a lifetime may become important when one's relations to others become of such a nature as to call forth the protective reaction of shutting out, washing away, and neutralizing. A man may then need to have his septum removed to allow more air to get through his nose.

The asthmatic person is closely akin in his pattern of reaction to the one who has trouble with his nose. Indeed, an asthmatic reaction seldom occurs without nasal involvement. It becomes evident by direct inspection that threatening topics cause the mucous membranes of the bronchi to become redder, wetter, and the lumen to become smaller. During a series of observations, topics calling forth feelings of bitterness, regret, and failure also precipitated asthmatic attacks.

Sensations of "air hunger," tightness in the chest, and "butterflies in the stomach" are sometimes experienced under stressful circumstances. Tight, unpleasant feelings of pressure in the middle of the chest may be mistaken for pains originating in the heart. These may result from a cramp of the diaphragm, a sheet of muscle separating the lungs and heart from the contents of the abdomen. When an X-ray picture of the diaphragm of a person in a relaxed and tranquil state is compared with that of his diaphragm when he is anxious, the latter shows a contracted state which would make it difficult to take in more air. There may be a fluttering sensation and sometimes cramps just underneath the heart.

Specificity of Reactions to Stress

When presenting a protective or adaptive reaction, people do not necessarily exhibit the whole of the reaction pattern; fragmentation of the pattern is characteristic. If one wished to shut out an unattractive experience, one could close off the entire airway system, but, actually, the reaction involves a small part of the pattern—that involving the nose. If one did not want to take something into the stomach, one could close the mouth, shut off the gullet, and vomit, but, actually, only a piece of the pattern, such as the closure of the gullet, may be exhibited.

Also, there is specificity as regards reactions during stress. Any kind or amount of stress doesn't evoke just any or all kinds of reactions. Observations were made by a distinguished physician in Holland who, during the bad years of Holland's occupation by the Germans, was able to examine a number of patients with ulcers of the stomach. He attended their medical needs before the Germans came and attended them also after they were put in concentration camps because of their religion. Before the war they were wealthy, comfortable, and successful merchants. They suffered a good deal with their stomachs. In the concentration camps their plight was horrible; they never knew in the morning whether they would survive that day. Life was filled with much stress, yet these people lost all manifestations of their peptic ulceration. The ironic aspect of it is that many of them regained their peptic ulcers and symptoms when they returned to "Main Street." The specific type of stress which had engendered the ulcer in their stomach lining was absent during the terror of their stay in the concentration camp.

A group of people with intense and frequent headaches were missionaries in Japan. During the heyday of their missionary activity they suffered considerably, even though esteemed and presumably effective. When these people were put into Japanese concentration camps, with all the deprivations entailed, they lost their headaches. When they were freed at the end of the war, the headaches returned. These instances indicate that danger has to have a specific meaning to a person in order to produce specific changes.

People may exhibit one and sometimes two of these protective or adaptive patterns. You may at one time have vascular headaches and at another time peptic ulcers; sometimes you may have them both together. Certain combinations, such as ulcers of the large bowel occurring with ulcers of the stomach, are uncommon.

Thus tissue derangement may be considered a part of an adjustment which was meant to protect the individual, including swelling, edema, reduction of blood supply to tissue, tenderness, inflammation, erosion, hemorrhage, ulceration, pus formation, changes in secretion, and lowering of the pain threshold.

Over-all Mobilization Patterns

So far, considerations have included patterns involving portals of entry—the mouth and airways—and portals of exit—the rectum and anus. Under certain circumstances the organism may exhibit general mobilization for action. If a man runs upstairs or exercises vigorously, he increases the output of blood from his heart with each beat: his heart rate is increased, his blood pressure goes up, and the amount of resistance offered to the flow of blood by the minute vessels in the tissues of the body is decreased. Such reactions, by insuring a good supply of blood to muscles, serve to make his actions more effective.

Similarly, in an interview in which some important relationship to another person is discussed which causes you to be frankly anxious and frightened, you act just as though you were running upstairs, or preparing for battle. A patient came to us in a tense, anxious state, complaining of pounding heart and breathlessness. Climbing a certain number of steps caused his already augmented stroke volume (the amount of blood ejected by the heart per beat) to be further increased. The heart rate also was increased. As the patient's general life adjustment improved, his circulation gradually improved, so that ten months later the same effort produced a minimal but effective response. At this time his state was relatively tranquil and relaxed.

A man ostensibly loved but actually hated his mother, although he never admitted this even to himself. He presented a bland exterior during an interview, but his blood pressure rose and the resistance offered to the passage of blood by blood vessels of many of his organs mounted. His blood became much stickier and coagulated more readily. During the interview concerning his relations with his mother, his blood pressure went up sharply and, as a part of his generally increased resistance to the flow of blood, the amount of blood that went through the kidneys was much decreased. With the increased stickiness and clotting proclivity of the blood, he might have damaged organs further. This clotting device serves presumably to help the animal stop bleeding during mortal combat, but when it is used every time a person comes in contact with his mother, it follows that he might appreciably damage his kidneys and perhaps his brain. Again, a device that serves to protect and prolong life is called into action so inappropriately as to threaten a man's very existence. On the other hand, a patient with elevated blood pressure did, by a restoration of self-esteem and by changing attitudes toward his environment, gradually, over a period of a year and a half, bring down the level of the blood pressure to the average.

Another feature of the mobilization reaction to threats results in backache. The amount of an individual's muscle contraction is indicated by the firmness of the muscle when it is felt. It can be shown also by a record of the electrical disturbance in the muscle, which roughly parallels in amount the magnitude of contractions. While a man was exposed to a discussion aimed to bring into focus feelings of hostility and anxiety, contraction of the big muscles of his back and legs increased, presumably in readiness for action, for fight, or flight. Being thus contracted for long periods, but not actually associated with movement which brings also relaxation, they began to hurt. When topics that interested him and brought him esteem and satisfaction were discussed, the muscle activity was reduced, but with a reconsideration of the threatening matters, the muscle contraction was again increased and again he had backache.

Similar painful contraction occurs in the muscles of the head and neck. Headaches can persist for days, weeks, or months, due to the sustained contraction of the sheet of muscle at the top of the head and neck when an individual is exposed to an environment which calls forth the need to be on the alert against assaults that may never come but always threaten. Electrical records of these muscles were recorded during such a headache and showed much contraction. A few weeks later, after the patient had had an opportunity to express something of his anxieties and fears and had adopted another attitude, the sheet of muscle was no longer contracted and the headache ended.

Blood vessel headaches, such as migraine, constitute a most important bloc of man's discomfort. A person with migraine headache may exhibit large, swollen blood vessels on the side of his head. A woman suffering with many headaches of high intensity came to the doctor on the first of September. She had had bad relations with her child and, frightened by the intensity of her anger, feared she might injure her child. She had no headache for nine days after telling this story to an understanding physician. However, the matter was rediscussed with her on the tenth day, and inadvertently her feelings of guilt and hostility were roused again, and a headache was precipitated. The headache was ended by the introduction of an agent which causes swollen blood vessels to come back to their original shape.

A similar headache was induced in a woman by an interview involving her husband, concerning whom her hostile feelings were barely suppressed. During

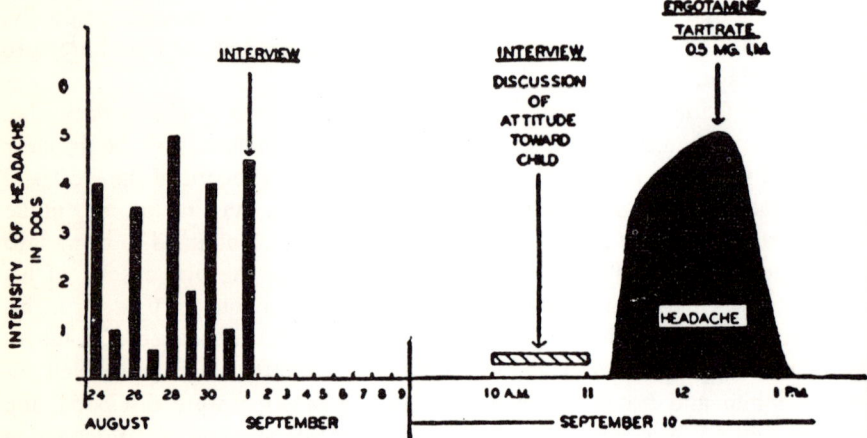

Precipitation of a migraine headache in a woman following a stressful interview concerning her feelings of guilt and resentment toward her child, which evoked anger.

discussion of this topic a headache developed as the large arteries of her head began to swell and painfully to pulsate. Instead of using an agent causing the blood vessels to constrict, this woman's faith in her doctor was utilized. When an intravenous injection of neutral salt water solution was then given, the vessels constricted and her headache stopped. In other words, normal salt was capable of terminating this woman's headache just as would an active, constrictor agent.

Stock Factor and Organ Inferiority

Why don't we all have the same bodily reactions during stress? Why do some of us get high blood pressure, others peptic ulcer, still others ulcerative colitis, others asthma, and others headache? We might as well ask: "Why are we different? Why do we look at the same assault or threat differently?" And in this rests the answer. In looking at it differently, we are prepared to meet it differently. These reactions represent our individual ways of meeting a threat. Do we run toward it? Do we run away from it? Do we try to avoid it? Do we try to act as though it didn't exist? Do we wish to fight but dare not? All these and more are possible ways of dealing with a threat. Now why is it that individuals of some families have headache, hypertension, or stomach trouble? Again, we might as well ask: "Why do dogs of certain breeds easily learn to retrieve birds, or fight fiercely, or follow scents? Why do beavers construct dams? Why do squirrels hoard nuts?"

The implication is that there are proclivities handed down; its easier for a bird dog to learn to be a bird dog. It doesn't follow that the proclivity leads to disease, it only means that it's easier for an individual to meet his problems in some ways rather than in others.

Thus he has inherited a proclivity which makes it easier for him to use a particular pattern. In addition, a way of dealing with life is shown every day by parents, and the child gradually takes it on as his way. For example, the individual whose parents have headaches would be likely to have a headache when the going is tough. But it doesn't mean that his life needs to be given over to headaches if he understands his nature, his way of looking at things, and how much of the latter he has learned from his parents, and that he can learn other ways, too.

Moreover, the repeated or prolonged participation of a given organ in a protective pattern cannot be construed as evidence of the weakness or inferiority of that organ, even though, because of such participation, it fails to maintain its structural integrity. The individual may be said to be in a weak or vulnerable state, but the organ can hardly be said to be weak and, indeed, may be especially well developed and strong for long periods before it finally fails.

Culture and Stress

It is doubtful if man has ever considered himself under more stress than he does today. A most conspicuous feature of our time is rapidity of change in values and customs. Cultures with opposite emphases, as, for example, Japanese and American, concerning parents, property, and relations with children exhibit the same disorders; thus the cultural values alone cannot be the prime factor. But in any rapidly changing culture a man's faith in his customs, habits, intuitions, his leaders, teachers, and parents is shaken.

With a cultural emphasis upon the desirability and need to face a "changing world," a man is mistakenly led to believe that long-term values and basic human relationships are also changing. Undoubtedly rapid and relatively superficial changes in mores bewilder those who cannot separate the wheat from the chaff. To be sure, there have been rapid changes in attitudes toward property and possessions; women's place politically and economically, and in manners. Also subject to rapid change have been the amount of social mobility, the precise symbols of power and prestige, the desirability or amount of "outdoing" one's neighbor. But there is no change in such basic elements in human societies as belief in man and in the desirability of his survival; recognition of his tribal nature and his responsibility to the group; certain aspects of a man's relationship to his mate; acceptance of adult and parental responsibility and the giving of effective support during childhood.

Two persons out of three exhibiting stress manifestations can be significantly relieved. The thoughtful doctor can do much to indicate that first things come first and to give support while the individual reorients himself. A responsible person of authority who helps the sufferer regain his self-esteem and change his attitudes can help him restore his body to more appropriate patterns of functioning. Certainly we can get courage from the knowledge that when we pursue a goal, we pay a price. If we know what the price is, we may then decide whether the goal is worth the cost. There are aims more important than comfort, and occasionally even more important than health. But when you know what price you are paying for your goals, you may decide that your values are poor and, by changing your attitudes, restore yourself.

Epitome

The stresses to which man is exposed include assaults by many living forms that aim to invade as parasites or to destroy; by meteorologic and climatic crises; by mechanical, electrical, and thermal forces that operate upon man merely in terms of his mass and volume, and by elements of the earth's crust that man manipulates for his comfort and delight or to satisfy a passion for destruction.

Man is further vulnerable because he is so constituted that he reacts not only to the actual existence of danger, but to threats and symbols of danger experienced in his past which call forth reactions little different from those to the assault itself. Since his adaptive and protective capabilities are limited, the response to many sorts of damaging agents and threats in any given man may be similar, the form of the reaction to any one agent depending more on the individual's nature and past experience than upon the particular injurious agent evoking it. Finally, because of its magnitude and duration, the adaptive-protective reaction may be far more damaging to the individual than the effects of the noxious agent *per se*.

Also—most important—man is a tribal or group creature with a long period of dependence and development. He is dependent for his very existence upon the aid, support, and encouragement of other men. He lives his life so much in contact with men and in such concern about their expectations of him that he is jeopardized as well as supported by his fellows; indeed, he may feel more threatened by cultural and individual human pressures than by other environmental forces. He must be part of the tribe and yet he is driven to fulfil his own proclivities. These pressures and the conflicts they engender are ubiquitous and create a large portion of man's stress.

In other words, in times of stress bodily changes and feeling states are evoked, representing a reaction to something that threatens us. What is its meaning? What do we do about it? Do we run? Do we try to get rid of it by vomiting? Do we grimly hold on? Do we try to act as though it never was? Do we try to deal with it by non-participation? All of these action patterns are associated with bodily changes and concurrent feelings, and bring with them a degree of tranquillity. But when used too long, they damage tissue and threaten the life that they might have prolonged.

STROKE See *Apoplexy*.

STUTTERING AND STAMMERING Modern views of stuttering point to the concept that it is a nervous condition based on some mental conflict. The stutterer has a tenseness and spasm of the muscles involved in speaking. He is unable to co-ordinate them properly. Back of his failure to co-ordinate is a state of the nervous system involving some mental conflict. History shows that stutterers are in good company. Among the great names in history of people who stuttered are Aristotle, Aesop, Demosthenes, Virgil, Charles Lamb, Erasmus, Darwin, Moses, Mendelssohn, and several of the kings of England and France.

Although stuttering may be largely mental in causation, physical factors are sometimes associated and may act to aggravate the stuttering. The doctor therefore makes certain that adenoids, abnormal length of uvula, abnormal size of the tongue, and improper development of the mouth are not present. Such defects are not, however, found with great frequency as the primary cause of stuttering.

The stutterer usually has most trouble with p, b, m, and w, which are the sounds made by the lips. The stutterer does not, however, always stutter on the same sound. His emotional status at the time of speaking may be a factor in determining the particular word or phrase that is associated with stuttering.

Often children who stutter develop behavior changes due to a lack of confidence with the fear of appearing ridiculous. Some children who stutter are even considered to be mentally retarded because of their speech defect.

Because stuttering is primarily a mental affliction, treatment directed to the mental conflict is of the greatest importance. When the nature of the conflict is discovered and revealed to the stutterer, self-confidence returns and there may be a readjustment toward life in general.

Since all people who have difficulty in speaking display disturbances of the normal rhythm of breathing and speaking, training is useful in developing the power of speech. This has been observed through the fact that many people get along without stammering when they whisper or sing or recite poetry or speak to a large audience but have difficulty under other conditions. Musicians who stutter sometimes become blocked in playing certain notes. This means that they stutter in their thinking as well as in their speech.

The re-education of the person who stutters requires training in relaxation, in breathing, in vocal gymnastics, and in phonetics. Such training is, of course, combined with proper mental study designed to release the block that occurs in the mind. The first task is to break down the spasm of the unco-ordinated muscles and liberate the imprisoned voice. This requires teaching in the relaxation of the muscles. The stutterer must be made to forget his problem by exercises in relaxing the muscles of the body, the head, the tongue, the throat, and the vocal cords. Excess effort toward speaking brings about wrong action of the diaphragm. The stutterer tries to talk while he is inhaling. This, of course, is difficult if not impossible. Therefore exercises are given in proper breathing and in control of breathing in relationship to speech.

Because of the difficulty in speaking stutterers form bad speech habits that need correction. These habits affect particularly the articulation of certain sounds. It becomes necessary to teach them how to articulate the sounds with which they have trouble.

Dr. John A. Glassburg has described a routine of approach to speech which is useful

1. Before you speak, think, inhale, and visualize the words.
2. When you speak, never go back, never repeat; lengthen your vowel sounds.
3. Always speak quietly, slowly, and calmly.

There is a good deal of trouble trying to distinguish between stuttering and stammering. Some people say that stuttering is reduplication of sound and stammering is hesitation in speaking. Some define stuttering as difficult speech and stammering as incorrect speech. This merely confuses a condition which has been considerably confused for a variety of reasons. For all practical purposes the average person may consider stuttering and stammering as the same kind of difficulty.

STYES See discussion under *Eye*.

SUBACUTE BACTERIAL ENDOCARDITIS (See also discussion under *Heart*) The proper name scientifically for a condition also called malignant endocarditis.

SUICIDE Every year about 20,000 people in the United States kill themselves. Suicide is not, therefore, an exceedingly prominent cause of death. Nevertheless, suicides are always attracting attention because of the natural drama associated with them.

Why do three and a half times as many men as women attempt suicide? Why is the tendency to commit suicide greater among older than among young people? It seems that suicide results chiefly from the discouragement and hopelessness of later years of life. During war the suicide rate always drops.

People differ as to the methods by which they commit suicide. The agents most frequently used are firearms and poisons, which account altogether for about one half of all suicides. Then there are asphyxiation and hanging. These four technics account for 83 per cent of all suicides.

People who commit suicide represent a group who are easily upset emotionally. They break down under strains which other people manage to surmount. Sometimes the strain arises from economic conditions, sometimes because of trouble with friends and relatives.

The psychologists are convinced that there is a steady progression of the tendency to self-destruction long before the self-destruction is finally consummated. Obviously, therefore, there is time when such a tendency is discovered to undertake corrective action with a view to overcoming the desire.

The ability to adjust oneself emotionally to one's surroundings is perhaps most important to the prevention of suicides. The conditions that influence people, such as poverty, unemployment, ill-health, mental abnormality, physical suffering or handicaps, may lead people to thoughts of self-destruction. Loss of honor and prestige, disappointment in love, failure in achieving one's ambitions, or any other failure in adequacy may result in thought of suicide.

Obviously the way to prevent suicide is to develop a proper attitude toward life in the young. This is the responsibility of the entire community as well as of the home. Young people must be given a proper mental and emotional outlook. They must learn to act properly toward the difficult situations that invariably arise in the human life.

SUICIDE—mental patients to be guarded from: See MENTAL, article NERVOUS AND MENTAL DISORDERS.

SUMMER CARE FOR BABIES (See also, *Child Care*) Nowadays we do not hear much about "summer complaint." Once great numbers of babies, nursed successfully at the breast during their first summer, died during the second summer because of infection from contaminated food, water or milk. Mothers believed that the second summer was somehow destined to be fatal to babies. Now we know that summer is no more dangerous than any other season of the year for a baby that is properly protected against infection, properly fed with food and drink that are clean, properly clothed to meet the heat, bathed frequently and given sufficient sunlight and rest.

Food—Children do not require quite as much food in summer as in colder weather. With very small babies the concentration of the feeding is lessened by adding more water. The total amount of the feeding of older babies may be reduced one-fifth to one-sixth. In hot weather babies need more liquids because of increased evaporation of water from the surface of the body.

The food of the child in summer should contain less fats because fats are particularly heat producing foods. If the baby is receiving eight ounces of whole milk at each feeding, the strength of the mixture may be changed by adding two ounces of boiled water to six ounces of whole milk. Of course, the mother who is being guided by her own doctor will follow his advice. The intelligent mother consults the doctor at frequent and regular intervals about the care and feeding of her baby. That is good preventive medicine.

The first signs that the baby may be having difficulty with food are such symptoms as diarrhea and vomiting. When this occurs, all food should be stopped immediately, the physician should be consulted, and plenty of plain boiled water given until the symptoms stop. Then milk diluted with half to two-thirds of the amount with plain boiled water may be used.

Remember also that milk must be kept in the refrigerator. In summer it is safer for the health of the baby to boil all milk even if it has been pasteurized. Boiling will more certainly destroy any harmful germs in the milk.

Clothing—A baby is much more sensitive to high temperature than is an older child or adult. Babies should never be overclothed, particularly in summer. In very hot weather the thinnest type of cotton undervest and diaper are sufficient. If the child is wearing too much clothing its skin will be constantly moist, soft, easily macerated, and therefore subject to irritation and infection.

During the cool mornings and evenings the baby should be protected against chilling. Sudden chilling is associated with congestion in the nose and throat and with colds. During cooler periods of the day additional clothing may be used and the baby may be protected with a light blanket.

If the child is going to play outdoors it may be in a play pen with a floor. The child should not play on the bare ground but may be kept on a blanket, a rug, or a large towel spread for the purpose.

Bathing—On hot days the baby should have its morning bath and usually one at night also. In fact the baby may be refreshed by bathing several times during the day. If everything is in order for the purpose this will take only a few extra minutes of the mother's or the nurse's time. When sponging the child, a solution of one teaspoonful of baking soda to a pint of water helps to prevent irritation of the skin. The bran bath is also a helpful preventive of prickly heat. A large handful of bran added to the water will serve the purpose. The baby should not have a cold bath even in exceedingly warm weather. A lukewarm bath is just as cooling.

SUN- AND HEAT STROKE

After the skin of the baby is dry, it may be powdered liberally with any of the many good baby powders. Then the child can be dressed in its sun-suit or in a light cotton undervest and diaper and play under suitable conditions until time for its nap.

SUNLIGHT AND FRESH AIR—Sunshine is not only beneficial but absolutely essential to healthful growth. However, sunlight, like every other influence on health, has possibilities for harm with overdosage. I have seen children seriously sick with redness and blistering of the skin, fever and even delirium and prostration from too much exposure to the sun.

On hot summer days the best hours for airing the baby outdoors are in the morning and late in the afternoon. Usually exposure of the child should be restricted to five minutes of reflected sunshine. Do not put the child in the direct rays of the hot sun. Gradually the amount may be increased by two minutes daily until the baby is receiving from one-half to one hour of exposure to reflected sunshine each day.

Older children, suitably dressed in sun-suits or play suits, may play in the sunshine for a longer time. Children seldom suffer from sunstroke because most of them have sense enough to get away from the sunshine when it begins to be uncomfortable. Many a grown person falls asleep or dozes on a beach while the sun insidiously burns and blisters the skin. Gradual acquiring of a sun tan helps to prevent sun burn.

SUN- AND HEAT STROKE (See also *Heat Sickness*) Sunstroke, as the term is popularly understood, is not the result of the light of the sun, but of the infrared, or heat, rays. The same symptoms may occur as the result of exposure to heat and humidity in a laundry, a steel mill, a fireroom, a deep metal mine, or any other industry. Among the more severe manifestations are symptoms of complete exhaustion and the occurrence of heat cramps.

When heat stroke occurs, the temperature-regulating mechanism of the human body is thrown out of order. Usually there are premonitory symptoms such as headache, dizziness, and nausea, but sometimes the worker goes on without paying much attention to the minor symptoms, to be stricken as by a flash of lightning, and to die suddenly before anything worth while can be done to save his life.

Among the symptoms of exhaustion are physical weakness, profuse perspiration, a moderate amount of fever, although sometimes the temperature may be lower than normal, and sometimes severe cramping pains in the abdomen or in the arms and legs. In the more severe cases the patient promptly becomes unconscious, his pulse gets very rapid, his breathing gets deep, and the pupils of the eye dilate.

Usually if the person afflicted lives through the second day of his attack he gets better, so that the most important measures are those taken promptly to meet the emergency and to permit the patient to survive the first shock.

In the case of heat exhaustion the first thing to do is to get the person into a cool place and absolutely at rest, flat on his back. If the temperature is high, sponging with cool water will help to control it. It may be necessary to give stimulation such as can be had from stronger drugs or from coffee in order to help the patient over the acute stage of the condition.

In the case of heat stroke with the more severe symptoms prompt action is even more necessary than in heat exhaustion. In such cases the body may be washed in ice water; cold sprays and injections of cold water may be used to bring the fever down rapidly.

The effects of the stroke on the

heart should be watched by a physician who may remain constantly in attendance until the heart action is satisfactory. He can give supportive drugs that will control the heart and this may make the difference between life and death. Sometimes congestion may be great and it may be necessary for the doctor to permit some blood to flow from the veins in order to relieve the congestion.

Many industrial plants and many golf clubs are now providing their employees and their patrons with little tablets made of common table salt. Special dispensers have been developed which are placed beside the drinking-water fountain. In the industrial plants the employees are encouraged to take one of these tablets every time they take a drink of water. It has been found by actual studies that this helps to eliminate the occurrence of heat stroke or heat exhaustion.

The human body is unable to adjust itself satisfactorily to high temperatures for a long time. The workers who are most likely to develop heat stroke or heat cramps are miners, firemen, laundry workers, and kitchen workers, but many a golfer who tries to play thirty-six holes of golf in a day may collapse halfway around because he failed to realize that the human body needs help in such a situation.

Some years ago a study was made of the miners in Boulder City, Nevada. It was found that heat cramps which occurred in these miners were associated with disturbances which resulted from a lack of salt in the body. A British investigator named Haldane found that miners at work may lose as much as five and a half pounds in an hour. A person in a Turkish bath may lose two pounds in an hour.

When large amounts of salt solution are taken into the body, the effects of heat cramps and heat stroke disappear.

The blood of a person suffering from heat stroke is found to contain less salt than normally.

In some industries all of the drinking water is modified by the addition of salt. This serves to protect even those workers who will not realize the importance of taking a salt tablet at fairly frequent intervals. In Great Britain miners are supplied with salted beer and are told that the food which they take daily should be salted liberally.

Our number of cases of sunstroke, heat stroke, and heat exhaustion is relatively slight for the year as a whole, but in the summer the number of cases rises quite definitely. The number of deaths from heat stroke vary, of course, with the severity of the temperature during the summer, but it has reached as high as 4000 in one year.

Sun Stroke—See article Occupation and Health.

Heat Stroke—first aid: See article First Aid.

SUNBURN As with every other disease, the doctors have coined a special name for ordinary sunburn. It is known as erythema solare, which merely means that it is an inflammation caused by the sun. The same term can, of course, be used to apply to an inflammation of the skin caused by ultra-violet rays from other sources.

The inflammation that develops varies from a slight flush to the severe burn that results in blistering and loss of skin. Immediately after burning there may be a sensation of heat which is followed in a few days or a week by itching and by peeling of the skin. Usually if the person protects the skin and avoids further sunburn, healing occurs promptly. Sunburns seldom produce scars unless there is a secondary infection of the damaged area.

If the sunburned area is very extensive, the effects of absorption of the material that has been damaged may be shown by dizziness, headache, fever, vomiting, and other symptoms of a constitutional disturbance.

Most people have at one time or another suffered the effects of sunburn and know just about what to do. The application of ordinary cold cream or any similar medication will stop the sensation of burning and dryness that results from the exposure of nerve endings. In the very severe cases it is necessary, however, to apply treatment exactly as if the surface of the body were burned by any other burning agent.

The dangers from sunlight are chiefly the effects of the ultraviolet rays. These are the short rays rather than the longer heat rays.

When doctors use sunlight in the treatment of disease, as, for example, tuberculosis, they carefully regulate the dosage of the rays that are given and also gradually accustom the person concerned to the sunlight. It is customary to apply the sun bath in a succession of short periods, particularly at the beginning, because these brief and repeated exposures to the sun enable us to escape any inflammation of the skin and the subsequent blisters, burning, and nervous reactions which result in loss of sleep.

Certain skins are much more delicate than others. Blonds, particularly with thin skins, react so quickly that even a short exposure may bring about a reaction to the heat and even the symptoms of sunstroke. The skin of the infant is much more delicate than that of the adult and will burn and become inflamed much more promptly.

A person of intelligence can determine for himself how much sunlight he ought to have, but the infant is certainly not able to settle such a question for himself.

Repeated sunburn is said to be associated with an increased susceptibility to cancer of the skin. Ninety per cent of cancers of the skin occur on areas habitually exposed to the sun. Usually the sequence is sunburn, then hardened patches such as occur on the skin of old people, and finally the appearance of what is called basal-cell cancer. The

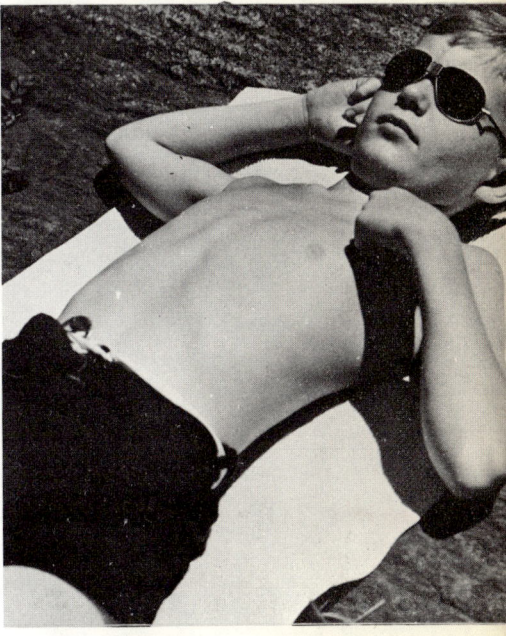

Overexposure to sun may cause severe sunburn, sunstroke or heat exhaustion. Sunburning should be done gradually. Exposure times can be increased by ten to fifteen minutes each day. Persons with fair complexions should be extremely careful because their skin absorbs more of the sun's rays than does that of darker persons.
Hygeia

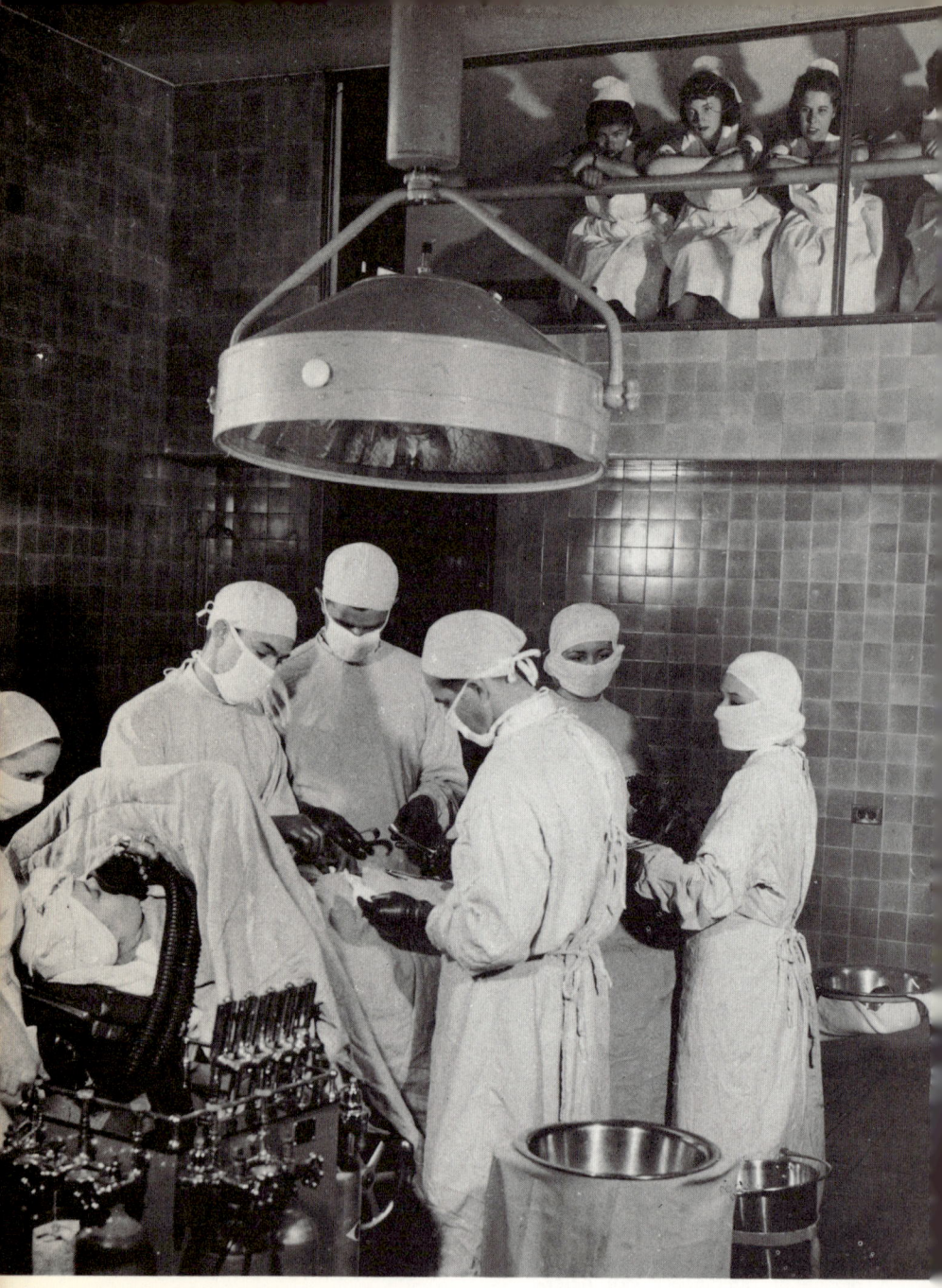

Scene in the operating room showing the surgeons and nurses busy at the operative site while the anesthetist keeps a close watch on the patient. Note the student nurses observing the operation from the gallery.

Ewing Galloway

condition is found most frequently in people of Scotch, Irish, English, and northern-Europe ancestry and mostly in blue-eyed persons. In the United States skin cancer is much more prevalent in the South than either the North or West. A drug called para amino-benzoic acid is a useful filter for the sun's rays; it is often used in sunburn ointments. However, there are other effective protective preparations for use by sailors, farmers, and others who are exposed a great deal to the sun.

SUNBURN—See SKIN, article THE SKIN.
SUNBURN—albuminuria may result: See KIDNEY, article THE KIDNEY: ITS DISEASES AND DISTURBANCES.
SUNBURN—drugs to use: See MEDICINE CHEST, article THE FAMILY MEDICINE CHEST.
SUNBURN—lupus erythematosus: See SKIN, article THE SKIN.
SUNBURN—pellagra mistaken for: See article DEFICIENCY DISEASES.
SUNBURN—protection: See SKIN, article THE SKIN.

SURGEON Formerly, a surgeon undertook anything that was to be done which involved the use of the knife on the human body. Now operations are so technical and the associated care of the patients so involved and intricate that surgery has broken up into a great number of specialties. These include surgery of the brain and nervous system, surgery of the heart and the associated blood vessels, surgery of the stomach and the intestines, surgery of the lung and chest, orthopedic surgery, genitalurinary surgery, gynecological surgery, plastic surgery and rehabilitative surgery. In many large schools and hospitals today, there are divisions for each of these surgical specialties. Moreover, the American Board of Surgery· which certifies a surgeon as to his qualifications, has recognized some of these specialty branches as sub-divisions of surgery with special examining boards. The training of the surgeon has become long and arduous in the United States requiring not only a degree in medicine but also general internship followed by a surgical residency and sometimes an assistantship of many years before the surgeon undertakes to practice alone. In the hospital or clinic the surgeon no longer functions merely with the aid of an anesthetist and a nurse but is now associated with a large group of persons known as a surgical team. Such a team might include the surgeon, the anesthetist, the surgeon's assistant, the surgical nurse and often associated personnel to take care of blood transfusion, the use of various fluids and resuscitation.

SURGERY (See also *Surgeon, Aneurisms, Surgery in; Blood Shunting, Surgery for; Surgery, History of; Diaphragmatic Hernia, Surgery in; Embolism, Surgery for; Gallbladder, Surgery of the; Open Heart Surgery; Hydrocephalus, Surgery in; Kidney Removal, Surgery in; Lungs, Surgery of the; Parkinson's Disease, Surgery in; Pulmonic Stenosis, Surgery in; Spleen Removal, Surgery and; Stomach, Surgery of the*) On the vast stage of life in which medical science performs its miracles, the part of leading man has always been played by the surgeon. Indeed the various earliest medical writings such as the Ebers and Edwin Smith papyri are devoted chiefly to records of surgical cases. Not until the time of Hippocrates does description of an illness or diagnosis come to mark the progress of medical science. Strangely, however, the great advances that have been made possible in surgery are actually dependent on medical · discoveries such as anesthesia discovered by William T. G. Morton and Crawford Long in 1847;

the prevention of infection during surgery which benefitted chiefly by the work of Pasteur and Lister with such a simple innovation as the wearing of rubber gloves which was introduced by Halstead. More recently, use of blood transfusion, the control of the fluid in the body, the feeding of patients by a variety of techniques and the use of drugs for controlling various symptoms have aided success in surgery.

Less than fifty years have passed since the time when few surgeons dared to invade the interior of the body as a

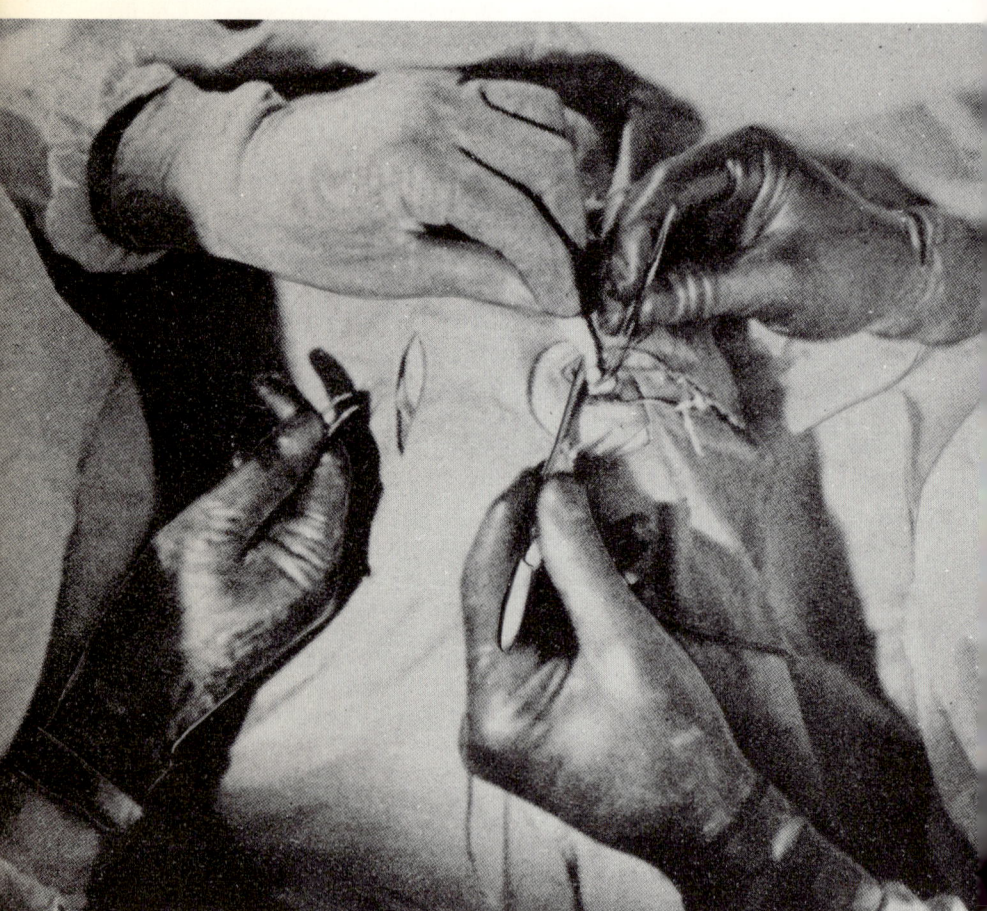

Two surgeons operating on an eye. The rest of the head and body is covered to prevent contamination. The eye is so intricate and delicate that extensive knowledge about the organ and precise operative technics are mandatory before surgery is attempted.

Postgraduate Medicine

whole, let alone the brain. Today there is no portion of the human body that is not invaded successfully. Previously the surgery was largely mutilating, involving the removal of diseased organs or tissues. The surgery of today is called physiological surgery and is aimed at restoring normal function of various organs and tissues when these functions have failed. Under these circumstances, the surgeon today does procedures which would have been called highly radical just ten years ago. Examples are removal of almost all of the organs of the pelvis for the treatment of cancer, the removal of the esophagus or swallowing tube because of the presence of cancer, the complete removal of

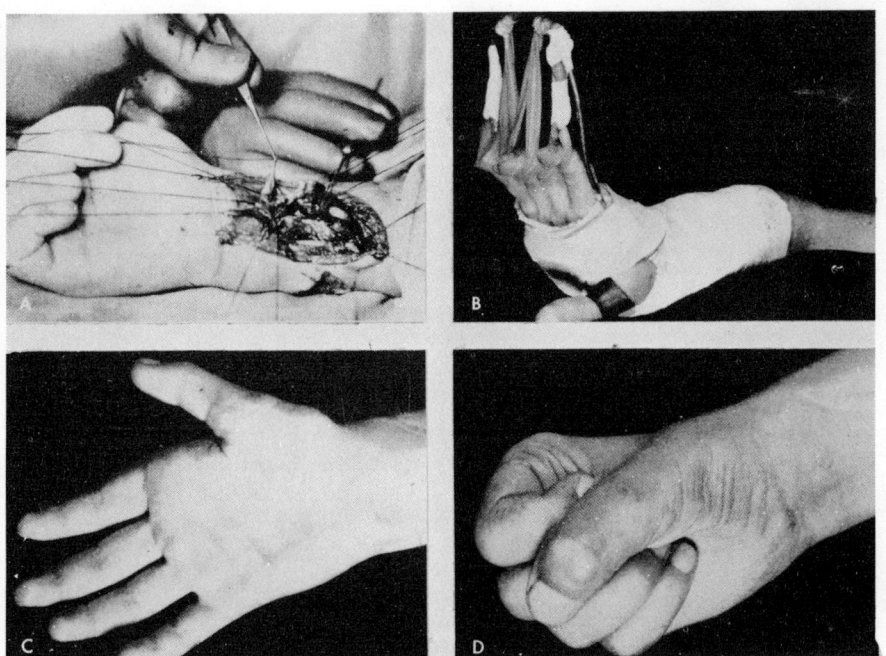

A—Injury to the wrist which cut the nerves and tendons. Surgeons are shown approximating and suturing the ends of nerves and tendons.

B—The surgery is complete and the hand has been placed in a splint. The splint will prevent movement of the joints, thus giving the hand and wrist a chance to heal.

C—Picture of the hand showing healed areas and full, active extension of the fingers.

D—Photograph of the same hand demonstrating the patient's ability to make a fist and exert strength.

Postgraduate Medicine

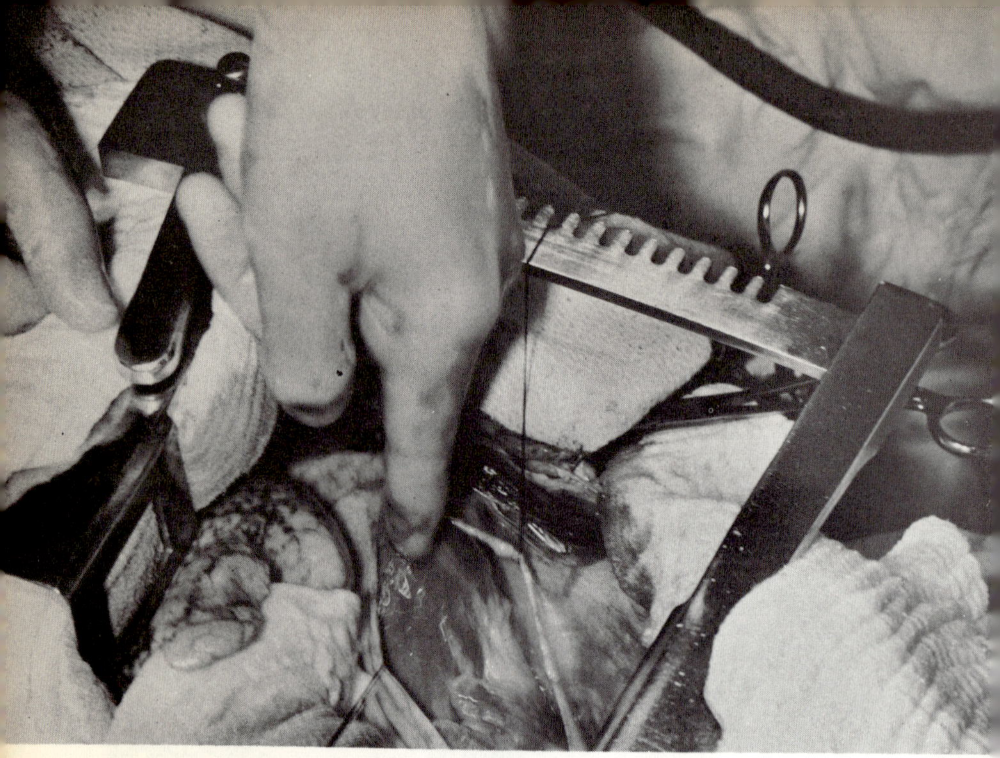

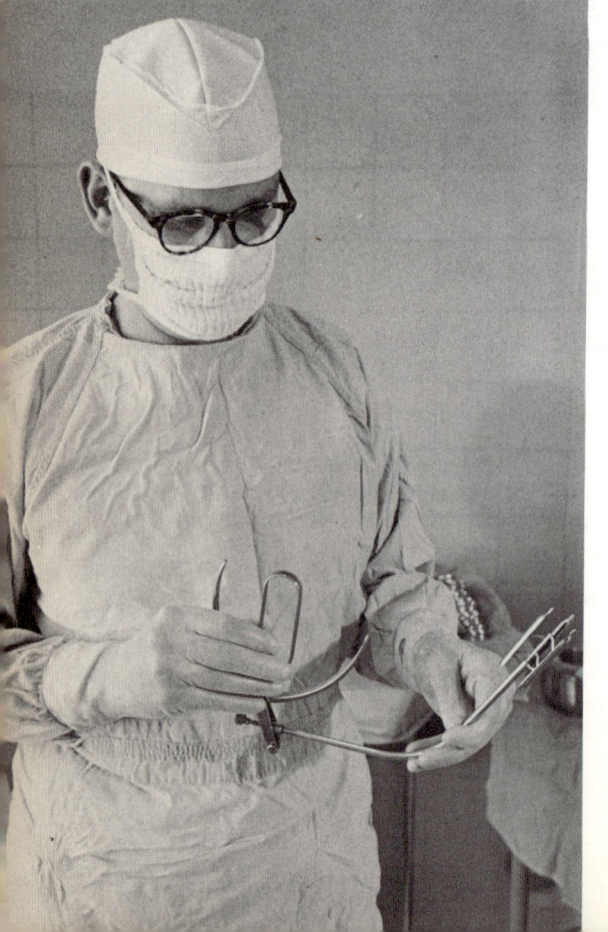

A—Photographs taken during actual surgery on the heart. Strictures of the aortic and mitral valves of the heart are being widened. Left side of the heart has been opened and the ribs are held back to expose the heart.

B—The aortic valve is to be dilated first. Surgeon is shown testing the aortic valvulotome which will be inserted into the ventricle. When the dilating mechanism is compressed the bars expand outwardly, widening the valve.

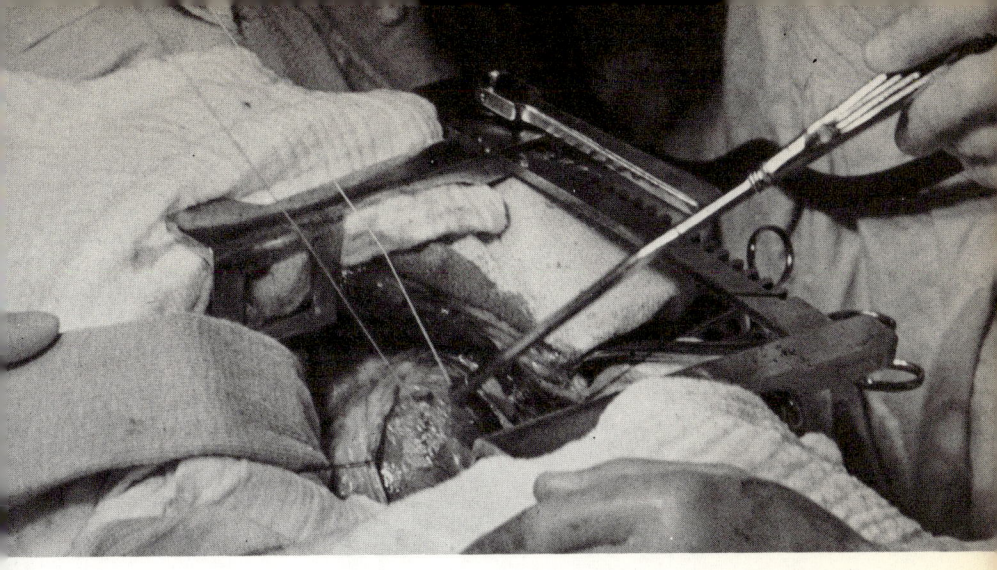

C—Purse-string suture is place in the myocardium of the left ventricle.

D—Surgeon holds his left finger over the stab wound just made at the center of the purse-string suture. The valvulotome, in the closed position, is introduced into the aortic valve. The valve will be opened when the mechanism is expanded.

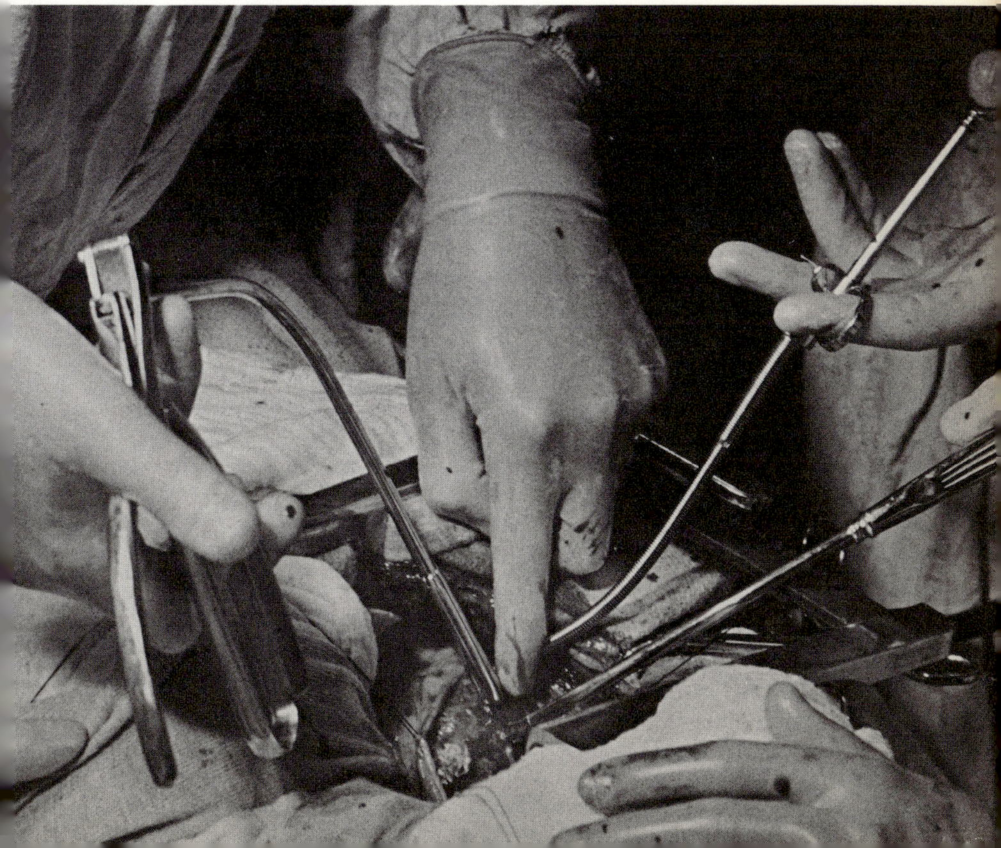

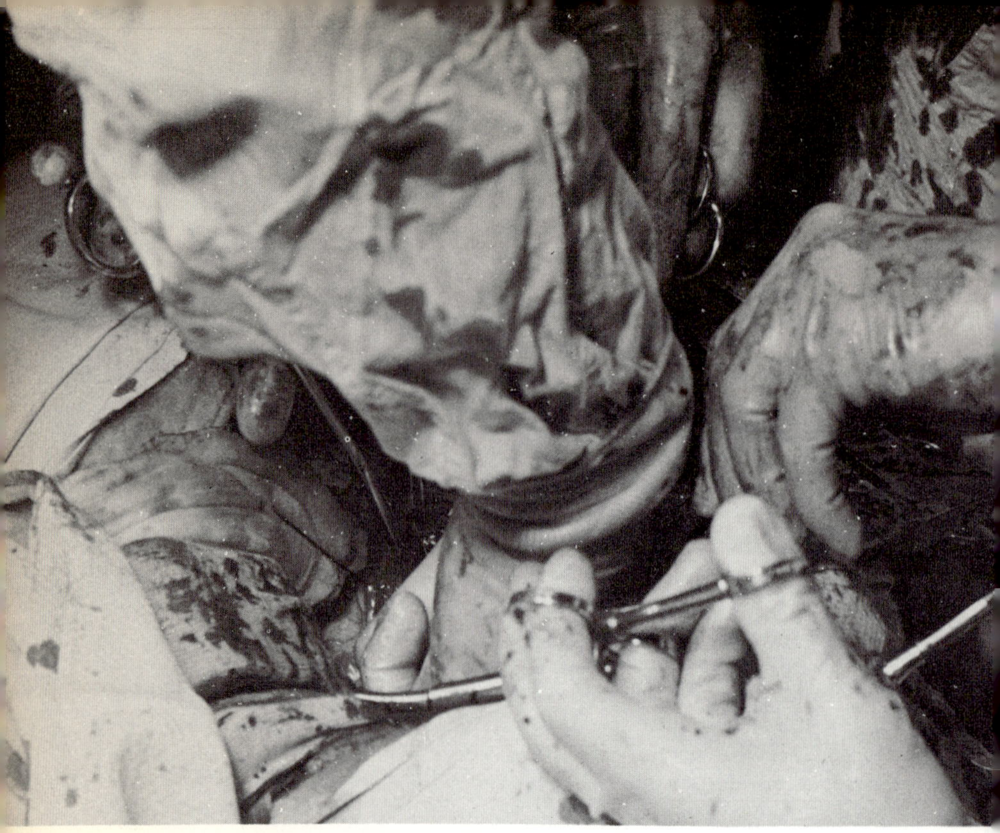

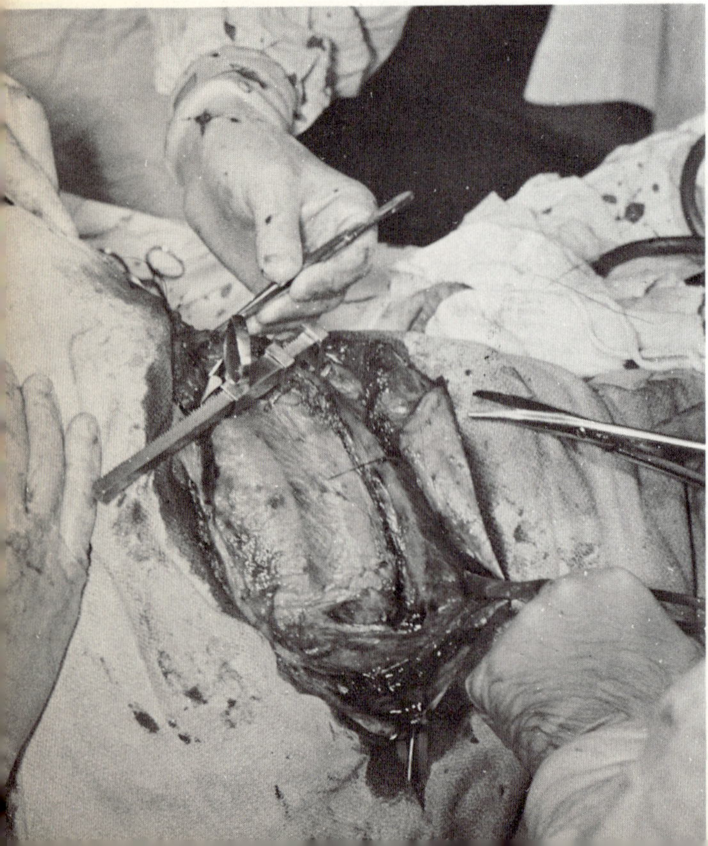

E—The mitral valve is being opened. The finger is introduced into the valve and the sides split to widen the opening. The technic is called "finger fracture."

F—The surgical procedures are completed and the chest is being closed.

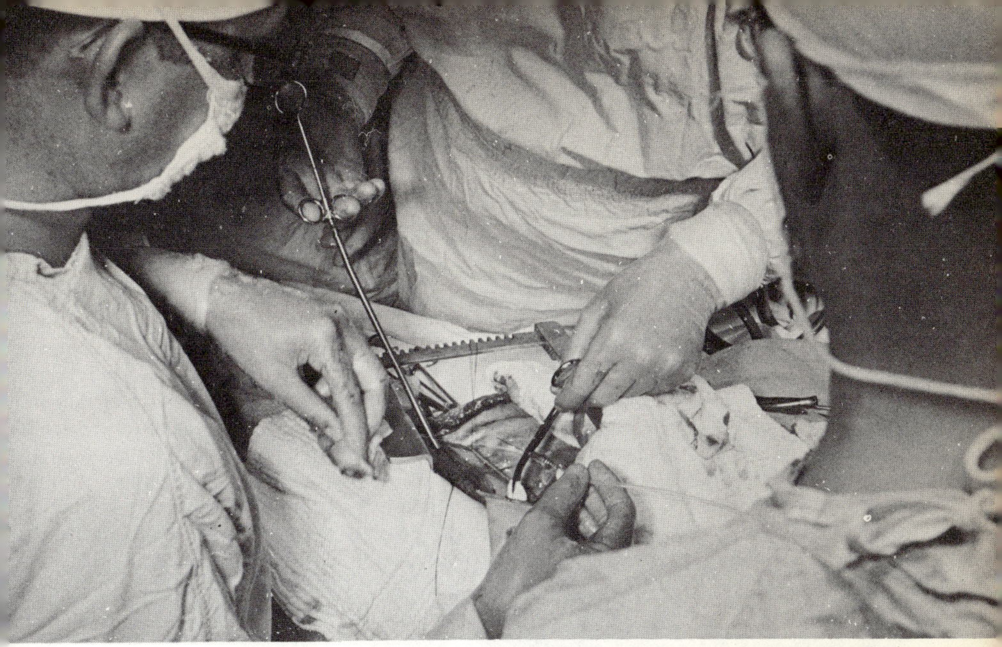

3—The doctors are taking pressure readings by means of a manometer connected to a needle which is inserted into the left heart chambers.

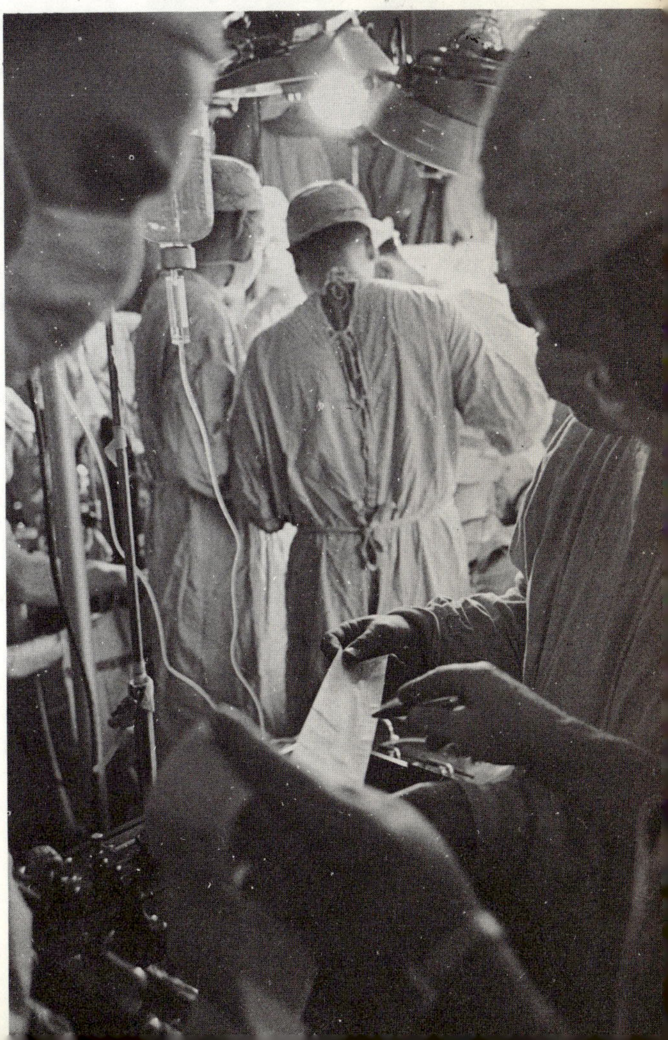

4—The pressure readings are being compared with those taken before surgery. Reduced pressures would mean that the surgery had been successful in relieving, at least partially, the stenotic valves.

Chas. Pfizer & Co., Inc.

the stomach, the removal of the breast with all of its associated lymph glands, the removal of the colon because of chronic ulcerative colitis or the appearance of polyps and diverticuli which may be related to cancer. This does not include the operations that have been done on the heart or removal of the lung in whole or in part and the extensive operations on the brain and other portions of the nervous system.

SURGERY, HISTORY OF The rise of surgery depended upon the knowledge of such fundamental sciences as anatomy, physiology, pathology and anesthesia. Just as the stethoscope is the sign of the physician, the scalpel or surgical knife is the token of the surgeon. The first scalpel ever seen in an illustration appears in the Temple of Esculapius on the Acropolis in Athens and dates back to 300 B.C. Scalpels continue to be modified in shape and form and as to their handles continuously and the final important modifications were made with relationship to ease of sterilization. Handles with ivory

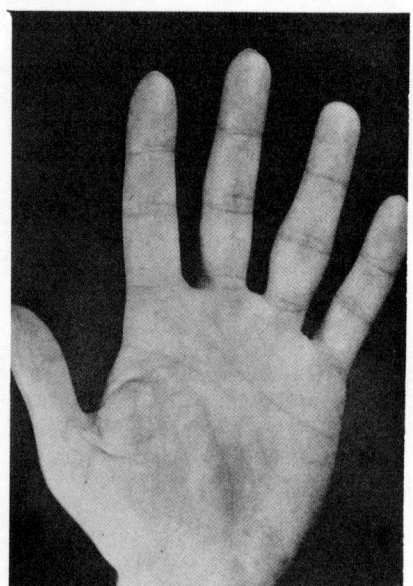
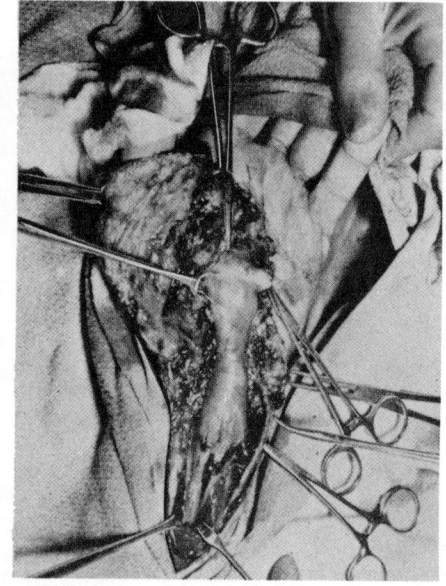

Tumor of the left hand, located just below the thumb in the palm area. In the picture on the right the tumor is being removed. Incision has been made and the interior of the palm is well exposed. Edges of the wound are held apart by retractors, and the tumor is freed from the surrounding tissues. The scissors-like instruments are hemostats which are used in clamping blood vessels to prevent hemorrhage. Hemostats have blunt points, do not cut and are self-locking.

Postgraduate Medicine

and boned wood and tortoise shell went out with the coming of Lister.

Ligatures for tying off blood vessels and for stopping hemorrhage were known as far back as the time of Galen, in Rome around 150 A.D. Apparently the saw has been known to man since before the birth of history and is supposed to have been conceived from studying the teeth of fish and such animals as the sawfish. Saws for surgery were modified continuously until the time of the modern saw which is electrically operated. Trepanning and opening of the skull was employed by the ancient Incas of South America. The practice was freely engaged upon in the time of Hippocrates and the ancient Egyptians.

Devices for dilating various openings of the body in order to permit the entrance of instruments and hands go back also to the ancients but the modern devices are far superior both as to perfection, as to the fit and to illumination. The discovery of electric light and its adaptation to surgical and medical instruments may be considered among the greatest of medical discoveries and new devices are introduced every year for such procedures.

Tapping for the release of fluid from the cavities of the body was performed by the ancient Greeks and Romans and the new devices which are known as trocars also are continuously modified with the introduction in more recent times of air suction and the use of the x-ray for indicating the area where a trocar is to be inserted.

Even as late as 1954 and 1955 new discoveries were made in relationship to the operating table which began with a simple board and four legs and which now has reached the stage of tables that can be adjusted to any position, tables which provide for the anesthetist and the nurses and for holding arms and legs and various portions of the body exactly as needed. There are tables which permit the head to be dropped backward for operations on the nose and throat and indeed special devices for brain surgery.

SURGERY OF OLDER PEOPLE

(See also discussion under *Aging, Degenerative Changes, Senescence*) An analysis of surgical operations done on older people at Johns Hopkins Hospital showed that, under modern conditions, surgery is performed on the aged with little risk; this is especially true when it is done as an elective operation rather than as an emergency. Much emergency surgery on older people could be avoided if chronic conditions requiring surgery were cared for before emergencies developed. Postponing an operation saps a patient's strength and increases the risk of shock and other complications.

SWEAT See *Perspiration*.

SWIMMING POOLS Hot weather means to the doctor an increasing number of infected ears and noses because people are careless about the places where they swim and bathe.

There are in the United States at least 6000 indoor swimming pools. No one knows how many beaches there are along the shores of lakes, rivers, and oceans. Great numbers of golf clubs have added swimmng pools as a special accessory for summer enjoyment. In 1900 there were said to be only 67 swimming pools in the United States.

The chief diseases that are transmitted through swimming pools are inflammation of the eye, boils and other infections in the ear, chronic inflammation of the nose and the sinuses, sore throat, various infections of the skin (including particularly the so-called athlete's foot), and, finally, infection of the bowels with dysentery. All swimmers who enter public swimming pools should be free from visible infections or acute disease at the time they enter the pool. Most managers now require a shower bath before each person enters the pool. This means at least one shower bath for every forty bathers and adequate comfort facilities for men and women as an accessory.

Drinking water near swimming pools must be controlled. The common use of drinking cups, towels, combs, hairbrushes, and other toilet articles should be strictly prohibited.

Most American swimming pools provide for the use of chlorine in the water as a means of keeping it pure, although the ultraviolet ray has also been developed as a useful technic for this purpose. Regular draining of the pool and the removal of sediment and infectious material also help to maintain sanitation. If a swimming pool is submitted to proper sanitation, there is less likelihood of infection for a swimmer unless he happens to come in contact with a heavy dose of germs from some person who should not be using the pool.

Few cases of infection develop from swimming in the ocean or in rivers or lakes where the people are not packed together. On crowded beaches, where there is hardly room to move the arms, people are constantly exposed to the excretions and secretions of their neighbors. This kind of crowding must bear the burden for infection of the respiratory tract and for dysentery.

Another important measure for use around swimming pools to prevent infection of the feet is to insist on a protected walk next to the pool to be used only by bathers who have previously had a shower and thus have cleansed their feet. This protected walk should be forbidden to visitors who are walking in their shoes and who thus carry infectious organisms and put them down where they come in contact with the naked feet of the bather. Such surface contamination may also be washed into the pool.

Scientific health standards demand that the germs in swimming pools be counted at fairly frequent intervals in relation to the total amount of water used. Large city engineering departments have facilities for conducting such studies.

SYMPATHETIC NERVOUS SYSTEM

Many functions carried on by the human body go on without any conscious activity by the brain. For instance the glands regularly secrete the glandular substances necessary to life. The blood is formed in the appropriate tissues. Associated with many of these necessary activities is the function of the sympathetic nervous system, also called the autonomic nervous system.

The nerve tissues of the autonomic nervous system go to practically all of the important organs of the body, to the sweat glands in the skin and the salivary glands. The nerves of the autonomic nervous system run alongside the spinal cord. Some of them are associated with important nerves affecting the eyes and ears. Certain drugs are known to influence particularly the sympathetic nervous system, although of course they do not affect that system alone but are likely to affect other portions of the body as well.

The blood supply to any part of the body can be increased by interrupting the sympathetic nerves that go to that part. This can be done by a surgical operation. It sometimes becomes necessary to undertake procedures of this kind in certain diseases. Nothing is to be gained by trying a procedure of this sort when the walls of the blood vessels are permanently hardened so that they cannot carry a greater blood supply.

One of the operations on the sympathetic nervous system that is sometimes used is the operation for high blood pressure, the idea being to increase the flow of blood into the abdominal area and the lower limbs and thus to decrease the pressure. Many cases are reported now in which this operation has been useful.

Occasionally interruption or treatment applied to the sympathetic nervous system has been used in conditions affecting the heart, like angina pectoris, or in severe pain involving the uterus. Operations have been done even to aid the activities of the bowel and the bladder and to control serious disturbances of the sweat glands.

In certain conditions that seem to be almost wholly emotional, the manifestations appear through activities of the sympathetic nervous system. This occurs, for instance, in shell shock, nervous breakdown, and in other conditions of the type called psychosomatic.

SYMPTOMS OF DISEASE (See also *Understanding Symptoms*) When people consult the doctor they do so because they have had feelings and sensations that are disturbing and uncomfortable. Perhaps they have had reactions in various portions of the body which are quite different from the usual. For instance, symptoms may include pain, weakness, shortness of breath, cough, or itching. One may notice a sudden increase of weight, or loss of weight. The hands and feet may seem to be cold and numb. Indigestion may occur with dizziness or vomiting or diarrhea. Because of jaundice the skin may develop a yellow appearance. All these are included in the signs and symptoms of disease; they are a warning that an investigation of the cause is needed.

People who are emotionally disturbed are likely to feel pain sooner and more intensely than are people in general. With the reaction to pain may come other changes brought about through functioning of the sympathetic nervous system. These include rapid beating of the heart, sweating, rise in the blood pressure and disturbances of digestion.

PAIN—Pain is described as burning, sticking or pricking, sharp, dull, throbbing or knifing. Different parts of the body feel pain in different ways. The skin reacts easily. Muscles may not feel puncture by a needle but ache when they are in spasm or suffer cramp. Compact bone may be cut without pain but porous bone may be painful when injured. The brain tissue may not be sensitive but the blood vessels have nerve connections and anything that pulls or stretches the blood vessels in the brain will give pain in the head. Pain from the intestines may be due to injury of the intestinal wall, stretching of the muscles in the wall or pulling on the tissues that hold the intestines in place.

HEADACHE—When you have a headache the doctor will want to know about the location of the pain, its quality, its intensity, the time when it comes on, and the way it is influenced by moving, reading, noise, and other factors. Usually a headache is a dull, aching pain, that arises from the structures within the skull. Sometimes a headache may be associated with a disturbance in the sinuses, or the eyes, or in the bones in the upper part of the spine.

Sensitivity to pain in the head varies in different people and in the same person at different times. The worst headaches are those associated with inflammations or infections of the meininges, which are the tissues that cover the brain. When a sudden, sharp pain affects the head the sensation may be due to a branch of the facial nerve. Usually headaches last longer, for minutes or even hours. When the headache is described as throbbing the effect comes from transmission of the pulse in the blood vessels.

A headache may be associated with exposure to cold. Other headaches may develop in healthy people during periods of great fatigue or emotional stress. Such headaches occur towards the end of the day; they begin as a dull ache in the forehead and spread towards the temples or towards the back. These headaches disappear when the person concerned has some good rest or sleep. Fear and worry seem to make headaches worse. Some headaches come from tenseness of the facial muscles which in turn may be caused by pain or anxiety or strain.

Psychologic disorders or mental disturbances may also be reflected in pains which are referred to the head. Such people complain of pressure on the head, of a tight fitting band which squeezes the head, or with a pain that presses on the very top of the head.

PAIN IN THE CHEST—Pain in the chest may come from the ribs and the tissues related to the ribs; from organs in the abdomen; from the heart or from other organs in the chest.

The muscle of the heart has to have oxygen and when this essential is not provided the muscle responds with pain. Angina pectoris is a pain of this type which is usually continuous and which is provoked by walking, or an emotional strain, or any other factor that increases the work of the heart. The pain tends to be relieved when the burden is removed. Interference with the flow of blood carrying oxygen through the coronary arteries into the heart will bring on an attack of pain. The pain of angina pectoris and that of coronary thrombosis are about the same. Usually that of coronary thrombosis is more severe and lasts longer. Occasionally, however, thrombosis may occur with little or less severe pain.

I should like to caution about jumping to conclusions relative to pain in the heart. Some people complain of pain over the heart, or in the heart area, who do not have the slightest sign of any real disturbance of the heart. Doctors call this a cardiac neurosis and credit it to abnormal anxiety about the heart. Such pains are not related to effort or work of the heart. They are usually accentuated by fatigue and emotional stresses.

Other pains in the chest may come from disturbances of the large blood vessels, from the nerves that reach the linings of the chest cavity, and from growths or abscesses behind the breast bone.

Heartburn probably arises from constriction at the bottom of the esophagus or swallowing tube, because material has been regurgitated from the stomach into this tube.

ABDOMINAL PAIN— Abdominal pain is usually lumped by most people into the common term "stomach ache." Just as the organs in the abdomen may transmit pain to the chest, so also may chest-organs transmit pain to the abdominal area. As a result of pain in the abdomen a person will have a look of pain on his face, walk slightly bent over and avoid motion when possible. Many people try to overcome abdominal pains by putting a finger down the throat to provoke vomiting; go repeatedly to the toilet and strain to empty the bowel; take enemas or purges. They will lie with the knees drawn up. Abdominal pains are described as colicky, sharp or knifing, continuous or steady.

The doctor inquires particularly about abdominal pains to find out when the pain began in relation to the taking of food. Then the doctor will try to locate the exact spot or the diffuse area where the pain appears.

One of the most important pains is that which follows the sudden rupture of any of the organs in the abdomen, like the gall bladder, the spleen, the liver, the uterus or the appendix. This is a sudden, sharp, terrifying pain, that seems to disappear soon; nevertheless it it a warning of extreme danger and the doctor should be called immediately to make certain what is wrong. Pain associated with inflammation is made worse by pressure on the abdomen.

Ileus is a name given by doctors to obstruction of the passage of material through the gastrointestinal tract. Such obstruction is a source of great danger to life itself. The blocking may come from many causes. The doctor gets important clues from the location of the pain, its waxing and waning, its frequency or continuity, and the amount of distention associated with the trouble.

PAIN IN THE BACK—Strangely one of the most difficult of all the diagnoses that a doctor has to make concerns the cause of a pain in the back. Excluding the pain that comes with breaking the bones of the spine or twisting the spine completely out of line, a number of different conditions may be responsible for different kinds of pains in the back.

Infections may attack the tissues of the back as they do other parts of the body. Rheumatoid arthritis may select the many joints of the backbone as a place in which to locate. The little cartilages or discs that act as cushions between the bones may be crushed or slip out of place. The ligaments which attach to the bones of the spine may be pulled to the point where they are painful with every movement.

Careful study by an experienced physician reveals the cause of pain in the back and indicates the type of treatment to be followed. This may vary from changing the shoes and wearing a specially designed brace or corset, to instructions for reducing weight, improving the posture or even a surgical operation. A recent postural instruction sheet designed by Dr. Paul C. Williams says:

When standing or walking, toe straight ahead and take most of your weight on the heels.

Sit with the buttocks tucked under so that the hollow in the low back is eradicated.

When possible elevate the knees higher than the hips while sitting.

Sleep on your back with your knees propped up or on your side with one or both knees drawn up. Bed should be firm.

Never bend backwards.

Avoid standing as much as possible.

Learn to live 24 hours a day without a hollow in the lower part of your back.

Avoid sleeping on the abdomen.

PAINFUL ARMS AND LEGS—Burns, frostbite, and cutting of the arms and legs may be painful. Similarly arthritis, abscesses in the bones and soft tissues, tumors and damage to the nerves may result in severe pain.

From the limbs of the body the nerves pass along until they connect with the roots in the spinal cord. Pressure, irritation or damage to these nerves at any point along their course may result in pain that is felt in the limb itself.

Pain may also be transmitted to the limbs from impulses arising elsewhere in the body. For instance, pain from the hip may be transmitted to the knee. Pain from the deep muscles of the back or from the small bones of the spinal column may be felt in the legs. Pain from angina pectoris or coronary thrombosis of the heart may be felt along the inner sides of the arms.

Various disturbances of the blood supply to the limbs may result in pain. This applies particularly to blocking of the circulation so that the tissues do not receive a proper amount of oxygen. As the blood supply becomes blocked there is a feeling of numbness and finally difficulty of movement. You say "My leg has gone to sleep." Blocking the blood to the arm causes the fingers to get quite numb in about twelve minutes, and then they are painful when touched. As the blood returns a sensation of tingling is felt, which is due to renewed activity of the nerves of the arm. If an arm or leg is moved while the circulation is blocked severe pain may be felt. This may be called a cramp, although actually the muscles are not in spasm but flaccid.

After a limb has been amputated pain may be felt as if it were in the limb. This is called phantom limb pain.

In diagnosing the causes of pain in the extremities the character and location of the pain are most significant.

SYNDROME Whenever a number of symptoms occur together regularly, the group of symptoms is called a syndrome. There are a wide variety of diseases that are known as syndromes, most of them named after the physician who first observed the occurrence of the symptoms as a group. Among the best known of these conditions, for example, is the Cushing syndrome, which is a series of symptoms due to certain tumors of the brain; the Christian syndrome, which is associated with the condition called diabetes insipidus.

SYNOVITIS The membranes which line the joints are known as synovial membranes. The fluid in a joint is known as synovial fluid. Inflammation of these membranes is known as synovitis.

SYNOVIAL MEMBRANE—See article ARTHRITIS, RHEUMATISM, AND GOUT.

SYPHILIS The word "syphilis," coined in 1530 by an Italian physician, has attained recognition.

Known to the world for many centuries, this disease gradually has developed increasing prevalence and prominence simply because one of its methods of transmission made its discussion taboo.

If syphilis were transmitted by a fly or mosquito, we could long since have stamped it out. It happens, however, to be spread in the vast majority of cases by contact between human beings, and by a form of contact which itself has been taboo as a subject for general discussion.

Through years of research the medical profession learned that the disease is caused in every case by an organism known as *Spirochaeta pallida*. Literally this means "pale coil of hair." It refers to a germ which appears under the microscope as a spiral germ of pallid coloring. One of these germs is about as long as an ordinary red blood cell.

IMITATES OTHER DISEASES—Were it not for the fact that this germ is susceptible to sunlight and air, and also to fairly mild antiseptics, syphilis might long since have destroyed human life upon this earth.

When the germ gets into the body, it multiplies quickly and gradually invades every organ and tissue. Some germs are limited largely to the lungs, others to the throat, and still others to the intestines, but the syphilis germ attacks any kind of tissue, and it has been said that because of this syphilis can imitate every other disease.

One of the most famous physicians, Sir William Osler, once said: "Know syphilis in all its manifestations and relations and all other things clinical will be added unto you."

IT CAN BE CURED—Until 1903 it was thought that syphilis occurred only in human beings. In that year it was first transmitted to monkeys, and since that time it occasionally has been transmitted to rabbits and white mice. Transmission of the disease to these animals has enabled us to study it on a larger scale and as a result has made it possible for us to say that syphilis can be cured.

Cure means not only elimination of the first lesion that the disease causes on the skin, but even the elimination of the organisms and their poisons from the entire body.

Clearing the germ from the body also halts secondary eruption on the skin, damage to internal tissues, and the germ's invasion of the brain. When syphilis attacks the brain, there results the condition called general paralysis of the insane and locomotor ataxia.

DEVELOPING TREATMENTS—The advance against syphilis has depended largely on certain epoch-making, world-famous discoveries. When the organism that causes the disease was discovered by Schaudinn in 1905, a great step forward was taken.

Wassermann's description of the test by which infection can be determined was another tremendous advance.

The final, most significant advance was the development of the product called 606, salvarsan, or arsphenamine, by Paul Ehrlich. This was important not only for its own value but also as a stimulus to subsequent discoveries which have led to the development of other drugs of great importance in the treatment of this disease.

Especially significant have been the new developments in relationship to the use of mercury, the determination of the germ of syphilis in the brain, and the development of bismuth and heat treatment and of penicillin in most recent years.

Syphilis can be transmitted from parents to their children. In these cases the germ that causes the disease passes from the mother to the child and infects the organs of the baby.

Usually the tissues that connect the mother to the baby act as a filter and keep back the germs of most diseases, including those of tuberculosis, but the germs of syphilis seem to be able to find their way through.

BIRTH TOLL IS GREAT—After a baby has been infected, he may die, and syphilis is recognized today as one of the important causes of premature birth of dead babies and stillbirths.

It is also recognized that babies born either prematurely or at the right time may be so enfeebled by syphilis that they will die while they are very young.

Moreover, if these enfeebled babies survive the first few months of life, they may later develop sores that leave ugly scars, deformed bones, bad teeth, blindness, deafness, paralysis, or even mental disturbances, as a result of the syphilis that has been transmitted to them.

It has been estimated that three out of every one hundred babies born have syphilis which they acquired in the period before they were born, and it has been stated that out of all of the babies who die before they are twelve months old 40 per cent die before they reach the age of one month, with syphilis outstanding as the cause of such early deaths.

EARLY TREATMENT BEST—The saddest fact in relationship to this misfortune is that this is all preventable but that modern social organization and science have not yet found the way to make prevention the practice.

Most important step in this prevention is the examination of every prospective mother, including the making of a Wassermann test. If the mother is found to be infected, arrangements must be made immediately for her to take treatment of the most active kind in order to prevent the birth of an infected child.

The best time to cure the disease is before the baby is born. If the mother begins treatment during the first three months of her expectant period, infection of the baby can be prevented. Treatment will drive the germs out of her blood so that they cannot travel from her circulation into that of the baby. But even if the treatment is not started until the fourth or fifth month, she still may have a healthy baby.

If treatment of the mother has been insufficient or if she has had no treatment before the birth of the child, then the immediate treatment of the baby after his arrival is of the utmost importance. This can be arranged without much difficulty because of new methods of administering the necessary drugs and other treatments important in controlling this disease.

It is commonly estimated that from 8 to 10 per cent of the American people have syphilis. That means that from 10,000,000 to 12,000,000 are infected.

It has been estimated that 21,000,000 working days are lost by infected men. Allowing for this at the rate of $4 per day, there is an immediate loss of $84,-000,000. This does not take into account time lost by women. It has been estimated that the annual bill for treatment of syphilis in New York State is more than $23,000,000.

The amount of infection seems to vary according to the status of society and the occupations of those who are concerned. Women of the "red-light" districts are said to be infected invariably sooner or later.

Among criminals in penitentiaries as many as 20 to 40 per cent have been found infected. Among men of better families the amount of infection seems to vary from 2 to 10 per cent.

Active Death Cause—The number of people who die from syphilis is not definitely known, because there is a disinclination to report syphilis as the main cause of death, and also because it is covered up by other more important causes.

If it is remembered, however, that syphilis is the real cause of death in all cases of general paralysis and locomotor ataxia, in many cases of epilepsy, and in a considerable number of other diseases, the importance of the condition as a cause of death is more easily estimated.

Life insurance companies are not likely to be willing to insure people who have syphilis. The sickness and death rates of those who have had the disease are likely to be higher than those for other people in the community.

If insurance companies do accept for insurance those who have had syphilis, they are likely to want a higher rate. Some companies will, however, insure people who have had a thorough course of treatment and who have been without symptoms for some three to five years.

Marriage Precautions—In many states syphilis is a bar to marriage. Twenty-two states demand a physician's certificate or a statement or affidavit from one or both candidates that they are free from venereal disease.

In Michigan and Oklahoma marriage by a person with venereal disease is expressly stated to be a felony. In Utah a marriage under such circumstances may by annulled.

Doctors everywhere warn people in the early stages of syphilis against marriage, and in every instance when syphilis has not been cured it is the duty of the doctor to warn the prospective partner against marriage until cure has been accomplished.

No one can possibly estimate the cost in money represented by the damage that syphilis does to human health and life. The amount is so tremendous that the figures stagger the imagination.

There are some records of syphilis infection by accident when a person with a sore on his finger has come in contact with syphilitic material on the body of another person.

There are records of infection from kissing, and babies have been infected from wet nurses. These secondary types of infection are, however, so unusual in comparison with the ordinary methods of spread of infection that this fact should not frighten anyone into a constant fear of this disease.

In the vast majority of cases syphilis is transmitted from one human to another during sex relationship.

Hotel beds, public lavatories, bathtubs, doorknobs, books, dishes used in restaurants, and similar materials are not easily infected. It is necessary for the germ to get into the body through a sore or through an easily infected spot if it is to invade the body generally.

USUAL SYMPTOMS—As has already been said, the organism that causes syphilis is killed by drying and is susceptible to soap and water. Thorough washing is an important factor in preventing the spread of the infection.

The first sign of the disease usually is a sore at the point where the germ has entered the tissue. The doctor who finds this sore will make his diagnosis by studying the material from the sore under the microscope, either fresh or after staining.

He also takes some blood from the veins and tests this blood with what is known as the Wassermann test or with the Kahn test. These tests determine usually at a fairly early stage whether or not a person has been infected with syphilis.

If the disease is not promptly treated, it will spread to the interior of the body, ultimately causing eruption on the skin, and all of the other serious conditions that have been mentioned.

MAY BE OTHER CAUSES—There are a few simple facts that everyone ought to know about syphilis:

This disease does not cause pimples.

It does not cause itching conditions of the skin.

It may cause ulcers of the legs, but more frequently these are due to varicose veins.

It may be responsible for failure to produce children, but there are also other conditions which may produce such failures.

It is not a form of blood poisoning. Testing of the blood will show whether or not the patient has syphilis.

It is not responsible for the vast majority of cases of baldness, but some cases of loss of hair not only of the head but of the entire body may be due to syphilis.

It has not been established in any way that syphilis is the cause of cancer or that these two conditions are in any way related.

BASIC RULES—There are a few simple instructions which were widely circulated during World War II to all soldiers who were found to be infected with this disease:

If you have any sore on your genitals, no matter how small, or if you think you have syphilis, consult your physician.

Do not under any conditions rely on the "blood medicines" that promise to eradicate syphilis, and do not be caught by advertising doctors—quacks—who try to get your money by promising to cure you quickly.

Do not let druggists prescribe for you; they are not qualified to treat syphilis.

Do not hesitate to tell your doctor or dentist of your disease. Later in life, if you get sick at any time, you should tell your doctor that you have had syphilis, since this fact may furnish a clue to treatment on which your cure depends.

Live temperately and sensibly. Do not go to extreme in any direction in your habits of life.

Try to get a reasonable amount of sleep—eight hours is the amount needed by the average person. And as a safeguard to others, sleep alone.

Take good care of your teeth. Brush them two or three times a day. If they are not in good condition, have them attended to by a dentist. But when you go to him, tell him that you have syphilis.

Don't Spread Trouble—Do not have sexual intercourse until you are told by your physician that you are no longer contagious. It will interfere with the cure of the disease, and it is criminal, for it is likely to give the disease to your wife.

You must not marry until you have the doctor's consent, which cannot be properly given until at least two years have passed after cure seems complete. If you do, you run the risk of infecting your wife and your children with syphilis.

Early in the course of syphilis, while it is contagious, the greatest danger of infecting other people is by the mouth. Because of this danger do not kiss anybody. Particularly do not endanger children by kissing them.

Do not allow anything that has come in contact with your lips or that has been in your mouth to be left around so that anybody can use it before it has been cleaned. This applies to cups, glasses, knives, forks, spoons, pipes, cigars, toothpicks, and all such things. It is better to use your own towels, brushes, comb, razor, soap, et cetera, though these are much less likely to be contaminated than objects that go in your mouth.

If you have any open sores—you will not have any after the first week or two, if you are treated—everything that comes in contact with them should be destroyed or disinfected.

As a result of the examination of 10,000,000 men in World War II, it has been found that the incidence of syphilis varies in different parts of the United States.

Early in the war men with a positive Wassermann test were eliminated from military service. Later it was decided to take these men into the service and to treat them. As a result syphilis is now being brought much more definitely under control.

In the modern treatment of syphilis, technics have been developed for shortening the period of treatment. These include an intensive treatment, occupying ten weeks, using principally the arsenical drugs; also a five-day treatment carried on in the hospital, in which the patient is given intensive, continuous treatment with drugs put directly into the veins. Sometimes there is combined with this a long period of heat treatment, using special devices known as hypertherms that have been developed for the purpose.

More recently syphilis is being treated with penicillin and other antibiotics. By giving penicillin either continuously over a period of five days or by repeated intramuscular injections one may stop the progress of the disease and change a positive Wassermann test to a negative Wassermann test inside of a week. The percentage of relapses with this treatment is relatively slight, being certainly well under 4 per cent of all the cases. The method has been found useful not only in the treatment of early syphilis but in halting the progress of syphilis of the nervous system.

Because of the great success of these methods of treatment many authorities now predict that syphilis may be completely eliminated from the United States within the next generation.

Syphilis—See Skin, article The Skin; Venereal Diseases, article The Venereal Diseases.

Syphilis—aorta: See Heart, article Diseases of the Heart and Circulation.

Syphilis—attacks every organ and tissue: See Infectious Disease, article The Prevention and Treatment of Infectious Disease.

Syphilis—blood test: See Blood, article The Blood and Its Diseases.

SYPHILIS—cause determined: See INFECTIOUS DISEASE, article THE PREVENTION AND TREATMENT OF INFECTIOUS DISEASE.

SYPHILIS—eye infection: See EYE, article THE EYE.

SYPHILIS—foot deformities may result: See FOOT, article THE FOOT.

SYPHILIS—hair loss: See HAIR, article THE HAIR.

SYPHILIS—heart: See HEART, article DISEASES OF THE HEART AND CIRCULATION.

SYPHILIS—hypertension may be aggravated by: See article BLOOD PRESSURE.

SYPHILIS—nephrosis: See KIDNEY, article THE KIDNEY: ITS DISEASES AND DISTURBANCES.

SYPHILIS—paresis caused by: See MENTAL, article NERVOUS AND MENTAL DISORDERS.

SYPHILIS—rat-bite fever treated similarly: See article TRANSMISSIBLE DISEASES.

TABES See *Locomotor Ataxia.*

TACHYPHAGIA The word "tachyphage" is another one of those long medical words composed of two Greek words: "tachy," meaning rapid; and "phage," meaning to eat. A tachyphage is a rapid eater, and the United States is full of them. A tachyphage is likely to wake up in the morning with a tight feeling in the abdomen at the thought of the day that is before him. He lies in bed too long thinking about his troubles, skips his bath, rushes through his dressing, grabs a glass of orange juice and a cup of coffee and runs for the train chewing on a piece of toast. Then he is troubled with discomfort in his abdomen most of the morning. At noon he bolts his luncheon, eating it off the corner of a desk or speeding through service at a luncheon club so that there will be time for the speaker. He gets home just in time to bolt his dinner so that he can be off to a movie or a bridge game.

Sooner or later the constant discomfort in his interior gives him an anxious look. He begins to think that he has hyperacidity or a gastric ulcer—and maybe he has. Thereafter he takes large quantities of baking soda an hour or two after each meal.

Most of the trouble is due to the fact that he eats too rapidly. Because of his mental state he has trouble in digesting what he eats. The chief step in his cure is the establishment of regular hours for his meals, insistence on spending enough time to eat the meal slowly, and, finally, the avoidance of all business discussions and telephone conversations or other anxieties during the meal.

The woman worker is no advance on

the big businessman when it comes to being a tachyphage. She gulps her lunch, including a sandwich and a cup of coffee, with possibly also a piece of pie, in five or ten minutes and spends the remaining time in gossip or shopping. Such a luncheon is of little use either for nutrition or the satisfaction of hunger. Therefore it is supplemented all day long with candy, soda-fountain drinks, and similar items.

Not long ago a number of the New York literati formed a Three-Hours-for-Lunch Club. That was probably a reaction against the establishment of tachyphagia as a universal American disease.

TALIPES (See also discussion under *Clubfoot*) Talipes is a deformity of the foot in which it is twisted out of shape or position. The common name for this condition is clubfoot. The condition has been classified according to the direction in which the foot is twisted. Sometimes when the foot stands on the toe the condition is called talipes equinus because it is like the foot of a horse. If it is twisted to the side, it is called talipes valgus. These conditions can be controlled by care given exceedingly early in life by an orthopedic surgeon.

TANTALUM This new metallic element has been found to be non-corrosive and malleable and is, therefore, used not only as a plate to replace areas lost from the skull by injury but also for the making of sutures to sew together damaged tissues.

TATTOOING With every outbreak of war and recruitment of men into military service tattooing becomes prominent. Then when the war ends, great numbers of men and even some women begin asking specialists in diseases of the skin how to get rid of the pictures.

In the process of tattooing mineral and vegetable substances are introduced into the skin by means of needles. Primitive savages pigmented the skin and tattooed the body largely in connection with religious worship. Soldiers and sailors apparently indulge in tattooing as a form of obtaining a permanent souvenir of some country that they have visited or some person whom they want to remember. Sometimes it is difficult to explain just why anyone has himself tattooed. One soldier had a tombstone in black tattooed on his forearm and below this in red letters "To the Memory of My Mother." A sailor from Liverpool had sixteen girls' names tattooed on his back. Fifteen out of thirty men with tattoo pictures had mermaids as the perdominating figure in their personal art galleries.

Tattooing of the skin sometimes occurs accidentally, as in the case of powder stains, in which particles of powder are deposited in the skin. Miners sometimes have permanent discoloration due to the imbedding of coal dust in scratches. Other metals which have been deposited in the skin with the effect of tattooing are silver and iron.

In the tattooing process the moistening is sometimes accomplished by the saliva of the tattooer. By this technic various diseases, including tuberculosis, erysipelas, bacterial infections, and even venereal diseases have been transmitted from the tattooer to the subject. Occasionally tattooing sets up reactions in the skin which result in the development of tumors.

Among the methods known for removing tattoo is the peeling of the skin by the use of caustic substances. This is quite dangerous, and even specialists in diseases of the skin dislike to attempt its use. It is, of course, possible to cut away entirely the tattooed area if it is not too large and to take care of the defect that is thus developed by grafting new skin from another portion of the body. A new successful method involves sterilizing the area with antiseptics, then sandpapering the tattooed skin off its base, controlling the bleeding and encouraging healing.

TEETH (See also *Dentifrices*) Thousands of years ago men, without the advantages that we possess today, recognized the importance of teeth. Human beings who have to get along without knives and forks—for instance, the Eskimos—learn to use the jaws and teeth in a manner in which civilized men never have used them. Eskimos will bite through bone and tear tough meats with their teeth.

The ancient Egyptians, Greeks, and Romans used abrasives to keep their teeth clean. They made gold supports to hold loose teeth in the mouth and even tried to replace lost teeth with teeth taken from sheep or calves. They endeavored to make their teeth more beautiful by inserting diamonds and other ornaments. There are still people who decorate their mouths in this manner, but most of us prefer porcelain or similar material, which gives the teeth as normal an appearance as possible.

The famous artist Leonardo da Vinci was among the first to recognize that the teeth in a normal mouth are of different shapes and different sizes in order to perform special functions. In the normal mouth there are thirty-two permanent teeth. These permanent teeth are preceded by baby teeth which must also be protected if the permanent teeth are to come in properly.

Until modern dentistry was developed in the United States, the care of the teeth was a side line for blacksmiths and goldsmiths. Decayed teeth were pulled and false teeth were made of gold, bone, and ivory. They were not the same size and shape as natural teeth.

The teeth George Washington wore were held in his mouth by spiral springs which often jammed and would not work. Washington's teeth were made about 1790. Ten years later a Frenchman in Philadelphia discovered how to keep false teeth in the mouth without springs.

About that time also the celebrated physician, Benjamin Rush, one of the signers of the Declaration of Independence, pointed out that infected teeth could bring about diseases in other parts of the body.

The first school of dentistry was established in Baltimore in 1840. Other dental schools were established promptly thereafter. Today dentistry in the United States leads all the world.

There is no known diet that alone will insure good teeth. A diet that contains the right proteins, carbohydrates, fats, mineral salts, and vitamins is a good diet for the teeth as well as for the

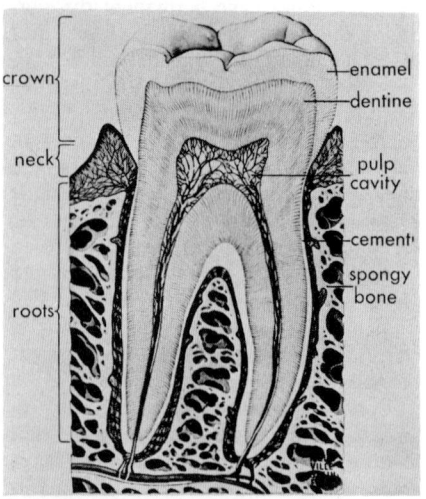

Cross section of a tooth showing the crown, neck and roots and internal structures. Within the pulp cavity can be found nerves and blood vessels.

American Medical Association

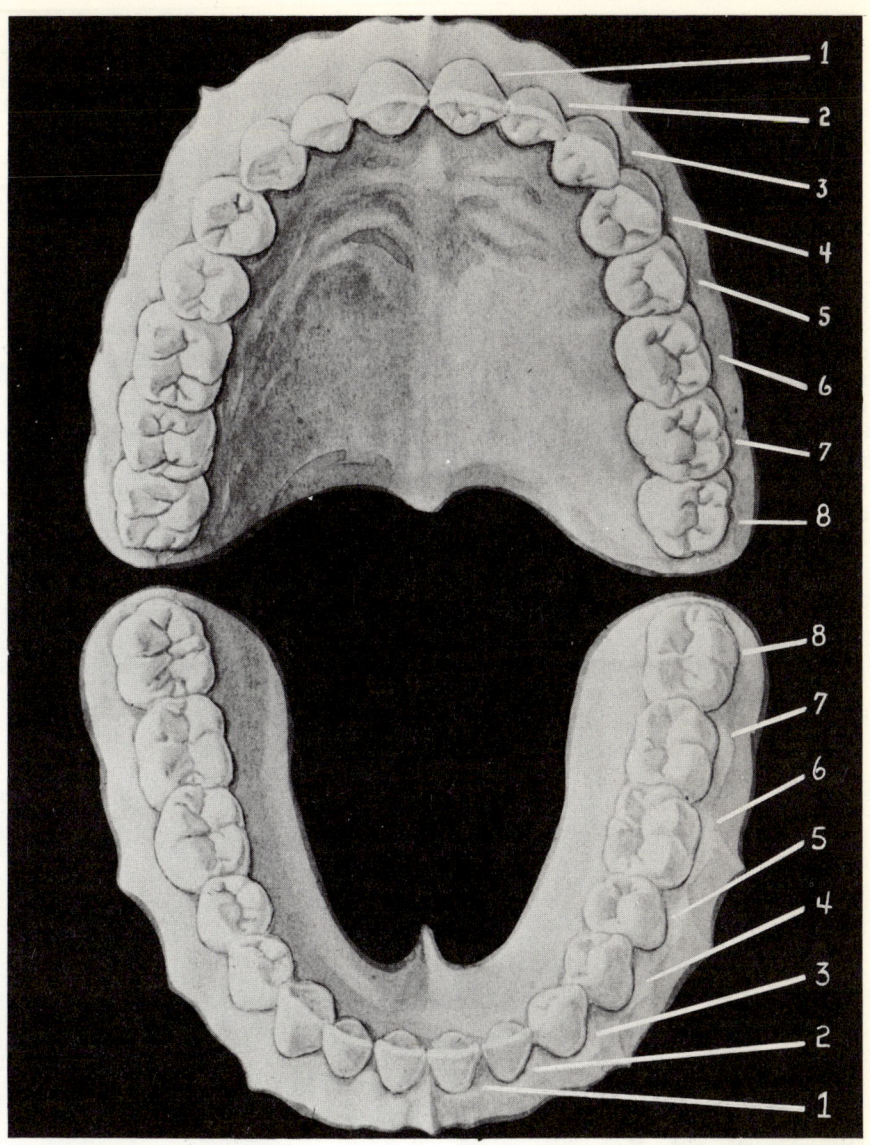

A full set of permanent teeth, 32 in number. Upper jaw: (1) central incisor, (2) lateral incisor, (3) cuspid, (4) first bicuspid, (5) second bicuspid, (6) first molar, (7) second molar, (8) third molar. Lower jaw: (8) third molar, (7) second molar, (6) first molar, (5) second bicuspid, (4) first bicuspid, (3) cuspid, (2) lateral incisor, and (1) central incisor.

rest of the body. However, teeth need minerals, like calcium and phosphorus, and these are found to best advantage in milk and milk products. If, however, you happen to be sensitive to milk, or if the milk acts unfavorably for your digestion, remember that other foods also provide these minerals.

These minerals are found in the leafy green vegetables. Moreover, the whole-grain cereals and the flesh of fish are also rich in phosphorus. In order that the calcium and phosphorus may be usable by the body for the production of sound teeth and bones, it is desirable that we take regularly enough vitamins A, C, and D. The use of the right amounts of cod-liver oil or halibut-liver oil helps to supply vitamins A and D.

The ultraviolet rays of the sun help the body to make vitamin D. The juice of tomatoes, oranges, and grapefruit and other citrus fruits provide plenty of vitamin C.

The dentist says give your teeth plenty of chewing exercise. If you eat the foods that require chewing, you are more likely to get the chewing exercise than you are if you try to get along with soft foods only. People who live largely on a liquid diet fail to remember that chewing is important for the preservation of their teeth.

In the first place the mouth provides saliva which contains a ferment capable of digesting sugars and starches. In the second place chewing benefits the teeth, the jaws, the nasal and breathing passages, as well as the stomach. The jaws should be well developed not only be-

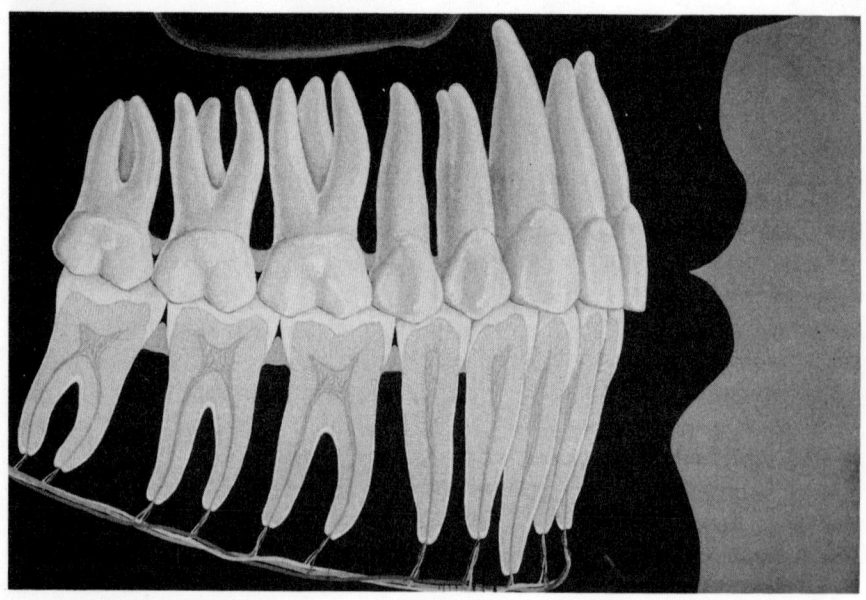

Adult dentition, showing right side of the jaw. From left to right: third molars, second molars, first molars, second biscupid, first bicuspid, cuspid, lateral incisor, central incisor.

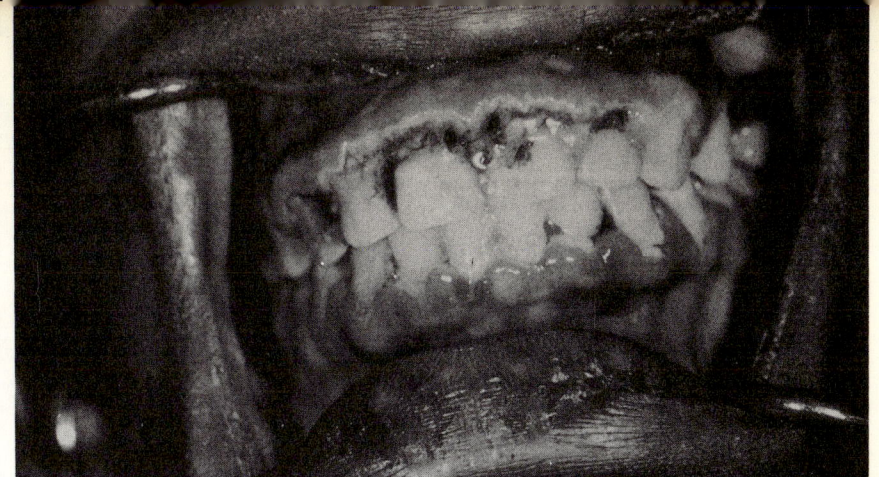

(B)

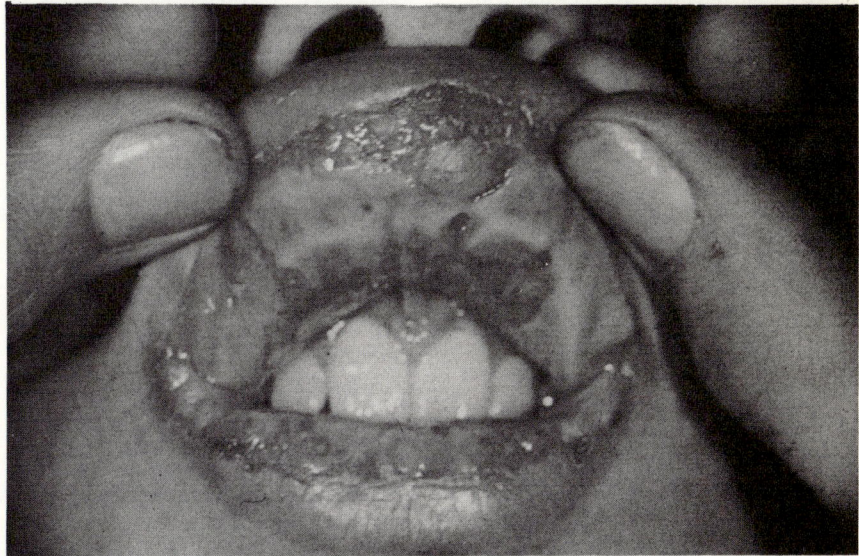

Good nutrition and oral hygiene help prevent diseases of the oral mucosa. Above are three photographs showing lesions of the gums and lips. (A) Vincent's gingivostomatitis; (B) Herpetic stomatitis; (C) Erythema multiforms.   Chas. Pfizer & Co., Inc.

(C)

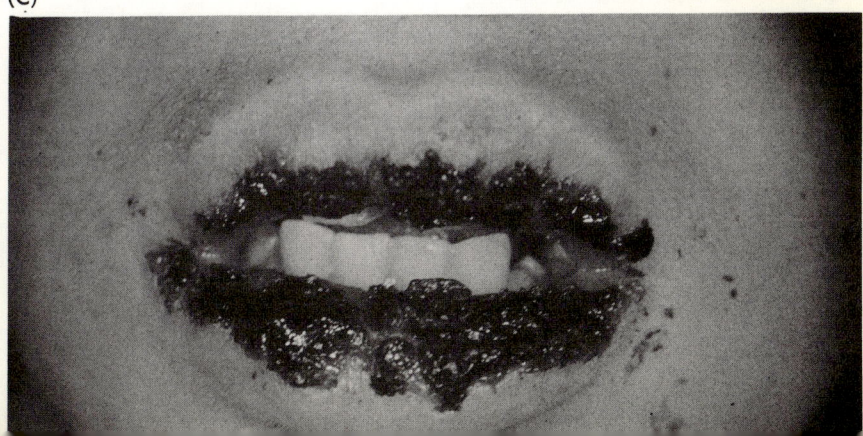

cause we have learned to admire a well-developed jaw, but also because a well-developed jaw gives the teeth plenty of room. When the mouth is not well developed, the teeth become crowded together and get out of line. That makes chewing more difficult—in short, a vicious circle.

Chewing can be performed not only by chewing gum, which exercises the teeth and jaws and helps to keep the teeth clean, but also by chewing fruits and vegetables with fiber, such, for instance, as carrots, apples, the hearts of cabbage and celery.

Your dentist says, "Keep your teeth clean." This can be made a habit. The dentist says, "Brush your teeth the way they grow." Since the upper teeth grow down, brush them down, and brush the lower teeth upward, and do not forget the surface between the teeth. Brush all the teeth—not just the front ones.

Once you form the habit of brushing your teeth, at least morning and evening if not after each meal, you will learn to relish the sensation of clean teeth.

Your dentist may not say that you ought to see him three times a year, but the facts are that small cavities appear in the teeth and persist and grow larger if they are not promptly cared for. It is, therefore, to your advantage to have your dentist look your teeth over three times a year.

Remember these four rules:

1. Eat the right food.
2. Give your teeth plenty of chewing exercise.
3. Brush your teeth at least twice a day.
4. See your dentist for an examination and cleaning of the teeth three times a year.

ABSCESSED TEETH—diabetics should have extracted: See article DIABETES.

ABSCESSED TEETH—hypertension may be aggravated by: See article BLOOD PRESSURE.

TEETH—adults: See TEETH, article THE CARE OF THE TEETH.

TEETH—brushes: See TEETH, article THE CARE OF THE TEETH.

TEETH—caries: See article DEFICIENCY DISEASES; TEETH, article CARE OF THE TEETH.

TEETH—cavities: See TEETH, article THE CARE OF THE TEETH.

TEETH—decay: See TEETH, article THE CARE OF THE TEETH.

TEETH—deciduous: See INFANCY, article CARE AND FEEDING OF THE CHILD.

TEETH—delayed in eruption by rickets: See INFANCY, article CARE AND FEEDING OF THE CHILD.

TEETH—dentures: See TEETH, article THE CARE OF THE TEETH.

TEETH—diet: See TEETH, article THE CARE OF THE TEETH.

TEETH—digestive role: See DIET, article ADVICE ON THE DIET.

TEETH—false: See TEETH, article THE CARE OF THE TEETH.

TEETH—first: See INFANCY, article CARE AND FEEDING OF THE CHILD.

TEETH—gaps should be filled to help digestion: See article DIGESTION AND DIGESTIVE DISEASES.

TEETH—halitosis: See TEETH, article THE CARE OF THE TEETH.

TEETH—malocclusion caused by thumb sucking: See INFANCY, article CARE AND FEEDING OF THE CHILD.

TEETH—mouth washes: See TEETH, article THE CARE OF THE TEETH.

TEETH—orthodontia: See TEETH, article THE CARE OF THE TEETH.

TEETH—pastes: See TEETH, article THE CARE OF THE TEETH.

TEETH—powders: See TEETH, article THE CARE OF THE TEETH.

TEETH—pregnancy care: See BIRTH, article CARE OF MOTHERS BEFORE AND AFTER CHILDBIRTH.

TEETH—pyorrhea: See TEETH, article THE CARE OF THE TEETH.

TEETH—scarlet fever: See CHILDHOOD DISEASES, article INFECTIOUS DISEASES OF CHILDHOOD.

TEETH—tartar deposits: See TEETH, article THE CARE OF THE TEETH.

TEETH—vitamin D: See SKIN, article THE SKIN.

TEETH—wisdom: See EAR, article THE EAR, TONGUE, NOSE, AND THROAT.

The Care of the Teeth

BY

MORRIS FISHBEIN, M.D.

Former Editor, *Journal American Medical Association,* Chicago; Editor, *Excerpta Medica, Bulletin World Medical Assn.; Post-graduate Medicine.*

THE CARE OF BABY'S TEETH

Few mothers realize that the first attention to the teeth of the child must begin before it is born. The mother should visit the dentist early, keep her teeth clean and well cared for, and eat the proper food so that the child's teeth will be properly developed. The proper foods include plenty of milk, fresh vegetables, eggs, fresh and cooked fruits, the coarser cereals, and a sufficient amount of calories to provide energy. Foods to be avoided are the sweets in excess, meat in excess, pastries, and highly seasoned foods.

During the early months it is not necessary for the expectant mother to eat more than her usual amount of food, but during the last four months the amount of food must be increased slightly in order to provide a sufficient amount of material for building the tissues of the child.

There used to be a notion that it was not safe for a prospective mother to visit her dentist, but it is now realized that the dentist can do the necessary dental work without serious harm or shock, and that it is better to take care of the teeth immediately than to permit bad conditions to go on for months.

Of special importance for building sound teeth are vitamins C, D, and A. Vitamin C is found plentifully in orange and tomato juice and in the fresh vegetables; vitamins A and D particularly in cod-liver oil and egg yolks. The physician should see the prospective mother just as soon as she knows that she is going to have a child and advise her regarding the taking of cod-liver oil or of excess vitamins in the form of concentrates.

The baby that is nursed by its mother gets the best food a baby can get. If it is not nursed by the mother, it will have to have a diet arranged so as to include the necessary substances. The basis of all baby diets is milk, but milk is deficient in certain necessary substances, and these the doctor can provide for through modifications of the diet. He will tell the mother when the baby is to have orange and tomato juice and cod-liver oil and the amount of each it should have. The vegetables are the first foods to be added to the baby's diet, and they should be started slowly in very small quantities. By the time the child is one year of age it can eat most vegetables; it can also be having fresh milk, fruit, and Zwieback or toast.

Many physicians and dentists believe that coarse foods strengthen the jaws and help in hardening the gums. When a new tooth is about to come in, the coarse foods serve as a resistance against which the gums may work in order to permit the tooth to cut its way through. If the child is excessively irritant when the teeth are coming in, it is wise to have the advice of the dentist or family physician.

The first teeth come in at the front of the mouth between the fifth and eighth months, as a rule. If they happen to be a little early or late, there is no cause for worry. The next teeth come in between the eighth and tenth months, and the others about the time of the first birthday. Until the first teeth appear, the mouth of the child does well if let alone. After the first teeth appear, the gums and teeth may be wiped daily with a soft clean cloth dipped in water to which a little salt has been added. It is well to be exceedingly gentle.

About the eighteenth month a soft toothbrush may be substituted for the soft cloth, and as soon as the child is old enough it should learn to brush its teeth for itself. If the child likes the taste of toothpaste, it may have toothpaste. If it prefers the water with added salt, it may have that. Most physicians and dentists are convinced that a toothpaste is of service only in cleaning and polishing the teeth and has little, if any, special value for preventing infection or counteracting acid.

The chief reason for preserving the baby teeth is to keep the mouth in the right shape for the second teeth. All of the twenty teeth that are called temporary teeth are usually in the mouth by the time the child is three. Behind the first set is the second set. In order to have the second set properly developed, the food must be right and the mouth free from infection. The only certain way to control infection is to have dental care when it appears.

The most important permanent tooth comes in between the fifth and sixth year of life and is known as the six-year molar. It comes in six teeth back from the one in the front of the mouth in center.

There are four six-year molars, one on each side of the upper and lower jaws. They should have the most careful attention. Once gone, they are not replaced except with artificial teeth. If they decay and are removed without proper dental attention, the entire expression of the face and of the mouth may change. In the absence of the proper molars, food is not sufficiently ground before entering the stomach.

Every child should see a dentist following the appearance of the six-year molars. Only a generation has passed since dentists first began to give special attention to the teeth of the child. Now the subject is so important that there are many dentists who specialize exclusively in children's teeth. They are concerned with seeing that all of the teeth are straight, that they fit properly against the opposites in the other jaw, that they do not grind off surfaces that are meant to stand, and that they remain firmly and are not pushed into the wrong positions.

With the help of the X-ray, the dentist is able to see that the teeth are sound at their roots. By personal inspection he finds tiny spots which indicate the beginning of decay. These can be filled and polished and their decay stopped. The additional cost of the X-ray pictures means future saving. Preventive dentistry done early is cheap. Curative dentistry, done after decay has proceeded far, after the teeth have gotten into wrong positions, after some teeth have been lost, may be expensive and can be prevented.

Many communities are now adding fluorides to the community water supply as a means of preventing dental caries. There seems to be no doubt that this helps prevention though other causes persist and cases appear even when all children get fluorides.

ORTHODONTIA

Within recent years a new specialty has arisen in dentistry and in medicine called orthodontia. The word means "straight teeth." It means literally to arrange crooked teeth in a more harmonious and symmetrical curve so that they will function better and improve the facial appearance. It is, of course, necessary to realize that back of all health are proper nutrition and growth. Unless the child has a diet which contains a sufficient amount of calcium, phosphorus, vitamins A, C, and D particularly, it is not likely to have good teeth.

Unless the baby teeth have been suitably controlled and well taken care of, the teeth that come in thereafter will not be properly developed and distributed. Dentists are convinced that there are a considerable number of bad habits that are associated with development of malocclusion, which means improper closing of the teeth and jaws. Breathing through the mouth, sucking the thumb, and similar bad habits may be associated with bad formation of the teeth, the bones of the jaw and the muscles which control them.

The twenty baby teeth of infancy begin to disappear around the age of six, at which time also the four big six-year molars appear. Unless there is a full number of healthy teeth in the mouth at each age, they will not be properly arranged nor will they close properly. Each tooth depends on the one next to it for support. If any groups of teeth are pushed out of position, the whole set becomes irregular.

The orthodontist is a specialist in producing regularity of the teeth. Through gradual changes exercised at certain points the teeth are brought into proper position. This is done by the use of wire and of gold, and must be done slowly and carefully so as not to destroy the teeth in the process. It is a specialty within dentistry which concerns the ordinary care of the teeth. It is no longer necessary for any girl to appear in public after she has grown to mature age with teeth crossing over one another or with the protruding snaggle teeth that gave so many women a comical appearance in the past. Science in this way does much for human happiness.

The Care of Adults' Teeth

The care of the teeth in the adult involves not only a suitable diet, but also a certain amount of simple dental hygiene. The popular slogan that a clean tooth never decays is probably correct if associated with the right definition of a "clean tooth." It is equally true that millions of unclean teeth never decay. Of course, unclean teeth are not desirable, because they permit the growth of bacteria that are usually associated with foul breath, they are unesthetic in appearance, and they are associated with irritations of the gums, cheeks, and tongue that may be serious.

About 1890 it was shown that certain acids formed by the action of mouth bacteria on a substance containing sugar when held in contact with enamel of the teeth for a certain number of hours would cause the enamel to fall apart and open the way to destruction of the softer dentine substance beneath.

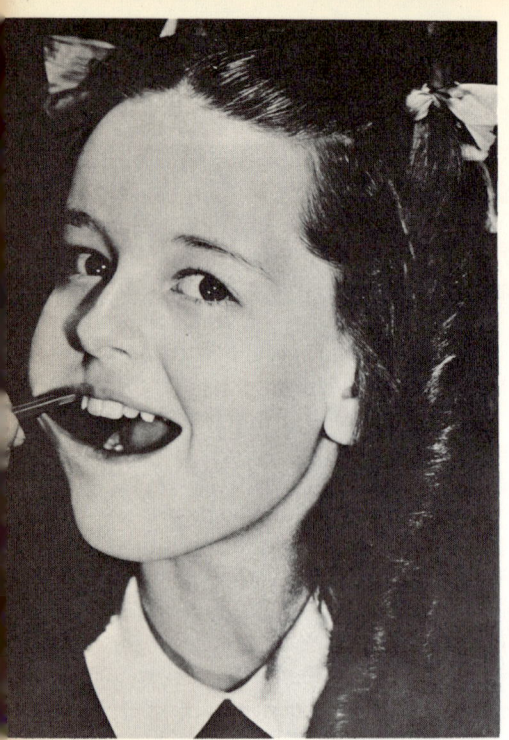
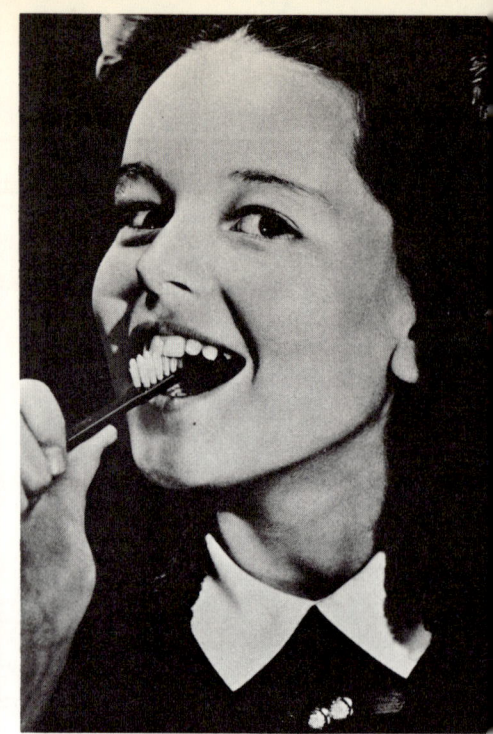
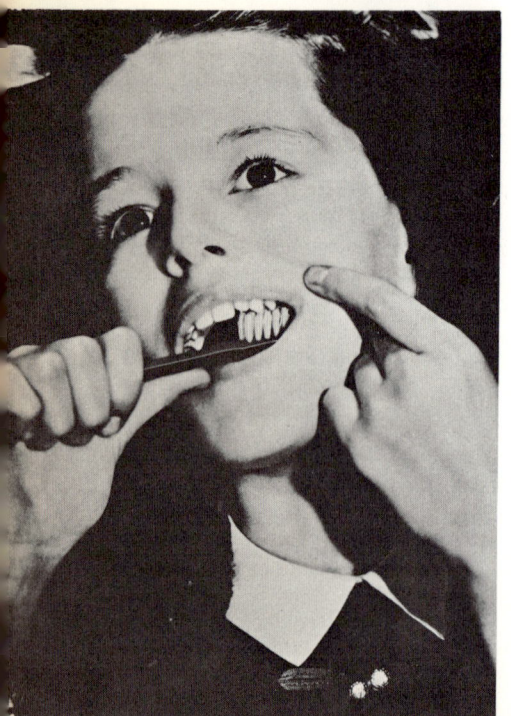

Series of photographs demonstrating the proper method of cleaning the teeth. Brushing up and down, rather than across from left to right, removes food particles more effectively. The backs of the teeth and the molars situated in the back part of the mouth should not be neglected.

American Medical Association

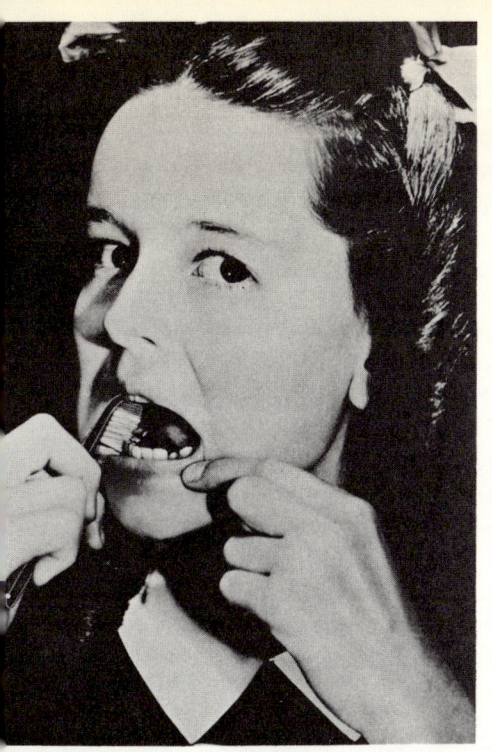
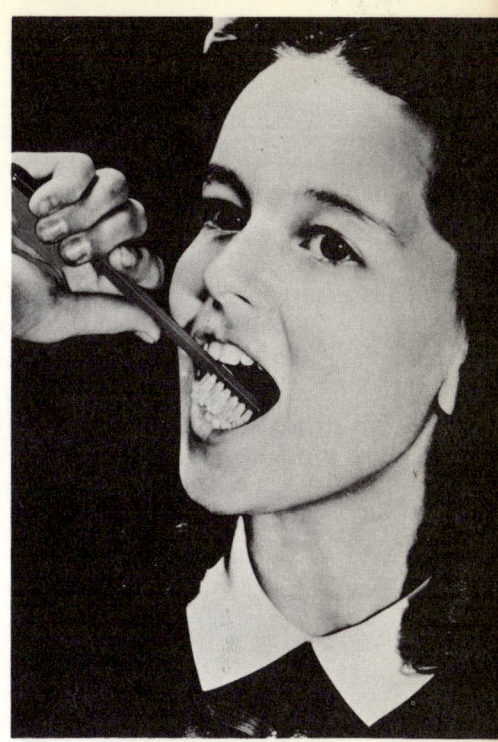
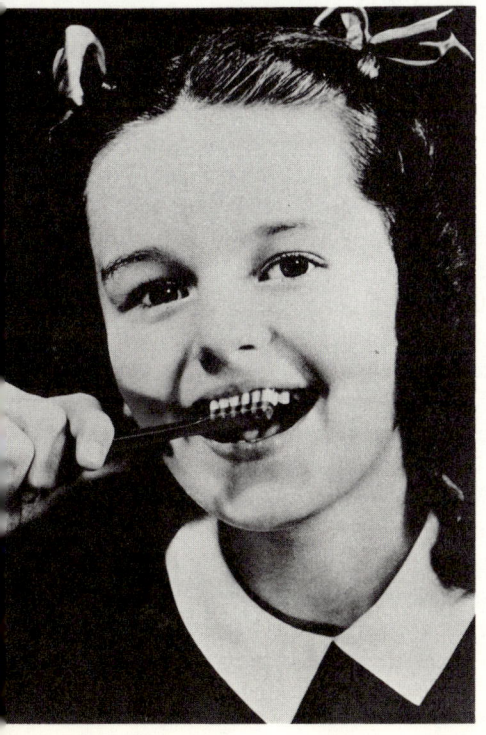
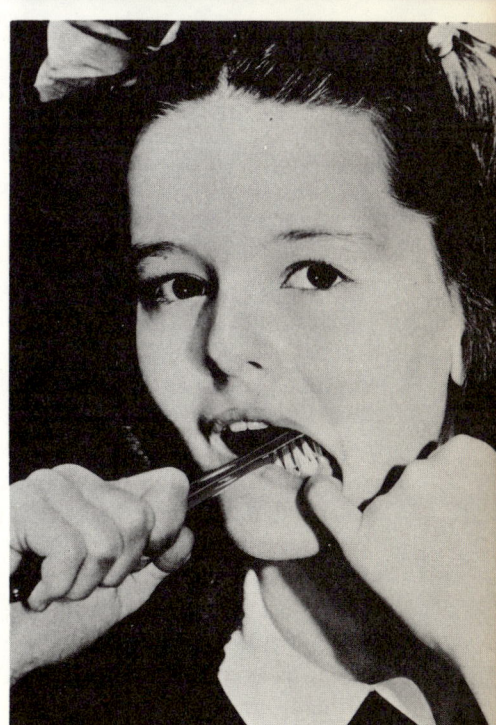

Since the acid must exist in concentrated form in order to do such work, the process usually goes on only in the tiny pits, fissures, or other defects in the enamel, or in the spaces between the teeth. The exposed surfaces of the teeth seldom decay because the natural movements of the lips, cheeks and tongue help to keep them clean.

Associated with the cause of tooth decay are errors in the diet. It is useless to take in large amounts of calcium unless the calcium is assimilated. Apparently phosphorus, the products of certain glands, ultraviolet rays, and the vitamins are involved in the use of calcium by the body and must be taken in the diet in order to permit the process to go on satisfactorily.

Once decay begins, once the enamel of the tooth is broken down, bacteria, constantly present in the mouth, aid the destruction. Chemical changes occur that are disastrous. The most that anyone can do is to keep teeth clean by the best methods possible, to overcome acids by the use of proper alkaline washes or pastes, and to see that the diet is of the proper nature to keep the teeth in a state cf satisfactory nutrition.

Tooth Decay

The University of Chicago summoned four experts who have been devoting themselves to research on teeth to discuss the problem of constant decay of the teeth which is a disease of our modern civilization. Apparently people who live in remote areas of the globe under native or natural conditions are more free from tooth decay and have fewer cavities than do civilized men. When these people come into contact with the civilization of the white man and adopt his manner of living and his diets, their teeth begin to decay immediately and apparently tooth decay progresses rapidly.

The United States now has a national institute of dental research which is under the direction of the United States Public Health Service. Dr. H. T. Dean who is director of this institute of dental research says that the acids of the mouth have a great deal to do with the amount of decay. However, modern medicine and dentistry have apparently failed to find any specific method of changing the reaction of the material around the surfaces of the teeth or of making the surfaces of the teeth more resistant to the actions of the acids. Several methods have been suggested, including various technics for getting rid of the bacteria in the mouth, but apparently none of these is yet well established. Dr. F. J. Orland who is assistant professor of dental surgery in the University of Chicago has made a special study of the bacteria of the mouth and he is convinced that the acids created by these bacteria can harm the enamel of the teeth.

Dr. Conrad A. Elvehjem of the University of Wisconsin, who is widely known as an authority in the field of diet, pointed out that the bacteria in the mouth break down sugars into acids and he believes it is the acid that causes the trouble. He says that a good diet will prevent dental decay.

Dr. J. R. Blayney, professor of dental surgery of the University of Chicago, said that the chief problem is the development of a technic that will check the decay of teeth, and that the three conditions necessary for decay include a susceptible tooth, foods in the mouth that are constantly present, and bacteria. The discussion proceeded along the lines of these three factors. No one knows now just why the teeth of some people seem to be much more susceptible to decay than are the teeth of others.

TOOTHBRUSH

In cleansing the mouth a good toothbrush is necessary. Most of the toothbrushes sold today are too large for efficient brushing. There are all sorts of shapes available with many strange distributions of bristles, but so far as is known it is impossible to make a toothbrush that will conform exactly to the shape of the dental arch inside and outside. Some toothbrushes are made with bristles higher in the center and low at the ends, some with the bristles high at one end and low at the other end, some with bristles lower in the middle and high at both ends.

This seems to make little difference, the only necessity being that the brush be small and that the handle be such that it can be manipulated so that the bristles will reach the front, back and sides of every tooth. The toothbrush demands proper care to give it long life and to prevent its acting as a carrier of infections rather than as a preventive.

When a toothbrush is split, when bristles begin to break off and come out, the toothbrush should be thrown away. A new toothbrush should be put in a strong salt cold-water solution for two hours before using. Cold water should be used to moisten the brush before using and to rinse it thoroughly after the teeth are brushed. The brush should then be hung in the open air in such position that the bristles will not come in contact with anything else for twenty-four hours before the brush is used again.

Obviously, therefore, persons should have two brushes, one for morning and one for evening use. If a toothbrush is kept moist for too long a period of time or kept in an airtight container, the bristles are quickly destroyed. Most important, however, is the fact that bacteria grow on warm, moist toothbrushes, and that the use of the brush before it has dried thoroughly will merely add new bacteria to those taken from the mouth in the previous washing.

TOOTHPASTES, MOUTH WASHES, AND TOOTH POWDERS

One of the most debatable questions in medicine and dentistry today concerns the exact value of toothpastes, mouth washes, tooth powders, and similar mixtures for the health of the mouth and the teeth. Many physicians and dentists are convinced that the most any toothpaste can do is to keep the teeth clean and polished, and that therefore any good soapy preparation that tastes well serves the purpose. However, the preparations that are available are complex in their formulas and extraordinary in their claims.

Some toothpastes are widely advertised because of their alkaline content, since it is urged that alkalis tend to counteract the tendency of the mouth to become acid. It has not, however, been proved that there is any serious tendency in this direction, nor that an opposite tendency is especially valuable.

Another preparation is sold with the argument that it duplicates normal saliva and that the presence of normal saliva prevents tooth decay. It has been argued that sugar helps to cause decay of the teeth and that food particles between the teeth increase dental caries. The disadvantage associated with food particles and sugar is that these provide mediums on which bacteria grow and that bacterial products are injurious to the teeth.

Some toothpastes are sold with the special claim that they kill the germs in the mouth on contact, but most physicians realize that the first mouthful of food or the first breath of air will bring new germs into the mouth. Some toothpastes contain abrasive substances which scratch the enamel, and this is bad, since anything that makes a scratch or an abrasion may produce a spot in which germs may enter more easily.

Another toothpaste is sold with the claim that it contains a substance which digests away food particles and mucus, and another is sold with the claim that it contains enough of certain antiseptic to sterilize the gums and keep them sterile. The important thing for the average person to remember is the fact that most of these preparations are kept in the mouth not longer than a few seconds and that any effects which they may accomplish are quite temporary.

Most recent additions to toothpastes are ammonia preparation for preventing decay and chlorophyll for preventing odors. The evidence in support of these additions is not generally convincing to most scientists.

Pyorrhea

Pyorrhea means a flow of matter. However, the flow of matter or, to speak of it scientifically—pus—is not the most significant thing about this disturbance of the mouth and teeth. The important fact is that the condition becomes chronic and that as a result of this the tissue of the gums separates from the roots of the teeth. When they have once separated they are not likely to become attached again. Moreover, a constant presence of infectious matter leads to secondary disturbances in the body which may be exceedingly serious.

The blood picks up the germs from the pus pockets around the teeth and carries them to other parts of the body, where they set up new infections. Because the teeth are loose and the mouth is foul, the person with pyorrhea is likely to lose his appetite. He is unable to chew food satisfactorily, his digestion is interfered with, and he becomes in general much sicker than he would be with a clean mouth cavity.

Because the mouth is easy to get at, because the gums are tough, and because the saliva keeps the mouth constantly lubricated, the tissues stand a great deal of punishment before the condition becomes so severe that it is impossible to delay attention. For this reason, pyorrhea is usually a chronic rather than an acute disease.

For this reason also it is necessary to remind people again and again that the mouth should be looked at by a competent dentist at least once in every six months in order that such conditions may be detected early and given adequate care before they become so serious that the only hope lies in removal of all of the teeth, surgical attention to the gums, and the provision of artificial plates.

Among the causes of infections of the gums are continuous irritation from the edge of rough crowns or of fillings. A good dentist will see to it that a crown or a filling is absolutely smooth and continuous with the surface of the tooth to which it is applied.

Food particles may accumulate between the teeth and set up spots of local irritation and decay. The regular use of the toothbrush and of dental floss is necessary to prevent such an occurrence. Toothpicks, and especially pins, knives, forks, or other objects used in lieu of toothpicks, do severe damage to the delicate tissues when manipulated by a careless hand.

Tartar deposits are just as irritant as rough fillings. Moreover, they are easily susceptible to the accumulation of bacteria. Pyorrhea is one of the most menacing diseases known to man, and its prevention depends on constant vigilance.

Fortunately, antibiotic drugs, applied locally to infected mouths and also taken internally, help to eliminate pyorrhea.

Halitosis or Bad Breath

Bad breath, now politely referred to as halitosis, is offensive. There is little excuse for anyone to permit himself to become obnoxious for this reason to everyone around him, since it is possible to prevent the presence of such odors. The most frequent cause is related to the teeth, which may be subject to cavi-

TEETH

article - THE CARE OF THE TEETH

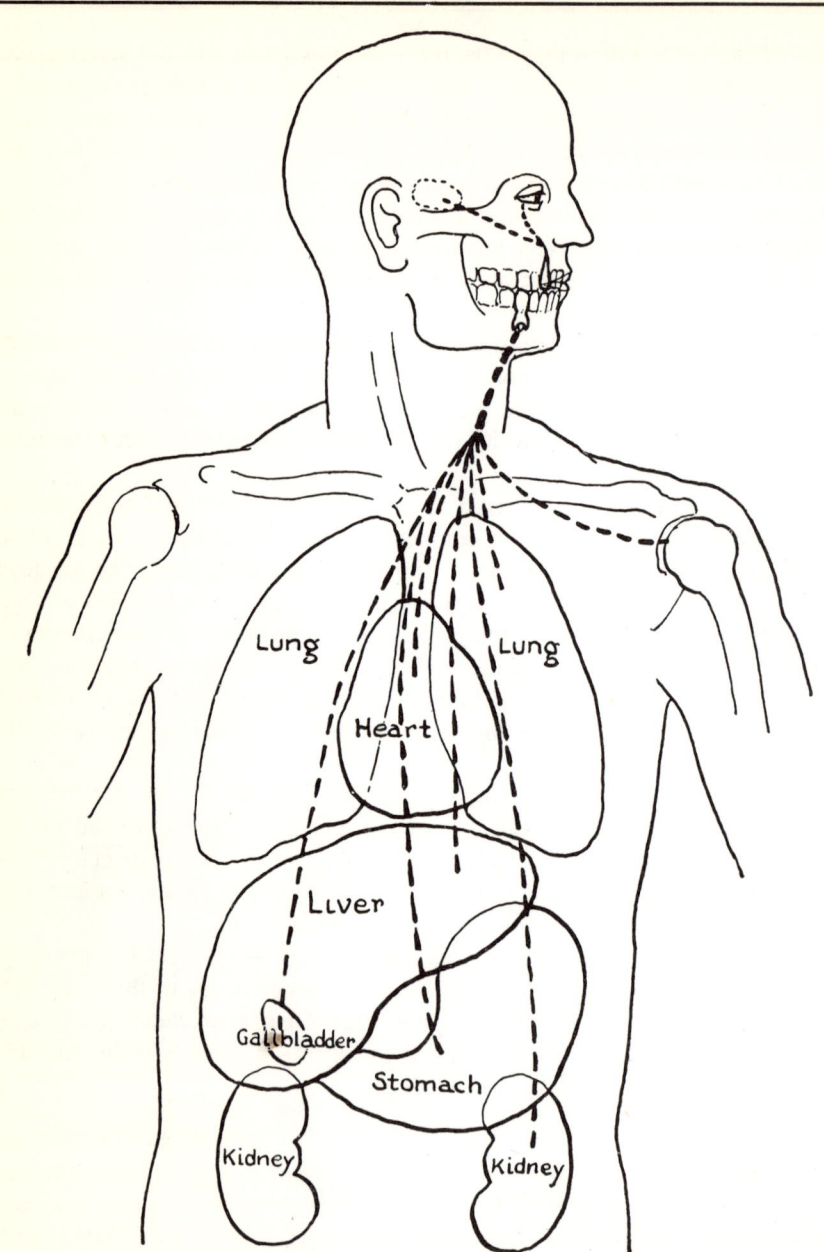

Effects of abscessed teeth.

ties or which may simply be surrounded with accumulations of decaying food products. Cavities should be filled and tartar deposits should be removed at least once every six months. The teeth may be kept clean by the use of dental floss and by the regular use morning and evening of a toothbrush with proper powder or paste. A high fat diet may be related to halitosis.

There are innumerable mouth washes containing antiseptics, alkalis, or acids, that may be used after the teeth have been brushed. Weak hydrogen peroxide solutions are sometimes of value. It is best to use strong solutions only on the advice of a competent physician or dentist.

After the teeth as the cause of bad breath have been eliminated, the tonsils must be examined as to the presence of infection. Another frequent cause of bad breath is infection in the nose or in the space behind the nose. The formation of crusts and of accumulations of infected material is bound to produce foul odor of the breath. Halitosis may also result from chronic disturbances of the stomach and of the intestines. If the tongue is constantly coated, if there is eructation of sour material from the stomach, the person concerned should consult a physician. Claims are now made that chlorophyll preparations control all sorts of body odors but the claims still need to be verified. Most recent evidence fails to support the claims for chlorophyll.

False Teeth

The person who is compelled to wear any form of removable appliance in the mouth to replace natural teeth has special problems to which dentists have been giving concern. False teeth, artificial teeth, removable bridges, and plates are included in this category.

The person who is going to lose his natural teeth by extraction because of infections or due to any other cause should have a thorough study by the use of the X-ray before any natural teeth are removed. The dentist who is going to make the artificial denture can then advise intelligently which teeth may be saved and which should be extracted. This is particularly important because he wants to restore the patient's natural appearance, and he wants to retain everything possible to permit the making of the most suitable denture.

To do this, he takes impressions of the mouth, makes a record of the patient's profile and facial contour, studies the natural color of the teeth and similar factors. It is sometimes possible in making an artificial denture to correct deformities or abnormalities of the lower portion of the face. When a person is fitted with an artificial denture his experience is similar to being fitted with a suit or a dress. It may not be exactly right the first time, and some adjustments may be necessary.

When the work is completed the patient should not assume that it is permanent. The human body is a growing and changing organism which differs from year to year. This means that dentures should be studied from time to time if they become uncomfortable so that old ones may be refitted or new ones substituted. If this is not done there actually may be changes in the appearance of the face, deep lines and wrinkles being associated in some instances with the constant wearing of unsuitable dentures.

Artificial plates and teeth must be given even more care than natural teeth. They should be brushed carefully and thoroughly after each meal and on going to bed at night. In this cleaning, cold or lukewarm water should be used—never hot water. It is just as important to be careful about handling dentures as handling expensive eyeglasses. The dentists suggest that when removing the dentures from the mouth the wearer should lean over a washbowl filled two-thirds full of water and hold the plates close to the water when brushing them. Then the water will break the fall if he happens to drop the artificial plate.

It is not advisable to try to crack nuts with artificial teeth. Biting threads, eating hard candy, and chewing on bones are sometimes responsible for ruining expensive dentures.

Just as soon as the teeth are secured, the person will do well to go into a private place and practice reading aloud in order to get used to the feel of the teeth and to their weaknesses. When the false teeth are first inserted, the facial expression may seem to be changed, but this is due to the effort of the muscles to take care of the plates. Just as soon as the false teeth become properly adjusted, the effort will disappear, and the expression will become natural again.

Naturally, the hardest thing to do with the false teeth is to eat. The person who has the teeth thinks that he has to manipulate both the teeth and the food. He will, therefore, do well to begin with food that requires little chewing and to avoid steaks and chops for the first few days. Small bits of food chewed slowly will easily be taken care of. Big masses of food may cause trouble. Until one learns to manipulate the teeth, and until the gums and the ridges have become hardened, one need not expect to eat everything and anything that is offered. If there are spots in the gums and the ridges have become excessively sore, the dentist should be consulted immediately to make the necessary changes and to prescribe the necessary treatment.

Artificial teeth, when out of the mouth, should be kept moist. The best arrangement is to put them in a salt solution, boric acid, or some favorite mouth wash.

TEMPERATURE AND INFECTION (See also, *Fever*) FEVER—By far the vast majority of instances of fever result from infection. There are, however, cases in which fever occurs and in which the exact cause cannot be easily determined. Certain principles have been established by years of experience for the handling of fever.

Rest in bed is the number one step for any person with fever. Under such conditions the work of the heart, kidneys, and liver is reduced. The sense of fatigue is lessened. The blood flow to the kidneys and liver tends to be better in the lying-down than in the standing position. The disadvantages of bed rest include less stimulation to breathing, a sluggish blood flow in the legs, and a noticeable diminution in muscular strength. Bed rest should always be used in association with a certain amount of activity suited to the condition of the person concerned. This may involve simply encouraging him to move, turn and sit up in bed, but might include controlled exercise or even moving of the patient's limbs by the attendant nurse or member of the family. In the nursing of those with fevers, special attention must be given to getting plenty of fluids.

The fever patient usually loses appetite and needs to be encouraged to eat, and if necessary, must be fed by the nurse. Dryness of the mouth can be helped by the use of suitable mouth washes or the nurse can cleanse the mouth by a piece of gauze wrapped around the finger. Profuse sweating may make necessary frequent changes of bedding and night clothes. The patient's skin must be protected against the formation of ulcers. If the sheets are kept dry and free from wrinkles, if alcohol rubs are used and if a suitable powder is applied, the skin is helped greatly. For dry skin baby oil is preferable to any other system of softening. Movement of the joints by the nurse is helpful against stiffening.

People whose temperature gets above 102 degrees need at least three quarts of water a day. If there is vomiting and diarrhea, the amount must be increased

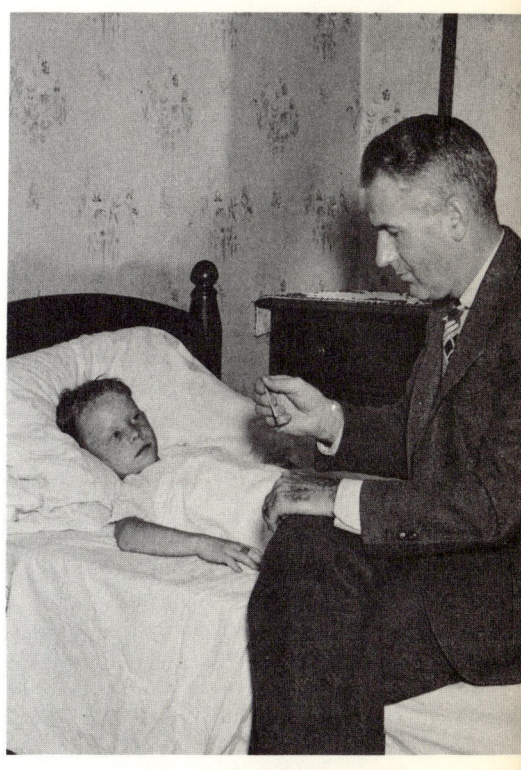

The normal body temperature is about 98.6 degrees Fahrenheit. When there is some disturbance or infection in the body the temperature rises. In some illnesses the temperature may be raised only slightly, but in severe infections it may move up to or even above 104 degrees.

Hygeia

by the amount of fluid lost in this way. If patients resist the taking of plain water, they can have fruit juice or vegetable juice, carbonated sweet beverages, milk, soups and similar fluid drinks.

The bowels become less active when there is fever and a person remains long in bed. The choice of a proper technic for getting rid of the waste material from the body is up to the doctor who understands the condition and the nature of the disturbance. He will have to prescribe the cathartic that is to be taken, whether something as strong as the salts or something like mineral oil or other lubricants or perhaps even a soapsuds or water-and-glycerine enema.

The doctor can always prescribe drugs which are known to be valuable in bringing down serious fevers. He can also prescribe sponges with alcohol or tepid water which do a great deal towards controlling temperature through aiding irradiation of heat from the surface of the body. Cold compresses and ice bags are other types of cooling.

THE ATTACK ON INFECTION—Only a few decades have passed since physicians confronted with cases of many serious infections could only apply a sort of general treatment. This involved putting the patient to bed, stimulating the action of the bowel and kidneys, aiding the action of the heart and controlling the fever with drugs that have a tendency to reduce fevers. Medicine has had for only a few years powerful remedies called chemotherapeutic remedies or antibiotic drugs which definitely control the growth of germs or viruses or other organisms in the human body.

The use of drugs to suppress the growth of organisms that damage the human body is one of the greatest accomplishments of modern medicine. Naturally the drugs must be able to stop the growth of the foreign invader without injuring the sick person. The new drugs attack germs in various ways. Quinine is a fine example of the way in which a drug can attack a single organism since it is practically a pure specific against the plasmodia which cause malaria. Some of the new antibiotic drugs can attack a great number of different germs of many different species. Some chemical substances damage certain cells of the human body and may interfere with their growth. Out of this fact may come eventually some new and effective treatment for cancer.

The sulfonamide drugs and the antibiotics act by interfering with the ways in which the germs themselves live. In deciding which drug to use the doctor must know its effect on the patient. For instance some patients do not react well to penicillin. In other instances the patient's germs have become accustomed to penicillin. Fortunately we now have streptomycin, chloromycetin, aureomycin, terramycin and other antibiotics, for each of which there is a long list of germs which it is capable of attacking successfully. Sometimes the medicine attaches itself to the tissues of the body and the germs cannot attack while the medicine is there. Sometimes the medicine relates itself to the way in which the germ feeds and grows.

The doctor chooses the remedy according to the dose he wants to give, the frequency with which the dose is to be given, whether or not the remedy can be taken by mouth or must be given by injection, whether it needs to be given by injection into the blood, into the muscles or under the skin or for a number of other reasons.

TEMPERATURE, BODY The ordinary fever thermometer has a red arrow at 98.6 degrees Fahrenheit, which is supposed to be the normal body temperature.

The human being is built with a thermostat device that controls his temperature. He is kept at the normal temperature by a regulating device in the body which gets rid of excess heat or produces extra heat if it is needed. When we perspire, water evaporates from the skin, and the temperature of the body is lowered. When we shiver or move our muscles, heat is produced and the temperature of the body is raised.

The sensation of heat or cold is not due to a change in the temperature of the body but to a change in the temperature of the skin. When the skin feels cold, a message is sent to the brain; the brain turns loose the mechanisms that

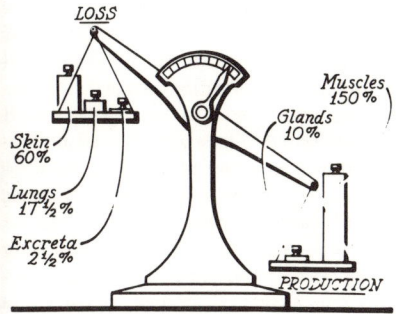

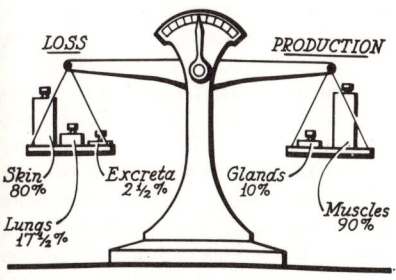

When the body's chemistry operates normally, the heat produced by muscles and by glands is lost by way of the skin, the lungs, and the excreta. When there is fever, the loss is unable to keep up with the production.

arrange for the temperature to be raised or lowered as needed. In the brain there is a little mechanism that works just like the thermometer that turns the oil heater on and off in your home. About four o'clock in the morning your body temperature as recorded by a thermometer in the mouth is likely to be 97.3 degrees Fahrenheit. About four o'clock in the afternoon it will probably be recorded as 99.1 degrees Fahrenheit.

If you are sick with a fever, the temperature may move up to 104 degrees or even higher. In severe infections at the time of death the fever may reach as high as 107 to 109 degrees. The average fever thermometer has a top of around 110 degrees. Above that temperature human beings usually die. Above 110 degrees conditions occur which affect the cells of the body generally and which are incompatible with life.

Cases are recorded of people who died of heat stroke and who had temperatures over 110 degrees. In one group of 14 cases 6 died and the remainder recovered.

When people report temperatures over 110 degrees lasting beyond a momentary or brief rise, it may be taken for granted that somebody is malingering or manipulating the thermometer.

Repeatedly it has been said that chilling of the human body is bad for health. Some people are much more susceptible to chilling than others. In general it is believed that chilling is more serious for a person with chronic infections of the nose and throat than for a person who is in excellent health. Some people are so sensitive to chilling that they suffer even after having a haircut, after washing the hair, from the coolness of the evening air or any other chilling process. Their response to the chilling is congestion in the nose and sinuses, and the appearance of a condition like a cold. Investigations have shown that people can be especially sensitive to either heat or cold and respond with symptoms of the type described.

TEMPERATURE, BODY—infants: See INFANCY, article CARE AND FEEDING OF THE CHILD.

TEMPERATURE, BODY—normal: See INFECTIOUS DISEASE, article THE PREVENTION AND TREATMENT OF INFECTIOUS DISEASE.

TEMPERATURE, BODY—rectal method more reliable in children: See HEART, article DISEASES OF THE HEART AND CIRCULATION.

TEMPERATURE, BODY—response to germs: See INFECTIOUS DISEASE, article THE PREVENTION AND TREATMENT OF INFECTIOUS DISEASE.

TEMPERATURE, BODY—resistance to disease decreased by temperature changes: See INFECTIOUS DISEASE, article THE PREVENTION AND TREATMENT OF INFECTIOUS DISEASE.

TENIA (See discussion under *Worms*) Tapeworm.

TENNIS HEEL (See also discussion under *Feet*) A person with "tennis heel" has a tender spot under one heel toward the front and middle of the pad of the heel. He feels pain when walking or standing. The most common cause of "tennis heel" is repeating bruising while walking on a hard surface with light footwear. The condition is relieved by using sponge rubber in the heel of the shoe, by building up the heel of the shoe, or by strapping the foot with adhesive to take weight off the heel. Taking of cortisone has also been effective.

TESTICLES See discussion under *Orchitis*.

TETANUS People used to think that tetanus or lockjaw was caused by scratching oneself with a rusty nail. This belief still prevails among many people, although the germ that causes lockjaw was isolated in 1886. The disease was known more than two thousand years ago and was described by Hippocrates.

The poison that is produced by the germ of tetanus is one of the most powerful poisons known. When the germ gets into the body, it sets up inflammation of nerve tissues. These germs have a special predilection for nerves. Some types of wounds are, therefore, more likely to be associated with tetanus than others. Most important are deep, penetrating, lacerating or crushing wounds which contain particles of foreign material. The soil of many areas contains the tetanus germ. The germs of tetanus seem to live preferably in the intestinal tract of cattle, horses, and man. In this way soil is contaminated. The germs live much better in the absence of oxygen; in deep wounds, therefore, they multiply more rapidly than in shallow wounds.

Tetanus begins about seven days after a wound which permits the germs to get into the tissues. The first signs are a sense of drawing pain in the wound with a twitching of muscles near by. Also there is irritability, headache, chills, and fever. Then comes the stiffness of the muscles of the jaw and neck which gives this disease its name. Serious spasms and convulsions ensue. In some cases there may be from three to forty spasms in an hour. All of the muscles of the body may be involved, including those of the bowels and of the bladder.

Even with the best of treatment patients with lockjaw may die because of the poisonous nature of the secretions of this organism. Fortunately medicine now has a preventive of tetanus so efficient that we are able to say that there was not one death from tetanus in the armed forces in World War II.

For the prevention of tetanus people who have been wounded, particularly when the wound is contaminated, should receive immediately an injection under the skin of the specific antitoxin against tetanus. Another injection may be given one week later. The physician who treats the case will open the wound widely, remove any clothing, soil, or other visible contamination that may be present, and treat the wound with appropriate antiseptic substances. Under the best of treatment it is possible to save the lives of one half to two thirds of the people who are infected.

TETANUS—See article TRANSMISSIBLE DISEASES.

TETANUS—cause determined: See INFECTIOUS DISEASE, article THE PREVENTION AND TREATMENT OF INFECTIOUS DISEASE.

TETANUS—contaminated nail: See article OCCUPATION AND HEALTH.

TETANUS—deaths: See article TRANSMISSIBLE DISEASES.

TETANUS—from fireworks: See article FIRST AID.

TETANUS—incubation period: See article TRANSMISSIBLE DISEASES.

TETANUS—nervous system: See INFECTIOUS DISEASE, article THE PREVENTION AND TREATMENT OF INFECTIOUS DISEASE.

TETANUS—prevention: See article TRANSMISSIBLE DISEASES.

TETANUS—skin reaction: See SKIN, article THE SKIN.

TETANUS—transmissible disease: See article TRANSMISSIBLE DISEASES.

TETANUS—treatment: See INFECTIOUS DISEASE, article THE PREVENTION AND TREATMENT OF INFECTIOUS DISEASE; article TRANSMISSIBLE DISEASES.

TETANUS—vaccination: See article ALLERGY.

THERMOMETER The thermometer is used in medicine to ascertain the temperature of the human body. The temperature is usually reported in terms of Fahrenheit, which makes the normal temperature 98.6 degrees when taken with the thermometer in the mouth, a degree higher when the temperature is taken inside the rectum, and a degree lower when the temperature is taken under the arm. Temperatures are also sometimes reported in centigrade according to the decimal system. In the decimal system 37 degrees corresponds to 98.6 degrees Fahrenheit as a normal temperature. A good thermometer registers the temperature in two or three minutes. Even if the thermometer is marked one minute, it is well to leave

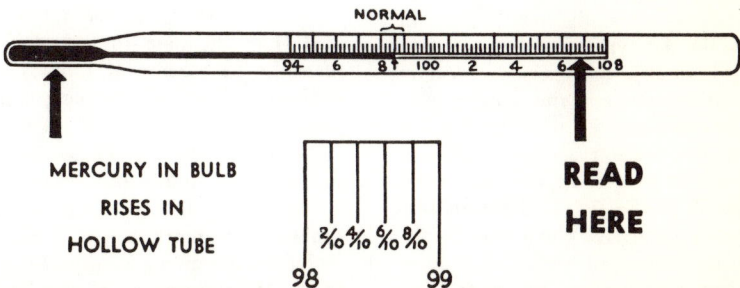

The normal range of temperature is between 98 and 99 degrees Fahrenheit. To read, look along the sharper edge between the numbers and the lines.

it in place two or three minutes for an accurate recording.

THERMOMETER—how to read (fig.): See RESPIRATORY DISEASES, article THE RESPIRATORY DISEASES.

THERMOMETER in medicine chest: See MEDICINE CHEST, article THE FAMILY MEDICINE CHEST.

THIAMIN DEFICIENCY (See also, (*Vitamin*s) The chief symptoms of a disease called beriberi are due to a lack of one of the portions of the Vitamin B complex called thiamin. Thiamin is soluble in water, damaged by heat and found chiefly in whole cereals, peas, beans, lean meats, nuts and yeast. Refined sugar, milled rice and low extraction flour have lost most of their thiamin.

People whose diets are low in protein and high in carbohydrates are likely to show symptoms of thiamin deficiency. In the United States the condition is seen often among chronic alcoholics who get insufficient amounts of the right foods because of their displacement by alcohol.

The chief damages to tissues of the body seen in thiamin deficiency are found in the nerves and in the heart and blood vessels. Often these tissues become swollen with water. After about three months on a diet really deficient in thiamin the symptoms begin to appear. Gradually the person becomes tired and irritable and the muscles, particularly those of the calf of the leg become painful. Later serious inflammations of the nerves appear and these may go on to the point of loss of sensation and paralysis. When neuritis becomes so prominent the doctor must make sure that it does not result from some other cause since lead or arsenic poisoning or various infections may also cause neuritis.

As soon as a sufficient intake of thiamin is assured the patient begins to improve. Thiamin is now available in the form of tablets or capsules that can be taken internally and also in forms that can be injected into the body when prompt action is desired. If treatment is begun sufficiently early most patients recover rapidly and completely. If treatment is delayed until actual destruction of nerve tissue has occurred, results are doubtful.

THROAT There are general inflammations of the throat associated with redness, swelling, and excessive discharge of mucus due to many different causes. Most common, of course, is exposure to cold, an extension of inflammation from the tonsils, the adenoids, or the nose.

Excessive use of tobacco, excessive exposure to dust, smoke, irritating fumes, and sudden changes in temperature, excessive dryness, and similar atmospheric conditions may cause irritation of the throat.

People who are sensitive to certain food substances sometimes react with blisters on the tissues of the throat, which become secondarily infected and produce irritations and inflammation.

There may be severe pain associated with swelling and inflammation of the throat, including pain in the ears because of blocking of the tubes which lead from the nose to the ears; there may also be a sense of fullness or obstruction, with much hawking and spitting.

The first thing to know about any inflammation of the throat is its cause. If the condition happens to be due to diphtheria, prompt action is necessary, including the giving of diphtheria antitoxin. If, however, it is due to some other type of germ, other methods of treatment are employed.

The pain of an inflamed throat is best relieved by use of an ice bag filled with cracked ice. Most doctors are now convinced that gargles seldom go deep enough in the throat in sufficient quantity or strength to permit them to have much effect in killing germs or in curing disease.

To have a definite effect from any antiseptic in the throat, it is necessary to apply it directly to the infected or inflamed part. This is best done by spreading material with a cotton swab or by using an atomizer properly. In order to get the antiseptic into the back of the throat, it may be necessary to hold the tongue or to use a tongue depressor.

The primary purpose of a mouth wash or throat wash is to clean and soothe. A good cleansing mouth wash is merely salt solution made by adding a fourth of a teaspoon of salt to a half glass of warm water. If there is much mucus, the addition of a quarter of a teaspoon of bicarbonate of soda or ordinary baking soda may be beneficial.

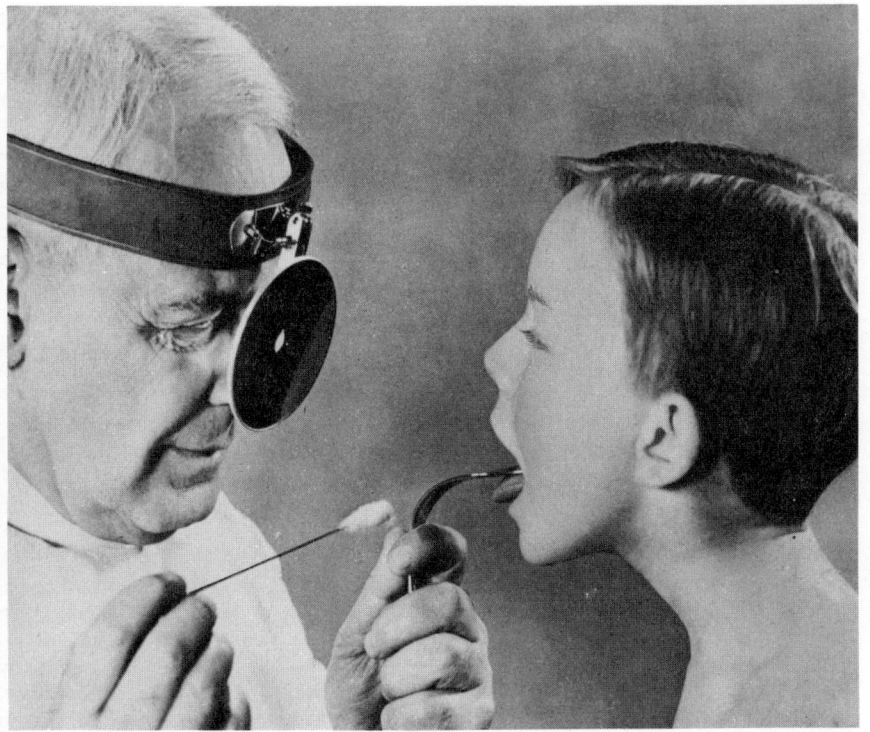

Inspection of the throat is an important part of physical examination. Changes in the throat or a sore throat may be symptoms of infection or a disease in another part of the body. To treat an infected area in the back of the throat the doctor uses a tongue depressor and applicator.

THROMBO-ANGIITIS OBLITERANS See *Buerger's Disease*.

SORE THROAT—See EAR, article THE EAR, TONGUE, NOSE, AND THROAT.

SORE THROAT—beginning of diphtheria: See CHILDHOOD DISEASES, article INFECTIOUS DISEASES OF CHILDHOOD.

SORE THROAT—beginning of infectious disease: See INFECTIOUS DISEASE, article THE PREVENTION AND TREATMENT OF INFECTIOUS DISEASE.

SORE THROAT—chicken pox: See CHILDHOOD DISEASES, article INFECTIOUS DISEASES OF CHILDHOOD.

SORE THROAT—gall bladder may be affected: See article DIGESTION AND DIGESTIVE DISEASES.

SORE THROAT—scarlet fever: See CHILDHOOD DISEASES, article INFECTIOUS DISEASES OF CHILDHOOD.

THROAT—See EAR, article THE EAR, TONGUE, NOSE, AND THROAT.

THROAT—foreign bodies, first aid: See article FIRST AID.

THROAT—infections: See INFECTIOUS DISEASE, article THE PREVENTION AND TREATMENT OF INFECTIOUS DISEASE; and entry COLDS.

THROMBOCYTOPENIA (See also discussion under *Atomic Energy, Granulocytopenia, Luekocytes, Surgery* and *Spleen Removal, Quinidine*) People who bruise and bleed easily and who develop purple spots on the skin are often suffering with a condition called idiopathic thrombocytopenic purpura. This means that there is a deficiency of blood platelets in the blood and that the cause is not known. The condition may develop as a result of an infection or after the taking of various drugs. These drugs however affect only few people in this way. The condition they cause usually disappears a few months after the drug is discontinued.

Chronic cases of this condition persist with ups and downs over the years. A new theory is that a chronic case is a result of a change in the person's blood in which the blood develops a substance which attacks its own platelets. This view has been confirmed by recent experiments which involved injection of the blood from a person who had the disease into a normal person. Such an injection made the number of blood platelets in the normal person decrease. The injection of normal platelets into people with thrombocytopenic purpura resulted in destruction of the normal blood platelets. Quite recently, ACTH and cortisone have been used in some of these cases with remarkably successful results. In fact the proper diagnosis of the condition and control treatment of this condition with ACTH and cortisone has been so successful that the operation which involved removal of the spleen as a life-saving measure in such cases has come into greatly diminished use. The emergency operation for removal of the spleen is now done in only the most severe cases which do not react favorably to the use of either ACTH or cortisone or both.

THROMBOPHLEBITIS See discussion under *Phlebitis*.

THROMBOSIS The formation of a clot in a blood vessel is called thrombosis. Clots form in all sorts of places and the thrombosis may be described in relationship to the place where it is formed. In various types of inflammation of the blood vessels, thrombi may form. When a portion of the thrombus breaks away and floats in the blood stream, the condition is called embolism.

THROMBI—kidneys: See KIDNEY, article THE KIDNEY: ITS DISEASES AND DISTURBANCES.

THROMBOSIS, CORONARY—diabetes: See article DIABETES.

THROMBOSIS, CORONARY—hypotension following: See article BLOOD PRESSURE.

THROMBOSIS, CORONARY—resulting from hardening of coronary arteries: See article BLOOD PRESSURE.

THRUSH Children become infected by various fungi which attack the tissues of the mouth. This condition is called thrush.

THRUSH—in infants: See INFANCY, article CARE AND FEEDING OF THE CHILD.

THYMUS GLAND The thymus gland lies in the chest in front of the windpipe, between the lungs and above the heart. Its nature is not yet fully understood.

During the first period of growth the thymus gland and a small gland in the brain called the pineal gland are greatly concerned. The thymus gland is large during the first eight or nine months of life, after which it gradually gets smaller and finally disappears. If it fails to get smaller and continues to send its secretion in large amounts into the body, changes may occur that are serious for life and health. If, however, the thymus gland fails to act during the early years of life, the results are also serious.

If the gland becomes quite large, its situation is such that it may cause difficulty in breathing and in the circulation of the blood in infants. In the condition called status lymphaticus sudden death sometimes occurs, apparently due to the enlargement of the thymus gland. If a physician finds the condition of enlargement on examination, he may wish to expose the gland to the X ray and in that way bring about a reduction in its size.

If the thymus gland continues to secrete beyond the time when it should have stopped, the skin of the person concerned becomes soft, smooth, and velvety. In fact the skin develops a "peaches and cream" complexion. When a boy with this condition becomes a man, he may find that it is unnecessary for him to shave or perhaps he will have to shave only once a week. Persons with persistent thymus glands appear younger than they are; the hair over the body is scanty, and the teeth rather a bluish-white in color. Moreover, they may have a low blood pressure and be easily fatigued.

If, however, the thymus gland discontinues to function too soon, the person concerned seems to grow old a little too soon. Such people are short in stature, the body hair develops early and is thick, and the blood pressure is usually too high.

Recently investigators have been injecting animals with thymus extract. They find that there is marked precocity in the offspring of the animals in the second generation. In the second generation the young animals show increased growth and development. The young of the third generation also grow and develop physically, sexually, and psychically at an unbelievable rate. They do not, however, become giants because the rapid rate of growth decreases from the second month on.

Some investigators believe that the thymus may control to some extent the mental make-up as well, namely, that those in whom thymus action persists remain childlike, self-centered, and simple in their mental processes and initiative, whereas those in whom the thymus disappears too soon become easily aroused to anger and are resentful. While they seem quite advanced when young, they never seem to mature completely.

It should be emphasized that work on the thymus gland is still in an exceedingly early experimental stage. The thymus gland seems to influence to some extent the growth of the skeleton. It

THYROID

seems to be concerned with calcium utilization by the body and also with the development of the sex glands.

THYMUS GLAND—See article ENDOCRINOLOGY.

THYMUS GLAND—location (fig.): See article ENDOCRINOLOGY.

THYROID (See also *Goiter*) The gland in the throat in front of the windpipe which secretes an internal secretion called thyroxin. Simple enlargement of the thyroid is goiter; excessive action is hyperthyroidism, also called Basedow's disease, Graves' disease, or exophthalmic goiter.

THYROID GLAND—See articles ENDOCRINOLOGY; BLOOD PRESSURE.

THYROID GLAND—adolescent girl's should have attention: See WOMEN, article HYGIENE OF WOMEN.

THYROID GLAND—age affects: See article OLD AGE.

THYROID GLAND—basal metabolism test to check function: See article ENDOCRINOLOGY.

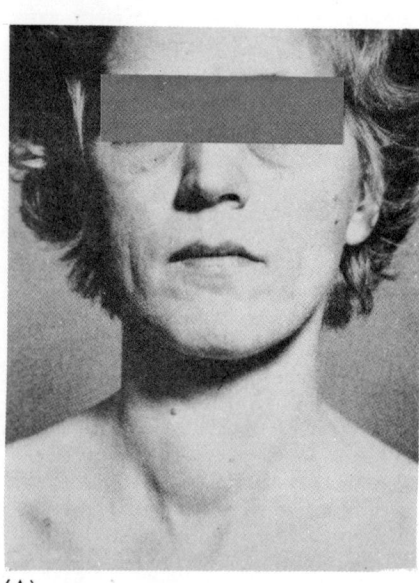

(A)

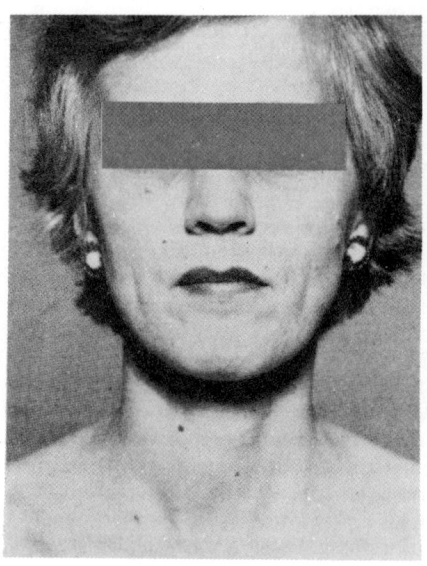

(B)

(A) Moderate enlargement of the thyroid gland caused by a noninfectious disease. This type of inflammation affects men much less frequently than women. The gland enlarges gradually and one area may be more prominent than another.

(B) Photograph taken two months later, showing regression of the enlargement. Patient was treated with desiccated thyroid, a substance made from the thyroid of sheep. Desiccated thyroid is used to cure certain thyroid conditions affecting human beings.

Postgraduate Medicine

THYROID GLAND—diabetes affected by: See article DIABETES.

THYROID GLAND—enlarged: See WOMEN, article HYGIENE OF WOMEN; article ENDOCRINOLOGY.

THYROID GLAND—function increased during pregnancy: See BIRTH, article CARE OF MOTHERS BEFORE AND AFTER CHILDBIRTH.

THYROID GLAND—goiter is enlargement: See article ENDOCRINOLOGY.

THYROID GLAND—hair growth: See HAIR, article THE HAIR.

THYROID GLAND—hormones made artificially: See article ENDOCRINOLOGY.

THYROID GLAND—iodine deficiency leads to enlargement: See DIET, article ADVICE ON THE DIET.

THYROID GLAND—location (fig.): See article ENDOCRINOLOGY.

THYROID GLAND—nail brittleness caused by deficiency: See HAIR, article THE HAIR.

THYROID GLAND—pituitary stimulates: See article ENDOCRINOLOGY.

THYROID GLAND—skin affected by: See SKIN, article THE SKIN.

THYROID GLAND—toxic: See HEART, article DISEASES OF THE HEART AND CIRCULATION.

THYROID AND THE HEART (See also discussion under *Goiter*) Of all the glandular functions that may disturb the heart, overactivity of the thyroid is most important since it speeds up the heart and may result in enlargement and eventually even in heart failure. Fortunately, the condition is now readily determinable by the use of various devices. The activity of the thyroid is measurable by the old basal metabolism test and by the use of radioactive iodine. When the excessive action of the thyroid is recognized, there are drugs which can control the action including the administration of radioactive iodine and also the possibility of surgical removal of portions of the thyroid gland to lessen its activity. When the gland is removed, in case thyroid function is deficient, it may be compensated by the giving of thyroid extract. Thus the evil effects of excessive thyroid are controlled.

TIC Any spasmodic movement or twitching, particularly of the face, is called a tic. People can develop tics as a habit, under which circumstances they are called habit spasms. Most serious of all tics is an actual neuralgia involving the facial nerves called tic douloureux. This condition is treated usually with certain drugs which are known to have an effect in many cases. Occasionally, however, all drug treatments fail, so that the condition has to be treated by injection of a substance that will paralyze the nerve or by surgical operation on the nerve or the ganglion cell.

"**TIN EARS**" (See also, *Ear*) One of the most common forms of injury to the external ear is the development of what the pugilist calls a "tin ear." Repeated pounding on the ear results in the pouring out of blood into the tissues of the ear and surrounding areas. At first such swellings are bluish-red; they feel to the touch like dough. In the worst cases surgeons open the tissue and remove the clot of blood to prevent permanent thickening and swelling. They also apply special bandages to mold the ear and hold it in shape while repair is taking place.

TOBACCO Today the American people spend more for tobacco than for education, religion, or health. The smoking of tobacco is a social habit which has become so firmly established in the American system of living that it represents a fixed charge on the expenditures of every family. The consumption of tobacco has gradually risen as our habits have changed.

Since 1905 the public taste has shifted largely from cigars to cigarettes. The consumption of large cigars dropped from 8,500,000,000 in 1920 to 5,500,000,000 in 1952. In the same period of time the consumption of cigarettes increased from 50,409,000,000 to over 400,000,000,000 cigarettes.

During this period of time doctors and psychologists have been seriously concerned with the study of the effects of tobacco consumption on the nation's health and welfare. The psychologists particularly have been concerned with the question as to why people smoke. A serious scientific questionnaire showed that sociability, relaxation, and steadying of the nerves are among the most significant of the reasons given. Less significant were the effects of smoking on hunger and the pleasures associated with the sight of the smoke, the feel of the cigarette, and the social charm associated with the habit.

From the point of view of the effects of tobacco on the body, the smoking of nicotine affects the nervous system and the blood vessels. Most serious of the effects of tobacco are its effects on the circulation of the blood. Thus the smoking of tobacco is definitely related to the increase in the condition called Buerger's disease or thrombo-angiitis obliterans. Especially important is the possible relationship of excessive cigarette smoking to cancer of the lung.

Secondary effects on the digestion and on the throat and lungs have also been established. These vary, however, in different people, depending on the amount of tobacco smoking that is done. Among the symptoms credited to excess smoking are irregular neuralgias, vague gastrointestinal discomfort, headache, insomnia, disturbances of the bowels, palpitation of the heart, and diseases of the circulation of the blood.

However, the records of thousands of persons who have smoked considerably over long periods of time indicate that, on the whole, the habit of smoking is not nearly so harmful as the sound of this list of symptoms would indicate. There is a tendency for the individual smoker to establish a certain amount of tolerance to the use of tobacco.

TOBACCO—adolescents: See WOMEN, article HYGIENE OF WOMEN; article SEX HYGIENE.

TOBACCO—cancer: See articles CANCER; OLD AGE.

TOBACCO—gastritis: See article DIGESTION AND DIGESTIVE DISEASES.

TOBACCO—hypertension: See article BLOOD PRESSURE.

TOBACCO—leukoplakia: See article CANCER.

TOBACCO—lung cancer: See article CANCER.

TOBACCO—occupational hazard: See article OCCUPATION AND HEALTH.

TOBACCO—poisoning: See article FIRST AID.

TOBACCO—pregnancy: See BIRTH, article CARE OF MOTHERS BEFORE AND AFTER CHILDBIRTH.

TOBACCO—syphilitics should not use: See VENEREAL DISEASES, article THE VENEREAL DISEASES.

TOBACCO—tuberculosis: See article OCCUPATION AND HEALTH.

TOBACCO—ulcers: See article DIGESTION AND DIGESTIVE DISEASES.

TOBACCO—Vincent's angina: See article TRANSMISSIBLE DISEASES.

TONGUE Doctors of a previous generation always looked first at the patient's tongue. A tongue that is dry, dark, and furred indicates disease. A tongue that is moist and clean reflects a normal condition.

A healthy tongue can be moved quickly or slowly in all directions. Various diseases modify the movements of the tongue. In people who have overactivity of the thyroid gland, the tongue moves quickly and snappily; those who have underactivity of the gland are likely to have a sluggish tongue. People who are weak or exhausted and those in a stupor or in a coma will put the tongue out just a little and leave it out until they are told to put it back.

Paralysis that affects only one side of the tongue results in having the healthy side push the tongue toward the paralyzed side. This sign is seen especially in people who have had a hemorrhage into the brain or who have lost the function of one side of the brain from some other cause.

Among the most common of the peculiar sensations that disturb many people is a burning feeling in the tongue. The tongue, like all of the other tissues of the human body, is connected with the nervous system. A burning sensation in the tongue is reflected through its nerves. Many investigations have been made of this symptom. Sometimes the tongue is inflamed by coming into contact with the edges of rough teeth or by the wearing of unsatisfactory false teeth. In some cases of pellagra or pernicious anemia there are burning sensations in the tongue. The symptom is also found occasionally associated with difficulties of the digestive system. When, therefore, a patient complains of a burning sensation in the tongue, the physician will want to make a complete examination, including particularly a study of the digestive system and of the blood.

In a few instances burning and even ulcers of the tongue have been found to be due to the fact that metals of different electric potentials are used to fill the teeth on opposite sides of the mouth. There are, of course, instances in which the tongue is itself infected by germs, also cases in which the tongue may be subject to cancer or other specific diseases.

Sometimes the surface of the tongue, instead of being smooth, becomes marked by deep furrows and elevations. As a result, it looks like a relief map. This condition is called geographic tongue. Sometimes the condition can be improved by the use of mouth washes, mild antiseptics, and the adoption of a diet that is rich in vitamins and anti-anemic substances like iron and liver. The exact cause of geographic tongue has not been definitely determined.

TONGUE—See EAR, article THE EAR, TONGUE, NOSE, AND THROAT.

TONGUE—coated, See article DIGESTION AND DIGESTIVE DISEASES.

TONGUE—location (fig.): See EAR, article THE EAR, TONGUE, NOSE, AND THROAT.

TONGUE—scarlet fever: See CHILDHOOD DISEASES, article INFECTIOUS DISEASES OF CHILDHOOD.

TONGUE—strawberry: See CHILDHOOD DISEASES, article INFECTIOUS DISEASES OF CHILDHOOD.

TONGUE DISTURBANCE (See also *Leukoplakia*) Doctors who look at the tongue describe its appearance as a sore or inflamed tongue, a glazed tongue, and a shiny tongue. These conditions of the tongue are associated with such conditions as vitamin deficiencies, pernicious anemia, or the effects of taking antibiotic drugs. Furring of the tongue is usually associated with delayed action of the bowels, and a change to a rougher diet usually clears the tongue. Other changes in the tongue are those associated with scarlet fever, called strawberry tongue, and with the condition called leukoplakia, which is a chronic form of irritation, often associated with excessive smoking.

TONSILS Why do we have tonsils? Apparently they serve some purpose in taking care of infectious germs that come into the throat. They respond to infection with swelling and inflammation associated with pain, soreness, difficulty in swallowing, swelling of the glands in the throat, fever, a rapid pulse, and illness generally.

The list of diseases that have been attributed to infection through germs of one kind or another attacking the tonsils is like the index of a medical book. Definite relationships have been traced between infection of the tonsils and infections of the ears, eyes, diseases of the skin, the heart, and the joints. In cases in which there is such inflammation or infection it has been found that removal of the tonsils has a good effect on the general health. Moreover, there are subsequently fewer disturbances of the throat and of the nose and chest.

The child who breathes constantly through the mouth because of the presence of tonsils or adenoids will be found after their removal to breathe through the nose. This has an excellent effect not only on the child's frame of mind but also in aiding sleep and improving the child's appearance.

An enlarged tonsil is not necessarily an infected tonsil. Enlargement may, however, be the result of repeated infections which subsequently heal.

Many hundreds of thousands, if not millions, of people have had their tonsils removed, and it is now possible for the doctors to draw some positive conclusions as to the desirability of removal of the tonsils in certain instances. The modern operation for the removal of the tonsils has been so well perfected that complications are exceedingly rare, and an occasional fatality even rarer. When the operation for the removal of the tonsils is properly performed, preferably in a hospital, with the anesthetic either general or local properly controlled, the operation is likely to be completely successful.

In very old people or in instances of heart disease or in other cases when the taking of an anesthetic is not possible, tonsils are sometimes treated with the X ray. The X ray is also used occasionally to treat fragments of tissue that may be left after removal of the tonsils. The experts consider this technic as suitable only in exceptional cases rather than as a routine.

Tonsils—diphtheria germs sometimes persist until removal: See Childhood Diseases, article Infectious Diseases of Childhood.

Tonsils—earache: See Ear, article The Ear, Tongue, Nose, and Throat.

Tonsils—endocarditis: See Heart, article Diseases of the Heart and Circulation.

Tonsils—eye may become infected: See Eye, article The Eye.

Tonsils—halitosis may be caused by: See Teeth, article The Care of the Teeth.

Tonsils—infected, diabetics should have removed: See article Diabetes.

Tonsils—infected, hypertension may be aggravated by: See article Blood Pressure.

Tonsils—location (fig.): See Ear, article The Ear, Tongue, Nose, and Throat.

Tonsils—lymph nodes: See Blood, article The Blood and Its Diseases.

Tonsils—nephritis: See Kidney, article The Kidney: Its Diseases and Disturbances.

Tonsils—normal, should not be removed: See Heart, article Diseases of the Heart and Circulation.

Tonsils—removal: See Respiratory Diseases, article The Respiratory Diseases; Heart, article Diseases of the Heart and Circulation; Ear, article The Ear, Tongue, Nose, and Throat.

Tonsils—rheumatic fever: See Heart, article Diseases of the Heart and Circulation.

Tonsils—sinus infection associated with: See Ear, article The Ear, Tongue, Nose, and Throat.

TONSILS—white spots may indicate diphtheria: See CHILDHOOD DISEASES, article INFECTIOUS DISEASES OF CHILDHOOD.

TORTICOLLIS When a person's neck appears to be twisted, so that the head leans or is tilted toward one shoulder or the other, the condition is called wry neck, twisted neck, or torticollis.

There are various causes for this condition. Sometimes an accident of birth is responsible. Many people tilt their heads to one side as a habit. In cases of wry neck that have lasted a long time, the tissue on the short side of the neck becomes shortened to accommodate itself to the twisting. The face as well as the skull may become deformed, giving it a slanting appearance. There may even be twisting of the spine to compensate for the twisting of the head.

In the ordinary case of wry neck the application of heat and the use of drugs to overcome the pain will frequently bring about relief. In every such instance, however, the doctor must make a thorough search to find out whether or not there are infections elsewhere in the body, since failure to overcome sources of infection may bring about repeated instances of twisting of the neck.

Occasionally wry neck occurs as the result of a nervous or mental disturbance associated occasionally with overwork or mental strain. This is called a functional nervous disorder and is treated by mental methods.

Wry neck sometimes occurs as a result of infection of the lymph glands in the neck. In still other cases it may be associated with damage to the spine or the spinal cord.

In the difficult chronic case of wry neck a surgical operation may be desirable to prevent secondary deformities such as those that have been mentioned. In this operation ligaments are cut and occasionally muscles are operated on to permit placing of the head in proper alignment to the neck. By the use of suitable braces or casts the head is held in this position until complete recovery has occurred. Regular exercises and massage are useful in the postoperative period to bring about better results.

TRACHEA The scientific name for the windpipe is the trachea. It is often involved in infections of the throat and the bronchial tubes. Any virus or germ that can produce inflammation of the respiratory tract can also cause the lining of the trachea to become infected. It is possible for the experts to see the lining of the trachea by the use of the bronchoscope.

In World War I there were many instances of severe inflammation of the lining of the trachea due to mustard gas poisoning. When the lining of the trachea becomes inflamed, the most typical symptom is the cough. These coughs are non-productive, hacking, and metallic. They tend to be worse after the person goes to bed and during the night. An acute inflammation of the trachea is accompanied by rawness, tightness, and discomfort, sometimes even pain, in the lower part of the neck and behind the upper part of the breastbone, or sternum. As the inflammation goes on, there is mucus and finally a good deal of sputum and mucus may be expectorated. If the infection is purulent, as with the staphylococcus or streptococcus, the material coughed up will be a mixture of mucus and pus.

These conditions can be helped by the usual treatment that is given to other inflammations of the respiratory tract. That means going to bed for a few days, applying warmth, and producing rest by the use of appropriate remedies which the doctor prescribes. Often inhalations of warm vapor treated with medicated oils help to bring relief.

In some instances the acute inflammation of the trachea becomes chronic. In such cases the cough is irritating and frequent. When these symptoms are present, it becomes necessary for the doctor to make certain that the patient does not have tuberculosis or any other condition affecting the lungs. In such cases it is customary to prohibit smoking. Often residence in a warm, dry climate is advisable. The use of anti-infectious remedies such as the sulfonamides and penicillin are important in eliminating infection.

TRACHEOTOMY—See article ALLERGY.

TRACHOMA One of the most widespread diseases of the world is an inflammation of the eyes called trachoma, now believed to be due to a specific virus. The condition is so common in Egypt, Palestine, and India, except among the upper classes, that it is almost a universal disease.

The infection is carried by the transfer of the secretions from the eyes through the use of the hands, towels, handkerchiefs, pillows, or even by sneezing. It has been thought indeed that in some areas the infection is carried by flies.

In this condition the eye becomes inflamed and red; then blisters and crusts form. The scarring and injury may change the shape of the eyelids. If the infection of the cornea of the eye becomes sufficiently severe, the eyesight may be destroyed.

This infection should be avoided with every possible effort. People who are in an area where trachoma is common should be exceedingly careful about the use of common towels and about rubbing the eyes with the hands.

The modern treatment of trachoma, using the sulfonamide drugs and aureomycin has been helpful in stopping the progress of the disease.

In treating the symptoms of trachoma, including the inflammation and the secretion, attempts are made to check and remove the granules and to overcome the enlargement of the tissues of the conjunctiva. This is accomplished by the application of caustic substances like sulfate of copper or nitrate of silver and by mechanical and surgical methods such as scraping or cutting away the excess material. This demands the utmost judgment and care on the part of the physician, since overirritation demands soothing treatment, so that there is no routine. Each patient must be treated according to the condition that exists at the time he is examined. It becomes necessary to keep the eyes clean for some time by the frequent use of solutions of salt or alkaline washes or other preparations which the physician may prescribe.

In the United States at least 10 per cent of the entire Indian population are said to be affected. Since the development of new methods of treatment, the condition is gradually being eliminated even from our Indian tribes.

TRACHOMA—See EYE, article THE EYE.

TRANQUILIZING DRUGS The new tranquilizing drugs—Chlorpromazine, Resperine, Frenquel, Miltown, Equanil, Atarax, Suavitil, Placidye, etc. are proving their value in the treatment of disturbed psychotic patients. These drugs affect the brain though exactly how is not clearly established. Some evidence indicates that a neurohormone called Serotonin is involved. When there is an insufficient amount of Serotonin, abnormal behavior may be observed. Although the therapeutic values of these new drugs have been widely corroborated, they are not a complete answer; no one drug is able to ameliorate the condition of all patients and none of these drugs is as efficacious for melancholia as is electric shock.

Various combinations of new with old drugs have been tested, such as combinations of Reserpine with various sedative drugs of the barbiturate series and with other active ingredients. In another study Reserpine and Chlorpromazine were given in combination with certain advantages claimed over therapy with Reserpine alone.

Miltown has been found to be the most potent anticonvulsant in the meprobamate series to which it belongs. Among the special qualities listed for this drug are as an agent in anxiety and tension states and muscle relaxant, particularly in fibrositic rheumatic disorders and in such conditions as torticollis and also back pain, for control of spasticity in such conditions as cerebral palsy and as a sleep inducer of a different order from the hypnotic or sedative drugs. Reports have also indicated its effectiveness in certain cases of petit mal and its desirability in what are commonly called tension states but which might include psychoses, psychoneuroses, and personality disorders as well as a wide variety of conditions classified as psychosomatic, including headaches, dysmenorrhea, hypertension, motion sickness, peptic ulcers, and a variety of skin disorders. Few allergic reactions have been reported, all of which responded to therapy with antihistamines.

Transmissible Diseases

BY

MORRIS FISHBEIN, M.D.

Former Editor, *Journal American Medical Association,* Chicago; Editor, *Excerpta Medica, Bulletin World Medical Assn.; Post-graduate Medicine.*

TYPHOID FEVER

IF THE CASE RATES and death rates for typhoid fever that existed in 1890 prevailed now, the city of Chicago would have in 1955, 60,000 cases of typhoid fever and approximately 6,000 deaths. Instead, the city of Chicago has had in recent years regularly less than 20 cases and seldom as many as 5 deaths. In Chicago from April 1, 1890, to April 1, 1892, there were 2,372 deaths from typhoid fever representing approximately 24,000 cases. Compare that figure with the population of that day to the great population of Chicago at present and the low incidence of typhoid. What a tremendous benefit modern scientific preventive medicine has been for all of mankind.

In an earlier day, the family doctor claimed that he could smell typhoid fever. His guess was likely to be accurate, since one out of five seriously sick people whom he saw was likely to have typhoid fever. There was a time when any doctor could definitely count on the financial returns from typhoid fever, and they were usually sufficient in amount to permit him to send all his children to college.

Typhoid fever is an acute infection caused by a germ which used to be known as the typhoid bacillus and which is now called *Salmonella typhosa*. The germ can be found in the blood of a person seriously sick with the disease, and in 80 per cent of the cases is found in the stools or excretions of the sick. The germ is spread from the sick person to those who are well by means of the excretions, by soiled food and clothing, particularly by contaminated water and milk, and to a large extent by people who carry the disease; that is to say, they themselves have been sick and have recovered, but they still have in their bodies germs which reside frequently in the intestinal tract and also in the gall bladder, and which may get out of those places and infect other people.

There was a time when cases of typhoid fever occurred from the use of ice made from water in polluted streams. Today the vast majority of ice used in this country is made artificially from clean water, and there is no danger of typhoid. Milk used to be a common source of typhoid germs; and milk products such as ice cream, butter, buttermilk, and cheese were also known on occasion to carry the germs. Once the eating of infected oysters was a prominent cause, because the oysters were developed in contaminated water. In fact, the best fattening grounds for oysters were known to be in and around sewers. Now the control of oyster breeding in uncontaminated water, and suitable methods of storage and transmission for oysters, have largely eliminated the shellfish as a source of contagion. Cases have been reported due to the eating of raw vegetables which had been fertilized with contaminated materials or watered with contaminated water.

It was thought for a while that flies were more responsible for spreading typhoid fever than any other cause, but today it is not believed that transmission by flies is important, however, the fly does feed filthily and may transmit any condition associated with the filth on which it feeds.

Typhoid fever used to follow a long and serious course once a person became infected with it. After a person gets the germs in his body, from three to twenty-one days elapse, known as the incubation period, during which the germs develop and liberate their poisons. The average length of time is ten and a half days. The condition begins with the usual symptoms of infection, such as headache, pains in the body generally, a feeling of exhaustion and loss of appetite. Sometimes there are chills. Quite frequently there is nosebleed, and almost invariably there is disturbance of the action of the bowels in the form of constipation or diarrhea. With the coming of modern methods of treatment using chloromycetin the duration of the disease has been shortened and its severity diminished. The fever is brought under control in a few days.

In addition to the loss of appetite, there is a tendency to the formation of gas with bloating of the body; and sometimes, because of the ulcers in the bowels and the bloating, sudden severe hemorrhages from the bowel. Sometimes the infection and the poisoning affect the nervous system so that there is delirium and even the appearance of mental disturbance during the course of the disease.

The physician who examines a patient with typhoid fever makes his diagnosis from the history of the case and from the appearance of the symptoms, and also by careful studies of the blood. It is possible to examine specimens of the blood and to determine by the use of a test, called the Widal test, after the Frenchman who discovered it, whether or not the condition is quite certainly typhoid fever. Any serious complications such as hemorrhage, perforation of the bowel, and changes in the heart action and in the nervous system, demand prompt and careful attention by a competent physician.

A person who has typhoid fever must be kept alone and preferably cared for by an experienced nurse. The room should be screened if the condition occurs during the summer, when flies are a common pest. Because the person with typhoid may remain long in bed in severe cases he should have a bed with a firm mattress, and arrangements must be made to change the bed linen any time it is soiled. The patient must be bathed at least once a day and the back and buttocks kept clean in order to prevent secondary infections. It is also important to see that the mouth is kept clean and rinsed each time after food is taken.

There was a time when it was thought advisable to starve patients with typhoid fever. The condition interferes with the nutrition of the patient, so that present methods involve the giving of a diet of from 3,000 to 3,500 calories. Then the patient will not lose weight during the course of the illness.

A vaccine made of the killed germs of typhoid fever is of value in preventing the disease. This was quite certainly proved during World War II. Anyone who is likely to be exposed to the taking of contaminated food or water ought to be vaccinated against typhoid fever. In the entire American army during World War II there were only slightly over one thousand cases of typhoid fever among something like five million enrolled troops. If the rate for typhoid which prevailed during the Spanish-American War had existed, there would have been approximately a million cases.

It is customary to give three injections of the vaccine against typhoid fever at ten-day intervals, although the intervals between injections may be shortened in time of necessity. Obviously, the giving of such vaccines is the work of a physician or of a trained nurse, since the average person cannot inject himself and does not understand the technic of preparation. Only rarely indeed are there reactions of a serious character following the injection of ordinary doses of antityphoid vaccine.

Persistent attention to water supplies and disposal of sewage, pasteurization of milk, education of the public in hygiene, and the control of typhoid carriers will eventually eliminate typhoid fever entirely throughout the civilized world. Means are now available in most states for proper control of carriers when they are discovered, but the discovery of a carrier demands expert bacteriological investigation.

The rates for typhoid fever have been falling steadily. With antibiotic drugs complications are controlled and chloromycetin, also called chloramphenicol, has proved especially valuable in this condition. Some research has shown even more rapid improvement with combined use of cortisone and chloromycetin.

Erysipelas

The condition called St. Anthony's fire is an acute inflammation of the skin caused by the streptococcus, an organism of the same type as that which causes scarlet fever and many other infections. Apparently, the condition was known in the time of the ancient Greeks and Romans. In fact, the greatest writers of those days, Hippocrates, Galen, and Celsus, all described this condition and credited it to living under unhygienic conditions. Finally, in 1882, a German investigator proved the specific character of the disease by isolating the germs.

Erysipelas occurs most often during the months from October to March, and in fact reaches its highest frequency in March. The disease is not so common in children as in persons between the ages of twenty to sixty. Men apparently have erysipelas more often than do women, perhaps because men are more frequently exposed to physical injuries and bad weather conditions during the winter months.

Erysipelas starts most often in a wound, abrasion, or rubbed place on the skin, and particularly in those places where the mucous membranes, such as those which line the nose and the mouth, join the outer skin. In hospitals, in the past, there were frequently epidemics of erysipelas because the infection was carried from one patient to another by attendants. Nowadays the great danger of erysipelas in a surgical ward has been recognized, and a person with erysipelas is promptly put in a room by himself and attended by a nurse who is not attending other people. In cases which occur in homes under ordinary conditions it is necessary to make certain that the other people in the family do not come in too close contact with the patient. The spread of this disease is almost always by the hands of the person who is taking care of the patient.

Erysipelas usually begins with a severe fever and a chill and associated with this all of the usual symptoms of an acute poisoning of the body such as headache, loss of appetite, vomiting, and, in the case of a high fever, perhaps some delirium.

The disease usually lasts from five to ten days, the average being eight days. When the erysipelas affects large areas of the body it may continue for as long as fifteen days.

Usually erysipelas begins on the face and extends from day to day, so that it eventually covers the entire side of the face, including the eyelids, which become enormously swollen and filled with fluid. Sometimes the swelling is sufficient to close the eye completely. Then the disease spreads onto the ear, which thickens tremendously, and finally reaches the line of the hair, where it stops abruptly. In other cases it may spread down the back. In many instances the condition begins on the bridge of the nose and spreads rapidly to each side so that it forms what is called a "butterfly" pattern.

Often any natural boundary such as the hair line, the nape of the neck, and places where the skin is tight over the cheek bones, will stop the spread of the disease.

When the inflammation of the skin stops, the fever begins to drop. Sometimes the skin peels where it has been greatly swollen. If the disease occurs again and again, almost a permament thickening may develop, which is, of course, exceedingly unsightly.

The doctor is able to diagnose erysipelas certainly by studying its general character and also by examining the blood in which the white cells are found to have been increased tremendously.

The most serious complication in erysipelas is a secondary infection. Under such circumstances the swelling changes to abscess. In the vast majority of cases erysipelas is not a fatal disease. In young infants and in old and sickly people it may be exceedingly serious, but in general it causes a death rate per year of about three people for each hundred thousand in the community.

Numerous remedies have been developed for the treatment of erysipelas, including the use of ultraviolet and X rays, antiseptics, antitoxins, and all sorts of drugs, especially sulfanilamide and antibiotics. Doctors used to attempt to control the disease by painting on iodine, silver nitrate, and similar preparations, but modern authorities feel that these accomplish little, and besides may so hide the spread of the disease as to interfere with its control. Sulfonamides, which are now available in many forms, prevent the growth in the blood of the germs that cause erysipelas. These should be prescribed by the doctor. If the eyelids are involved, it is customary to drop some mild antiseptic solution, which the doctor will supply, directly into the eyes. The new drugs like penicillin control the disease in most cases.

Dr. Konrad Birkhaug recommends the use of compresses soaked in an ice-cold solution of magnesium sulphate (or Epsom salts). If these cloths are kept cold and applied repeatedly, they offer great relief by lessening the tightness of the skin and diminishing the burning pain and swelling. This will not, however, stop the spread of the erysipelas.

Since erysipelas is caused by a streptococcus, the condition is now controllable by the use of the antibiotics, particularly penicillin, aureomycin **and** tetracyclines and by the use of sulfadiazine. These new remedies have made unnecessary the use of biologic preparations like antitoxins. The manifestations on the skin are treated with direct application of specific remedies. Since erysipelas arises in most instances from a small beginning, early and prompt treatment of scratches and minor infections has greatly reduced the total number of cases of erysipelas. Cold compresses are often soothing and some physicians recommend moistening the compresses in a mild solution of aluminum acetate (Burow's solution, 1:1000).

Because erysipelas, like other infectious diseases, tends to break down the blood and weaken the patients generally, it is well to give people who are sick with erysipelas plenty of fluids, actually forcing them to drink not less than ten and as many as sixteen glasses of water daily. It is also well to have the food easy to digest and nourishing, in fact, what is ordinarily called a nutritious soft diet. There is danger in using too much cathartic because of irritation of the bowels during the presence of a serious infection.

A person who has once had erysipelas is likely to have it again. Such people should be exceedingly careful about picking the nose or scratching the ear. If these parts of the skin are irritated, they should be kept covered with mild ointments or cold cream.

Tetanus or Lockjaw

The ancient Greeks knew about lockjaw. Indeed, the father of modern medicine, Hippocrates, described it and made some statements about the likelihood of recovery which are still good. It was not, however, until 1865 that it was thought to be infectious. The germ was not described until 1886. Today it is possible to isolate the germ, to grow it artificially, and to produce lockjaw in animals by injecting the germs into their bodies. The germ is called *Clostridium tetani*.

The poison produced by these germs is one of the most powerful poisons known. Most people used to think that tetanus, or lockjaw, was always caused by scratching the skin with a rusty nail. Today it is known that the rusty nail produces the disease because it is contaminated with material containing the germ of tetanus.

When this germ gets into the body by any means whatever, it sets up inflammation of nerve tissue. Because these germs have a special predilection for certain nerves, the condition called lockjaw is produced.

Certain types of wounds are more likely to cause tetanus than others. Most important are wounds which are deep, penetrating, lacerating, or crushing and which, because of that fact, permit particles of foreign matter containing the germs of tetanus to go deeply into the tissues and to remain there. This germ lives much better in the absence of oxygen. When it is pushed deep into a wound it is without oxygen and therefore is under the best possible conditions for its growth. The effects are produced more by the poisons produced by the germs than by the germs themselves. Indeed, it is believed that the poison, or toxin, is transported by the lymphatics and that in this way it reaches the nerve tissues.

The germs of tetanus seem to live preferably in the intestinal tracts of cattle, horses, and man. Because the germs are fairly widespread it is remarkable that the disease is not more common. Apparently, however, it is necessary for the germs to get deep into the tissue through a wound in order to multiply and produce the disease.

In the United States somewhere around one thousand to thirteen hundred deaths occur each year from tetanus. The number is less now than formerly because of the disappearance of horses and manure from city streets, because of the diminution of Fourth of July accidents associated with explosives, and because of the use of new methods of prevention which were not formerly generally available.

Tetanus usually begins about seven days after the wound which permits the germs to get into the tissues. It may, however, come on somewhat later or, rather rarely, earlier. The first signs are a sense of drawing pain in a wound with the twitching of muscles near by; also the usual signs of infection such as irritability, headache, chilliness, and fever. Then comes the stiffness of the muscles of the jaw and neck which gives the disease its name.

It becomes more and more difficult to open the mouth, and finally the jaws may be clamped shut and the neck rigid. Attempts to open the mouth intensify the spasm. Due to the fact that the muscles of the face are contracted, the corners of the mouth are drawn back and the eyebrows raised. This gives the person a typical grinning appearance which is described by the scientists as *risus sardonicus*—in other words, a sardonic expression.

Eventually, of course, other muscles and nerves are involved so that there are serious spasms and convulsions. In fact, there may be from three to forty spasms in an hour. The whole body may be involved, including even the muscles of the bowels and of the bladder. Of course, when the heart and the breathing muscles are involved, the condition is fatal.

Even under the best of treatment, patients with lockjaw may die because of the potency of this poison. Much depends on the time at which the antitoxin is given and on the amount. Of greatest importance is the prevention of lockjaw through the proper treatment of people who have been wounded, at the earliest possible moment. It should be taken for granted that a wound acquired in localities where the soil is likely to be contaminated, such as wounds acquired in fields, stables, and farmyards, or such as gunshot and powder wounds, are infected.

A physician who treats such a case will probably open the wound widely, removing any clothing, soil, or other visible contamination that may be present, and then treat the wound with proper antiseptics such as tincture of iodine or hydrogen peroxide to destroy the germs that can be reached. The opening of the wound is especially important, because this germ multiplies in the absence of air. Opening of the wound permits air to be present. It also permits removal of contamination, and it allows the antiseptics to reach the infectious material.

It is also important at this time to inject under the skin the specific antitoxin against tetanus, and perhaps to give another injection one week later.

If the disease develops in spite of preventive treatment, the patient should be placed in a quiet room, preferably in a hospital. The room must be kept darkened, and all noises or vibrations prevented, because they may serve to stimulate spasms. It may be necessary even to use an anesthetic to prevent these spasms. In order to feed the patient it is sometimes necessary to pass a narrow tube through the nose and down into the stomach, because the jaws may be so tightly clamped as to make it impossible to get food into the body otherwise. Someone must be constantly with the patient to prevent injury from convulsions and to guard against sudden death from paralysis of the breathing.

Several reports have appeared on beneficial effects of combined treatment using antibiotics such as penicillin or terramycin with antitoxin.

In no condition is the constant and immediate attention of a competent physician, and at the same time good nursing, so important. This makes the difference frequently between life and death. The antitoxin which opposes the poison must be given early in the disease and in large doses. Because of the great irritability of the patient it is sometimes necessary to put him to sleep in order that the antitoxin may be given. Under the best of treatment it is possible to save the lives of from one half to two thirds of the people who are infected.

Rabies or Hydrophobia

The word *"rabies"* is Latin for madness or rage. "Hydrophobia" means fear of water and thus defines what seemed to be the most significant symptom of the disease. It is one of the oldest of the diseases definitely classified by man. Around 100 A. D., Celsus recommended cauterization of wounds produced by mad dogs. As early as 1804, long before the nature of the disease was discovered by Pasteur, it was known that the saliva of a person or of a dog that had the disease would transmit it. Since, however, no means was known for preventing its spread, sufferers at that time were sometimes put to death by strangulation or smothering because people so greatly feared the disease. Until the time when Pasteur made the great discovery which freed mankind from fear of hydrophobia it was customary, as a means of treatment, to burn with a redhot iron the flesh of a person who had been bitten by any mad animal.

Some strange superstitions about hydrophobia still remain. One is that it commonly occurs in the "dog days." It has been believed that the danger from mad dogs was greater at that time than at any other. There is no evidence to support this view, because the bites of mad dogs occur at any time. They are likely to be more frequent from April to September than from October to March because dogs run loose more often and more generally in the spring and summer than they do in winter.

When a mad dog bites another animal or a human being the disease is transmitted by the saliva, which contains the poisonous virus. It is called a virus because it is so small that it will pass through the pores of a clay filter. The time when the disease attacks is from fourteen days on. There are wide variations in the period of incubation, in fact from ten days to twelve months, but in the vast majority of cases the onset follows the bite in from twenty to ninety days. It is rarely less than 15 days or more than 5 months.

During this period of incubation the person may show only signs of restlessness and apprehension, sometimes of irritation or tingling and pain at the site of the bite. However, when the disease begins, the horrible symptoms which give it its name reach their peak. A slight huskiness of the voice and a sense of choking are followed by severe spasms of the muscles of swallowing and breathing. There is shortness of breath. So severe are the symptoms following any attempt to swallow that the affected person will refuse to take water. This, of course, gave rise to the name hydrophobia, or fear of water. Eventually the convulsions and spasms may affect almost the whole body, and the nervous system is so sensitive that the slamming of a door or a sudden draft of wind will bring on an attack. Finally, the spine may stiffen and bend and death result from paralysis of the apparatus of breathing.

Because the affected person or animal is unable to swallow, thick saliva accumulates and drips from the mouth. Because of the paralysis of the muscles of breathing the breath comes in harsh gasps. The person who is infected does not necessarily foam at the mouth or bark like a dog, but the nature of the symptoms is such as to give people this impression.

Because of the great danger associated with this disease, everything possible should be done to prevent its spread. At times when hydrophobia, or rabies, is prevalent in any community the lives of both dogs and children may be freed from menace by protecting them from exposure to the bite of a mad animal. Homeless animals should be picked up and disposed of by the usual methods.

A failure to enforce the laws regulating the control of homeless animals represents nothing in the way of friendship for the animal and exposes innumerable human beings to the danger of one of the most serious of diseases.

The dog that is kept in a good home is usually watched carefully, kept from contact with savage dogs, and is not so likely to be involved as the one that runs free. However, any dog may suddenly bite a human being, under provocation or sometimes without provocation. Because of the terrible possibilities of rabies, there is only one course to follow after a dog bite. The animal should be penned up or kept secured for at least ten days, during which time it will either die or develop the symptoms of hydrophobia, if it has that disease.

Far too often, when police are called to kill a dog suspected of hydrophobia, the dog is shot in the head or the head crushed with a club. This should not be done, because it is difficult for a laboratory to examine the brain of the dog when it is too severely injured.

The diagnosis of hydrophobia is made by examination of the brain of the animal under the microscope. When this disease is present the brain contains certain substances known as Negri bodies, which can be seen by the investigator. If there is the slightest suspicion that the dog which has bitten a person was mad, the Pasteur treatment for the prevention of hydrophobia should be begun immediately. If there are bites on the face or even on the hands it is wise to commence immediate treatment because of the short time which usually elapses when bites occur in these places. Otherwise it may be safe to delay for a few days to make sure that the animal was rabid or mad.

The wounds should be immediately cauterized with carbolic or fuming nitric acid. The Pasteur treatment is administered by any private or state laboratory. Moreover, it is available to physicians in any village or town through material that can be supplied by pharmaceutical houses. In the Pasteur treatment a special vaccine is used which is prepared from the brains of rabbits that have been injected with the disease. In these tissues the virus has been attenuated by passage through many animals and by other treatment, such as drying. There are no contra-indications to the use of this treatment.

The success of the Pasteur treatment for preventing hydrophobia is almost certain. Failures occur in less than one half of one per cent of the cases in which it is used. Notwithstanding the fact that information concerning this disease has been widespread for many years, there are still more than one hundred deaths annually from the disease in the United States. These are preventable deaths. Once the disease has developed, the physician can do much to relieve suffering and should be in constant attendance for this purpose.

Control of rabies includes measures which prevent dogs from biting, licensing of dogs, seizure and destruction of stray dogs, quarantine or muzzling of dogs during outbreaks of rabies and subjection of all imported dogs to six months quarantine. These measures eliminated rabies from England and Canada. Vaccination of dogs against rabies is recommended where quarantine cannot be enforced or where the disease prevails among wild animals.

Vincent's Angina

In 1898 a French physician named Vincent described an infection of the mouth and throat due to a peculiar spiral organism called *Treponema vincentii* and *Borrelia vincentii*. Apparently the disease occurred only in man, was accompanied by slight general disturbances with but a small increase in temperature, but there was pain on swallowing, enlargement of the glands, and a yellowish gray membrane in the mouth and throat. Because of this membrane, the disease was often mistaken for diphtheria until the differences were clearly established.

Sometimes the germs responsible for Vincent's angina were found in mouths that were not infected, but which were in bad condition. Occasionally also the disease appeared to be especially favored by fatigue, chill, exposure, improper food, or the excessive use of alcohol or tobacco. During World War I the disease spread widely among the soldiers and was given the common name of trench mouth, a name which has persisted.

In this common infection penicillin has already been established as especially curative. With good dental care and suitable application of such remedies the condition is controllable. Penicillin is taken by injection, as an application to the infected areas and in troches dissolved on the tongue. Bacitracin troches have also been used successfully.

When the disease is once established, it may be treated by the repeated use of solutions of hydrogen peroxide or by the application of a paste of sodium perborate, as the physician or dentist may advise. In severe cases treatment includes injections with sulfanilamide or neoarsphenamine and also local application of drugs. For prevention it is also advisable to have the teeth clean and smooth and to discontinue tobacco as long as any evidence of the disease remains.

Undulant Fever or Brucellosis

Years ago, British soldiers quartered on the island of Malta developed a disease in epidemic form which was called Malta fever. Later, as the disease spread about the world it became known as Mediterranean fever. Finally, it was called undulant fever because of its intermittent character; that is, the fever went up and down in waves. Three types of organisms are now known as causative including *Brucella melitensis, Brucella abortus* and *Brucella suis*. The condition is related to contagious abortion of cattle.

The menace of undulant fever is not the menace of epidemics of yellow fever or even of influenza. The disease insidiously creeps into a population and gradually affects increasing numbers of people. Fortunately, it is likely to spread slowly, if at all, in American communities, because milk is the most important medium in transmitting the disease. Since 1900, milk supplies in the United States have been controlled through suitable public health laws and measures. Milk is made safe for human consumption by pasteurization, in which the milk is heated for a sufficient length of time to destroy dangerous germs.

Before 1927, undulant fever was regarded as a curiosity when it occurred in a human being in the United States. Since that time cases have appeared in practically every state of the union. In the great majority of cases the taking of raw milk containing the germ, which is identified also as the one which causes contagious abortion of cattle, was demonstrated to be the source of the infection. Apparently the condition is more likely to be spread by goat's milk than by that from cattle, particularly since the goat's milk is not usually as well controlled in its assembling and distribution as is the milk of cows. Moreover, the infection is more generalized among goats than among cattle.

From ten to thirty days after the person becomes infected with this disease he has the usual symptoms associated with an infectious disorder—weakness, tiredness, chilliness, loss of appetite, general aching, chills and fever. The condition develops slowly, so that frequently weeks may pass before the person who is infected considers himself sick enough to call a physician. He is inclined to believe that he has something like a persistent cold or rheumatic condition and that it is hard to break up.

Eventually, the symptoms of a person who has contracted undulant fever develop with sufficient fullness and persistence to make him realize that he is subject to a serious complaint. The physician who examines the blood of a patient with this disease finds that changes have taken place in the blood, and it is possible for a laboratory to make the kind of test that is made on the blood in typhoid fever and to determine with certainty that the patient is infected with undulant fever.

The disease resembles many other infectious diseases, such as typhoid, tuberculosis, malaria, or almost any other infectious disorder. In a few instances, perhaps two out of every one hundred cases, death may occur as a result of the seriousness of the infection or from secondary complications.

Of course, the way to avoid undulant fever is to avoid milk that has not been properly pasteurized. Men who work in packing houses where they come constantly in contact with infected animals should, of course, take the necessary precautions in their work. Men with wounds or abrasions on their hands should be certain to wear gloves and perhaps to clean their hands thoroughly at frequent intervals.

The real control of this disease will rest on the ability of government bureaus and of the veterinary industry to eliminate the condition from domestic animals.

The patient who has undulant fever must be handled in much the same way as one who has had typhoid. He must be put into a separate room; the health authorities must be notified; all of the excretions and secretions must be sterilized before they are disposed of in any way. This means either burning, boiling, or the use of proper antiseptic solutions. The patient, of course, must remain in bed and be properly fed to overcome the loss of weight, the anemia, and the weakness that are due to constant chills and fever. The wearing effects of such conditions on the body are extremely serious in producing changes in the nature of degeneration of important organs.

A treatment with sulfadiazine and streptomycin or with aureomycin or chloromycetin or terramycin has been found most effective in treating undulant fever. The drugs are administered by the doctor. There is also a vaccine which is occasionally helpful. Artificial fever treatment is now recommended alone and combined with drug treatment.

Amebiasis and Dysentery

Since the outbreak of amebic dysentery, from a source in two Chicago hotels during 1933, the world has become increasingly aware of the menace of this disorder, which was formerly considered a tropical disease. Instead of being caused by an ordinary germ, this condition is caused by a large type of organism known as the *entameba histolytica*. This organism gets into the large bowel, and once there sets up symptoms that are exceedingly serious. Moreover, the organism may spread to the liver particularly, or to other organs of the body, and there set up secondary places of infection which are also a menace to health and life. Although this condition was formerly unheard of in the northern portions of the United States, more recent evidence indicates that from five to ten per cent of all the people of this country are infected.

The organism which causes this disease multiplies in the bowel and gives off daughter cysts. These cysts are passed out of the body with the excretions, and if they reach food or drink in any way are naturally swallowed. They pass through the stomach and small intestines and then get into the upper portions of the large intestines. Here they divide up and multiply organisms which invade the walls of the bowels.

Ordinarily, the entameba histolytica which infects mankind comes in food or drink that has been contaminated in the manner suggested. After a person has had the disease and recovered, he may carry the organisms in his bowel for long periods of time, and as a carrier of the disease is constantly able to transmit it to other people. These carriers, who apparently are healthy or who have mild symptoms of the infection, are the ones most concerned in transmitting the disease.

Occasionally, however, the disease is transmitted by impure water supply. It has been shown that the cysts of the entameba histolytica may live for days and several weeks in water, depending on the temperature of the water and the number of bacteria in the water. It was thought in the past that these methods of transmission were of comparatively little importance in this country, except in the rural districts where people deposit their excretions on the soil, and where wells and springs are the chief sources of the water supply.

More recently, it has been found that any severe contamination of the water supply in a large building may result in the spread of amebic dysentery.

In China and Japan human excretions are frequently used as fertilizing material for vegetables. This is a serious menace to health, because it has been shown that the cysts of this parasite will remain alive in the moist excretions for as long as two weeks, and when they contaminate the vegetables, they may in this way transmit the disease.

It has also been shown that it is possible for the fly, which feeds on excretions, to carry the organism and deposit it on food. The most common method of transmission of this disease, however, is through the contamination of food and drink by food handlers who happen to be carriers of the entameba histolytica. The food handlers concerned may be waiters, cooks, dish washers, or any other kitchen personnel in a family or in a large hotel.

Inasmuch as the organism may live in the intestines for months or years without producing serious symptoms, it is not possible to say just how long a time is required for infection to develop. However, there is some good evidence that the swallowing of the cysts of entameba histolytica is followed in from ten to ninety-five days, with an average period of 64.8 days, by the beginning of the symptoms which are characteristic in this disease. Usually the disease comes on suddenly, but often it begins with mild diarrhea which gradually becomes worse. When the disease begins suddenly, there is severe abdominal pain with nausea and vomiting and a chilly sensation. The irritation of the bowel becomes acute, and the patient tries to evacuate the bowels repeatedly. This irritation may be so constant that the number of actions of the bowels will vary from six to eight in twenty-four hours to as many as thirty to forty actions of the bowels in twenty-four hours in severe cases.

As a result, the patient becomes exhausted, complains of aching in the back and great weakness in the legs, and is likely to be mentally depressed. There may be little or no fever; even in severe cases the temperature reaches at most from 100 to 102 degrees, but in very severe cases may go higher.

As a result of the extensive action of the bowels, such patients have tenderness in the abdomen, the skin appears sallow and jaundiced, and the patient loses weight rapidly. The doctor will want to examine the blood to find out how much the red cells of the blood have been injured and also whether or not there is any significant rise in the number of white blood cells. Frequently the distinction between this condition, appendicitis, and peritonitis will depend on a careful examination of the blood.

In times when amebic dysentery is prevalent and physicians are naturally on the lookout for it, they are likely to check up the cases. However, in the past physicians have not been particularly aware of this disease; certainly not in the northern parts of the United States. Since the diagnosis is made with certainty only after the excretions have been examined under the microscope in order to determine whether or not entameba histolytica is present, it is not safe to make a diagnosis until such a microscopic study has been made. At the same time, the man who makes the laboratory study must make certain that the ameba is the real entameba histolytica and not a form of the other amebas that live in the bowels without causing symptoms. He must also distinguish between the dysentery that is caused by the ameba and the dysentery which follows infection with some bacteria.

There are certain ways in which the community may protect itself against amebiasis. Much depends on having a properly guarded water supply, on the proper disposal of sewage, the protection of food from flies, and on suitable examinations and treatment of waiters, cooks, dish washers, and other food handlers in public eating places.

Chlorination of water will sterilize it so far as bacteria are concerned, but it takes one hundred times as much chlorine to kill the cysts of the entameba histolytica as it does to kill bacteria in water. In fact, the addition of this amount of chlorine to water would make the water unfit for drinking. Therefore, whenever water is heavily contaminated with entameba histolytica, the only way to make it safe is to boil it: obviously a difficult matter for any city water supply.

In controlling food handlers, it is necessary that they be examined at fairly frequent intervals, and that their excretions be examined in the laboratory to rule out the presence of the organism.

Fortunately, there are now available several methods of treatment which have been established as useful in controlling amebic dysentery. All of the remedies concerned are potent. Since they are powerful remedies, they are dangerous if taken in excessive dosage and should never be taken except under the advice and control of a physician. Among the remedies most commonly used today, and proved to be valuable, are chiniofon, carbarsone, and vioform, also milibis and various combinations. The drug called emetin, which is much used in this condition, is especially valuable in controlling the symptoms of the disease and is usually given early in order to bring about prompt recovery of the patient.

Aureomycin, chloramphenicol and terramycin have all been used successfully. Amebiasis is difficult to cure and relapses are frequent.

TULAREMIA

For the last thirty years market men have known about a condition called "rabbit fever." About 1911 cases were described under the name of deer fly fever. Finally, in 1912, investigators of the United States Public Health Service found a plague-like disease among the squirrels in one of the counties of California and discovered that this disease was caused by a germ which they named in honor of Tulare County, Calif., the *bacterium tularense* now called *Pasteurella tularensis*. Then, Francis, another investigator from the United States Public Health Service, found in 1919 that this germ which caused both the plague-like disease of rodents and deer fly fever could infect human beings with a condition which was named tularemia. Francis later examined the livers of a thousand rabbits offered for sale in the markets of Washington, D. C., and found at least one hundred seventy of these rabbits infected with the same germ.

While the disease caused by the bacterium tularense is not an especially serious disease, seventeen out of four hundred twenty people who had it died. The human being who becomes infected with this germ usually does so in the handling or dressing of rabbits sick with the disease. The rabbit sick with tularemia is not likely to be active. Health authorities warn particularly against eating rabbits that can be knocked over with a stick. If the rabbit gives a good chase and has to be shot with a gun it is probably not a sick rabbit.

The person who has tularemia develops swellings of the skin with the formation of abscesses, swelling of the lymph glands and nodules, and small spots of infection in the internal organs. The typical history of such a case is that the man in question or the woman in question dressed wild rabbits, that he or she had at the time a sore on the finger, and that shortly thereafter the sore developed into an ulcer; then the glands became involved, and finally other organs of the body.

Rabbit meat, even from rabbits infected with this condition, is harmless as a food if it is thoroughly cooked, since a temperature of 133 degrees F. will kill the germ. It is safer, however, for everyone who is dressing rabbits for use as food to wear rubber gloves during the process.

This condition can be transmitted from one animal to another, including the human being, by means of deer flies, wood ticks, rabbit ticks, and lice;

and such creatures as the sheep, the coyote, the cat, the quail, and the grouse may be infected, as well as rabbits and squirrels. However, as far as is known, the horse, cattle, dogs, and chickens have not been infected with this disease. In the Eastern states it is most likely to occur during November, December, and January.

Most people who become infected with tularemia have to go to bed from ten days to three weeks, and sometimes recovery is slow. There is no specific serum. The discovery of streptomycin provided a new specific treatment for tularemia that is quite effective. Aureomycin, chloramphenicol and terramycin are also effective.

Sometimes it is necessary to put hot packs on the spots of infection and then to open the abscesses in order to relieve the pressure of the broken-down material. In this infectious condition, as in every other, it is wise to convalesce slowly, since any disease with considerable fever and infection throws a strain on the heart and the circulation.

Malaria

Authorities in medicine have attributed the fall of the Roman and Greek civilizations to the development of malaria among the population. Certainly, malaria can devitalize any person.

Any community that is willing to spend sufficient money to stamp out the disease can do so. Malaria is becoming less prevalent in the United States each year. Nevertheless, a million people in the United States constantly suffer from malaria. Possibly one-third of the people in the world are infected. Malaria has been called the greatest single destroyer of the human race.

The physician diagnoses malaria by the characteristic symptoms, which include regularly recurring attacks of chills and fever, the presence of an enlarged spleen, and the presence of the malarial parasite in the blood of the sick person. He must not only diagnose malaria but also the special form that is present.

The plasmodium, as the organism which causes malaria is called, was discovered by the famous scientist Laveran, who received the Nobel Prize for this discovery. Ross and Grassi, a British and an Italian investigator, proved that the organism of malaria is transmitted from one human being to another through the bite of the anopheles mosquito.

Although malaria has practically disappeared as one of the great medical problems in large cities, the disease is still to be found in many rural communities, particularly in the southern portions of the United States.

In river valleys and creek bottoms malaria has been found to be highly endemic, averaging fifteen cases for every one hundred persons. The wors infection is always found in the immediate vicinity of some lake, pond, or marsh which could be the natural habitat of the malaria mosquito. The district extends about a mile in every direction from the pond, which marks the range of flight of the mosquitoes.

Country club ponds must be watched particularly, as these artificial pools have been found frequently to be excellent breeding places for the mosquito.

The malaria mosquito bites most frequently at dusk. If it has fed on a sick person and then bites a well one, the latter is likely to be supplied with some malarial infection. In summer resorts where the population is mixed, including people coming from all sorts of localities, the chance of infection is greater.

One of the means used to destroy the mosquitoes that carry the malaria organisms is to stock all lakes, ponds, and sluggish streams with the variety of fish that lives on the larvæ of the mosquito. The routine for mosquito control should include the clearing of the edges of the ponds of willows, cattails, water grasses, and floatage. Thus the bank of the pond is left sharp and clean, so that the fish can swim close to the bank and feed on the mosquito wiggletails.

The fish that has been found to be most active in feeding on the mosquito larvæ is the little top minnow *Gambusia affinis,* also called the pot-bellied minnow. This little fish swims in the most shallow waters.

The drainage of small ponds or marshes and the use of oil sprays are methods suitable to areas where it is not necessary to preserve the pond for decorative or for amusement purposes. Adult mosquitoes can be destroyed by DDT.

As long as the adult parasites are present in the blood of the individual in sufficient quantities to infect the mosquito that bites the individual, the person is a possible conveyor of malaria. Since the parasites remain in the blood for months, providing that the individual is not properly treated, anyone who is not undergoing regular treatment is a menace to those around him.

Children suffer more severely with the disease than do adults. Negroes apparently are less affected than are the white people. Malaria has been practically stamped out of northern communities, and cases are rarely seen even in large charity hospitals in the northern part of the United States.

In the more serious types of malaria not properly treated, anywhere from 10 to 30 per cent of the people die. The milder forms of the disease become chronic, and the fatality rate may be less than 5 per cent.

In controlling malaria, patients who are sick with the disease are protected from the bites of the mosquito. It has been established that the regular use of sufficient doses of quinine will control the condition. Many varieties of antimalarial drugs are now available. Quinine and atabrine are best known. Primaquine and pyrimethamine are newest. Paludrine and Camoquin can arrest the full blown development of the disease. Chloroquine or Aralen is used both for suppression and treatment.

RAT-BITE FEVER

When human beings are bitten by animals of the rodent type, including incidentally not only the rat but the weasel and the pig and occasionally, as will be seen later, even the cat, they are sometimes infected with a peculiar organism called a *Spirillum* which produces a disease of the whole body. This disease is characterized by short attacks of fever alternating with periods without the fever, and also an eruption on the skin. Such cases have been known in the United States for a century, and medical journals have reported approximately one hundred.

The usual course of such a case is as follows: After the person has been bitten, the wound heals promptly unless a secondary infection occurs. From one to three weeks after the date on which the patient was bitten, the spot of the bite becomes red and swollen, and the person who is infected develops the usual symptoms of infections in general: namely, headache, general pains and fever, sometimes a chill and a general feeling of sickness. Finally an eruption appears, at first most prominent in the region of the wound, but later spreading over the body.

From this time on, attacks of fever will occur every five or six days, sometimes less frequently. Gradually the person loses weight and may become exceedingly sick due to the loss of nutrition and general health. Somewhere between 6 and 7 per cent of the people who are infected eventually die of the disorder, but the tendency is for the majority to recover.

There have been instances reported in medical periodicals of children who have been bitten by rats when left alone by their parents, particularly when they live in basement homes or poverty-stricken tenements. Of course, a cat may become contaminated through its hunting of the rats.

The doctor makes his diagnosis of this condition not only by the symptoms that have been mentioned, but also by finding the germ which causes the disease in the wound, and sometimes in material taken directly from lymph glands near the wound. There are also cases in which people have been bitten by rats and become infected, not with this organism but with the usual germs that cause infection, such as the staphylococcus and streptococcus.

Formerly this condition was treated like syphilis, with salvarsan or arsphenamine or, as it was more popularly known, "606." Now penicillin seems to be fully effective in rat-bite fever, as in syphilis.

Rocky Mountain Spotted Fever

As was shown years ago in investigations made by Dr. Theobald Smith, many diseases of man are transmitted by the bite of a tick. Among the most serious of these is the condition called Rocky Mountain spotted fever, an infectious disease seen frequently in eastern Idaho and the Bitter Root Valley of Montana, but also occurring in most western states and occasionally in eastern portions of the United States. This condition occurs most commonly in men because of their occupations as surveyors, foresters, hunters, fishermen, sheep herders, or cowboys. These occupations expose them to the bite of the tick. If bitten, women and children are just as likely to become affected.

The tick is found on the rodents in the areas mentioned, and from these rodents picks up the organisms which it then transfers to man when it bites. From four to seven days after he is bitten, the man comes down with the disease. At first there are loss of appetite, general aches and pains, and slight fever. Then suddenly there is a chill followed by a high fever. This may reach 104 or 105 degrees. At first there are severe headache and backache with pains in the muscles. Even the skin may be tender. Eventually the nervous system may be involved, with restlessness and lack of sleep and even disturbance of the action of the bowels.

About the third to the seventh day, the infected person breaks out with tiny pinkish spots which generally appear first on the wrists and ankles, and which give the disease its name—spotted fever. In serious cases the spots run together. Since they are due to blood, they gradually turn purple. The fever remains high for a week to ten days and, if recovery occurs, falls gradually. In the fatal cases death occurs from the seventh to the tenth day, with high fever.

The physician is able to make his diagnosis certain by examining the blood, in which he finds not only changes in the blood cells but also specific reactions which are certain evidence of the presence of the disease. This condition resembles the old typhus fever, or jail fever, as it was called when jails were almost universally unsanitary, which is transmitted by the bite of a louse.

The use of paraminobenzoic acid has been recommended and also aureomycin, terramycin and chloromycetin. The diet should be nutritious and high in carbohydrate. Plentiful liquids are given. Most serious complication is pneumonia.

The obvious method of preventing this disease is to avoid the bite of the tick which causes it. This has been attempted in some places through eliminating rodents and through dipping cattle. As a method of prevention this has not, however, been extremely successful.

Investigators of the United States Public Health Service have developed a vaccine made of the ground-up bodies of the ticks. This is found to be a protection against infection with this disorder and can minimize severity.

Glanders

Most farmers think of glanders as a disease affecting horses and mules, but occasionally it attacks human beings. It has been reported also in cats, rabbits, sheep, mice, and various wild animals of the cat tribe.

Because the disease is commonly transmitted by horses and affects horses more frequently than any other animal, it is now rarely seen in large cities, from which horses have practically disappeared.

In the first twenty years of the present century there were seven cases of glanders in the wards of the Bellevue Hospital, New York City, but since then, not a single case has been seen.

Glanders is caused by a germ known as the bacillus of glanders. From three to five days after the germ gets into the body, the symptoms first appear. There are the usual symptoms of infection, such as nausea, headache, vomiting, chills, and some fever. Quite soon, however, nodules appear on the skin, associated with inflammation of the lymphatic ducts and glands near the places where the abscesses are located. Sometimes a hard nodule develops which ulcerates and breaks down, discharging a profuse, sticky substance. If the disease attacks the lungs it gives symptoms like those of pneumonia.

Nowadays, a diagnosis of glanders is hardly likely to be made unless the condition described happens to occur in someone who is constantly working around horses. The acute infection is very serious in the human being, and most of the patients die.

In the control of a disease like glanders, everything depends on stamping out the source of the infection in the animal which transmits it. Hence, it is recommended that practically every animal with glanders should be promptly destroyed and the stables thoroughly disinfected, including all harness and watering buckets. All animals that have been exposed should be examined for the infection and kept under observation until well past the time when there is any likelihood that the infection may develop in them.

A doctor who takes charge of such cases treats them usually by the surgical method of opening the abscesses and draining away the infectious material.

Psittacosis or Parrot Disease

In 1904, three cases of psittacosis or "parrot disease" were reported in

Boston. In the fall of 1929 an outbreak of this disease was reported in Buenos Aires, and more outbreaks have since been reported in the United States. In Hamburg, Germany, twenty-eight cases, with five deaths, occurred in the fall of 1929. In the epidemic of psittacosis which occurred in Paris in 1892 there were forty-nine cases and sixteen deaths, and it was reported that the infection had been caused by parrots brought from South America.

When psittacosis occurs it begins with a chill and fever, with a good deal of weakness and depression, and usually some inflammation of the lungs.

"Parrot disease" is essentially a medical curiosity and need occasion little alarm among the people of the United States. The symptoms resemble those of other infectious diseases, and one should be certain that the disease is actually psittacosis and not pneumonia or other infection of the lungs.

Obviously, the first step is to get the suspected parrot and to find out whether or not it contains the germs which are responsible. In addition to parrots many other bird pets occasionally become infected, including love birds, cockatoos and parakeets.

The occurrence of this condition is another demonstration of the fact that we are likely to contract diseases from all sorts of contacts and that it is not safe to demonstrate too much fondness for our animal neighbors.

Psittacosis has been known for a long time as a disease of parrots, but the first cases of pneumonic infection traced directly from parrots to man were described in 1879 in Germany.

The proof of the fact that human infection has come from the parrot depends on isolation of the germ from both the parrot and the affected human being.

In parrots, psittacosis is highly fatal, killing from 50 to 95 per cent of the infected birds. The disease can be transmitted from one parrot to another by infected feathers, food, water, dishes, or the soiled hands of attendants. Mice or insects may carry the infection from one cage to another. When a parrot becomes infected it gets weak, loses its appetite, has diarrhea, and is likely to die in a few days. Then the germs will be found in practically all of its organs.

As might be expected, a disease that can pass from parrot to man may also infect chickens, rabbits, mice, and guinea-pigs. It is interesting that this disease which chiefly infects the intestinal tracts of birds strikes the lungs in man. In many instances the infection is due to the fact that the parrot is fed by the mouth-to-mouth method. Not infrequently, however, it occurs merely from handling the sick birds, and not infrequently the person in a family who becomes sick passes the disease on with infected hands to other members of the family.

Fortunately, this disease is rare in civilized communities, probably because parrots are not nearly so frequent as pets as are other animals and birds, and probably also because the disease kills the parrots so rapidly that the likelihood of infection is lessened.

The occurrence of cases of psittacosis in the United States is new evidence of the fact that methods of transportation, exchange of products among various nations, and the complete abolishing of boundary lines between peoples make it impossible any longer for a nation to be isolated. The disease of one people will sooner or later appear among others.

The sulfonamide drugs help to stop the growth of the virus. Aureomycin and terramycin are also effective in checking the disease.

Epidemic Encephalitis

No one knows when the first epidemic of lethargy associated with fever and destruction of brain tissue first afflicted mankind, but several observers have pointed out that Hippocrates, the famous father of modern scientific medicine, himself described an epidemic of this character which appeared in the spring and continued on into the autumn, at which time it was more fatal. It was suggested that there were similar epidemics in the sixteenth century in various parts of Europe. At the end of 1890, such an epidemic occurred in southern Europe and was described under the name of *nona*.

The modern condition called epidemic encephalitis was described in Vienna in 1917, during the World War, and was given the name *encephalitis lethargica* because it is an inflammation of the brain associated with drowsiness and somnolence. The disease spread to England and to the United States and Canada; it seems possible, however, that there were individual cases in the United States before 1915.

Encephalitis means inflammation of the brain. Now many different causes of such inflammations are recognized. Transmitted by insects are St. Louis encephalitis, Japanese B, Australian X, Western equine, Venezuelan equine and Russian tick borne encephalitis. These are distinct from the condition called *nona* or epidemic lethargic encephalitis.

Epidemic encephalitis occurs most frequently in February and March but may occur at any time of the year. The condition is caused by a virus and at least seven different types of virus more or less closely related to each other have been distinguished. Principal varieties include the so-called eastern type and western or St. Louis type. The disease seems to have been more common in the United States and in Europe than on other continents. It is quite mildly contagious, but outbreaks have been reported in schools, asylums, and barracks in which large numbers of people are housed.

There has been much research in an attempt to find a preventive serum based on the discovery of virus. The virus may be transmitted to humans from lower animals like birds, rats, horses or domestic pets. Such conditions as the louping ill of sheep, X disease of Australia, "B" virus disease in monkeys, and other virus diseases are believed to be related in a group.

In most cases of encephalitis the disease occurs in three stages: first, the beginning, which is sudden; second, a milder condition following the first acute condition; and, finally, a sort of chronic condition in those who recover. In the acute stage there are the usual symptoms of infection, such as fever, weakness, headache, and running of the nose, but in addition in these cases there are quite frequently double vision and emotional disturbances indicating that the brain has been affected. Most of the patients become lethargic or sleepy at the beginning of the disease and remain in this condition until the recovery from the acute stage has taken place. There are, however, other cases which actually have insomnia, and there are some who are lethargic in the daytime and awake at night.

While these patients seem to be completely unconscious, there are recorded instances in which the patient who apparently slept was aware of everything that went on in the room. The brain was affected in such a manner that the patient could not speak or let other people know that he heard what was being said. In association with the somnolence or lethargy in many of these cases there is a delirium in which the patient may have emotional outbursts, delusions, or periods of depression. An exceedingly interesting phenomenon is the development of what is called occupational delirium, in which the person who is affected dwells constantly on the occupation; the orator continually makes speeches, the teacher lectures, the accountant adds figures.

In association with the primary symptoms that have been mentioned are many other symptoms indicating that the nervous system has been involved, such as paralyses, convulsions, tremors, and similar disorders.

After the patient has recovered from the first stage, which may have been slight—in fact, so slight as hardly to have had medical attention—comes the second stage of this disease, in which the patients are weak and say that they have been sick since an attack of influenza. They remember that they were drowsy, but they never feel well, and they are likely to be called neurasthenic or hysterical or simply plain lazy by their families. However, the condition is likely to go on to the time when anyone can realize that these patients are seriously sick, since they begin to develop symptoms like those of Parkinson's disease, or the shaking palsy. In this condition the face is mask-like, the arms and legs are held rigid, the movements are slow, the speech monotonous, and the thumb and forefinger move rather constantly in a pill-rolling movement.

In association with this there may be an apparent oversupply of saliva with some drooling from the mouth because of the changes in the muscles of the face.

There develop frequently in the later stages difficulties of behavior in children who tend to become moral imbeciles. These children are cruel, disobedient, destructive, abusive, rather filthy in their habits, and may actually become a menace from the point of view of their lack of sanity. Without a recognition of the disease which is involved such children are frequently brought before the courts and treated as criminals rather than as invalids. In the same way adults occasionally develop strange mental conditions following encephalitis and constitute a problem for those responsible for their care.

None of these patients are actually sleeping over months or years, but the mentality is seriously disturbed, and the rhythm of sleep may be changed.

Unfortunately, scientific medicine has not yet developed any specific method of treatment that will prevent this disease or arrest its progress. It does, however, attempt to aid these patients by what is called symptomatic treatment, treating each of the symptoms as it develops by well established methods. A number of serums and vaccines have been tried. These patients have been injected with non-specific proteins in the form of typhoid vaccine; malaria germs have been injected to produce shock and artificial fever; and artificial heat has been tried, but thus far the results are quite inconclusive, and no one can say definitely that any of these methods of treatment actually stops the progress of this disorder.

During 1938 outbreaks of a form of brain inflammation or unconsciousness called encephalitis broke out in North Dakota, Minnesota, Vermont and Massachusetts. In the same area at the same time there were numerous cases of a form of inflammation of the brain among horses called equine encephalomyelitis. The investigators proved that both conditions were caused by a virus of a certain type and that this virus is also to be found in a disease that affects the field mouse and other rodents, as well as partridges and pigeons. With an understanding of the nature of the disease which has thus been made available it only remains to find the chain of communication from the animals to man. Then it will be possible to prevent the further appearance of the disease among human beings.

These conditions are diagnosed by doctors through laboratory studies which demonstrate neutralizing or complement fixing antibodies in a patient's serum two weeks or more after infection. Both types of antibody persist for two years at least. After death the conditions found in the brain are not specific, but a diagnosis can be made by the demonstration of virus through intracerebral inoculation of mice with brain tissue. The virus is virulent for mice, monkeys, rabbits, guinea pigs, rats and sheep.

TREATMENT OF ALLERGIES

(See also discussion under *Allergic Conditions, Allergy, Allergy in Children, Cortisone in Skin Diseases*) Among the most important treatments developed for allergies has been the use of ACTH and cortisone and this is particularly the case with the development of the new substance called prednisone which is three to five times more powerful than hydrocortisone or cortisone. The advantage of prednisone is the lessened disturbance of water and salt metabolism in the body.

People should not however attempt to treat themselves with these powerful drugs and the doctor will try to reduce the drug as much as possible and even eliminate its use if that is possible in some of his patients. The drug is not a cure for allergy. It does temporarily control the symptoms. The cortisone drugs have been developed in many different forms for application to conditions of the skin that itch and burn, for inflamations of the eyes, and for severe reactions that may affect the bowel or the blood. Nose drops and sprays are available for nasal allergies.

TRENCH MOUTH See *Vincent's Angina.*

TRICHINOSIS

When the Jewish leaders prohibited the eating of pork around 1500 B.C., they probably did so because there had been trouble with infected pork. The infection that usually occurs is trichinosis, first recognized as a disease around 1822. The organism that causes trichinosis was not demonstrated, however, until 1835. This is a small, round worm, scarcely visible to the naked eye, quite slender and tapering. The organism multiplies freely in the intestines. After development it passes by way of the blood to the muscles, where it lives and causes pain and other serious symptoms. Occasionally considerable numbers of people are infected by eating pork that has been improperly inspected, insufficiently cooked, and improperly handled.

The United States Department of Agriculture requires storage of pork at a temperature of 5 degrees Fahrenheit or below for twenty days before it is used. This will destroy all the trichina organisms. Occasionally, however, meat of animals killed for home consumption is not properly controlled; then the people who eat the meat get the symptoms of trichinosis. A temperature of 137 degrees Fahrenheit for a sufficient period of time will destroy the organisms of trichinosis; therefore proper cooking of pork will help to prevent an outbreak.

In a typical case the symptoms begin with headache, chills, and a general feeling of illness. Then the eyes become swollen and painful. There may be sore throat and a general soreness of the muscles. Fever appears. Examination of the blood reveals the presence of great numbers of white blood cells and especially an increase of one type of white blood cell known as eosinophiles.

There is not much to be done in the way of specific treatment of the disease. After a while the tissues of the body surround the organisms and encapsulate them.

The way to avoid this disease is to make sure that all pork products are properly inspected, properly stored, and properly cooked. At the same time there must be a campaign of education as to the feeding of swine. Swine which are fed on garbage are infested with trichinae from three to five times as often as swine that are fed on grain. In some instances the infection gets into the hogs from the eating of rats. The feeding of garbage to swine may seem economical, but if it is to result in any considerable number of cases of trichinosis, it will prove far more costly than will the feeding of suitable material free from the possibility of infection.

TRIGEMINAL NEURALGIA (See also, *Neuralgia*) Given the French name of *tic douloureux*. In this condition there is severe paroxysmal pain in the various portions of the face to which the nerve from the brain reaches. The pain is sharp and usually lasts less than a minute. The pain can be caused by pressure on the angle of the mouth, the cheek, or a tooth, by eating, drinking, washing, shaving, or even by blowing on the face. Physicians have found that the injection of alcohol into the nerve will stop the pain, and a surgical operation has been developed for cutting the nerve away from the ganglion cell. This operation which is done by specialists called neurologic surgeons has now been proved to be successful in many instances.

TRYPSIN IN ALLERGY (See *Allergic Conditions, Allergy, Allergy in Children, Treatment of Allergies*) two groups of investigators reported to the American College of Allergists that the inhaling of a mist of trypsin, an enzyme that dissolves proteins, was a great help to people with conditions in which the lungs fill up with mucus. When inhaled, the vapor thinned down thick, sticky mucus making it much easier for the patient to cough up.

TUBERCULOSIS Tuberculosis has destroyed more human beings than any other disease. Today it is still seventh in the list of causes of death. It destroys life mostly in early and middle adult ages, at the time when people are most productive economically and most useful. It kills more men than women proportionately and attacks colored people much more seriously than it does the white race. Some 80,000 people die each year from this infection.

In 1910, 136 out of every 100,000 people in our country died from tuberculosis. In 1932 it was 56.4. Today the rate is near to 20. Nevertheless, our present death rate means that between 7,000,000 and 8,000,000 people now living in the United States will die eventually of tuberculosis unless some new discovery or wider use of present methods materially controls the condition.

The discovery of new drugs like streptomycin, paramino salicylic acid, and isoniazid has stimulated research. New methods are now being intensively studied. Combinations of various new remedies are so effective in treatment that many people are now treated while ambulatory instead of being placed in sanatoriums.

Tuberculosis is a germ disease. It is not an inherited disease. Usually it attacks children through contact of the child with some older person who has the disease or with an animal suffering from the disease or with food products or other materials contaminated by the germ. Sometimes the disease attacks not in childhood but later along in life. Modern methods of diagnosis reveal that the tendency is more and more for protection of the child against the disease until a later period in his life.

We now have tests which show whether or not a child has been or is infected with the germs of tuberculosis. These tests can be applied to large groups of children to determine the extent of infection. In some areas every child is examined by these methods. England has just arranged for their use on a large scale.

People seldom suspected tuberculosis in previous times until severe coughs with expectoration began with loss of weight and night sweats. With modern methods the disease is detected long before any such serious signs are present. The use of the X ray shows promptly changes which occur in the lung. The use of the tuberculin tests can demonstrate the presence of the disease. Many people now arrange to have their family doctor use such technics at regular intervals to find out whether or not children are in danger.

In the tuberculin test a small amount of material called tuberculin is applied to the skin or in some cases injected between the layers of the skin. If the skin reacts positively to this material, the significance is that the tissues have been sensitized to the material of the germ of tuberculosis. A positive tuberculin test means that the tubercle germs have entered the body and that somewhere in the body there is infection.

There may, of course, be cases in which the reactions are doubtful and other cases in which other possible evidence of tuberculosis cannot be found by any of the well-accepted measures. In most instances this should indicate, however, either the necessity for further testing or the necessity for continued watchfulness and further study to determine the point at which the infection is localized.

Not always will a person who has a positive tuberculin test become severely sick with this disease. Approximately 20 per cent of those who react positively to this test do present manifestations of the disease at some subsequent time. We do not, however, have any certain way of knowing which of those who react positively will fall into the 80 per cent of those who are going to be safe and which will fall into the 20 per cent of those who are going to be severely infected. The safe measure is, therefore, to examine carefully at regular intervals those who react positively to the tuberculin test.

CAUSE—Tuberculosis is caused by a germ, first described by the bacteriologist Robert Koch. There are different kinds of tubercle germs—those which affect human beings primarily, those which affect cattle, those which affect birds, and those which affect cold-blooded

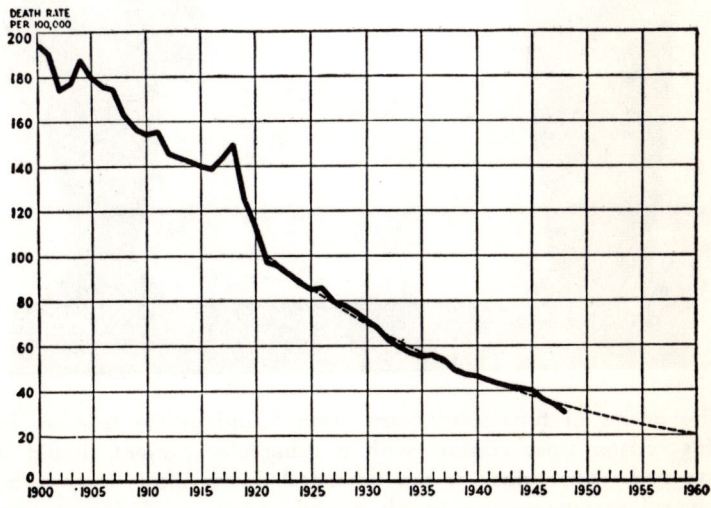

Decline in tuberculosis mortality in the United States since 1900.

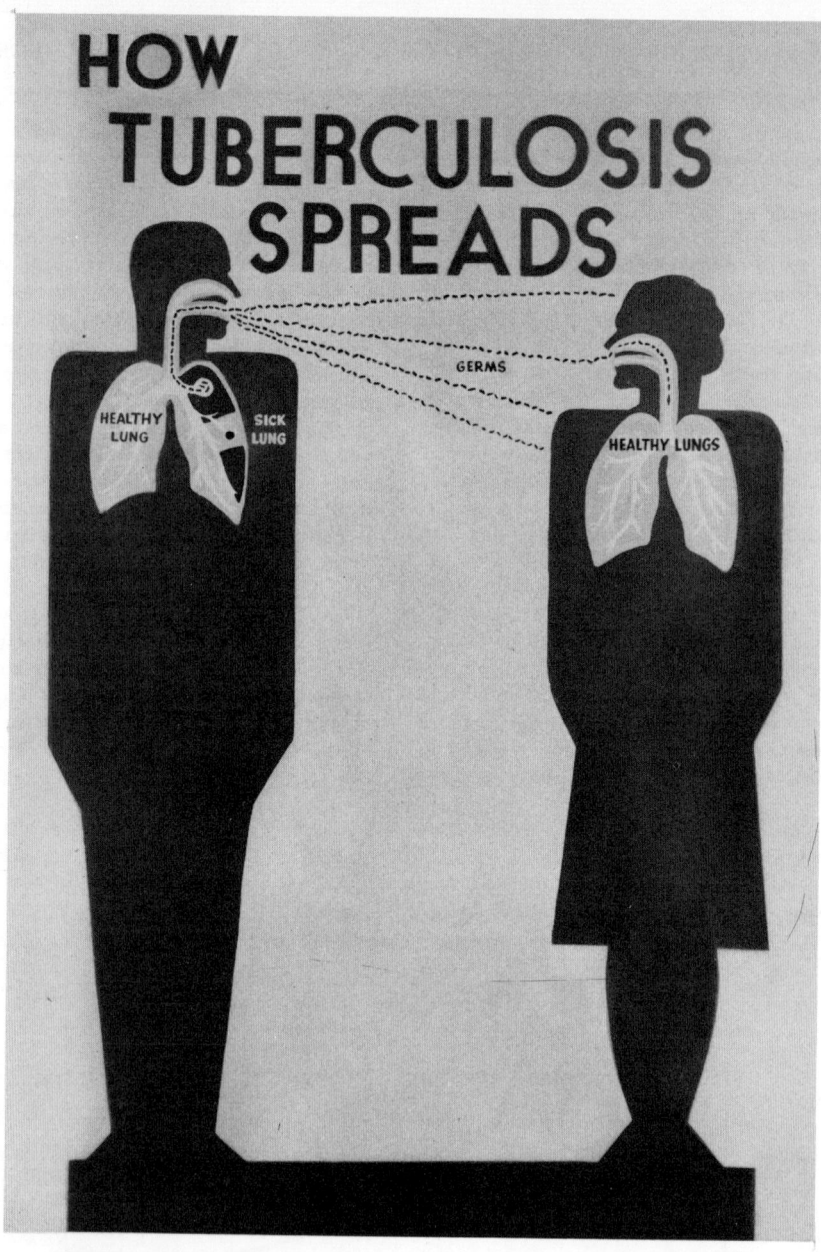

The germs of tuberculosis are often found in the sputum. For this reason close contact with a tubercular patient should be avoided. Tuberculosis is not inherited. Tuberculosis may attack several members of a family mainly because of close contact and greater opportunity for infection.   Cleveland Health Museum animals like the frog and the turtle. The ones which affect cattle are most like those which affect man, but the human type is more dangerous to a human being than it is to domestic animals, and the cattle type is more dangerous to domestic animals than it is to man.

The cattle type may, however, infect human beings, especially children. Indeed the bovine, or cattle, form of tuberculosis is known to be largely responsible for tuberculosis of the bones, joints, and lymph glands of children who have been in the past infected by drinking milk from cows infected with bovine tuberculosis.

As a result of the recognition of this menace to health milk supplies are controlled by submitting cattle to the tuberculin test and by eliminating from the herds of cows those which are found to have the disease. In the United States we have cut down the incidence of tuberculosis in cattle to the vanishing point. There are still countries in the world, however, including England, where tuberculosis, particularly of bones, joints, and glands, has not been well controlled. In the United States tuberculosis of the glands of the abdomen is exceedingly uncommon and, when it does occur, is mild. In other countries in which control of tuberculous cattle has not been so efficient, such tuberculosis continues to appear. In most instances tuberculosis of the glands of the abdomen is due to the swallowing of germs which have been coughed up from the lungs or to milk products containing the germs of tuberculosis.

One of the saddest forms of tuberculosis is that which causes a crippling of the spine. This condition is called Pott's disease after a British physician named Pott who first described it. When one of the bones of the spine becomes involved, the central portion of the bone is broken down and softened so that the muscles pull the bones together and produce the buckling of the spine which is characteristic of Pott's disease. Tuberculosis may also affect the hip joint or other joint or other bones, producing crippling injuries which are easily recognizable. Tuberculosis may affect the glands, the covering of the brain, the spinal fluid, the eye, and many other tissues as well as the lung. In each instance it is necessary for the doctor to make a suitable diagnosis and then to treat the condition according to the portion of the body that is concerned. It is quite possible for a person to have not only tuberculosis of the lung but at the same time some of the other forms of the disease that have been mentioned.

At one time it was thought necessary for every child to have tuberculosis in order to develop resistance against the disease. We now recognize that this was a view like the old belief that every child ought to be exposed to measles so as to have the disease and get it over with.

There now is in Britain a definite increase in bone and joint tuberculosis among children. Be sure that children get grade A pasteurized milk; that is insurance against milk as a source of tuberculosis.

PREVENTION—The truly extensive knowledge of tuberculosis which we now have should make its complete prevention an ultimate possibility. The disease cannot be stamped out overnight, but persistence can control it, as some states and cities already are proving. The first step is elimination of the exposure of young children to infection from adults with whom they come in contact. Today we are crowded together beyond anything that occurred in the past. The home has largely disappeared in our great cities. We have tremendous apartment houses, tenements, and barracks. These apartments are occupied by from three to a hundred families, where the children come in contact not only

NEWLY REPORTED ACTIVE* TUBERCULOSIS CASES PER 100,000 POPULATION, UNITED STATES AND TERRITORIES, 1954
(Provisional Data)

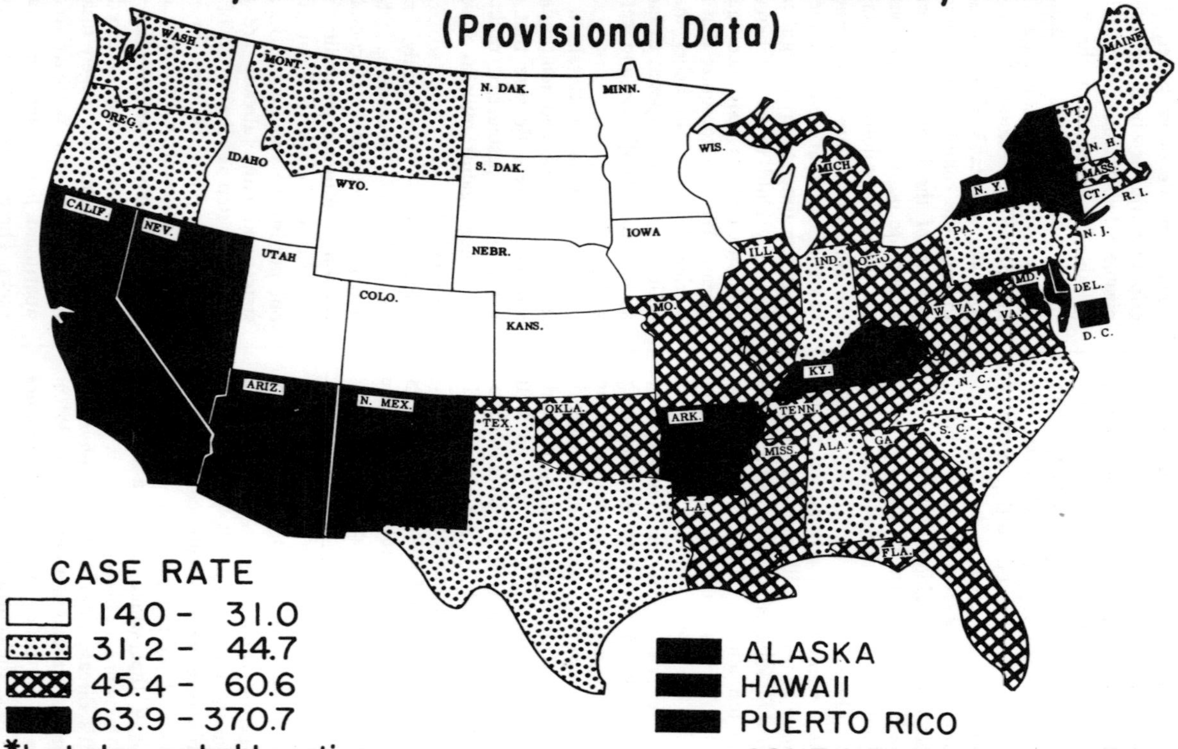

CASE RATE
- 14.0 – 31.0
- 31.2 – 44.7
- 45.4 – 60.6
- 63.9 – 370.7

*Includes probably active

ALASKA
HAWAII
PUERTO RICO
CONTINENTAL U.S. 49.1

with their own parents and relatives but with vast numbers of other children and other families. A child of an earlier day played in his own back yard until the age of six. Today the child goes early to nursery school or plays about with others while his mother is at work. Then he goes to kindergarten and afterward to assemble with other children in public schools. Human beings are crowded together in streetcars, busses, and elevators, and assemble in crowds of thousands in motion picture houses and in crowds of tens of hundreds of thousands at various public events. It is not possible for any person living in a modern city to avoid contact with other human beings.

We know that the people of many portions of the world did not have tuberculosis until it was brought to them by civilized human beings. We know, moreover, that the first infection coming into a population which has not been previously subjected to tuberculosis is far more destructive than an infection coming into a community in which there has always been tuberculosis.

The attack on tuberculosis must be not only a medical but also an economic attack. This is a disease associated with bad hygiene. It multiplies when there is an insufficient amount of food, rest, sunlight, and fresh air. It can be shown that a sudden drop in wages or financial depression will result in an increase of tuberculosis.

When the germ of tuberculosis gets into the body either by direct inhalation of germs or by inhaling dust containing the germs or by any of the other methods that have been mentioned, it tends to localize and to set up an infection. The infection may be a sudden, severe one or a slower and more chronic infection. It seems likely that sometimes a child is lightly infected with the disease, recovering quite promptly, but that it is thereafter sensitive to a new infection with the same organism.

The germs which establish themselves in the body form lesions or spots of infection which are typical of tuberculosis. These areas may become secondarily infected with other organisms which, of course, change the general picture of the disease.

Symptoms—The symptoms by which most people know tuberculosis include the cough, which is an indication of an infection of the lung, whether by tuberculosis or by some other germ. Any cough that lasts for three or four weeks is always suspect of the possibility that it presents a disease of the lungs. With the cough there is frequently expectoration. There is also in certain cases enough destruction of lung tissue so that the person with tuberculosis may expectorate some blood. Also there may be pouring out of fluid into the walls of the chest—an example of the attempts of the body to control the infection.

Because of the manner in which the disease attacks the human body, the person with tuberculosis is generally rather sick and complains of loss of strength and loss of weight. There may also be a slight afternoon rise of temperature or fever and associated with that an increase in the rate of the pulse. The night sweats are commonly found in the presence of tuberculosis, but they may be caused by many other conditions as well. When a physician finds symptoms and signs of this character in a patient, he then extends his examination promptly to take advantage of modern methods of diagnosis. Chief among these methods of examination is the use of the X ray. The X-ray pictures will show in many instances the extent of involvement of the lung. The doctor will also put to use all of the older systems of examination which have been proved valuable by many years of experience. These include a general examination of the chest to determine any changes that have taken place in its shape or its contour and also in its movements. The doctor puts his hands on the chest to find out whether or not there are spasms of the muscles or vibrations associated with the passing of air into the lung or out of it. He thumps the chest in order to find out by the sounds whether or not there is dullness, tympanic response, or increased resonance.

These and other signs indicate to the doctor the nature of the changes in the tissue of the lung. Next he listens with his stethoscope, because the various sounds made by the air passing into the lung indicate the presence of interference with the passing of the air, the presence of fluid, the presence of solid tissue, or other changes.

The sputum of the patient is examined for the presence of the germs of tuberculosis, and if these are found present by suitable straining methods, the evidence is well-nigh unimpeachable. The absence of the germs does not, however, exclude the disease because in the earlier stages of the disease they may be absent in as many as 35 per cent of cases.

The hope of successful treatment in this disease depends largely on the recognition of the disease at the earliest possible moment. Hence, whenever there is any question of tuberculosis, those concerned should have everything in the way of diagnostic aid that modern medicine can offer to prove the presence or absence of this disease.

TREATMENT—Once the doctor has determined the extent of the tuberculosis, the age of the infections, the portions of tissue involved, and other important factors, it is necessary for him to decide what to do about treatment and also to decide what to tell the patient about his future. The future of the patient depends on the extent of the disease at the time treatment is begun, the character of the disease—namely, whether it is a rapidly progressive or slowly progressive type—the extent to which other organs have been involved by complications, and the general condition of the body so far as relates to its nutrition and general existence.

Much depends on the amount of response that the patient may make to the proper treatment. If he responds favorably and promptly, he is much more likely to do well than if it is difficult to get any change. The age of the patient is also of great importance.

Generally speaking, the more advanced the disease happens to be at the time when the diagnosis is made, the poorer is the likelihood of recovery. In cases of tuberculosis that are far advanced recovery in more than 10 to 20 per cent of the cases is unlikely. Tuberculosis is more quickly fatal and more serious in the extremely young than in those who are older. Where living conditions are exceedingly bad, the likelihood of recovery is not so great. The temperament of the patient and his attitude toward the disease are important factors, because a patient without hope and without anxiety to recover will not give to his doctor or his nurse the kind of co-operation that is necessary in this disease. If the patient happens to have diabetes, heart disease, or some kidney disturbance in addition to tuberculosis, his chance of recovery is less.

Nowadays cases of tuberculosis are classified as minimal, moderately advanced, or far advanced. Another classification describes the cases as apparently cured, arrested, apparently arrested, quiescent, improved, or unimproved. A decision as to the exact status of the case rests in every instance on a complete study of the condition, using all of the best available modern methods of physical and laboratory examination.

One of the first measures to be considered formerly was a change of climate. Nowadays it is believed quite possible to get a suitable climate anywhere in the world. The only advantage in traveling to hunt a cure is the advantage that accrues from a change of surroundings.

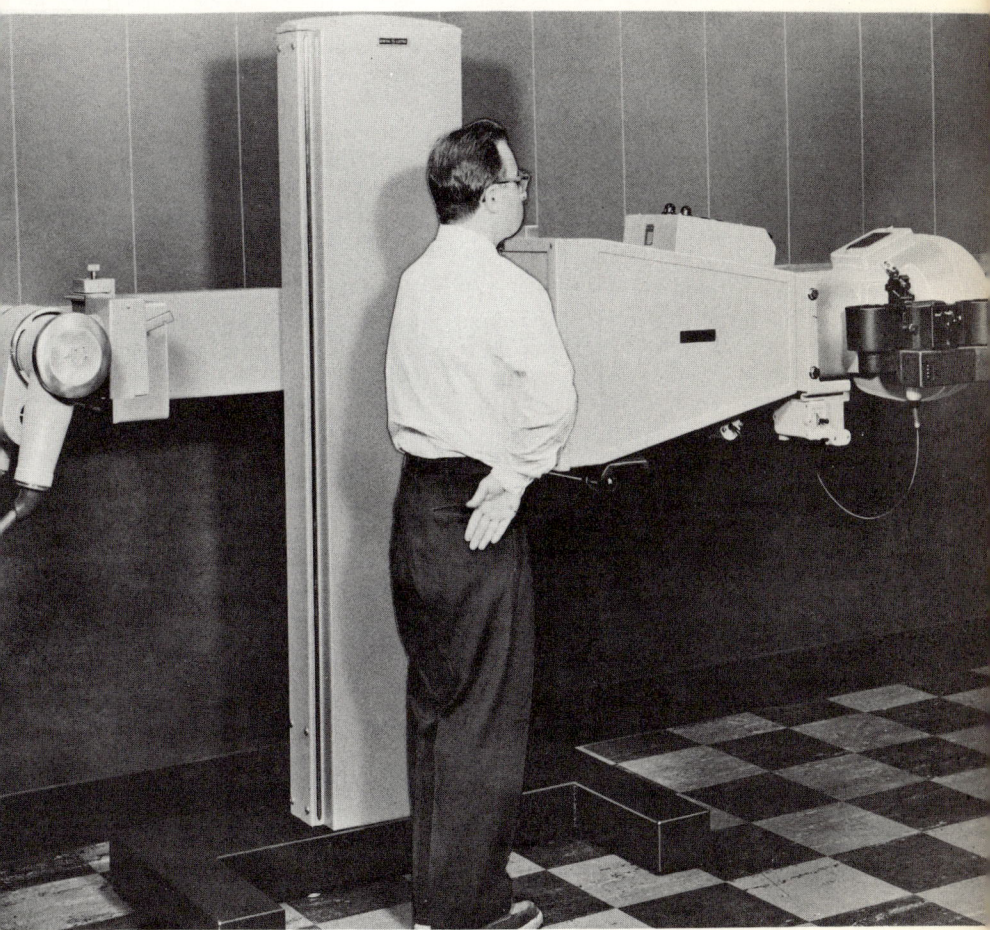

The annual chest X-ray has become a familiar experience for most of us. Special chest X-ray units like this one have contributed greatly to the speedy examination of large groups of people. Diseases, such as tuberculosis, can be detected earlier and treated more effectively. The person being X-rayed is leaning against the film plate, and the source of X-rays is the tube shown at the left. *General Electric*

In general it is well established that open air is helpful to the tuberculous and that it is most effective when the temperature of the air is cool and bracing. One authority points out that the favorable effect of rest in the open air on the toxic symptoms of tuberculosis is often striking. This measure of treatment may be begun promptly and developed until it becomes a habit. The patient can be out of doors during all of the daytime and in many cases sleep out of doors as well, although outdoor sleeping is not essential if plenty of air is available by use of screened porches or open windows. In general cold air seems to be helpful, but if the circulation of the blood is not good and the reaction to cold air is insufficient, exposure to cold air need not be a routine. In any type of outdoor life exposure to dust, wind, rain, and fog is undesirable. Heat or cold in great excess are dangerous to health. In general warm, moist climates are believed to have a depressing effect, and cool, dry climates to be stimulating. There is really no one best climate for all who are tuberculous. Proper treatment under scientific conditions is more important than climate alone.

New remedies such as streptomycin and neomycin and para-aminosalicylic acid have revolutionized the treatment of tuberculosis. They are used particularly for tuberculosis in the young, tuberculous meningitis, and tuberculosis of the larynx.

CLIMATE AND TUBERCULOSIS—There was a time when everyone who had tuberculosis immediately began traveling. Not long ago the United States Government, through the United States Public Health Service, protested against the shipping of patients to certain states when such patients did not have the means for the necessities of life after they arrived at the new location. The minimum costs of care approximate twenty-five to fifty dollars a week. Unless an invalid is able to provide from twelve to eighteen hundred dollars a year for his care, he cannot do himself much good by moving to another state in which neither his citizenship nor his residency is established. When the burden of providing for himself in a strange town is added to the burdens of the disease from which he suffers, the invalid loads himself with a handicap so great that it may mean the difference between life and death.

After a consideration of all of the various factors involved in the climatic factors of tuberculosis, Dr. James Alexander Miller summarizes the situation with ten aphorisms which follow:

1. The regimen of regulated rest and exercise, proper food, and open-air life is the fundamental essential in the treatment of tuberculosis. Suitable climatic environment makes this open-air life more easy, enjoyable, and beneficial.

2. When these essentials are assured, a change of climate is of definite value in a considerable number, probably the majority of cases, but with the proper regimen many cases will do well in any climate.

3. Any change of climate involving the fatigue of travel is contraindicated in acute cases with fever or hemorrhage, or in very far advanced and markedly debilitated cases. Absolute bed rest is the one essential here.

4. No patient should be sent away in search of climate who cannot afford to stay the reasonably-to-be-expected time and to have the necessary food, lodging, and care.

5. Competent medical advice and supervision are essential.

6. One of the most valuable assets of change is the education of the patient. This may, of course, be obtained in a suitable environment without reference to climate, as in a sanatorium near home.

7. Selection of a suitable locality is an individual problem for every patient, depending upon his temperament, tastes, and individual reaction to environment, as well as the character of his disease. The advising physician should have an appreciation of these as well as a knowledge of the particular environment to which the patient is being sent. Contentment and reasonable comfort are essential.

8. There is no universally ideal climate. For each patient there may well be a most favorable environment, if we are wise enough to find it.

9. There is a reasonable amount of evidence that certain medical types of cases are more favorably influenced by certain conditions of climate, everything else being equal. For example reasonably cold, dry, variable climate, such as is found in the mountains, for young or vigorous constitutions which will react well. Dry, sunny climates for laryngeal cases and those with marked catarrhal secretions. Equable mild climates at low altitudes for the elderly and those of nervous temperaments, as well as for those with arteriosclerosis, weak hearts, or marked tendency to dyspnea.

10. Successful selection of climate and environment for cases of tuberculosis requires wide knowledge of human nature, of places, and of the disease. This can only be acquired by patience, skill, and experience.

ARTIFICIAL PNEUMOTHORAX—Among the many ways in which the lung of the person with tuberculosis may be rested, that which has received the greatest consideration in recent years is the so-called application of pneumothorax, sometimes called collapse treatment. There are many different ways by which a lung may be collapsed so that the tissues may be quiet and out of use until they have opportunity to recover. The purpose of collapse is not only to give rest to the lung but also to hinder the spread of the disease from one portion of the lung to another.

The first of the procedures is known as artificial pneumothorax, and it seems to be applicable in anywhere from one fourth to one half of all cases, preferably those in which only one lung or a portion of one lung is involved rather than a considerable amount of both lungs. This method is not suitable to patients who have large amounts of fluid in the chest or those in whom there has been a great deal of pleurisy with attachment of the lung to the chest wall.

In brief the method of treatment involves the insertion of a needle into the chest cavity and the passing of air into the cavity from without in sufficient amounts to compress the lung tissue and to stop its motion. Some investigators have suggested the injection of mineral oil into the chest cavity instead of air, but this procedure has not been widely adopted.

It is also possible to put the lung at rest by cutting the nerve which goes to the diaphragm. Elimination of movement of the muscles of the diaphragm and of the chest on the side concerned causes the diaphragm to be rested and thus to diminish the amount of work in the chest cavity.

Another method is wholly surgical and is seldom used until after pneumothorax has been tried and failed or else has been found to be impossible to apply. In this method, known as thoracoplasty, there is an actual operation on the chest wall involving the removal of portions of the ribs, thus bringing about collapse and complete rest of the lung tissue.

In many instances the method of artificial pneumothorax fails because it is not applied soon enough. When the method of treatment is applied soon enough and in the proper manner, patients who would in previous years have been compelled to remain constantly in the sanatorium are actually given opportunity to go about their work. It cannot be expected, however, from this or any other method of treatment that the patient will recover immediately. In many instances the pneumothorax must be kept up for one, two, or three years before signs of healing appear as shown by the use of the X ray and other modern methods of investigation.

THE CHANGING CHARACTER OF TUBERCULOSIS was the subject of a report published by the Joint Tuberculosis Council of Great Britain. The declining death rate is associated with an apparent increasing longevity in survivors. Certain types of the disease—such as tuberculous laryngitis, enteritis, and cervical adenitis—are now infrequent. In pulmonary disease the focus is relatively more often detected than in the past.

Changes in the social pattern of tuberculosis, and of the types of disease seen in the individual patient, have been observed throughout the world. Though deaths have declined, laboratory and clinical studies do not support the view that the bacillus is becoming less virulent. New cases fall into two groups: young adults with primary infection progressing to overt disease, and older males in whom recrudescence of disease acquired earlier in life leads to breakdown in health. Public-health measures can reduce the risks of infection for young adults, but they have less effect in preventing disease in the older men. The pool of infection therefore tends to persist among the older section of the population, and the proportion of tuberculous patients in this age group is rising. In the United States the lower rate of infection among young people is showing itself in the results of tuberculin tests on recruits for the armed services. In 1949 and 1950 10.6% of the recruits (aged 17-20) joining the U.S. Navy and Marines were positive reactors, compared with 65.6% of the National Service men in Britain. By 1954 the percentage of positive reactors among the American recruits had fallen to 4.6.

The case fatality rate has improved since 1948. The risk of infection in the community is also diminished, for many chronic sputum-positive cases, though not healed by prolonged chemotherapy, may be rendered sputum-negative for long periods.

Tuberculosis, though declining, has become a more chronic disease. "The intrinsic character of tuberculosis has not altered since the time before the 1939-45 war, but the pattern of disease is being progressively modified by various factors.

TUBERCULIN TESTS—See RESPIRATORY DISEASES, article THE RESPIRATORY DISEASES; article ALLERGY.

TUBERCULIN TESTS—children: See RESPIRATORY DISEASES, article THE RESPIRATORY DISEASES.

TUBERCULOSIS—See article SEX HYGIENE; RESPIRATORY DISEASES, article THE RESPIRATORY DISEASES.

TUBERCULOSIS—ACTH contraindicated: See article ALLERGY.

TUBERCULOSIS—Addison's disease as one manifestation: See article ENDOCRINOLOGY.

TUBERCULOSIS—arthritis may result: See article ARTHRITIS, RHEUMATISM, AND GOUT.

TUBERCULOSIS—asthma mistakenly diagnosed: See article ALLERGY.

TUBERCULOSIS—beds available in United States: See RESPIRATORY DISEASES, article THE RESPIRATORY DISEASES.

TUBERCULOSIS—beryllium poisoning produces similar changes in lungs: See article OCCUPATION AND HEALTH.

TUBERCULOSIS—bleeding lungs, first aid: See article FIRST AID.

TUBERCULOSIS—bones: See INFECTIOUS DISEASE, article THE PREVENTION AND TREATMENT OF INFECTIOUS DISEASE.
TUBERCULOSIS—cattle: See RESPIRATORY DISEASES, article THE RESPIRATORY DISEASES.
TUBERCULOSIS—cause determined: See INFECTIOUS DISEASE, article THE PREVENTION AND TREATMENT OF INFECTIOUS DISEASE.
TUBERCULOSIS—climate in prevention and treatment: See RESPIRATORY DISEASES, article THE RESPIRATORY DISEASES.
TUBERCULOSIS—cortisone contraindicated: See article ALLERGY.
TUBERCULOSIS—death rate: See RESPIRATORY DISEASES, article THE RESPIRATORY DISEASES; article DIABETES; HEART, article DISEASES OF THE HEART AND CIRCULATION.
TUBERCULOSIS—detected early in diabetics: See article DIABETES.
TUBERCULOSIS—diabetes mortality lower: See article DIABETES.
TUBERCULOSIS—diabetes seldom complicated by: See article DIABETES.
TUBERCULOSIS—diet: See RESPIRATORY DISEASES, article THE RESPIRATORY DISEASES.
TUBERCULOSIS—disordered action of the heart classified as: See HEART, article DISEASES OF THE HEART AND CIRCULATION.
TUBERCULOSIS—endocarditis symptoms similar: See HEART, article DISEASES OF THE HEART AND CIRCULATION.
TUBERCULOSIS—eye: See INFECTIOUS DISEASE, article THE PREVENTION AND TREATMENT OF INFECTIOUS DISEASE.
TUBERCULOSIS—eye infection may accompany: See EYE, article THE EYE.
TUBERCULOSIS—foot deformities may result: See FOOT, article THE FOOT.
TUBERCULOSIS—health resorts, costs of: See RESPIRATORY DISEASES, article THE RESPIRATORY DISEASES.
TUBERCULOSIS—heart disease less expensive in cost of human lives: See HEART, article DISEASES OF THE HEART AND CIRCULATION.
TUBERCULOSIS—hypotension: See article BLOOD PRESSURE.
TUBERCULOSIS—incidence: See INFECTIOUS DISEASE, article THE PREVENTION AND TREATMENT OF INFECTIOUS DISEASE.
TUBERCULOSIS—joints: See INFECTIOUS DISEASE, article THE PREVENTION AND TREATMENT OF INFECTIOUS DISEASE.
TUBERCULOSIS—kidneys: See KIDNEY, article THE KIDNEY: ITS DISEASES AND DISTURBANCES.
TUBERCULOSIS—larynx: See RESPIRATORY DISEASES, article THE RESPIRATORY DISEASES.
TUBERCULOSIS—lungs: See article FIRST AID; INFECTIOUS DISEASE, article THE PREVENTION AND TREATMENT OF INFECTIOUS DISEASE.
TUBERCULOSIS—measles lowers resistance: See CHILDHOOD DISEASES, article INFECTIOUS DISEASES OF CHILDHOOD.
TUBERCULOSIS—menopause formerly believed to cause: See article SEX HYGIENE.
TUBERCULOSIS—nervous system: See INFECTIOUS DISEASE, article THE PREVENTION AND TREATMENT OF INFECTIOUS DISEASE.
TUBERCULOSIS—predisposition in children with congenitally defective hearts: See HEART, article DISEASES OF THE HEART AND CIRCULATION.
TUBERCULOSIS—renal albuminuria: See KIDNEY, article THE KIDNEY: ITS DISEASES AND DISTURBANCES.
TUBERCULOSIS—resistance reduced by chronic disorders: See INFECTIOUS DISEASE, article THE PREVENTION AND TREATMENT OF INFECTIOUS DISEASE.
TUBERCULOSIS—respiratory disease: See RESPIRATORY DISEASES, article THE RESPIRATORY DISEASES.
TUBERCULOSIS—retina changes: See

Eye, article The Eye.

Tuberculosis—rheumatism may result: See article Arthritis, Rheumatism, and Gout.

Tuberculosis—scalp changes: See Hair, article The Hair.

Tuberculosis—secondary invader in measles: See Childhood Diseases, article Infectious Diseases of Childhood.

Tuberculosis—silicosis: See article Occupation and Health.

Tuberculosis—skin reaction: See Skin, article The Skin.

Tuberculosis—symptoms produced by an allergy: See article Allergy.

Tuberculosis—tobacco: See article Occupation and Health.

Tuberculosis—undulant fever resembles: See article Transmissible Diseases.

Tuberculosis—whooping cough frequently precedes: See Childhood Diseases, article Infectious Diseases of Childhood.

Tuberculosis—young married couples: See article Sex Hygiene.

TULAREMIA Almost twenty years have passed since Dr. Edward Francis of the United States Public Health Service announced the discovery of a disease infecting human beings who had been in contact with diseased rabbits. Rarely the condition is carried to a human being by a tick. By far the most common source of infection is an infection of the hands of a person who has dressed the flesh of a diseased rabbit for cooking purposes. The rabbit meat thoroughly cooked is harmless as a food, since a temperature of 130 degrees Fahrenheit will kill the germ of tularemia.

When tularemia appears on the body, there is usually an ulcer at the point where the germs entered through the skin. The ulcer usually appears several days after the exposure to the infected rabbit. Following the appearance of the ulcer, there develop aching of the muscles and joints, weakness, chills, and fever, which may last for several weeks.

Tularemia, or rabbit fever, gets its name from Tulare County, California. Some years ago the wild game in Tulare County were found to be dying by the thousands because of a plaguelike condition that was spreading among them. The germ isolated was the germ of tularemia.

Chiefly it is the wild rabbit that is infected, although the past twenty years have brought to light cases of infection in almost every other type of small wild animal, including muskrats, opossums, and water rats, also squirrels, cats, and sheep.

During the year 1938, 545 cases of tularemia were found in a survey of twenty large cities with a total population of 20,000,000 people.

Men who hunt rabbits should be warned of the danger of bringing home for cooking any rabbit that can be knocked over with a stick. A healthy rabbit is one that can run like a "scared rabbit" when the hunter approaches. The animal that can be knocked down is one that is likely to be infected with tularemia or some other disease.

People who handle rabbits for any purpose ought to wear rubber gloves. If they do not, they should wash their hands thoroughly in some mild antiseptic solution and most thoroughly with soap and water after they have finished the handling of the rabbits. Never let a scratch, a cut, or a sore come in contact with the flesh of the rabbit or with the dish or pan in which rabbit meat has been kept. Wrapping paper which has contained the bodies of dead rabbits should be burned. The attention of the doctor should be called to every cut or sore just as soon as there is the slightest evidence of swelling or secondary infection.

TULAREMIA—occupational disease: See article OCCUPATION AND HEALTH.

TULAREMIA—transmissible disease: See article TRANSMISSIBLE DISEASES.

TULAREMIA—treatment: See article TRANSMISSIBLE DISEASES.

TUMORS A word describing any overgrowth of tissue. See discussion under *Cancer*.

GROWTHS—skin: See SKIN, article THE SKIN.

TUMORS—arthritis: See article ARTHRITIS, RHEUMATISM, AND GOUT.

TUMORS—described: See article CANCER.

TUMORS—ear: See EAR, article THE EAR, TONGUE, NOSE, AND THROAT.

TUMORS—jaundice: See article DIGESTION AND DIGESTIVE DISEASES.

TUMORS—keloids: See SKIN, article THE SKIN.

TUMORS—kidney: See KIDNEY, article THE KIDNEY: ITS DISEASES AND DISTURBANCES.

TUMORS—lymph node: See BLOOD, article THE BLOOD AND ITS DISEASES.

TUMORS—nose: See EAR, article THE EAR, TONGUE, NOSE, AND THROAT.

TUMORS—pancreas: See article ENDOCRINOLOGY.

TUMORS—pituitary: See article ENDOCRINOLOGY.

TUMORS—rheumatism: See article ARTHRITIS, RHEUMATISM, AND GOUT.

TUMORS—uterus: See article ENDOCRINOLOGY.

TUMORS—vascular: See SKIN, article THE SKIN.

TUMORS—X-ray used to detect: See article DIGESTION AND DIGESTIVE DISEASES.

TYPHOID FEVER Once typhoid fever was first in the subjects seriously discussed in textbooks of medicine. Today it has been relegated to a less important position because modern sanitary methods have practically eliminated the danger of typhoid fever in a modern community.

If the case rates and death rates that prevailed in Chicago in 1880 existed today, there would be 60,000 cases of typhoid fever and approximately 6000 deaths from that disease every year. Instead Chicago has seldom had as many as 200 cases with 10 deaths in any one year.

Typhoid fever is an acute infection caused by a germ known as the typhoid bacillus. The germ can be found in the blood of a person seriously sick with the disease, and in 80 per cent of cases the typhoid germ is found in the material that is passed by the bowels. The germ of typhoid fever is spread by means of the excretions of the body, by contaminated food and clothing, and by water and milk which contain the germs. The primary menace in typhoid fever today is the typhoid carrier, the person who has had the disease and recovered but who still continues to give off the germs.

Typhoid fever follows a long and serious course once a person becomes infected. From three to twenty-one days after the infection, which is known as the incubation period, the germs develop in the body and liberate their poisons. Typhoid fever begins with the usual symptoms of infection, such as headache, pains all over the body, the feeling of exhaustion, chills, and fever. Frequently there is nosebleed, and almost invariably there is serious disturbance of the bowels due to the fact that the typhoid germs produce ulcers in the bowels. As the disease goes on, the infected person becomes sicker and sicker; clots may form in the blood vessels; rose spots appear on the skin at the end of the first week or beginning of the second week. Because of the damage to the bowels, there is formation of gas with bloating and sometimes severe hemorrhages from the bowels.

TYPHOID FEVER

Occasionally the infection also attacks the nervous system, producing pains and even delirium.

The doctor who examines the patient with typhoid fever makes his diagnosis from the history of the case, the nature of the symptoms, and also by careful studies of the blood. A blood test called the Widal test is a means of determining with reasonable certainty that the condition is typhoid fever.

A person who has typhoid fever must be kept alone and preferably cared for by an experienced nurse. The room should be screened if the illness occurs during the summer when flies are common.

Because the person with typhoid is likely to remain in bed for a long time, he should have a firm mattress, and arrangements must be made to change the bed linen any time it is soiled. The patient must be bathed at least once a day and kept clean in order to prevent

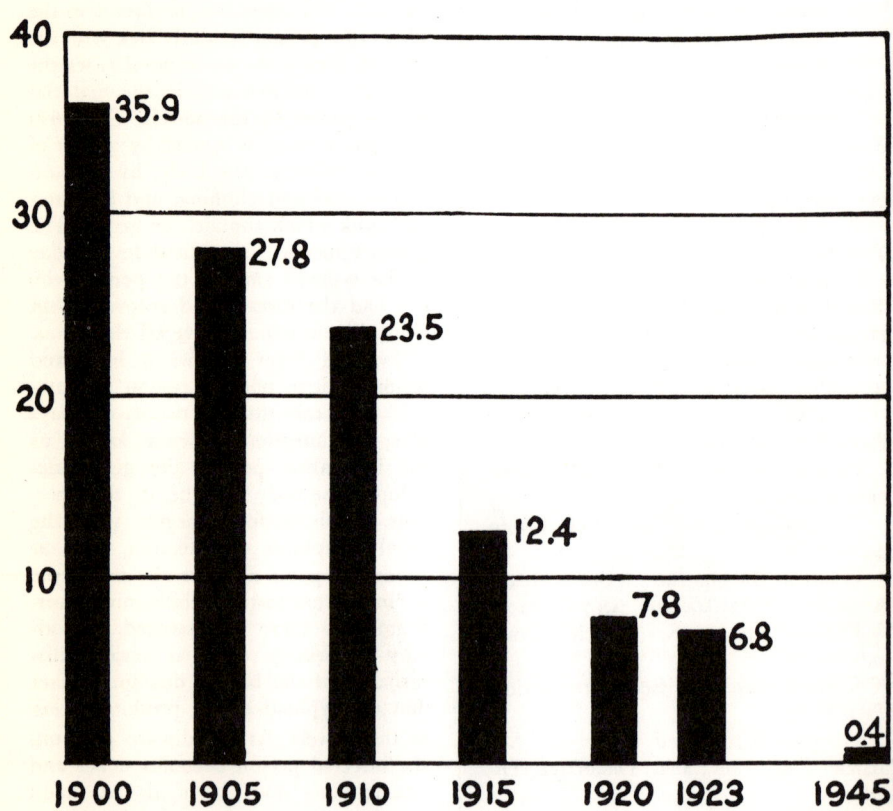

Typhoid fever is in retreat in the registration area of the United States. Modern sanitary methods, pasteurization of milk, control of typhoid carriers and immunization have practically eliminated the disease.

secondary infections. It is also important that the mouth be rinsed each time after food is taken.

There was a time when it was thought advisable to starve typhoid patients. It is now known that the condition is so serious as to break down the nutrition of the patient, so that present methods involve the giving of a diet of from 3000 to 3500 calories. Then the patient will not lose weight during the course of the illness.

It is well established that a vaccine made of the killed germs of typhoid fever is of value in preventing the disease. It is customary to give three injections of the vaccine at ten-day intervals, although the intervals between injections may be shortened. Obviously such vaccines should be given by a physician or a trained nurse. Only rarely indeed are there reactions of a serious character.

It is probable that persistent attention to water supplies and disposal of sewage, pasteurization of milk, education of the public in hygiene, and the control of typhoid carriers will eventually eliminate typhoid fever entirely throughout the civilized world.

In typhoid fever chloromycetin or chloramphenicol is effective.

Typhoid Fever—See article Transmissible Diseases.

Typhoid Fever—antibodies developed by vaccination: See article Allergy.

Typhoid Fever—arthritis can result: See article Arthritis, Rheumatism, and Gout.

Typhoid Fever—bacillus: See article Transmissible Diseases; Skin, article The Skin.

Typhoid Fever—blamable: See article Diabetes.

Typhoid Fever—carriers: See article Transmissible Diseases.

Typhoid Fever—chloramphenicol: See Infectious Disease, article The Prevention and Treatment of Infectious Disease.

Typhoid Fever—chloromycetin: See Infectious Disease, article The Prevention and Treatment of Infectious Disease.

Typhoid Fever—encephalitis treated with typhoid vaccine: See article Transmissible Diseases.

Typhoid Fever—febrile nephroses may result: See Kidney, article The Kidney: Its Diseases and Disturbances.

Typhoid Fever—gall bladder may be affected: See article Digestion and Digestive Diseases.

Typhoid Fever—germ isolated: See Infectious Disease, article The Prevention and Treatment of Infectious Disease.

Typhoid Fever—hair loss may follow: See Hair, article The Hair.

Typhoid Fever—incidence: See Infectious Disease, article The Prevention and Treatment of Infectious Disease; article Transmissible Diseases.

Typhoid Fever—incubation period: See Infectious Disease, article The Prevention and Treatment of Infectious Disease; article Transmissible Diseases.

Typhoid Fever—infants: See Infancy, article Care and Feeding of the Child.

Typhoid Fever—infected water most common source: See article Digestion and Digestive Diseases.

Typhoid Fever—inflammation of colon: See article Digestion and Digestive Diseases.

Typhoid Fever—intestines: See Infectious Disease, article The Prevention and Treatment of Infectious Disease.

Typhoid Fever—leukopenia: See Blood, article The Blood and Its Diseases.

Typhoid Fever—Osler's "Principles

and Practice of Medicine" indicates importance: See Respiratory Diseases, article The Respiratory Diseases.

Typhoid Fever—pneumonia frequently follows: See Respiratory Diseases, article The Respiratory Diseases.

Typhoid Fever—protection: See Infectious Disease, article The Prevention and Treatment of Infectious Disease.

Typhoid Fever—resistance reduced by chronic disorders: See Infectious Disease, article The Prevention and Treatment of Infectious Disease.

Typhoid Fever—rheumatism can result: See article Arthritis, Rheumatism, and Gout.

Typhoid Fever—"shots": See Respiratory Diseases, article The Respiratory Diseases.

Typhoid Fever—tongue inflammation: See Ear, article The Ear, Tongue, Nose, and Throat.

Typhoid Fever—treatment: See article Transmissible Diseases.

Typhoid Fever—ulcers in the intestines: See Infectious Disease, article The Prevention and Treatment of Infectious Disease.

Typhoid Fever—undulant fever resembles: See article Transmissible Diseases.

Typhoid Fever—vaccination: See article Allergy.

Typhoid Fever—white blood cells decreased: See Infectious Disease, article The Prevention and Treatment of Infectious Disease.

TYPHUS Typhus fever is one of the most important of all epidemics in the world today. An epidemic of this disease, which has in the past been called hospital fever, spotted fever, jail fever, camp fever, and ship fever, is devastating.

We know that the condition is spread by the body louse and that a similar condition is spread by the rat flea. There are other diseases like typhus—perhaps different forms of the same disease—that are spread by various insects in different parts of the world.

A Chicago physician named Howard Taylor Ricketts proved that the Mexican form of typhus fever called tabardillo is spread by the body louse. This disease has been named in his honor Rickettsia.

Usually typhus appears about twelve days after a person has been bitten by an infected louse. Prostration is one of the first symptoms. About five days after the first signs of illness a dark red, mottling eruption occurs, later changing to blood spots. In the form of typhus that occurs in civilian life away from war fronts, the condition begins like any other infectious disease with rapidly increasing fever. The eruption takes place on the fifth or sixth day. Then there may be a crisis with recovery or perhaps death.

The prevention of typhus fever involves measures associated with the elimination of lice and fleas. In time of war all of the clothing of our soldiers is sterilized in special delousing apparatus. One of the greatest discoveries of World War II has been the development of extracts of pyrethrum with which the underwear of soldiers may be treated so that a louse cannot live in contact with the underwear as long as six weeks after the underwear is first sprayed or dipped in the solution.

Another great development is DDT powder. By the liberal use of this powder the spread of typhus fever was stopped in Naples immediately after the American troops captured that city. The DDT powder is freely sprinkled in the clothing, particularly in the seams. The body lice cannot live in contact with this powder.

Finally, vaccines have been developed which are made by preparing emulsions of Rickettsia organisms. All of the American soldiers going into typhus-infested areas are given immunity against the disease with the vaccine.

By the use of all of these measures our troops were kept relatively free from typhus throughout the war.

There is always some typhus in various portions of the United States, and our health authorities are constantly on the watch for it. We have every reason to believe that the spread of the disease in this country can be halted by the methods known to modern medical science.

TYPHUS—lice carry: See SKIN, article THE SKIN.

TYPHUS—rats carry: See SKIN, article THE SKIN.

TYPHUS—Rocky Mountain spotted fever resembles: See article TRANSMISSIBLE DISEASES.

ULCERS Any open sore, other than a wound, is called an ulcer. The term is applied to a loss of substance inside the body. Ulcers may occur from infection, from injury to the blood supply, from damage to nerves, and from a wide variety of other causes. The occurrence of an ulcer is an indication for a physician to find out exactly what caused the ulcer. The method of treatment is definitely related to the cause.

PEPTIC ULCERS—gastritis resembles: See article DIGESTION AND DIGESTIVE DISEASES.
PEPTIC ULCERS—heartburn: See article DIGESTION AND DIGESTIVE DISEASES.
PEPTIC ULCERS—role of blood sugar in development: See article DIGESTION AND DIGESTIVE DISEASES.

ULCERATIVE COLITIS—effect of insecurity and anger: See article STRESS AND DISEASE.
ULCERATIVE COLITIS—functional significance: See article STRESS AND DISEASE.
ULCERATIVE COLITIS—polyps: See article DIGESTION AND DIGESTIVE DISEASES.
ULCERATIVE COLITIS—related to chronic bacillary dysentery: See article DIGESTION AND DIGESTIVE DISEASES.
ULCERS—See article DIGESTION AND DIGESTIVE DISEASES.
ULCERS—appendicitis confused with: See article DIGESTION AND DIGESTIVE DISEASES.
ULCERS—bichromates may cause: See article OCCUPATION AND HEALTH.
ULCERS—bowel, result of constipation: See article DIGESTION AND DIGESTIVE DISEASES.

ULCERS—cancer: See article DIGESTION AND DIGESTIVE DISEASES.
ULCERS—chrome: See article OCCUPATION AND HEALTH.
ULCERS—colitis: See references ULCERATIVE COLITIS above:
ULCERS—diet: See article DIGESTION AND DIGESTIVE DISEASES; DIET, article ADVICE ON THE DIET.
ULCERS—distinguishing from gall-bladder disease and appendicitis: See article DIGESTION AND DIGESTIVE DISEASES.
ULCERS—duodenal: See entry STOMACH ULCERS.
ULCERS—emotional tension may cause: See article BLOOD PRESSURE; MENTAL, article NERVOUS AND MENTAL DISORDERS.
ULCERS—eye: See EYE, article THE EYE.
ULCERS—gastro-intestinal allergy: See article ALLERGY.
ULCERS—kidney: See KIDNEY, article THE KIDNEY: ITS DISEASES AND DISTURBANCES.
ULCERS—peptic: See references PEPTIC ULCERS above.
ULCERS—polycythemia: See BLOOD, article THE BLOOD AND ITS DISEASES.
ULCERS—protective function: See article STRESS AND DISEASE.
ULCERS—reaction to stress: See article STRESS AND DISEASE.
ULCERS—stomach: See entry STOMACH ULCERS.
ULCERS—vitamin E: See SKIN, article THE SKIN.
ULCERS—X-ray used to detect: See article DIGESTION AND DIGESTIVE DISEASES.
ULCERS—zinc sulphate may cause: See article OCCUPATION AND HEALTH.

UMBILICUS See *Navel, Diseases of.*

UNDERSTANDING SYMPTOMS
(See also *Symptoms of Disease*)

WEAKNESS—People come to the doctor saying, "I'm weak." Or they may say "I get tired easily." People who are healthy have vim and vigor. Ben Hecht once said: "They have bounce." Elasticity in both mind and body is a sign of health. Those who lack energy and who are listless usually have something wrong. Such symptoms may be quite different from the loss of power in the muscles, which may be due to other causes. Just being unduly fatigued is also different from being faint or slightly dizzy.

Any physical or emotional disorder can be accompanied by lack of energy or listlessness. After an acute infection, following hemorrhage whether sudden or prolonged, or following long-continued subjection to cancer, this lack of energy may be a prominent symptom.

A severe emotional outbreak or upset leaves people weak, exhausted. Such outbreaks can also lead to depression or neurosis accompanied by anxiety.

Lassitude or languor may also be noted frequently as the result of insufficient action of the thyroid gland or from deficiency of secretion in the adrenal glands. However, excessive action of the glands can also lead to overstimulation and ultimate exhaustion.

Lassitude is often observed by the doctor in cases of chronic disease of the liver; in the old days people called this debility. Shakespeare says in *As You Like It,* "I did not woo the means of weakness and debility."

Various drugs, by their effects or actions on the body, can bring about lassitude, among these particularly bromides, alcohol, and the barbituric acid derivatives.

ASTHENIA AND FEEBLENESS—People who are old and those who have been confined in bed for a long time get weak. Their muscles seem to lose the power to act. In a disease called *myasthenia gravis* the muscles get weak but seem to recover strength after rest, becoming weak again almost immediately after the least exertion. During their action the muscles use up certain materials. Through actions of the nervous system the use of this material, called cholinesterase, is inhibited. The giving of drugs like neostigmine prevents the destruction of cholinesterase and thus helps these patients.

As in the case of lassitude a number of conditions can also produce asthenia. A long-continued infection, an excessive action of the thyroid with too rapid beating of the heart, severe anemia, nutritional deficiencies, or habitual taking of drugs or poisons may be a prime factor. The doctor has to make a thorough study using many laboratory tests to determine the cause with certainty.

Dr. Tinsley Harrison has said that nearly all patients with true asthenia have lassitude but the majority of patients with lassitude do not have asthenia.

When people are troubled by faintness, lightheadedness or dizziness a great variety of conditions must be investigated. Usually this symptom results from disturbance of the supply of blood to the brain. The difficulty may be in the blood vessels of the brain, in the power of action of the heart or in the quality of the blood. The symptom can occur also in epilepsy and in hysterical conditions. Sudden drop in the sugar in the blood also causes this symptom. This symptom makes people anxious although the conditions causing it are seldom fatal.

Coma or Unconsciousness—Persistent unconsciousness or coma is quite different from recurrent or repeated attacks of sudden fainting. The coma may be preceded by stupor or alternate with delirium. Among the common causes of coma are serious deficiencies of oxygen, sugar or vitamins; excessive amounts of sedative or hypnotic or narcotic drugs. Coma occurs from intoxications associated with diabetes, uremia or liver disturbances. Heat stroke or freezing may result in long periods of unconsciousness. Damage to the circulation of the blood and excessive pressure on the brain, such as that which follows fractured skull or concussion may be the cause of loss of consciousness that persists.

When the doctor examines a patient who has been long in coma he must find out first and as soon as possible the cause of the condition. The prompt application of treatment frequently means the difference between life and death, but proper treatment cannot be given unless the cause is known. Frequently unconscious people have been thrown into jail with a charge of drunkenness when the cause of their stupor was not alcohol but a skull fracture. The same thing has happened to people who had had too much insulin.

A person intoxicated by alcohol has the odor of alcohol on the breath; diabetic coma carries with it an odor like that of spoiled fruit and uremia has an odor to the breath like that of urine. An exceedingly high temperature may mean heat stroke.

The doctor may measure the patient's blood pressure as a clue to the cause of unconsciousness. An exceedingly high blood pressure may mean a stroke, or apoplexy, or uremia. An exceedingly low pressure may mean diabetes, drugs, drunkenness, or a hemorrhage.

Convulsions—Strangely almost any condition that can cause coma or persistent unconsciousness can also cause convulsions. No single mechanism is known that is responsible for all kinds of convulsions. Changes in the supply of oxygen reaching the brain, in the relationship between acid and alkali—called the acid-base-balance; changes in the amount of calcium, sugar or chlorides in the blood; disturbance of the fluid balance or equilibrium between salt and water in the body and associated changes in the pressure on the brain have all been related to convulsions. A great variety of conditions may develop in which these chemical changes in the tissues of the body occur.

By a series of careful examinations the doctor can often classify convulsions in relationship to a definite cause but there still remain great numbers of cases for which no specific cause can be determined. Where some positive factor is established—for instance, pressure on the brain from a growth, a gunshot wound or a fracture—some positive measures may be taken to control the epilepsy. Convulsions in young children are most often idiopathic epilepsy. In older people a definite cause may be found as a tumor, or a change in pressure on the brain from some other cause.

When a person has convulsions help should be given to keep him from injuring himself by falling against hard or sharp objects. A soft gag in the mouth will prevent biting or injuring the mouth and tongue. Doctors can prescribe or give by injection drugs that serve to induce quiet. However, any attack of convulsions should always be an indication or a warning that immediate steps must be taken to determine what is wrong.

PARALYSIS—Startling and frightening to any person is sudden loss of ability to move any portion of the body that one moves voluntarily. The anxiety associated with sudden loss of ability to see, or hear, or taste, or feel heat or pain, strikes terrible dismay. Yet these conditions are frequent enough to warrant the assurance that good medical care can do much to alleviate the difficulties and benefit people who have been stricken with paralysis.

The term "plegia" means paralysis. If one leg or an arm is paralyzed the condition is called monoplegia. If one side of the body is paralyzed the term is hemiplegia. If both legs are paralyzed, most frequently as a result of spinal cord disease, the condition is paraplegia. Weakness of all four extremities which occurs in a few severe and long standing conditions is a quadriplegia or four-way paralysis. Of course, such diseases as infantile paralysis or meningitis or encephalitis may damage only certain groups of muscles.

From the area involved and the symptoms associated the doctor may be able to tell the portion of the spinal cord or brain that is damaged. Much depends on whether there is just failure of movement or whether this is accomplished by wasting of the tissues, difficulty in circulation of the blood or other significant factors.

Harm may come to the nervous system from hemorrhages, infections, blows or injuries, tearing or breaking of the nerves. A nerve can be injured in an arm or leg which then affects only the muscles reached by that nerve. Since a knowledge of just where each nerve originates and goes is needed for a diagnosis, specialists with such knowledge are called neurologists.

SHORTNESS OF BREATH CALLED DYSPNEA—When people get so short of breath that the very effort of breathing is difficult and when breathing is harsh and labored, anyone can tell that something is wrong. Since respiration is necessary to life difficult breathing creates serious anxiety. Usually people breathe 18 to 20 times a minute and regularly. The breathing is effortless and without any special sensation. If breathing becomes irregular or if a severe effort has to be made to get enough breath pain may appear.

Anyone can get short of breath after severe work or exhaustive exercise. Shortness of breath occurs more often

UNDERSTANDING SYMPTOMS

in fat people than in thin ones, in old people than in young ones, and in women than in men. The response of the heart and the breathing to a measured physical effort may be used as an indication of physical fitness.

When shortness of breath is not accompanied by extra effort, the trouble may be more mental than physical. Anyone can imitate shortness of breath. Allergic conditions and asthma which narrow the bronchial tubes bring on "wheezing." Damage to the diaphragm, the lining of the chest cavity or the lungs may bring about trouble in breathing. In pneumonia when a portion of the lung is inflamed and congested, the breathing is labored. Severe anemia which lessens the supply of blood able to carry oxygen may result in quickened breathing to get the necessary oxygen to the tissues.

The most important causes of shortness of breath are diseases of the heart and lung, and disorders which in any way prevent air from getting into the lungs. As with every other part of the body, damage to the nervous system can also be reflected in serious difficulties with breathing.

WHEN YOU COUGH—Anything that irritates the surface of your breathing tract between the throat and the secondary branches of the bronchial tubes can make you cough. A cough has three stages: first you draw in air, then you compress the chest; then you expel the air. In order to expel the air with force you draw up your diaphragm while your chest cavity elongates and then by pressure of the abdominal muscles you drive the diaphragm up towards the chest like a piston.

In many common diseases cough is an outstanding symptom. In acute bronchitis one begins with a dry cough which becomes moist as secretion develops. In this condition the chest X-ray will not usually reveal any altered condition.

In chronic bronchitis cough and expectoration, usually much worse in the morning, are the chief symptoms.

Chronic bronchiectasis has symptoms like chronic bronchitis, but the volume of sputum is large. Some patients produce as much as a quart a day. The breath and the sputum usually have an offensive odor.

Tuberculosis is associated with cough and for this condition examination of the chest with X-ray is of utmost importance. The doctor makes a physical examination of the chest and may also send a specimen of sputum to the laboratory to search for germs of tuberculosis.

Heart failure, cancer, abscesses, embolus in the lung due to a clot that has broken loose somewhere in the circulation, and infection with parasites may be causes of cough. Some people develop a cough habit and then keep it up without any physical cause for the cough.

BLEEDING FROM THE LUNGS—HEMOPTYSIS—Blood coming from the lungs is usually bright red and frothy whereas that from the stomach may be dark red, brown or black and mixed with scraps of food. Vomiting is usually preceded by retching and nausea, but a hemorrhage from the lung may come quietly and without warning. Blood in the lung may be associated with severe coughing and ocassionally severe coughing may tear tissue so as to produce bleeding.

In the early stages of pneumonia a severe cough may bring up blood because the lungs are at that time heavily congested. Such blood has a rusty or prune juice color but may be bright red.

Among the commonest causes of blood from the lungs in the absence of tuberculosis is the passing of a clot elsewhere in the body into a pulmonary artery, the large blood vessel that supplies the lung with blood. The small blood vessels around the area become congested and the irritation causes a cough which may bring up blood.

In chronic bronchiectasis the surface tissue of the bronchial tubes may be torn with severe coughing so that blood appears in the sputum.

The hemorrhage from the lungs in tuberculosis is due to actual erosion or destruction of blood vessels by the disease. Cavities form in the lung in tuberculosis due to destructive action by the germs. The blood vessels in the walls of these cavities may be eroded. One of the dangers is spread of the infection by inhaling and by forcible expulsion of germs in severe coughing.

Among young people with hearts that have been damaged by disease, especially with narrowing of the mitral valve of the heart, the backing up of blood into the lungs causes swelling of the large and small blood vessels with occasional breaking and therefore a hemorrhage from the lungs.

Any time blood comes from the lungs the symptom should be taken as a warning that something serious has occurred.

PALPITATION OF THE HEART—Ordinarily we are not aware of the beating of our hearts. If you do become conscious of the heart's beating, the symptom may have significance but often is unimportant. Many letters come to doctors who write health colums from people who say they have noticed that their hearts were flopping, skipping, pounding, bumping or fluttering.

If you run too hard or engage in too much muscular activity an extra burden is put on your heart and you may feel it pounding. As soon as you have "caught your breath," the sensation disappears. When the heart beats too rapidly, as it does in excessive action of the thyroid or in other disturbances, you become aware of it. People seem to be conscious of sudden alterations in the heart rate. Different people respond differently to various conditions that affect the body. Those who are placid may pass unnoticed a situation that will seriously disturb a person who is sensitive to minor stimulations.

Palpitation may be due to sudden alterations of the heart rate, particularly in cases when the heart beats too rapidly; this condition in turn may be due to excessive action of the thyroid gland. Anemia, hemorrhage, fever, and a lessened amount of sugar in the blood are other conditions in which palpitations occur. In such instances an excess of epinephrine secreted by the adrenal gland may be basically responsible. Many people who complain of palpitation constantly swallow air while eating too rapidly; when the stomach is distended they become conscious of the beating of the heart.

Many people described as nervous and who have nothing physically wrong complain of palpitations. These people have a cardiac neurosis in which their minds are centered on their heart action. The suspicion that one has heart disease may set up or intensify such a neurosis. A doctor can find out the facts and thus cure both the neurosis and the palpitation which arises from it.

UNDERWEIGHT, HAZARDS OF

The first problem encountered in a consideration of the hazards of underweight is that of definition. What is underweight? As has been pointed out elsewhere [*Weight, Normal For Health*] the answer is not easy because of lack of certain knowledge of what constitutes normal weight. It is clear that normal weight will depend on age and sex. This everyone knows. It is clear also that it depends on height or size. The short person might be expected to weigh less than the tall person of the same age and sex. But this is not always true, and this brings in the factor of constitution, or body build, or conformation. All of us know the chunky, chubby, or tubby "type," the tall, lean, thin "bean pole," and the less extreme examples of these types.

In the absence of any actual knowledge of what constitutes the proper weight of any individual in relation to height, age, sex, or other characteristics dependence has of necessity been put on the average weights of groups of supposedly healthy persons of like age, sex, and height. These averages form standards with which the weight of a given individual can be compared. In some tables allowance is made for constitutional type, or body build, in use, and allowance is of necessity made for a permissible variation above or below the standard (average).

None of the standards available and in common use are altogether satisfactory, as was learned to our sorrow during the war when the weight of individuals in large populations became of great importance in problems of food supply, rationing, relief, and even survival. Variation between standards may exceed apparent limits of normality, and the range in some standards is so great as to make them of little value. Nevertheless, some weight tables, including that used in this book, are reasonably satisfactory for our present use.

What, then, is our criterion? When are we underweight? Disregarding as we must for the present the deficiencies in our standards, we can define underweight as weight more than 10 per cent below the standard for the individual. There are, however, certain modifying conditions which must be added if we are to avoid mistaking an individual characteristic for an abnormal condition. First, such underweight is more likely to be significant in children, and even more so if it persists and the child fails to increase in weight. It must be remembered, however, that growth, including increase in weight in children, is irregular and, to an extent, seasonal.

Second, underweight of this degree is much more likely to be abnormal and represent a state of ill health if it is the result of loss of weight in an individual previously of standard weight. Underweight in an individual who has always or habitually weighed below his standard and who is in good health is most apt to represent an individual variation from the usual and to be without sinister significance. In fact, it probably reflects a fortunate state conducive of longevity.

Third, as may be deduced from the above, underweight is much more likely to be significant to health if the individual concerned does not enjoy *good* health and complains of any one of many symptoms. Finally, underweight becomes more worthy of attention if it is the result of, or accompanied by, restriction of food intake, particularly voluntary restriction as may occur with reducing or other forms of dieting.

A better understanding of the hazards of underweight will be had if physiological and biochemical conditions accompanying underweight are discussed. When food intake is reduced below that needed to maintain the existing weight the body draws on its own tissues. With the exception of very small reserves of sugar and animal starch (glycogen) the body fat is the first to furnish this food or fuel. For those who are overweight this is not objectionable; in fact, it is desirable and, of course, the basis for reducing. For those who are at their physiological weight (healthful weight) or below it means the encroachment on, and eventual loss of, the protection of their vital body substance, protein. The time it takes to lose the fat and expose the protein to loss depends, of course, on how deficient the diet is. If it is only slightly deficient it will take a long time to deplete the fat. Inevitably, however, the fat is lost if the deficient diet is continued, and under many conditions of dieting or reduced food intake the fat does not last long.

Some idea of the speed at which weight is lost can be gotten from a study which showed the loss of weight in a group of experimental subjects eating somewhat over half of the food they required. The group lost on the average approximately thirty-four pounds, or nearly a quarter of their original weight, within sixteen weeks. It can be assumed that none were significantly obese at the start. Under these conditions the greater part of the body fat must have been lost early, to be followed by serious inroads on their protein tissues leading to protein deficiency.

The body's reserves of protein are small. Any unusual loss must come from our tissues and organs, and, because of the nature of protein, it even comes from the vital tissues of the body. Much of the protein-containing tissue is muscle, and the muscle tissues and organs contribute their protein to be burned. The skeletal muscles such as our biceps and similar muscles are only a part of our tissues. Many organs such as the stomach contain muscles on the integrity of which much of their function depends. Furthermore, such a large and important organ as the heart is a muscular organ, composed almost entirely of muscle tissue. Protein makes up a large part of the substance of such organs as the liver and tissues not commonly thought of as such—the blood, for instance. Finally, protein is a principal constituent of many important hormones, secretions, and protective substances, some of which are manufactured by the body in relatively small but vitally important amounts, such as thyroid secretion, insulin, and the various antitoxins. Others such as milk are produced in relatively large quantities.

The sequence of events then is this:
Amounts of food insufficient to maintain weight are eaten. The body then draws on its own tissues. Fat being expendable without ill effect is used first, but, except in the obese, is relatively soon exhausted.

Protein is then consumed. Protein being an indispensable tissue, a state of protein deficiency ensues, with the ill effects to be described below.

Perhaps the most evident and easily recognized effect of underweight is weakness. This is a direct result of the loss of muscle substance. The muscles shrink and become smaller, a change which can readily be observed. Actually a visible wasting of the exterior muscles of the body is one of the first signs of such nutritional deficiency. The weakness is most marked in terms of muscular endurance. Although strength for single muscular acts is somewhat lessened, it still is maintained surprisingly well in even rather extreme states of undernutrition. But sustained muscular effort such as holding, squeezing, and pulling are much less well performed. Perhaps the best common example is found in climbing stairs, an act which becomes increasingly difficult. With the weakness there is a disinclination to exertion, in part related directly to the increased effort needed, but, as we shall see, partly caused by other changes.

It is not only the skeletal muscles, however, which suffer. As previously pointed out, muscular tissue of all kinds all over the body is affected and, as it becomes smaller, displays evidence of its weakness. For instance, the heart becomes smaller and its contractions less forceful.

The weakening of the muscles of the front wall of the abdomen permits hernias or ruptures to develop more readily, and those which previously existed to a slight and insignificant degree may become enlarged to an extent which is disabling and requires treatment. From the esthetic point of view, there is a sagging and bulging of the abdomen with resulting sad effects on the figure. The muscles of the walls of the intestines weaken and allow the bowel to distend, diminish contraction and favor delayed passage of food through them.

One of the important structures to suffer with undernutrition is the blood. More than one of the elements of the blood is affected. Protein is involved in the formation of both the blood cells, red and white, and of the plasma (serum) in which the cells are suspended.

Anemia is a rather constant occurrence in underweight and undernutrition. This anemia, which is usually mild but may reach moderately serious proportions in severe and continued undernutrition, is the result of both a reduction in the number of red blood cells and the amount of hemoglobin. It is not the result of inadequate supplies of vitamins or minerals and appears despite an adequate supply of these substances. Its exact cause is unknown, but there is reason to believe that it, too, is related to the loss of protein. Protein is needed for both the manufacture of the red blood cells and the hemoglobin which they contain. Inadequate protein diets are known to impair blood formation in animals under experimental conditions. It is worth noting that recovery from the anemia of undernutrition is slow, even with a full and good diet. Restoration of the blood to normal may lay behind the recovery of body weight.

The white cells may be affected slightly. In the absence of intercurrent infections there is usually a slight-to-moderate decrease in their number. Changes in their character or in the proportion of the various cell types are not to be expected.

Another important constituent of the blood which may be affected is the serum, or plasma protein. There are two principal kinds of proteins in the blood plasma: albumin and globulin. Both serve the important function of holding water within the blood vessels, but in this the albumin is more important. Globulin is importantly concerned with immunity and resistance to disease as will be described below. Finally there is a small amount of a protein known as fibrinogen, which is required for the proper clotting of blood.

The quality of these proteins may be decreased as the result of undernutrition accompanying states of underweight, with resulting disturbance of the functions for which they are responsible. The reduction in the serum proteins may result in the condition known as edema, or dropsy, which under these conditions is spoken of as nutritional edema or dropsy. In the ordinary mild states of underweight such swelling is slight in degree, confined usually to the feet and lower legs and more pronounced toward evening, often disappearing by morning. It may be displaced during the night and appear as puffiness of the face and hands in the morning. Locally this dropsy may impair the vitality of the tissues and interfere with healing. It is only fair, on the other hand, to point out that a slight swelling or increase in fluid in the tissues may serve to hide the haggard appearance that follows a loss of subcutaneous and muscular tissue. Such swelling should be distinguished from the normal or physiological swelling of the feet and even ankles which comes at the end of the day as a result of long sitting or standing and the fullness of the hands which is sometimes noticed in the morning. Actually these normal and abnormal changes in the amount of water in the tissues are of essentially the same nature, differing only in degree. As a rough guide the abnormal swellings are detected by the persistence of "pits" in the tissue when pressed on by the finger, but the exact interpretation in cases of swelling should be left to the physician.

A number of undesirable, if not injurious, changes take place in the surface tissues, skin, and hair with underweight. The least of these is a looseness, a sagging, a wrinkling, an accentuation of lines particularly in the face as the skin loses its support of subcutaneous and muscular tissue. In effect the envelope becomes too big for the contents and becomes "baggy." In younger people this may be compensated for to some extent by the elasticity of the skin, which after a time readjusts itself to the change. In older people in whom the elasticity of the skin is naturally decreased this fails to occur. At the same time the skin itself becomes drier, thinner and tends to be somewhat rough and scaly as its turgor and the blood flow through it are decreased. With the latter there is apt to be some grayish pallor and decreased warmth. Finally it has been observed that undernutrition is apt to be accompanied by a blotchy, brownish pigmentation, especially on the face. The hair tends to be dry, rough, and of poor quality. It is possible that all of these changes are related to a diminished blood flow through the skin, though the whole process is a complex one involving a lowered metabolic rate, a decreased surface temperature, and diminished action of the sweat glands and possibly of the sebaceous glands. In people studied by Keys of Minnesota the eyes had a dull, glazed appearance, apparently because of decreased blood flow in the sclera or whites of the eyeball.

In underweight of a degree consistent with chronic undernutrition the basal metabolic rate is reduced. The reduction, though only slight-to-moderate, is significant. The basal metabolic rate is a measure of the amount of heat produced by the body in relation to the individual's age, sex, and size, and the reduction is assumed to be a compensatory mechanism to conserve body heat and the wasting of body tissues when the food intake is inadequate to maintain normal weight. Direct ill effects from this reduction are not serious, but there is apt to be some disinclination to physical activity and an unusual sensitiveness to a cool environment. As already indicated, this reduction probably contributes indirectly to other changes, such as those in the skin, by reducing blood flow.

Because the lowered basal metabolic rate is mediated through the thyroid gland, there is reason to believe that other glands of internal secretion are affected, all such glands being closely interrelated. That this occurs in severe malnutrition is well known, and evidence of disturbances in the structure and function of certain of the sex glands has been observed. However, in these instances the diets have been deficient in many nutrients, and it has been impossible to say that simple undernutrition, as represented by underweight, can cause such effects. Nevertheless, temporary stopping of menstruation or shortened duration and diminished flow are common in undernourished populations and have been observed to occur in association with dietaries which were apparently not deficient except in calories and perhaps protein. If this is, in fact, an effect of simple undernutrition it may be reasoned that possibly there is also an effect on conception. On the other hand very considerable losses of weight can occur in such diseases as tuberculosis without the amenorrhoea. Such occurrences illustrate the complexity of the situation and the many factors involved.

No special effects on the digestive tract are noted with underweight, with the possible exception of those described in association with the loss of muscular tones of the intestines. Unlike complete starvation in which the appetite is lost after a few days, under ordinary circumstances of *involuntary* restriction of food the appetite remains ravenous and the thoughts of food dominate the waking hours and even the dreams of night. But the factor of appetite is affected by so many factors, particularly psychological, that under many circumstances accompanying loss of weight, especially when the restriction of food is voluntary, appetite may actually be unaffected or diminished.

The effect of true underweight on the heart and circulation is, as stated above, a decrease in its size, a smaller output, a slowing of the pulse rate, especially during rest, and a lowering of the blood pressure. These changes, aided by others, cause a poor circulation through the skin and may lead to slight lividity, especially of the extremities. Such individuals often complain of giddiness or faintness. In themselves these cannot be considered serious ill effects and, in fact, such underweight and undernutrition has been used in the treatment of heart disease and high blood pressure. It is a well-known fact that the incidence of certain types of heart disease and hypertension become much less frequent and severe in populations which have been subjected to undernutrition.

On the other hand the secondary effects of undernutrition on the nutrition of the heart may be deleterious, and a certain number of patients with heart disease suffer from undernutrition. With loss of weight and loss of muscle substance there probably is first a reduction in the size of muscle fibers and, if it continues, presumably in the actual number of fibers themselves.

The only infectious diseases for which a definite relation between underweight and resistance to the disease seems to have been established are tuberculosis, pneumonia (lobar), and influenza. Underweight is associated with an increased mortality rate from tuberculosis at all ages, being more than twice that for those of normal weight. Furthermore, the increase in the mortality rate is even greater as the degree of underweight increases.

Formerly the death rate from lobar pneumonia was significantly higher in the underweights, but the introduction of new and effective drugs in the treatment of pneumonia has greatly influenced the situation. Deaths from influenza were more frequent among the underweight group in the pandemia of 1918-20. Although the evidence is not clear, it is probable that the effect of undernutrition on tuberculosis is on pre-existing but inactive infections, a state which may be found in a large proportion of adults. Lowered resistance to the initial infection with tuberculosis seems much less likely.

Theoretically the existence of diminished resistance to a large number of infectious diseases in states of underweight involving any significant degree of protein deficiency is highly probable. As has been pointed out, the antitoxins and other immune substances which our bodies manufacture as a protection against acquiring or succumbing to a large number of infectious diseases are made from protein, principally the globulin fraction. When protein deficiency exists there may be a defective or deficient manufacture of those substances and hence diminished resistance to those diseases, as has clearly been shown experimentally in animals. Practically this has been difficult to demonstrate unequivocally in man, but general observation on the incidence and mortality of many diseases such as typhus fever, diphtheria, and dysentery in undernourished subjects, except as modified by newer and powerful drugs, supports strongly the theoretical possibility. It is, however, to be pointed out that an exception must be made in many if not all diseases due to viruses in which undernutrition, at least in the sense of underweight, apparently exerts no unfavorable influence.

It might be thought that such solid and apparently indestructible structures as the bones and teeth would show no effect of the type of undernutrition and underweight being considered here. That is probably true of the teeth. It is also apparently true of the bones if the state of underweight is of relatively short duration, say several months. It may not be true with even rather mild underweight, however, if the condition is maintained over long periods. So-called hunger or famine thinning of the bones has been recognized and detected for many years. Usually the degree of undernutrition and underweight has been rather severe, but not always. Furthermore, it is now known that the bones are not the unchanging, static, almost inanimate things they were once considered to be but are dynamic, constantly changing structures with a continuous exchange of mineral salts and other evidence of a rather active metabolism. Thinning and demineralization of the bones occur associated with protein deficiencies and might be a cause under conditions which suggest long-continued, though mild, undernutrition. Though there is a loss of lime salts under such circumstances, the condition is not the result of a deficiency of calcium but more likely a protein deficiency. Particularly among the elderly it seems possible that the thinning and atrophy of the skeleton, although the result of other factors in many cases, may sometimes be the result of the chronic undernutrition and underweight not infrequent in these subjects.

Despite the occurrence of some actual structural changes in the nervous tissue in rather severe states of inanition and loss of weight it is unlikely that they are present in the milder degrees of underweight. Nor are they likely to be the cause of the mental changes which may develop. Included in this statement are the special senses, essentially nervous in structure and function, none of which show any significant effect with even severe loss of weight. The same is true of intellectual capacity, which remains unimpaired, although it may be unexercised because of the disinclination to exertion, physical or mental. This is not so true, however, of the personality and the emotions. As always, there are so many factors concerned with emotional responses and personality reactions that it is difficult to show that a single factor scuh as loss of weight and the undernutrition causing it are the causes of such changes, except under carefully controlled conditions which are difficult to have in ordinary living. For instance, the preoccupation with food and the emotional behavior associated with restriction of food which can be found in experimental subjects may be entirely lacking in the individual whose distorted thinking with regard to food and eating has been the actual cause of the underweight. The compulsive factor differs in the experimental subject and the individual who voluntarily or even on medical advice restricts his food intake. Nevertheless, the latter individual may suffer some of the effects on his or her emotional make-up and personality that have been shown to occur experimentally, even though they voluntarily stay underweight because of social custom or style. Such changes need not be extreme or even particularly evident. They consist of lack of interest, depression (though mild), and a trend to introversion. Irritability is perhaps the most common and noticeable. In the more severe restrictions there may be a trend to hypochondriasis and hysteria.

It will be apparent from what has been written that the dangers and impairments resulting from a moderate degree of underweight are not, with the exception of increased susceptibility to tuberculosis, serious. In fact, as already stated, a certain amount of underweight may be beneficial. However, there is here a rather fine distinction between what may be considered beneficial underweight and harmful undernutrition. The former refers to a state in which the weight is maintained slightly below the accepted standards but without progression downward and without encroachment on the healthy size or function of the organs and tissues. The latter refers to a state in which these structures have become actually deficient. With even the milder grades of the latter the effect on health, efficiency, and that precious asset, a sense of well-being, may be considerable.

UNDULANT FEVER Among the other names common for the condition called undulant fever are brucellosis, Malta fever, Mediterranean fever, abortus fever, and melitensis fever. These names represent the history of the condition and the investigator who first determined its cause.

Undulant fever has existed in the Mediterranean region from early times. It was first definitely studied on the island of Malta. A British physician named Bruce first isolated the causative germ. Then a similar organism was found to be responsible for contagious abortion in cattle.

The disease occurs as a natural disease of goats, sheep, and cattle and is commonly contracted in man by consumption of infected milk or milk products such as butter, cheese, and ice cream. Occasionally it may result from direct contact with infected animals. It may also spread through contamination of soil and water. Instances are known in which an infection has followed puncture of the skin by a contaminated needle, and it is conceivable that the condition may at times be carried by biting insects.

Somewhere from twelve days to three weeks after the person has been exposed to the condition the fever begins. It is of an undulating type, climbing like a stepladder with morning remissions of one degree. Then, having reached a level of 102 or 103 degrees, the fever will remain raised for a few days and gradually fall by a stepladder descent. Successive waves of fever and intermissions may go on in this way for weeks or months. With the fever come headache, disturbance of the bowels, principally constipation, and occasionally the cloudiness and dulling of the intellect which accompany continued fever. There are cases in which the fever is continuous. Instances also occur in which undulant fever is a very severe disease, rising to a sudden high temperature and not infrequently causing death.

Because of the nature of this disease it has at times been confused with typhoid fever, tuberculosis, malaria, and a variety of tropical diseases.

Before 1927 undulant fever was regarded in the United States as a medical curiosity. Now cases have been recorded in every state. In the Southwest the condition has been called goat fever, Texas fever, and Rio Grande fever.

Methods have now been developed for testing the blood of people who are believed to have this condition, using a test similar to that used for typhoid fever. These tests, carried out now by our state medical laboratories, aid the physician in confirming the diagnosis.

For many years little could be done for the person with undulant fever. Now, however, vaccines have been developed, made from the killed organisms, which seem to be helpful in some cases. The injection of foreign protein substances causes a fever reaction in the body, which helps in some cases. In some instances the sulfonamide drugs have been useful, particularly when combined with treatments in the hypertherm, or heat cabinet. Combinations of streptomycin and sulfonamides have been found effective in undulant fever.

UNDULANT FEVER—See article TRANSMISSIBLE DISEASES.

UNDULANT FEVER—arthritis can result: See article ARTHRITIS, RHEUMATISM, AND GOUT.

UNDULANT FEVER—cause determined: See INFECTIOUS DISEASE, article THE PREVENTION AND TREATMENT OF INFECTIOUS DISEASE.

UNDULANT FEVER—incubation period: See article TRANSMISSIBLE DISEASES.

UNDULANT FEVER—infected milk: See article OCCUPATION AND HEALTH.

UNDULANT FEVER—leukopenia: See BLOOD, article THE BLOOD AND ITS DISEASES.

UNDULANT FEVER—rheumatism can result: See article ARTHRITIS, RHEUMATISM, AND GOUT.

UNDULANT FEVER—symptoms: See article TRANSMISSIBLE DISEASES.

UNDULANT FEVER—treatment: See INFECTIOUS DISEASE, article THE PREVENTION AND TREATMENT OF INFECTIOUS DISEASE; article TRANSMISSIBLE DISEASES.

UREMIA If both kidneys are removed, the person concerned, or the animal concerned, will die in a few days because poisons formed in the body are not eliminated. This condition is called uremia. It begins with drowsiness, promptly followed by convulsions. Most cases of uremia occur as complications of inflammation of the kidney. Uremia may occur from conditions lower down in the urinary tract which block the flow of urine from the body.

One of the first signs likely to attract attention is severe headache. The headache may precede all other symptoms by weeks. If the headache is associated with constant nausea, occasional vomiting, and a good deal of restlessness and disturbance of sleep, the physician will probably suspect uremia. An immediate examination of the urine will help to determine whether or not satisfactory excretion is taking place.

As the materials that are toxic accumulate in the body, shortness of breath develops. Sometimes the shortness of breath resulting from this type of poisoning is difficult to differentiate from the shortage of breath due to weakness of the heart. Heart weakness is not uncommon in late forms of kidney disease.

Doctor's recognize various forms of uremia associated with different types of inflammation of the kidney. When the uremia is due to a retention of the toxic products in the body, the patient may become drowsy and apathetic and then pass into a quiet unconsciousness during which he may die. In other forms there may be a vast accumulation of fluid in the body. The patient gradually becomes short of breath due to pressure on the lung, and he also becomes increasingly sluggish in his thought and speech.

In children particularly, when inflammation of the kidney associated with acute infection occurs, the swelling of the face and of the tissues may appear suddenly and be followed almost immediately by a severe convulsion. These convulsions may come on so rapidly and continue so persistently that death follows. Therefore physicians are particularly watchful for the changes in the urine associated with conditions like scarlet fever, severe sore throats, inflammation of the tonsils, and pneumonia.

Whenever a patient shows signs of uremia, quick action is imperative. Everything necessary must be done to help out the action of the heart. Sometimes if the pressure on the brain and the spinal fluid is too great, the patient is helped by withdrawing some of the spinal fluid after puncture of the spine.

Headache, which is a warning symptom, should not be treated with sedative or hypnotic drugs. The patient should go at once to bed, and the diet should be kept under suitable control, the urine being examined regularly to determine the extent to which the kidneys are functioning. After the diagnosis is made, suitable drugs may be prescribed for the control of the headache in patients with chronic inflammation of the kidney.

UREMIA—See KIDNEY, article THE KIDNEY: ITS DISEASES AND DISTURBANCES.

UREMIA—mercurial nephrosis: See KIDNEY, article THE KIDNEY: ITS DISEASES AND DISTURBANCES.

UREMIA—polycystic kidneys: See KIDNEY, article THE KIDNEY: ITS DISEASES AND DISTURBANCES.

URETER The ureter is the tube that passes from the kidney to the bladder. It may be blocked by a stone; it may become twisted; it may become infected. Specialists in conditions affecting the urinary tract are known as urologists. Any serious condition affecting the ureter demands that kind of specialistic care. One of the first steps is to take an X-ray picture after injecting a substance which will cause the ureter to be visible.

URETERS—See KIDNEY, article THE KIDNEY: ITS DISEASES AND DISTURBANCES.

URETERS—absent: See KIDNEY, article THE KIDNEY: ITS DISEASES AND DISTURBANCES.

URETERS—double: See KIDNEY, article THE KIDNEY: ITS DISEASES AND DISTURBANCES.

URETERS—stones: See KIDNEY, article THE KIDNEY: ITS DISEASES AND DISTURBANCES.

URINATION (See also *Kidney, Uremia*) Ancient doctors used to attach even greater significance to examination of the urine than do moderns but actually they knew very little about it. They based their judgments largely on color, odor, and quantity which were easily determined.

Painful urination is usually associated with infection, irritation, or inflammation in the lower part of the urinary tract and to the passages of stones. Any obstruction to the flow of urine may be painful. Such conditions may also cause frequent urination but that may be due as well to excitement or anxiety. Hesitancy in urination may also be due to psychological causes. Failure to control the flow of the urine, which is called incontinence, may come in times of great fright or during unconsciousness, but children may fail to control the urine for a variety of both physical and mental causes.

Increase in the amount of urine associated with frequent urination may be due to increased intake of fluids, or to failure of sweating. A sudden change from warm to cold weather causes a rise in the volume because of lessened perspiration.

Certain diseases that affect the urinary mechanism, including conditions affecting the pituitary gland and diabetes, cause an increase in amount of urine. People with dropsy or collection of fluid in the body may respond to rest, or treatment with certain drugs that rid the body of large amounts of fluid through the urine. Similarly a diminished output may result from failure of the heart to put enough blood through the kidney and from collection of fluid in the tissues and cavities of the body.

Usually the quantity of urine is diminished during sleep. Anything that disturbs sleep may result in urination at night. Irritations along the tract may also cause awakening and urination at night.

URTICARIA See *Hives*.

UTERUS (See also *Hysterectomy, Pregnancy,* and *Prenatal Care*) This is the scientific name for the womb, the organ which carries the child previous to childbirth. The uterus is a muscular organ which has a lining of tissue from which the menstrual fluid comes each month. Like any other tissue of the body, the uterus may be infected so that its lining is seriously inflamed. An inflammation of the lining of the uterus is called endometritis. The opening of the uterus into the vagina is called the cervix. It is possible for the cervix to become infected by various germs. The cervix may also be injured during childbirth. An examination of the cervix and of the uterus at least once each year after the age of forty is recommended to every woman as a preventive against cancer.

Sometimes an irritation of the wall of the uterus results in damage to the tissues so that it becomes necessary to dilate the cervix and by means of the curette to scrape the lining of the uterus. The tissue thus removed is examined under the microscope for the presence of cancer or determination as to the nature of the disturbance in the tissues. The process of dilating and scraping, or curetting, is called dilation and curettage and is commonly spoken of around the hospitals as the "D & C" procedure.

UTERUS—See article SEX HYGIENE.
UTERUS—(figs.): See WOMEN, article HYGIENE OF WOMEN.
UTERUS—cancer: See articles SEX HYGIENE; CANCER.
UTERUS—congested in menstruation: See article SEX HYGIENE.
UTERUS—function in menstruation: See WOMEN, article HYGIENE OF WOMEN.
UTERUS—glands developed by estradiol and progesterone: See article ENDOCRINOLOGY.
UTERUS—periodic examination of womb for cancer: See article CANCER.
UTERUS—removal: See BIRTH, article CARE OF MOTHERS BEFORE AND AFTER CHILDBIRTH.

UVULA From the middle of the palate there hangs down into the throat a small fleshy mass which is known as the uvula. Rarely it becomes infected; otherwise it is best let alone. Seldom is it necessary to clip, cut, or treat it in any way.

UVULA—location (fig.): See EAR, article THE EAR, TONGUE, NOSE, AND THROAT.

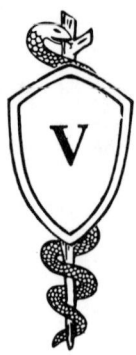

VACATIONS AND HEALTH When your head starts drooping about three o'clock in the afternoon, when you begin complaining of the heat, and when your work loses much of its usual interest you are about ready for your vacation. You may think you are doing better to stay home and work. Scientific studies show, however, that a vacation is an asset from the financial point of view, because you do more productive work afterward than you did before.

An old-time doctor was asked by a young assistant how to run his office successfully. The doctor gave him two suggestions for routine treatment. "First," he said, "ask your patients what they eat and order something else; second, find out where they are going on their vacations and send them some place else." The old doctor knew from common experience that most people do not pick their vacations properly for health and rest.

Any vacation should bring about a change from the routine of daily life, but rest is most important. In fact, hygienists have asserted that one of the greatest contributions of the Biblical code to hygiene was its emphasis on one day of rest in every seven. With the coming of the machine age the pressure has so greatly increased that a five-day week is likely in many industries, which means the regular disposal of two days each week for recreation.

Many organizations have become interested in proper disposal of this time, from the point of view not only of recreation but also of adult education. Executives who work under high pressure with great responsibility are likely to take both winter and summer vacations. If we live twice as fast as we used to we ought to rest twice as much and twice as often.

GET AWAY FROM YOUR YEAR-ROUND HABITS—A long and healthy life depends largely on the type of body you inherit from your ancestors and your freedom from infection. It depends also on the speed with which you use up your vitality and the amount of time that you take for recreation. There are many records in medicine of men and women who pushed themselves to the breaking point and who developed nervous breakdowns simply because they refused to rest.

One of the greatest British doctors said that the best test of the necessity for a vacation is to try one. The type of vacation you choose should be such as to cause you to forget your usual occupation and habits. Desk workers and clerks should preferably spend their vacations in some occupation involving muscular exercise. The manual laborer will probably find his vacation most profitable with suitable amounts of time in rest, flat on his back or perhaps in a hammock with a good book. The desk worker who spends his two weeks' holiday playing bridge in a hotel room or attending theaters in a crowded city is not getting the kind of rest he ought to have.

There is nothing as sad as a vacation that goes sour. The worst vacation is that of the businessman who loads his family into a big touring car and drives away to some resort. The demands on him during the travel and at the resort are greater than any single day in his office. He is forced not only to look after the family and to provide for them but to amuse them as well. It is unfair to ask the mother of a family, whose full time is spent in looking after the children, to spend her vacation looking after them under conditions far more difficult than those at home.

A vacation always should mean a change from routine. It should be a change not only from routine work but also from the routine of home and of recreation. It should be a change not only of surroundings but also of people. Everybody knows that some people can get on one's nerves. That type of person is no help on a vacation.

VACATION FOOD AND DRINK—In picking a place for your vacation always consider questions of health. Pure water, good sanitation, pure milk, and a good food supply are absolutely essential.

The motor vacation, which involves stops in numerous camps, demands particular watchfulness. The summer camp for children needs to be studied with these points in mind.

Any exposed drinking water is a possible source of danger. Seaside springs should be distrusted. Health authorities ought to cover them with concrete and arrange to discharge the flowing water into a river or a sewer. Any spring water properly filtered and treated with chlorine may be considered safe. Spring water in camps may be protected by suitable disposal of sewage. Water unfit for drinking is probably equally unfit for bathing in most instances. It is always wise to take some drinking water with you when you go on a camping trip.

Dishes may be washed in water taken from springs or rivers, provided the water is first thoroughly boiled. Most people who live in cities are so used to drinking water as it comes from the faucet that they forget to watch the water supply when they travel.

Be certain also that the food supplies you buy from wayside vendors are fresh and cleanly handled. Particular precautions must be taken in regard to milk. It is better to drink no milk than to take a chance on milk bought from a farm which does not use pasteurization or does not determine whether the cattle that supply the milk are free from infection. Modern cities demand that cattle be tuberculin tested and free from streptococci infection. These facts are determined by inspectors. When you buy milk from any farmer along the roadside you cannot be sure even of ordinary cleanliness.

It is safer to eat canned vegetables and fruits than to take a chance on vegetables sold at a roadsde stand without proper equipment for cleaning them. Improper handling of vegetables may be responsible for many kinds of illness.

Flies around eating places are a constant menace. Eating places should be guarded from flies by use of mosquito netting or screening.

Some persons traveling on vacations try to get along with a diet of bread, eggs, and coffee. Such diets are tiresome and lack the essentials of a well-balanced diet, which include fresh fruits, vegetables, and plenty of milk. A suitable diet is a great help to a healthful vacation. Many persons who go to American-plan hotels overeat and return from their vacations with digestion completely disordered by the extra strain they have borne during the weeks supposed to be given to rest. Remember that your internal organs need a rest, as well as the muscles and the brain.

A HEALTHFUL VACATION—Chief factors of a healthful vacation can be listed as follows: first, change of occupation; second, sunshine and the open air; third, plenty of rest at night and during the day; fourth, congenial friends and surroundings; fifth, freedom from social routine.

This, for instance, was the type of vacation long taken by Henry Ford, Thomas Edison, Harvey Firestone, and John Burroughs—all noted for hard work, success, and long lives. These representative notables used to travel about in a motor car, camping at night in the woods or in some convenient place. They were with congenial people who were not included in their usual environment. They had interest in conversation different from that of their daily lives. They spent much time in the sunshine and in the open air. They went to bed early at night and arose when they wished in the morning. They were not governed by any routine on their vacation. They did not have to dress for meals or for the evening but wore the most comfortable and roughest clothing that they had. Their vacations have become proverbial as representing the best in type.

Your vacation always should be selected according to your build and your state of health. The real vacation for the average city dweller is one in which he can have comforts suitable to the conditions of his body. For a real rest, a real bed with a real mattress is a help to weary limbs. A hot bath with a rubdown by trained hands helps to soothe the tired muscles.

Instead of attaining these comforts, many a worker who has had fifty weeks of office routine tries mountain climbing of playing thirty-six holes of golf daily, putting terrific stress on his blood vessels and his heart. Thereafter, instead of sleeping in a comfortable bed, he finds a strange bed with a mattress concocted from cotton, straw, or corncobs. Then he wonders why his back and his thighs hurt so much when he gets up the next morning.

Many a vacationist has been heard moaning for his own bed, his own hot bath, coffee cooked the way he likes it, and the morning paper with the news that interests him. Under such circumstances, there is no place like home!

TOURING AND CAMPING—The people who really have to worry most about their vacations are those who take to the road. It is astounding how much wreckage a family vacation in a motor car can bring about from a health point of view. Driving all day means that the calls of nature are ignored. Cinders fly in the eye; elbows and knees are bumped and rubbed. The digestion is disturbed and the muscles are cramped by hours of sitting in contorted positions. Children suffer from the glare of the sun, the dust of the road, the impossibility of getting the right kind of food, insect bites, bad meals and water. A baby should never be taken on such a vacation, and even children from two to six years of age are likely to suffer from such performances.

Fortunately, most of our states have taken over control of motor camps, so that you can be reasonably sure in such camps of suitable water and milk supplies. Smart tourists nowadays carry along twenty or thirty yards of mosquito neeting to fend off insects. There is little fear of infection from the average mosquitoes in the northern part of the United States, but a mosquito bite that itches or bleeds can spoil any vacation. A weak solution of camphor or a one-per-cent solution of menthol in a suitable lotion will stop the itching and give comfort.

Every camper ought to take along a spade and a first aid kit. The spade is used to bury remnants of food, empty tin cans, and bottles. These always should be buried twenty-five feet from any running stream or body of water. The spade also is used to cover fires.

The first-aid kit should contain, at least, a bottle of tincture of iodine, a cake of soap, two rolls of gauze, some cotton, and adhesive plaster. It should also carry some of the family's favorite laxative, vaseline or petrolatum, and a simple ointment for abrasions, chafing, and sunburn. Any ordinary zinc oxide ointment serves this purpose. There should be a cold cream for use on dry, chapped lips and perhaps a small amount of some antiseptic solution that is really antiseptic and will not act as a caustic on a burn.

Such a first-aid kit may save a life and is of great help in securing comfort and relief from pain in emergencies. Manufacturers now make such kits for use of motorists.

Nervous Breakdown—There seems to be an idea that anyone who suffers from nervous exhaustion or nervous breakdown will be benefited by a sea voyage. Such voyages do have the advantage of taking people away from their usual surroundings. But certain precautions must be taken.

If depression is a prominent symptom the intervals between ports should be short. People who are melancholic become more and more depressed by the sight of nothing but water for several days. People who have been ill and get seasick easily should not take a sea voyage for convalescence. A person who has had a nervous breakdown should never travel alone.

After all, the choice of a vacation is a relatively simple matter if you are reasonable, but it does demand a good deal of foresight. A good vacation is one during which you enjoy yourself thoroughly, in which you are rested when you return, and in which your mind selects a new groove. A good vacation is one without undue exposure to the sun, the rain, or the cold, or bad weather generally, particularly if you suffer from coughs or colds, hay fever or asthma.

A good vacation is one in which the persons who surround you are so congenial that you never lose your temper. A good vacation is one in which your health is benefited, as determined by effects on your digestion, your blood pressure, your circulation, and your nervous system. A good vacation is one taken in a place where there is pure water, pure milk, and a good food supply. A good vacation is one in which the muscles are exercised, but not to the point of exhaustion or danger to the tis-

VACCINATION

sue beyond repair. A good vacation is one in which you think of your business, but do not worry about it. A man who thinks so little of his business that he can forget it completely while on a vacation is not in the right business.

VACCINATION See *Diphtheria, Immunization, Smallpox, Tetanus,* etc.

VACCINATION—avoid during phase of allergic skin condition: See article ALLERGY.

VACCINATION—Calmette method: See RESPIRATORY DISEASES, article THE RESPIRATORY DISEASES.

VACCINATION—defined: See CHILDHOOD DISEASES, article INFECTIOUS DISEASES OF CHILDHOOD.

VAGINA The canal which in the woman extends from the outer sex organs to the uterus is known as the vagina. The outer organs are called scientifically the vulva.

VAGINA—(figs.): See WOMEN, article HYGIENE OF WOMEN.

VAGINA—See article SEX HYGIENE.

VAGINA—bleeding as a sign of cancer: See article CANCER.

VAGINAL TAMPONS—worn during menstruation: See article SEX HYGIENE.

VARICELLA See *Chicken Pox.*

VARICOSE VEINS

VARICOSE VEINS Once human beings were so modest that it was undesirable even to mention varicose veins. Now comedians crack jokes about them on the radio.

Most of the veins of the body are provided with valves which keep the column of blood going back to the heart from settling back in the veins. When the valves break down, the veins dilate.

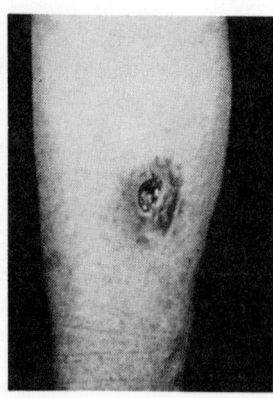 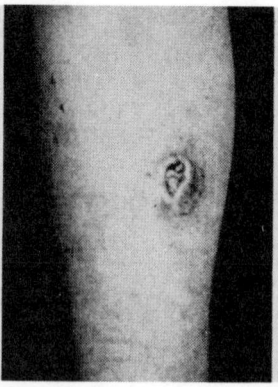 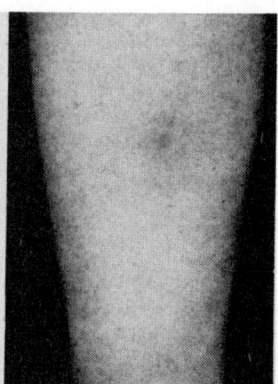

Veins which have lost their elasticity become enlarged and swollen. The weakened walls of the veins cannot withstand the pressure of the blood. The condition is called varicose veins. Varicose veins develop in the legs of middle-aged people, but the condition may appear in young pregnant women. Sometimes the skin over the veins develops an ulcer. Three photographs show the healing process of an ulcer under treatment for about five weeks.

Postgraduate Medicine

Such dilated veins are called varicose veins. When the veins dilate, they project above the skin in lumpy masses. If they get blocked, clots may form in the veins. Occasionally these become secondarily infected.

The veins of the legs are first affected, for the simple reason that the power of gravity has a stronger influence on the veins of the leg than on those higher up in the body. Varicosity of the veins around the bottom of the bowel produces hemorrhoids. Women who are pregnant are likely to develop varicose veins because of the blocking of the return flow of blood through the veins.

In the prevention of varicose veins the mechanism of causation must be kept in mind. If the veins have been blocked because of the wearing of tight belts or tight garters, discontinuance of such garments is indicated. After the birth of a child the pressure on the circulation is relieved, but the valves may be broken down, and they do not again recover. Excess weight may interfere with the action of the circulation and also with exercise. Hence fat people tend to have varicose veins more easily than thin ones.

Among the methods used to control varicose veins are the wearing of elastic bandages or stockings, removal of the varicose veins by surgery, and obliteration of the veins by the injection of caustic substances. If the procedure that brought about the varicose veins still operates, new veins will become varicose as older ones are blocked. In severe cases the physician may tie off a large blood vessel high up on the thigh so as to prevent the secondary effects that have been mentioned.

Ordinarily the injection method of treating small varicose veins is simple. The doctor, having located the extent of the dilated portion of the vein, frees the blood vessel of blood and then injects into it a substance which causes irritation of the walls of the blood vessel so that the walls will grow together. A variety of solutions are used for this purpose, the doctor determining in each instance the one which he prefers to use for the individual patient.

VARICOSE VEINS—bleeding, first aid: See article FIRST AID.

VARICOSE VEINS—old people: See article OLD AGE.

VARICOSE VEINS—pregnancy: See BIRTH, article CARE OF MOTHERS BEFORE AND AFTER CHILDBIRTH.

The Venereal Diseases

BY

MORRIS FISHBEIN, M.D.

Former Editor, Journal American Medical Association, Chicago; Editor, Excerpta Medica, Bulletin World Medical Assn.; Post-graduate Medicine.

THE VENEREAL DISEASES are among the most common that afflict mankind. They spread from person to person in response to satisfaction of the biologic demand of the glands of man, but also occasionally through perfectly innocent sources, such as contaminated utensils, towels, and other appurtenances intimately used by human beings.

One fact must, however, be constantly kept in mind: both major venereal diseases, syphilis and gonorrhea, are caused by germs. The germs must be transmitted in order to transmit the disease. Every case of either one of these diseases comes from another case. Until a patient with one of these diseases is satisfactorily treated and his infection brought under control, he is a menace to everyone around him, including his wife—if he is married—his children, his friends, or associates.

The diseases are not new with man. They have probably existed since the earliest times, certainly since the Middle Ages. Everyone should have knowledge of the nature of these diseases and means of transmission, means of prevention, and correct method of treatment. Proper dissemination of such knowledge seems to be the only hope for their ultimate control.

Syphilis

Whether or not syphilis existed previous to 1493 is not established with certainty. About that time it appeared in Barcelona among Spanish sailors who had returned from Haiti. It reached Italy with the army of Charles VIII, and from Italy spread throughout Europe. At first it was called "Neapolitan disease" or the "French pox." The name spyhilis was given to it in 1530 by a writer named Fracastorius. Since that time, physicians have studied the disease constantly. Even before the modern era doctors had learned to treat syphilis with a fair degree of success with mercury. However, it was the discovery of the organism of the disease, and later the discovery of specific methods of treatment, that offered the first promise of complete control. The organism of spyhilis, known as "spirochaeta" or "treponema," was definitely established as the cause of the disease by the investigator Schaudinn in 1905. The organism is seen only with the microscope, and is found in the sore which is typically the first sign of infection with this disease.

TRANSMISSION OF SYPHILIS

In the vast majority of cases syphilis is transmitted from one human being to another during sexual relations. There are, however, records of accidental infection, such as those which occur on the hands of surgeons and midwives who have not properly protected their hands during their work; such as occur on the lips from infection through kissing, and such as occur occasionally on the breasts of wet nurses. Occasionally also the child may be infected before birth from its mother, in instances even when the mother herself is not actively diseased.

These facts should not frighten anyone into a phobia or constant fear of syphilis, since the disease is not transmitted as easily as the description may seem to suggest. Hotel beds, public lavatories, bathtubs, door knobs, books, utensils used in public eating places are not easily infected. Moreover, the germs do not live easily in the presence of dryness. Finally, it is necessary for the organism to get into a sore or an easily infected spot in order to invade the body. In most instances, thorough washing with soap and water does much to remove danger of infection. When it seems likely that one has been directly exposed to the development of the infection with syphilis, the rubbing of mercury ointment into the exposed area has been proved to be a protective measure of great value. It is well, however, to emphasize again that syphilis is rarely acquired by those who observe the elementary laws of personal hygiene and who have sexual relations only with those who are free from the disease.

FIRST SIGNS OF SYPHILIS

The first sign of syphilis is usually the appearance of a sore on the genital area or on the finger or wherever the germs gain entrance into the tissues. These sores develop slowly. At the same time the lymph glands in the region near by become swollen. A physician who sees such a sore makes his diagnosis certain by taking some of the fluid from the sore and studying it under what is called the dark field microscope. By reflected light he is thus able to see the spirochaetes wriggling in the fluid. He may also spread some of the secretion on a glass slide and stain it with suitable stains which make the organisms visible with the ordinary microscope.

The healing of the primary sore or its removal will not, however, prevent syphilis from invading the body. Usually, by the time the organisms are found freely in the sore, the body has already been quite fully invaded and it is necessary to give general treatment to control the condition. If immediate treatment is given before the appearance of the secondary symptoms, these are not likely to appear. Hence, the physician urges emphatically that every case of syphilis be treated at the earliest possible moment; in fact, that every case diagnosed from the symptoms be treated even before getting the results of the Wassermann test, so as to be certain that the control will be brought about at the earliest possible moment.

The test known as the Wassermann test, and a similar test, known as the Kahn test, are means of examining the blood so as to determine whether or not it contains a substance opposing syphilis, which is present only if syphilis has invaded the body. These tests are positive in more than 95 per cent of cases in an early stage. By their nature they enable the physician to determine whether or not improvement is taking place, and later whether or not the patient has been cured.

Venereal diseases can be cured, provided treatment is given sufficiently early and with sufficient intensity and for a long enough period of time. Modern treatment is based on use of adequate amounts of penicillin or other antibiotic drugs.

The secondary symptoms of syphilis appear about the time when the first sore is disappearing. These symptoms represent invasion of the body as a whole. Now the person is usually sick, he may be jaundiced, and eruptions may appear about the body. Frequently the hair falls out in spots, and occasionally serious sores develop on the skin. There may even be inflammation of the eyes, of the mouth, of the joints, or of the nervous system in this stage of syphilis. Because these symptoms may come and go, some patients are inclined to neglect treatment in the second stage of syphilis. This, however, should never be done. It is easier to treat the condition in this stage than in the third stage, in which the brain and nervous system become involved.

In the secondary stage there has seldom been destruction of the tissues of the body, so that treatment in this stage is more likely to be effective. Under no circumstances should the patient believe that the gradual disappearance of the symptoms represents cure of the disease. He should have a definite statement by a competent physician after that physician has made sufficient laboratory tests to venture an opinion with reasonable certainty.

In the third stage of syphilis, there occur not only destruction of tissues, but growths within various organs of the body, inflammations of the blood vessels, hardening of some of the organs, and other serious changes. In fact, the lesions of this disease are so varied that Sir William Osler once said that one who knew all of syphilis really knew all of medicine. The third stage grows constantly worse unless sufficiently treated. Fortunately, the third stage of syphilis is not likely to be as dangerous to other people as are the first and second, because in this stage the lesions are buried deeper within the body, so that the organisms are not so easily transmitted outside the body.

In the later stage of syphilis, it affects the nervous system. As a result come those two exceedingly serious diseases which are responsible for much disability and death: locomotor ataxia or tabes dorsalis, and paresis, also called general paralysis of the insane and dementia paralytica. In these conditions, other methods of treatment are required besides those commonly used for syphilis in the early stages. It may be necessary to apply treatment directly to the spine or to the brain. It may be necessary to infect the patient with malaria, which has been found to have special virtue in the attack on general paralysis, or to use the heat treatment, which has come to be well established as a useful method.

FACTS ABOUT SYPHILIS

Among certain facts which should be known to everyone relative to syphilis are the following:

This disease does not cause pimples.
It does not cause itching conditions of the skin.

It may cause ulcers of the legs, but more frequently these are due to varicose veins.

It may be responsible for failure to produce children, but there are also other conditions which may produce such failures.

It is not a form of blood poisoning, but testing of the blood will show whether or not the patient has syphilis.

It is not responsible for the vast majority of cases of baldness, but some cases of loss of hair not only of the head but of the entire body may be due to syphilis.

It has not been established in any way that syphilis is the cause of cancer or that these two conditions are in any way related.

INSTRUCTIONS FOR THOSE WITH SYPHILIS

If you have any sore on your genitals, no matter how small, or if you think you have syphilis, consult your physician. Do not under any conditions rely on the "blood medicines" that promise to eradicate syphilis, and do not be caught by advertising doctors—quacks—who try to get your money by promising to cure you quickly. Do not let druggists prescribe for you; they are not qualified to treat syphilis.

Do not hesitate to tell your doctor or dentist of your disease. Later in life if you get sick at any time, you should tell your doctor that you have had syphilis, since this fact may furnish a clue to treatment on which your cure depends.

Live temperately and sensibly. Do not go to extreme in any direction in your habits of life.

Try to get a reasonable amount of sleep—eight hours is the amount needed by the average person. And as a safeguard to others, sleep alone. Avoid possible contamination of others by contact with your secretions or excretions.

Absolutely do not use alcoholic liquors. All experience shows that drinking —even moderate drinking—is bad for syphilis.

Take good care of your teeth. Brush them two or three times a day. If they are not in good condition, have them attended to by a dentist. But when you go to him, tell him that you have syphilis.

Do not have sexual intercourse until you are told by your physician that you are no longer contagious. It will interfere with the cure of the disease, and it is criminal, for it is likely to give the disease to your wife.

You must not marry until you have the doctor's consent, which cannot be properly given until at least two years have passed after cure seems complete. If you do, you run the risk of infecting your wife and your children with syphilis.

Early in the course of syphilis, while it is contagious, the greatest danger of infecting other people is by the mouth. Because of this danger, do not kiss anybody. Particularly, do not endanger children by kissing them.

Do not allow anything that has come in contact with your lips or that has been in your mouth to be left around so that anybody can use it before it has been cleaned. This applies to cups, glasses, knives, forks, spoons, pipes, cigars, toothpicks, and all such things. It is better to use your own towels, brushes, comb, razor, soap, etc., though these are much less likely to be contaminated than objects that go in your mouth.

If you have any open sores—you will not have any after the first week or two, if you are treated—everything that comes in contact with them should be destroyed or disinfected.

To live up to these instructions will only require a little care until you get used to them; after that, it will be easy. If you do live up to them, there is a good prospect that syphilis will not do your health permanent harm or cause injury to others; and you will have the satisfaction of knowing that, after your misfortune, you have acted the part of an honest man in your efforts to overcome it.

Remember, the antibiotic drugs, particularly penicillin, are now known to be efficient in controlling syphilis. Often the condition is fully controlled in a few weeks. The number of cases has dropped to one-tenth what it used to be. To insure future safety, treatment must be continued until every evidence of the disease has disappeared. For your own good, you must see to it that you do not neglect your treatment after the first few months.

Penicillin, terramycin, and aureomycin are most important in the treatment of syphilis. By intensive treatment, patients may be free from the danger of infecting others in a few days. In early cases, the disease is apparently brought under full control within a week or ten days. Treatment demands, however, complete control by the physician during the period of treatment. Penicillin taken by mouth or in other ways is not safe or efficient. Patients must return frequently for repeated examinations and tests to be sure the condition is completely controlled.

WHEN PEOPLE WITH SYPHILIS MAY MARRY

One of the questions most frequently asked by a patient with syphilis is whether or not he may marry. Most physicians are convinced that a patient should be free from all syphilitic symptoms for at least one year before marriage should be contemplated. In some American states the bridegroom is compelled to furnish a medical certificate to show that he has been examined and found free from venereal disease. This has been, for instance, the law in Alabama, Louisiana, North Carolina, North Dakota, Oregon, Wisconsin, and Wyoming. However, none of these states requires a certificate from the prospective bride. The marriage of a person who has a contagious venereal disease is forbidden in Delaware, Indiana, Maine, Michigan, Nebraska, New Jersey, Oklahoma, Pennsylvania, Utah, Vermont, Virginia, and Washington. However, there does not seem to be any good evidence that any of these states secures adequate evidence from those applying for a license to marry.

The treatment of this condition is one of the most intricate problems that can confront a physician. He must use his remedies in relationship to the reaction of the patient and the response of the patient to them. No one with the disease should ever discontinue treatment until he is pronounced by a competent physician free from danger of transmitting the disease and cured to the extent that the condition is brought absolutely to a halt in his body. Persistence in the use of the new remedies that are available under proper control will yield a successful result in the vast majority of cases.

Gonorrhea

Gonorrhea has existed certainly since Biblical times. Although it is a widespread and serious disease, it is not a killing disease. As a cause of ill health, it ranks among the leaders, but as a cause of death it is not especially prominent. Many people believe that gonorrhea concerns only the sex organs, whereas the germ which causes it, described by the investigator Niesser in 1879, may invade any part of the human body. Like syphilis, it is spread mostly by sexual contacts. However, there are infections of the eyes sustained during childbirth or in other ways which attack mostly infants at birth. There are infections of the tissues in women associated with the use of bathtubs and toilet devices not properly cleansed, which are accidental infections with this disease. Little girls are occasionally infected by soiled hands of mothers or nurses.

Gonorrhea is responsible for a considerable percentage of all cases of blindness. It is one of the common causes of infection in the female abdomen, resulting in necessary surgical operations and occasionally removal of the female organs. It is responsible for a considerable amount of sterility in men due to infections of the various parts of the sex tracts. It is found not only among the poor but in all classes of society.

FIRST SIGNS OF GONORRHEA

From three to five days after a sex contact with a person who is infected the first signs of the disease may appear. These usually are a feeling of burning or stinging at the time of urination, associated with redness and soreness, and associated also with the formation of pus or matter which drips from the sex organ. This material is highly infectious and should not be allowed to come in contact with the eyes or sex organs of any other person.

If a physician is consulted immediately, he may be able to stop the disease in these early stages, when it is confined to the lower portion of the sex organs. If, however, it is not stopped at this time, the germs get farther back into the glands of the male and into the organs and tissues of the female. To the extent to which these organs and tissues are involved, gonorrhea is a serious disorder. The physician may make his diagnosis by an examination of the matter under the microscope, in which case he can actually find the germs, and also by tests of the blood. Occasionally the condition affects the joints, and it is also largely responsible for painful heels, causing outgrowths on the large bone of the heel.

TREATMENT OF GONORRHEA

In treatment, the physician uses many types of remedies, including antibiotics such as penicillin and terramycin given by injection into the muscles or blood stream. Gonorrhea is now controlled in 48 hours. Military authorities prevent gonorrhea by giving penicillin to men going on leave.

ADVICE TO THOSE WITH GONORRHEA

Persist in treatment until your doctor tells you you are cured.

Do not try to treat yourself.

Do not use a patent medicine or some "sure shot" that may stop the discharges but will not cure you.

Do not let an advertising doctor—a quack—get your money, and do not let a drug clerk treat you.

If you have had gonorrhea and you suspect that it is not cured, report to your medical officer.

During the acute stages keep quiet and take little exercise. As long as you have any discharge avoid violent exercise, especially dancing.

In order to avoid chordee, while the disease is acute, sleep on your side, urinate just before going to bed, and drink no water after supper.

Never "break" a chordee. To get rid of it wrap the penis in cold wet cloths or pour cold water on it.

Except at night, drink plenty of water—eight or ten glasses a day.

Do not drink any alcoholic liquors; they always make the disease worse and delay its cure. Also avoid spicy drinks such as ginger ale.

Do not eat irritating, highly seasoned, spicy foods, such as pepper, horseradish, mustard, pickles, salt and smoked meats, or fish.

Always wash your hands after handling the penis, particularly in order to protect your eyes. Gonorrhea of the eyes is very dangerous; it will produce blindness if not at once treated, and the infection is easily carried to the eyes on the fingers.

Keep your penis clean. Do not plug up the opening with cotton or wear a dressing that prevents the escape of the pus from it. Wash the penis several times daily.

Burn old dressings, or drop them into a disinfecting solution.

Never use anybody else's syringe or let others use yours. While you are using a syringe keep it clean by washing it in very hot water, and, when you have finished with its use, destroy it.

Avoid sexual excitement. Stay away from women. Do not have intercourse. It will bring your disease back to its acute stage, and it is almost sure to infect a woman. Sexual intercourse while you have gonorrhea is a criminal act.

You are likely to obey instructions while your gonorrhea is acute, because it causes so much pain. Persist in them after pain is gone; by so doing you will prevent relapses, make your cure much easier and more certain, and expose no one else to the disease.

MODERN TREATMENT OF GONORRHEA

Penicillin is effective not only in venereal gonorrhea but also in gonorrhea affecting the eyes, the joints or the heart. Whereas this disease was formerly considered well nigh incurable, with penicillin cures seem to be almost 100 per cent.

MARRIAGE AFTER GONORRHEA

As regards marriage after an attack of gonorrhea, the patient should be examined at weekly intervals to determine whether or not any infection is present following treatment. The results should be negative three consecutive times before he can be considered definitely cured. It should be remembered that self-treatment with drug-store remedies is just as dangerous as complete neglect of treatment.

Prevention in gonorrhea is far better than cure. The chief factor in prevention consists in the avoidance of sex contacts when infection is present, and infection is likely to be present in any promiscuous woman, either commercial or private. There are various methods of protection against the possibility of infection, such as the use of rubber devices and injections of various antiseptics immediately after sex contact, these antiseptics being held in the organs until the antiseptics have sufficient amount of time to act.

VENTILATION While most people worry most about ventilation in hot weather because it is hard to keep cool, the real problems of ventilation are those of the winter. In summer you can always get fresh air by opening the windows; in winter a cold, drafty room is uncomfortable. A hot, dry room may be even more uncomfortable.

Most American homes are too hot and too dry in winter. The windows are closed, the steam heat is left at capacity, and people forget that air requires a certain amount of moisture to be comfortable for men and safe for furniture. If the air is too dry, it will pick up water wherever it can. Therefore the skin of the body, the membranes of the nose and throat become dry. The furniture becomes dry and brittle and cracks at night. The groaning and crackling of the furniture which is warping and pulling apart interfere with sleep.

Nowadays many types of air moisteners are available. However, many of the devices that evaporate fluid rapidly cause a sensation of dampness. The valves on radiators that are supposed to release moisture keep up a hissing noise and occasionally drop water on the floor, so that you have a choice between crackling furniture or hissing radiators. Pans of water placed over radiators help to put a certain amount of water into the air, but the water evaporates rapidly, and most people forget to keep the pans full. Among the efficient humidifiers are those with troughs of water and belts of cloth that pass through the water, a fan that blows the water, and a motor that operates the fan. This is a lot of machinery for a very simple purpose.

Experts in ventilation of the home are now agreed that the proper use of a barometer is the first important step. This will show the extent to which the air contains moisture. Careful use of the doors and windows, coupled with the cracks in the ordinary residence, will provide for circulation of fresh air. Good ventilation provides for the prevention of smoke, dust, and gases in the air. A comfortable house temperature in summer varies from 70 to 85 degrees Fahrenheit. The best temperature of the air in winter is from 65 to 68 degrees, with sufficient water vapor in the air to produce a relative humidity of from 30 to 60 per cent.

VENTILATION—colds affected by: See RESPIRATORY DISEASES, article THE RESPIRATORY DISEASES.

VERTIGO See *Dizziness*.

VINCENT'S ANGINA During World War I many of our soldiers suffered with a condition that was called trench mouth. In this ailment sores and ulcers occur on the lining of the cheeks and gums, sometimes also on the tonsils and in the back of the throat. The ulcers may become so large as to incapacitate the person who is infected. The gums become acutely inflamed and bleed easily.

Trench mouth is not, however, purely a war condition. A French physician named Vincent found that it was due to an infectious organism which has been called Vincent's organism.

The person who has Vincent's infection may spread it to other people by kissing, by contaminating eating utensils or drinking cups. Cases have been reported in which the disease has been spread by improper sterilizing of dental instruments.

The prevention of Vincent's infection demands constant watchfulness of the condition of the mouth, teeth, and gums. Persistent bleeding of the gums or the appearance of an unpleasant odor or the occurrence of ulcers in the mouth demands that the patient consult a competent dentist or physician at once. Control of this infection is much easier in the early stages than at a time when the condition has become chronic.

Vincent's infection occurs most frequently in those with bad teeth and with mouths that have been badly cared for. Regular, competent attention to the teeth and gums helps to prevent the spread of such infection. The removal of deposits around the teeth and proper attention to the cavities and crevices make it difficult for the germs to grow and persist around the teeth and in the gums.

Such conditions as scurvy, diabetes, lead or bismuth poisoning, and syphilis may produce damage to the mouth and gums and ulcers, to which Vincent's infection may be secondary. It is important, therefore, that in each instance the physician determine exactly what is wrong.

In the modern treatment of Vincent's infection drugs like hydrogen peroxide are used to remove the dead tissue and infected material. The drug called sodium perborate is believed to have a definite effect in destroying the germs of Vincent's disease. These drugs must be used with great care because they may cause chemical burns of tender gums and of the lining of the cheeks. It is known that the sulfonamide preparations are sometimes helpful. Materials constantly in contact with the teeth and gums have been developed, including solutions and the incorporation of the sulfonamides in chewing gum. The dentist or the physician who treats Vincent's infection may apply the drugs directly to the infected area and may by such technics keep the materials closely in contact with the area in which the germs are found. In some instances the use of arsenical preparations injected directly into the veins has been helpful.

Often Vincent's infection is a persistent condition, difficult to cure and demanding attention over long periods of time.

VINCENT'S ANGINA—See article TRANSMISSIBLE DISEASES.

VITAMINS VITAMIN A—A characteristic disease of the eyes, usually called xerophthalmia, results from a deficiency of vitamin A; one of the first signs of its absence is a condition called night blindness; a deficiency of this vitamin sometimes results in a condition of the skin which is called hyperkeratosis, meaning a thickening or hardening. There has been a tremendous amount of experimentation with vitamin A, with a view to proving that it has many other virtues. The Council on Pharmacy and Chemistry of the American Medical Association does not permit the claim that the giving of extra vitamin A to drivers of automobiles will diminish accidents from driving at night in any considerable number of people. Neither does the Council accept the view that the taking of extra amounts of vitamin A is of any value in preventing colds, influenza, or other respiratory infections. Neither is there proof that the taking of a sufficient amount of vitamin A or vitamin A in excess will prevent the formation of kidney stones in man. There does not seem to be any proof that vitamin A, either in normal amounts or in excess amounts, will help excessive action of the thyroid gland, anemia, degenerative conditions of the nervous system, sunburn, or ulcerations of the skin.

Vitamin A has fortunately gotten by without having affixed to it a popular promotional name. There was for a while an attempt to call it the anti-infective vitamin, but science caught up with promotion, and that name has gradually disappeared from both public and medical writing. Oleomargarine

VITAMIN VIRTUES

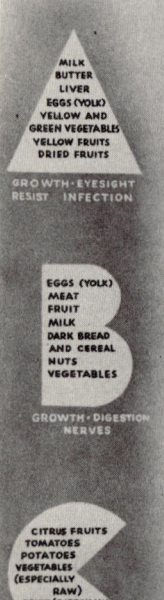

Vitamin A keeps the colds away
And tends to make meek people nervy.
B's what you need
When you're going to seed,
While C is specific for scurvy,
Vitamin D makes the bones in your knee
Tough and hard for the service on Sunday.
While E makes hens scratch
And increases the hatch
And brings in more profits on Monday.
Vitamin F never bothered the chef
'Cause that vitamin never existed.
G puts the fight
In the old appetite,
And you eat all the foods that are listed.
So now when you dine
Just remember these lines
If long on earth you would tarry.
Just try to be good
And pick out more food
From the garden, the orchard and dairy.

has been enriched with this vitamin to make it more nearly resemble the virtues of butter.

VITAMIN B COMPLEX—Vitamin B complex is the name for a group of substances which have been shown to be a part of what was once known as vitamin B. The list includes thiamine, riboflavin, nicotinic acid, pantothenic acid, pyridoxine, and most of the other substances which have been found to have some relation to nutrition of animals, but apparently little, if any, importance in human nutrition.

THIAMINE—The name "thiamine" for the vitamin once called B_1 was selected by Dr. R. R. Williams, who showed the chemical character of the substance. This factor was first isolated in 1927, but long before thiamine was isolated it was known that polished rice produced beriberi and that unpolished rice prevented that condition. Fortunately there is not much beriberi in the United States. However, thiamine is also of value in correcting and preventing the loss of appetite that is apparent in many digestive conditions.

There seem to be conditions in which vitamins, although taken into the body, are not properly absorbed. For instance when there is constant vomiting, when patients have to be fed with tubes, when there is a paralysis of the muscles associated with swallowing, when there is excessive alcoholism, it may be necessary to give thiamine in amounts beyond those ordinarily taken, and perhaps even by direct injection into the body.

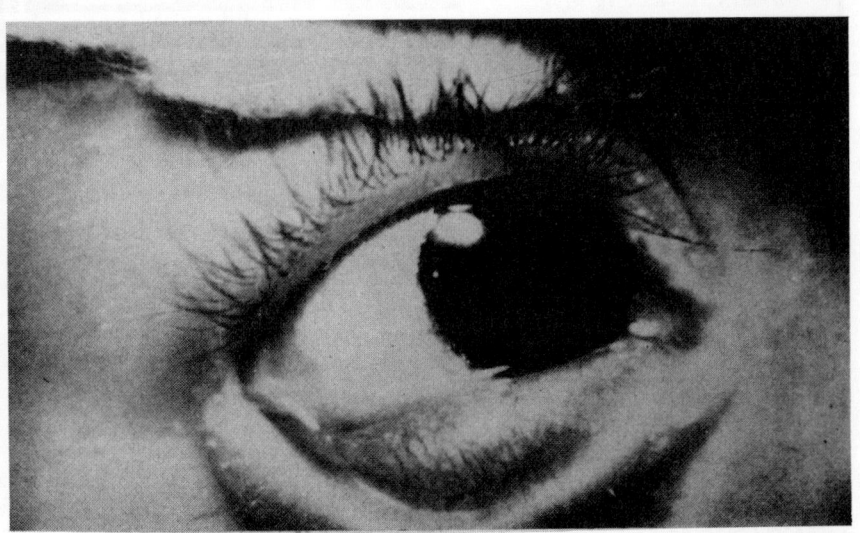

Affliction of the eye caused by a deficiency of vitamin A in the diet. Light yellow patches develop on the lining of the eyelid. The lining loses its moistness and luster and becomes dry like skin. The person is not able to see distinctly in bright light. Postgraduate Medicine

In animals disturbances of the heart and blood vessels are sometimes associated with lack of this vitamin. But few conditions, apparently, exist in human beings in which there is waterlogging of the system associated with lack of thiamine. We know that excessive action of the thyroid gland or fever or vigorous muscle activities use up more thiamine than is ordinarily available, and that people with these conditions need extra amounts of the vitamin.

RIBOFLAVIN—Another portion of the vitamin B complex is riboflavin. When it is absent, characteristic disturbances appear on the tongue, the lips, and the face. These conditions differ from those

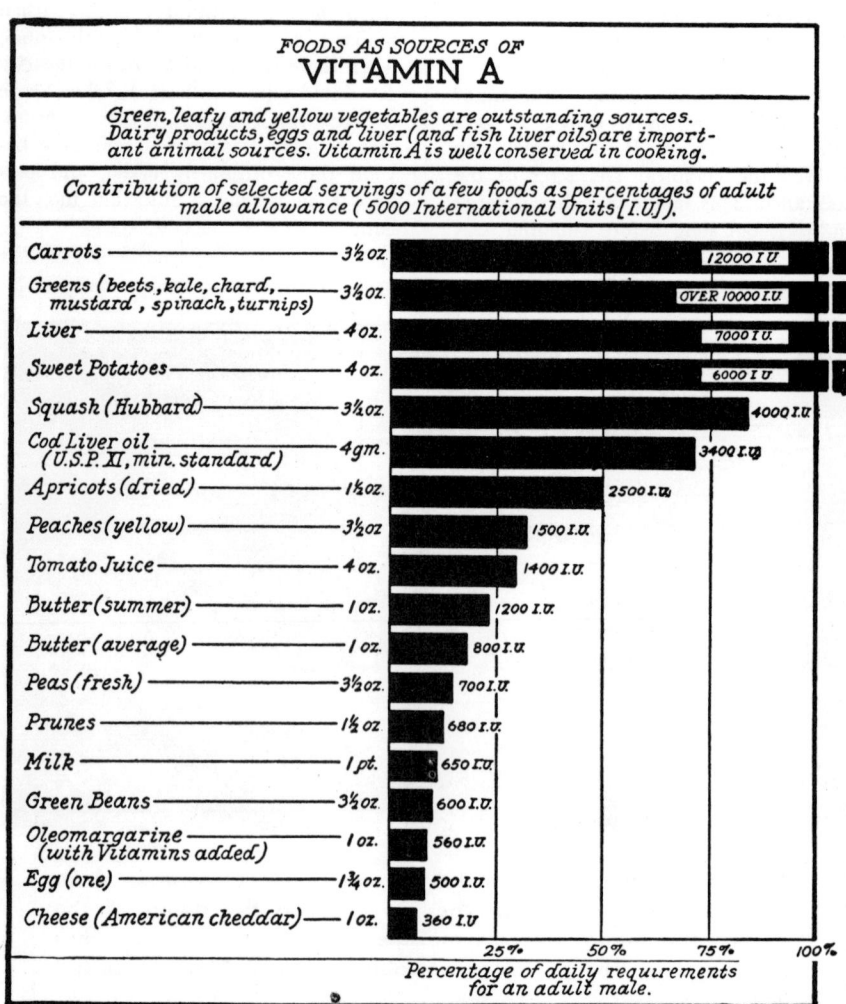

FOODS AS SOURCES OF
VITAMIN A

Green, leafy and yellow vegetables are outstanding sources. Dairy products, eggs and liver (and fish liver oils) are important animal sources. Vitamin A is well conserved in cooking.

Contribution of selected servings of a few foods as percentages of adult male allowance (5000 International Units [I.U.]).

Food	Serving	I.U.
Carrots	3½ oz	12000 I.U.
Greens (beets, kale, chard, mustard, spinach, turnips)	3½ oz	OVER 10000 I.U.
Liver	4 oz.	7000 I.U.
Sweet Potatoes	4 oz.	6000 I.U.
Squash (Hubbard)	3½ oz.	4000 I.U.
Cod Liver oil (U.S.P. XI, min. standard)	4 gm.	3400 I.U.
Apricots (dried)	1½ oz.	2500 I.U.
Peaches (yellow)	3½ oz	1500 I.U.
Tomato Juice	4 oz.	1400 I.U.
Butter (summer)	1 oz.	1200 I.U.
Butter (average)	1 oz.	800 I.U.
Peas (fresh)	3½ oz.	700 I.U.
Prunes	1½ oz	680 I.U.
Milk	1 pt.	650 I.U.
Green Beans	3½ oz	600 I.U.
Oleomargarine (with Vitamins added)	1 oz.	560 I.U.
Egg (one)	1¾ oz.	500 I.U.
Cheese (American cheddar)	1 oz.	360 I.U.

Percentage of daily requirements for an adult male.

Deficiency of vitamin A in the body can cause the skin to become rough, dry and scaly, as shown in this close-up. Green, leafy vegetables, carrots, squash, sweet potato, liver and cod liver oil are excellent sources of vitamin A.
Postgraduate Medicine

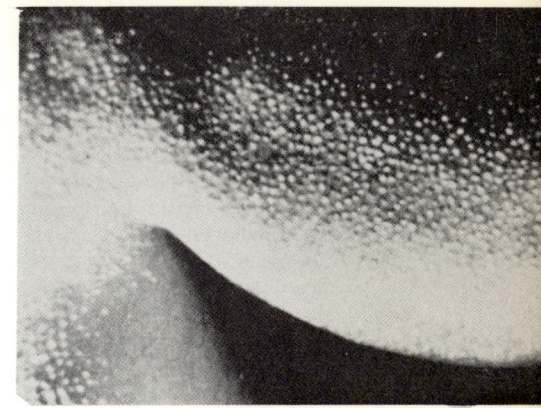

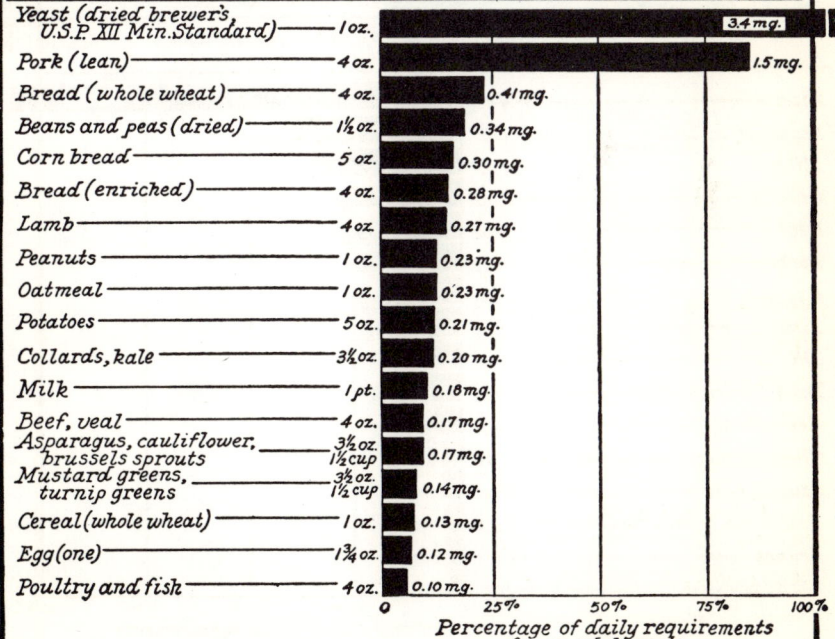

FOODS AS SOURCES OF
THIAMINE (Vitamin B₁)

Except for pork, common foods supply only small amounts of thiamine, the best sources being nutritionally unimpaired cereals and meats; some thiamine may be lost in cooking, either through destruction by heat or extraction by water...

Contribution of selected servings of a few foods as percentages of adult male allowance (1.8 milligrams)

Food	Serving	mg
Yeast (dried brewer's, U.S.P. XII Min. Standard)	1 oz.	3.4 mg.
Pork (lean)	4 oz.	1.5 mg.
Bread (whole wheat)	4 oz.	0.41 mg.
Beans and peas (dried)	1½ oz.	0.34 mg.
Corn bread	5 oz.	0.30 mg.
Bread (enriched)	4 oz.	0.28 mg.
Lamb	4 oz.	0.27 mg.
Peanuts	1 oz.	0.23 mg.
Oatmeal	1 oz.	0.23 mg.
Potatoes	5 oz.	0.21 mg.
Collards, kale	3½ oz.	0.20 mg.
Milk	1 pt.	0.18 mg.
Beef, veal	4 oz.	0.17 mg.
Asparagus, cauliflower, brussels sprouts	3½ oz. / 1½ cup	0.17 mg.
Mustard greens, turnip greens	3½ oz. / 1½ cup	0.14 mg.
Cereal (whole wheat)	1 oz.	0.13 mg.
Egg (one)	1¾ oz.	0.12 mg.
Poultry and fish	4 oz.	0.10 mg.

Percentage of daily requirements for an adult male.

that affect the same tissues in pellagra. Sometimes itching, burning, and a sensation of roughness of the eyes are associated with lack of riboflavin. But actually these conditions are so difficult to diagnose that the doctor tries to make certain first that the riboflavin in the diet is inadequate before he recommends extra riboflavin.

NICOTINIC ACID OR NICOTINAMIDE—The discovery that another portion of the vitamin B complex known as nicotinic acid or nicotinamide is specific in the treatment of pellagra is one of the greatest discoveries of modern medical science. When pellagra is present, the use of this substance will lead to the disappearance of the symptoms related to the skin, the digestion, and the nervous system. However, there does not seem to be much good evidence that extra amounts of nicotinic acid are good for the wide variety of conditions in which they have been tried and recommended.

VITAMIN C—Vitamin C is the antiscurvy vitamin. This has been established experimentally and proved on patients. However, a tremendous number of articles have been published about the use of vitamin C in a great many other conditions.

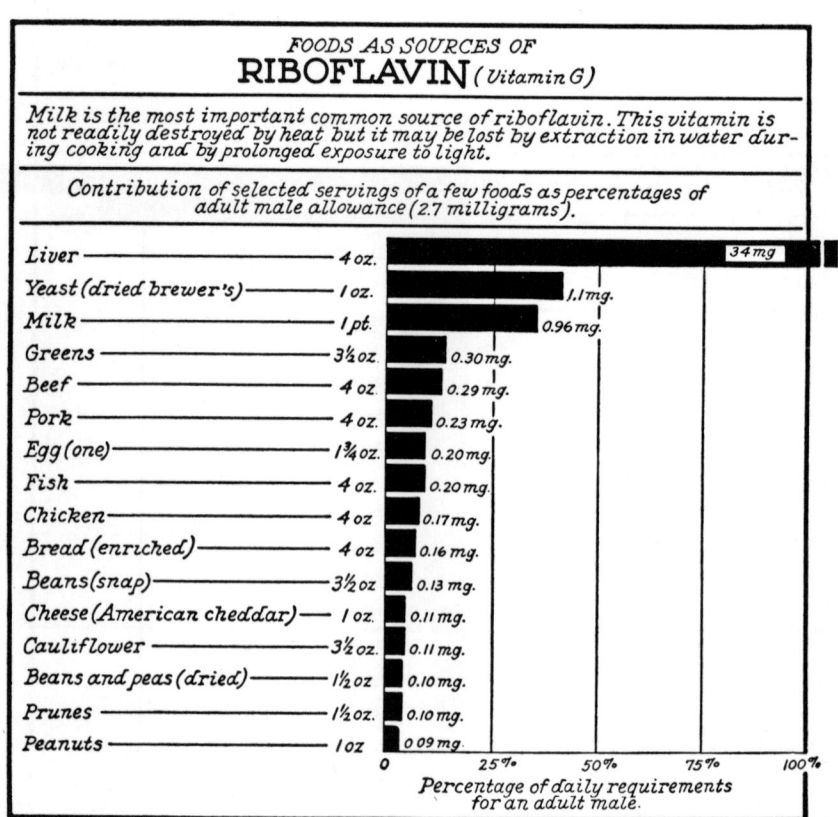

Apparently there are people who do not have outright scurvy, but something resembling scurvy. There are evidences that dental caries, pyorrhea, certain infections of the gums, loss of appetite, anemia, undernutrition, and infection are sometimes found along with insufficient amounts of ascorbic acid. However, again it would be desirable to prove always that there is a deficiency of this vitamin taken into the body and properly utilized, rather than to begin the treatment of such a wide variety of conditions by assuming in advance that the deficiency of the vitamin was responsible and that the giving of large amounts of ascorbic acid or orange juice or tomato juice would bring about a cure.

VITAMIN D—Vitamin D is known in many forms, of which at least two are definitely related to proper use of calcium and phosphorus by the human body. Reports have appeared claiming improvement in chronic arthritis and in some allergic conditions by use of massive doses of vitamin D. The statement has been made that massive doses of this vitamin will improve psoriasis. The Council on Pharmacy and Chem-

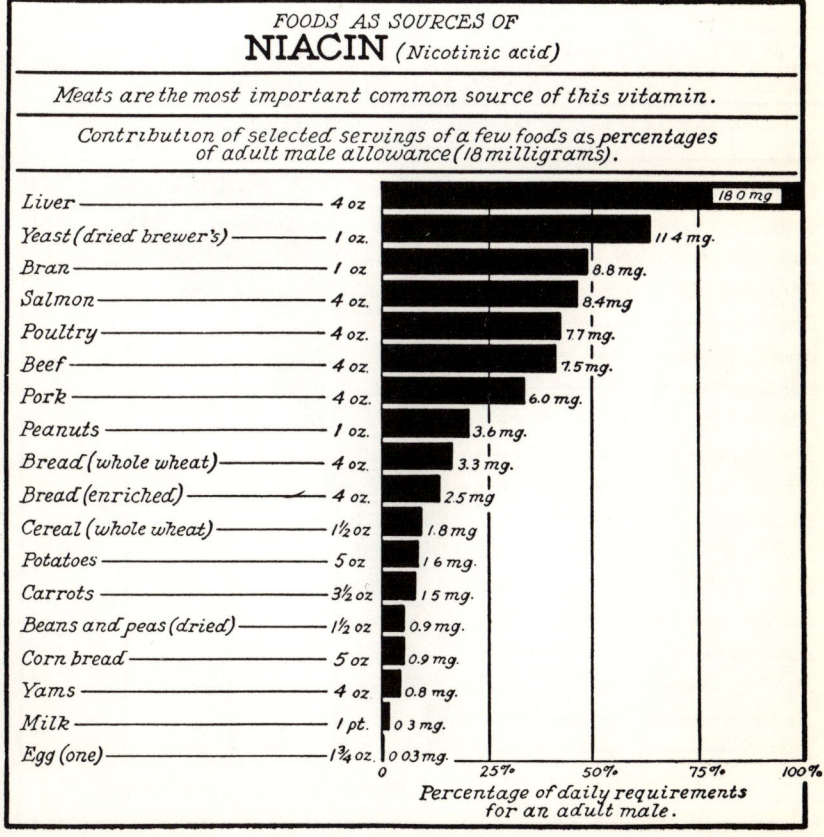

istry of the American Medical Association has held, however, that there is not sufficient evidence to prove either of these claims, although the Council does not discourage further experimentation.

VITAMIN E—For years it has been known that vitamin E must be included in the diet of the rat if there are to be little rats. In other words, this is the anti-sterility vitamin, as the imaginative boys of the press describe it. But the Council on Pharmacy and Chemistry, which talks very concretely on these subjects, simply says that vitamin E is of no value in the treatment of sterility. There are indications that it may be of value in case of habitual abortion, but further studies are necessary to clarify the picture.

VITAMIN B_{12}—This substance has cobalt as a chief chemical ingredient. The product is known also as Cyanocobalamin. This has blood-stimulating activity like that of the anti-anemia factor of liver. Therefore, it is used especially in

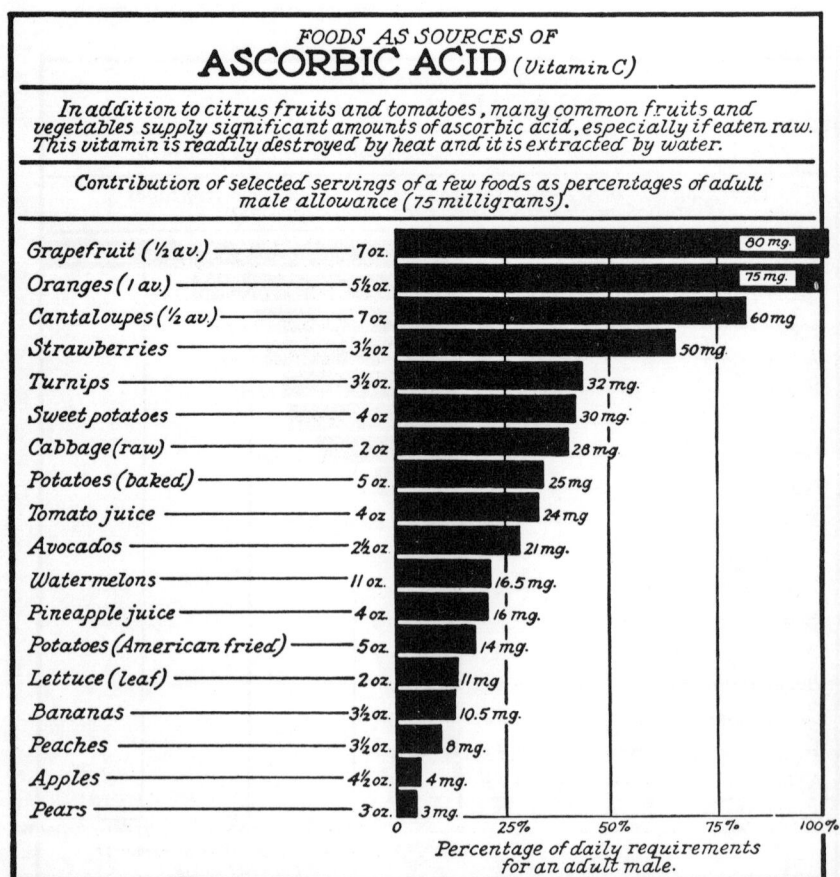

pernicious anemia. The drug is used also in sprue and in anemias resulting from vitamin B_{12} deficiency. Combined with material from the wall of the stomach, the mixture is effective in anemias with neurologic complications. These substances can be taken by mouth.

VITAMIN K—Vitamin K represents again one of the greatest discoveries of medical science. It is the anti-hemorrhagic vitamin. It is useful in obstructive jaundice, in hemorrhagic states associated with certain intestinal diseases, and in some hemorrhagic conditions of the newborn. The evidence is accepted that the mother should have some of this vitamin before childbirth and that the infant should have a normal amount of prothrombin in his blood at the time of birth.

VITAMIN A—absorption impeded by liquid petrolatum: See MEDICINE CHEST, article THE FAMILY MEDICINE CHEST.

VITAMIN A—cold-preventing diet: See RESPIRATORY DISEASES, article THE RESPIRATORY DISEASES.

VITAMIN A—daily requirements: See

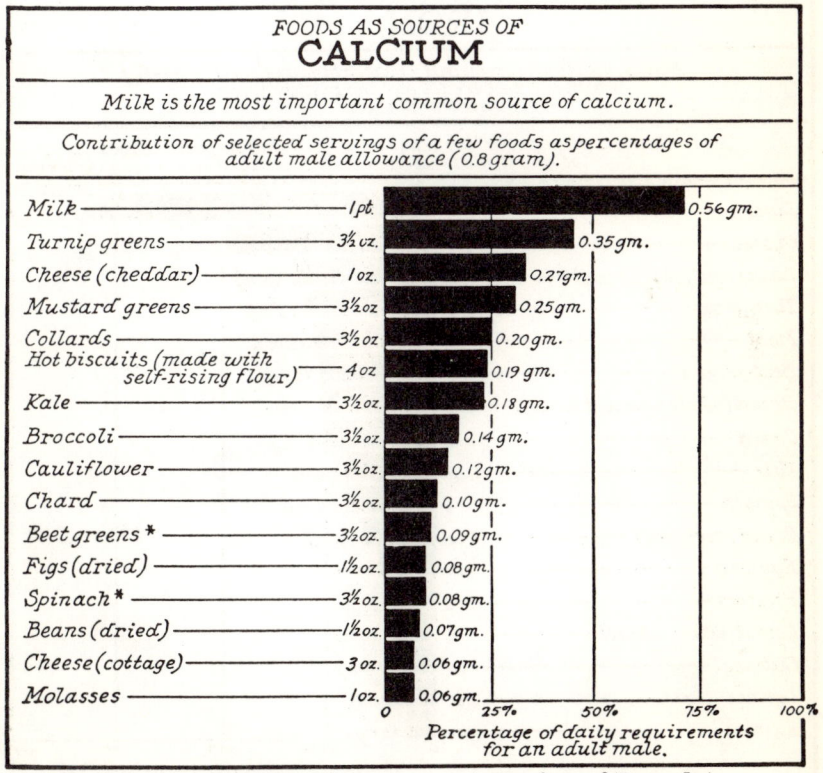

* The calcium in beet greens and spinach is in the form of the oxalate which is not assimilated by the body.

SKIN, article THE SKIN; DIET, article ADVICE ON THE DIET.
VITAMIN A—deficiency: See article DEFICIENCY DISEASES; SKIN, article THE SKIN; HAIR, article THE HAIR.
VITAMIN A—eczema: See SKIN, article THE SKIN.
VITAMIN A—foods as sources (fig.): See article DEFICIENCY DISEASES.
VITAMIN A—hair growth: See HAIR, article THE HAIR.
VITAMIN A—infant's diet: See INFANCY, article CARE AND FEEDING OF THE CHILD.

VITAMIN A—mineral oil depletes body's source: See SKIN, article THE SKIN.
VITAMIN A—nail brittleness: See HAIR, article THE HAIR.
VITAMIN A—optimal amount higher than minimal requirement: See article DEFICIENCY DISEASES.
VITAMIN A—resume: See article DEFICIENCY DISEASES.
VITAMIN A—skin: See SKIN, article THE SKIN.
VITAMIN B COMPLEX—bread: See DIET, article ADVICE ON THE DIET.

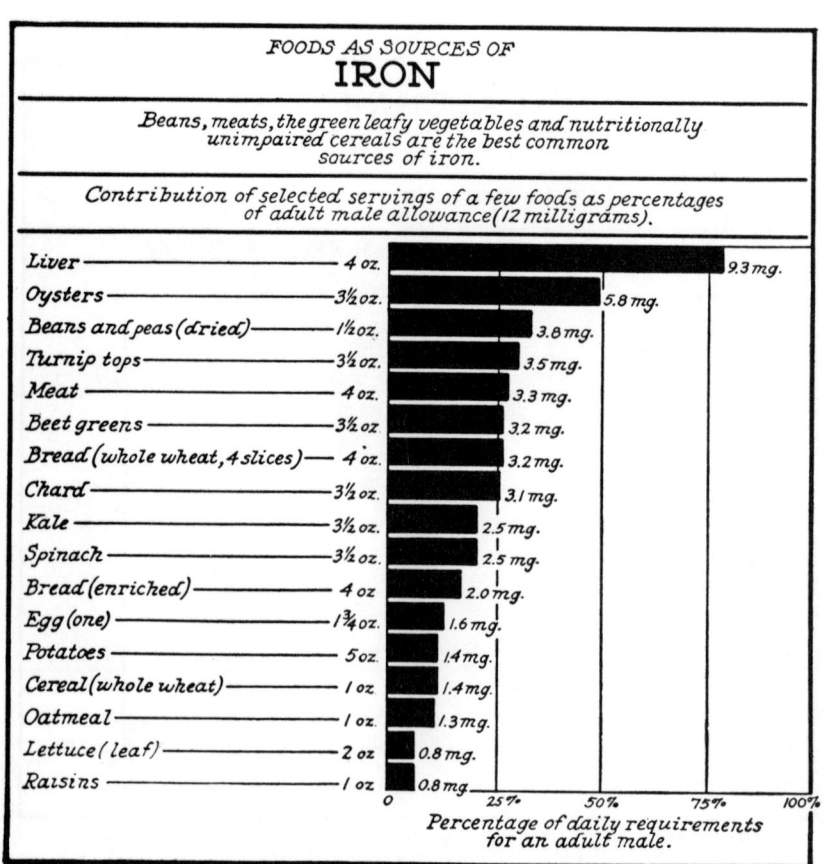

FOODS AS SOURCES OF
IRON
Beans, meats, the green leafy vegetables and nutritionally unimpaired cereals are the best common sources of iron.

Contribution of selected servings of a few foods as percentages of adult male allowance (12 milligrams).

Food	Serving	mg
Liver	4 oz.	9.3 mg.
Oysters	3½ oz.	5.8 mg.
Beans and peas (dried)	1½ oz.	3.8 mg.
Turnip tops	3½ oz.	3.5 mg.
Meat	4 oz.	3.3 mg.
Beet greens	3½ oz.	3.2 mg.
Bread (whole wheat, 4 slices)	4 oz.	3.2 mg.
Chard	3½ oz.	3.1 mg.
Kale	3½ oz.	2.5 mg.
Spinach	3½ oz.	2.5 mg.
Bread (enriched)	4 oz	2.0 mg.
Egg (one)	1¾ oz.	1.6 mg.
Potatoes	5 oz.	1.4 mg.
Cereal (whole wheat)	1 oz	1.4 mg.
Oatmeal	1 oz.	1.3 mg.
Lettuce (leaf)	2 oz	0.8 mg.
Raisins	1 oz	0.8 mg.

Percentage of daily requirements for an adult male.

Vitamin B Complex—cancer of esophagus: See article Cancer.

Vitamin B Complex—certain components destroyed by neutralizing agents: See article Digestion and Digestive Diseases.

Vitamin B Complex—components formed in intestine: See article Digestion and Digestive Diseases.

Vitamin B Complex—deficiency: See article Deficiency Diseases; article Cancer; Skin, article The Skin.

Vitamin B Complex—eczema: See Skin, article The Skin.

Vitamin B Complex—gastritis: See article Digestion and Digestive Diseases.

Vitamin B Complex—gray hair: See Hair, article The Hair.

Vitamin B Complex—infant's diet: See Infancy, article Care and Feeding of the Child.

Vitamin B Complex—milk diet deficient in: See Infancy, article Care and Feeding of the Child.

Vitamin B Complex—optimal amount higher than minimal requirement: See article Deficiency Diseases.

Vitamin B Complex—resume: See article Deficiency Diseases.

Vitamin B Complex—seborrheic dermatitis: See Hair, article The Hair.

Vitamin B Complex—skin: See Skin, article The Skin.

Vitamin B Complex—skin oiliness lessened by: See Skin, article The Skin.

Vitamin B1—See article Deficiency Diseases.

Vitamin B1—constipation: See article

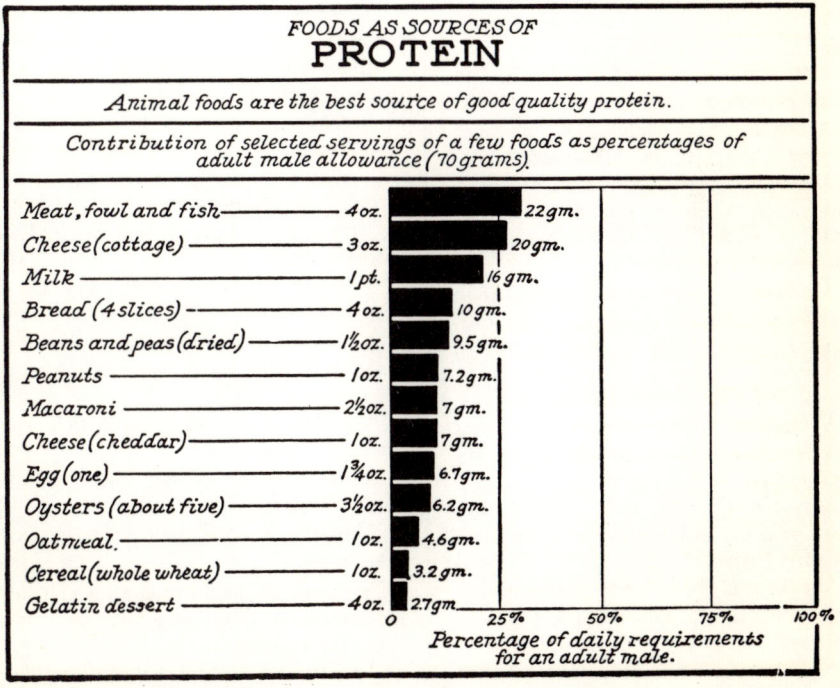

VITAMINS

Digestion and Digestive Diseases.

Vitamin B1—daily requirement: See Diet, article Advice on the Diet.

Vitamin B1—deficiency: See article Deficiency Diseases.

Vitamin B1—foods as sources (fig.): See article Deficiency Diseases.

Vitamin B2—See entry Vitamins.

Vitamin B2—daily requirement: See Skin, article The Skin.

Vitamin B6—See article Deficiency Diseases.

Vitamin B6—skin: See Skin, article The Skin.

Vitamin B12—See article Deficiency Diseases.

Vitamin B12—lack seen in patients with pernicious anemia: See article Digestion and Digestive Diseases.

Vitamin B12—maturation factor in pernicious anemia: See Blood, article The Blood and Its Diseases.

Vitamin B12—seborrhea: See Skin, article The Skin.

Vitamin B12—seborrheic dermatitis: See Hair, article The Hair.

Ascorbic Acid—See Infancy, article Care and Feeding of the Child.

Ascorbic Acid—deficiency produces scurvy: See article Deficiency Diseases.

Vitamin C—daily requirement: See Skin, article The Skin; Diet, article Advice on the Diet.

Vitamin C—deficiency: See article Deficiency Diseases; Ear, article The Ear, Tongue, Nose, and Throat.

Vitamin C—foods as sources (fig.): See article Deficiency Diseases.

Vitamin C—infant's diet: See Infancy, article Care and Feeding of the Child.

Vitamin C—milk diet deficient in: See Infancy, article Care and Feeding of the Child.

Vitamin C—nosebleed: See Ear, article The Ear, Tongue, Nose, and Throat.

Vitamin C—optimal amount higher than minimal requirement: See article Deficiency Diseases.

Vitamin C—resume: See article Deficiency Diseases.

Vitamin C—rheumatic complications: See article Arthritis, Rheumatism, and Gout.

Vitamin C—scurvy: See article Arthritis, Rheumatism, and Gout; Blood, article The Blood and Its Diseases.

Vitamin C—skin: See Skin, article The Skin.

Vitamin D—daily requirement: See Skin, article The Skin; Diet, article Advice on the Diet.

Vitamin D—infant's diet: See Infancy, article Care and Feeding of the Child.

Vitamin D—milk diet deficient in: See Infancy, article Care and Feeding of the Child.

Vitamin D—resume: See article Deficiency Diseases.

Vitamin D—rickets: See Infancy, article Care and Feeding of the Child; article Deficiency Diseases; Skin, article The Skin.

Vitamin D—skin: See Skin, article The Skin.

Vitamin D—skin produces: See Skin, article The Skin.

Vitamin D—tetany: See article Endocrinology.

Vitamin E—See article Deficiency Diseases.

Vitamin E—infant's diet: See Infancy, article Care and Feeding of the Child.

Vitamin E—resume: See article Deficiency Diseases.

Vitamin E—skin: See Skin, article The Skin.

Vitamin K—See article Deficiency Diseases.

Vitamin K—hemorrhages occur when not absorbed: See article Digestion and Digestive Diseases.

Vitamin K—infant's diet: See In-

FANCY, article CARE AND FEEDING OF THE CHILD.

VITAMIN K—resume: See article DEFICIENCY DISEASES.

VITAMIN-DEFICIENCY DISEASES—See article DEFICIENCY DISEASES.

VITAMIN G—foods as sources (fig.): See article DEFICIENCY DISEASES.

VITAMIN H—skin: See SKIN, article THE SKIN.

VITAMIN P-P—daily requirement: See SKIN, article THE SKIN.

VITAMIN P-P—skin: See SKIN, article THE SKIN.

VITAMINS—See DIET, article ADVICE ON THE DIET.

VITAMINS—anti-infective: See article DEFICIENCY DISEASES.

VITAMINS—anti-ophthalmic: See article DEFICIENCY DISEASES.

VITAMINS—antirachitic: See article DEFICIENCY DISEASES.

VITAMINS—anti-xerophthalmic: See article DEFICIENCY DISEASES.

VITAMINS—chart (fig.): See DIET, article ADVICE ON THE DIET.

VITAMINS—dangers: See DIET, article ADVICE ON THE DIET.

VITAMINS—function: See article DEFICIENCY DISEASES.

VITAMINS—infant's need: See INFANCY, article CARE AND FEEDING OF THE CHILD.

VITAMINS—measles diet: See CHILDHOOD DISEASES, article INFECTIOUS DISEASES OF CHILDHOOD.

VITAMINS—pregnancy diet: See BIRTH, article CARE OF MOTHERS BEFORE AND AFTER CHILDBIRTH.

VITAMINS—resume: See article DEFICIENCY DISEASES.

VITAMINS—scarlet fever diet: See CHILDHOOD DISEASES, article INFECTIOUS DISEASES OF CHILDHOOD.

VITAMINS—whooping cough diet: See CHILDHOOD DISEASES, article INFECTIOUS DISEASES OF CHILDHOOD.

VITAMIN C (See also discussion under *Child Care, Vitamins*) Vitamin C, the antiscurvy vitamin, is found most abundantly in oranges, lemon, tomato, black currant, but most of all in acerola, the Puerto Rican wild cherry. It is destroyed by cooking in open vessels. Synthetic vitamin C is now available. Many juices which are deficient in vitamin C such as pineapple and apple juice may be enriched by mixing with richer juices such as orange and acerola, or by adding the synthetic vitamin. The weekly production of vitamin C in the United States is about 15 tons, equivalent to the vitamin C content of 200 million oranges.

Both men and animals show an increased need for vitamin C (ascorbic acid) when they are exposed to cold, stress, or a shortage of oxygen. Some of the vitamins of the vitamin-B complex are also involved in the reactions of the human body to stress. Vitamin C is obtained mainly from citrus fruit and some of the green vegetables. It is also available in concentrate form. Recent surveys show that even at the American level of eating, the highest in the world, intake of vitamin C is generally below the optimum requirements.

VITILIGO In vitiligo the pigment in the skin entirely disappears from some spots on the skin, so that these appear quite white in contrast with the rest of the skin. Because of the absence of any pigment mechanism in these portions of the skin they are much more prominent when the rest of the skin is tanned or sunburned. The cause for the absence of pigment from some portions of the skin is not known.

When vitiligo occurs in Negroes, as it sometimes does, they appear to be turning white, and there are cases on record in which most of the pigment has disappeared from the skin of a colored person. Some of these also have been exhibited in museums and side shows.

Recently a drug called ammoidin was found in Egypt which seems to be able to control vitiligo. The drug is painted on the area involved and is also prescribed to be taken internally.

It has been suggested that those who are exceedingly sensitive have their skin painted with some of the cosmetic preparations now available so that the white spots will not appear so prominently.

Research on glands has revealed the presence in the pituitary gland of a hormone known as MSH or the melanocy stimulating hormone which seems to be definitely associated with pigmentation. Continuous studies are being carried on with this hormone to find out exactly the mechanism by which it functions and possibly to develop from it a preparation that will be useful in such cases.

Studies have been made on the skin in vitiligo in which pigment is absent. The chemistry of the skin indicates that the sulfhydryl content of the skin was 40% to 100% higher in areas without pigment than in normal skin. Apparently these chemicals act in the skin to prevent the deposit of the melanin pigment.

*Since 1949 a new treatment for vitiligo has been in use and is apparently effective in many cases. The Egyptians have long used a drug derived from an Egyptian weed known as *Ammi majus linn* which grows abundantly in the Nile Delta. Since the thirteenth century the Egyptians have used the powder prepared from the fruit of this plant for the treatment of vitiligo. The drug has been somewhat toxic so that people who took it had disturbing reactions in the stomach and some have also had inflammations of the kidneys. Between 1947 and 1949 the active principle of this plant known as ammoidin and ammidin were isolated. These were prepared in tablet form to be taken by mouth and also as an alcoholic paint which was applied to the areas without pigment. The combined treatment was used in many cases and results were reported from Egypt as being most effective.

Studies were then made in France and the French physicians found that the preparation had to be given intermittently for several months. The paint when applied to the skin was dried by irradiation with ultraviolet. Sometimes blisters appeared; however, in general this treatment was followed by the production of pigment at the edges of the patches and gradually darkening the entire area. Exactly how these drugs work is not known but the drugs are now being manufactured and being widely used so that much more information is likely to develop in the near future.

Vitiligo—See Skin, article The Skin.

VOCAL CORDS See *Laryngitis, Larynx.*

Vocal Cord—location (fig.): See Ear, article The Ear, Tongue, Nose, and Throat.

VOICE See *Laryngitis, Larynx,* and *Speech.*

VOMITING Two of the most common symptoms of all sorts of disease are nausea and vomiting. They occur not only in infections and disturbances affecting the nervous system, in diabetes and in kidney disease, but often from purely mental causes.

The doctor does not treat nausea and vomiting as if they were diseases. He controls them as symptoms and then endeavors to determine exactly what may be the underlying condition responsible. If a person vomits, something has happened to cause the stomach to wish to be emptied. Not much is to be gained, therefore, by pouring a lot of things into the stomach. There are, of course, instances in which the vomiting occurs because of irritation by poisons. In this event the drinking of a great deal of fluid, which is promptly vomited back, serves to wash out the stomach.

In the average case of vomiting the doctor is likely to recommend, first of all, that the patient take no food for at least twenty-four hours. It is necessary, however, to keep the body supplied with fluid, since vomiting serves to diminish the fluids in the body. The loss of fluid may, in itself, produce serious symptoms. If the fluid cannot be kept in the stomach, the doctor may recommend the injection of fluid into the body by other means.

The mechanism of vomiting has been studied under the X ray. First the valve at the bottom of the stomach through which the food passes from the stomach to the bowels closes. Next come a series of waves in the wall of the stomach which do not pass downward, as is the case ordinarily, but upward in a reverse order. As these waves continue, the person affected begins to breathe deeply; then there is a powerful contraction of the diaphragm and of the abdomen, so that the contents of the stomach are forced, as by an explosion, up the esophagus, into the mouth and out. Sometimes this takes place so rapidly that the material is evacuated through the nose, if the passage from the throat to the nose is not closed.

The initiation of the vomiting of seasickness probably takes place in the organs of the body that have to do with maintaining its balance.

A severe pain associated with conditions affecting the heart may produce reflex vomiting. The severe pain associated with a violent blow on the abdomen may cause vomiting. The sight of an unpleasant or revolting object, a fetid smell, or even an unpleasant sound or an insulting word may be followed by vomiting.

Often there is a feeling of dizziness preceding the vomiting, which itself is a part of the accumulated nerve impulses that bring about the emptying of the stomach.

VOMITING—anemia: See BLOOD, article THE BLOOD AND ITS DISEASES.

VOMITING—anthrax: See article OCCUPATION AND HEALTH.

VOMITING—appendicitis: See article DIGESTION AND DIGESTIVE DISEASES.

VOMITING—arteriosclerosis of kidneys: See article BLOOD PRESSURE.

VOMITING—bacillary dysentery: See article DIGESTION AND DIGESTIVE DISEASES.

VOMITING—bowel cancer: See article DIGESTION AND DIGESTIVE DISEASES.

VOMITING—diabetic coma: See article DIABETES.

VOMITING—dysentery: See articles TRANSMISSIBLE DISEASES; DIGESTION AND DIGESTIVE DISEASES.

VOMITING—dyspepsia: See article DIGESTION AND DIGESTIVE DISEASES.

VOMITING—erysipelas: See article TRANSMISSIBLE DISEASES.

VOMITING—gall-bladder disease: See article DIGESTION AND DIGESTIVE DISEASES.

VOMITING—gallstones: See article DIGESTION AND DIGESTIVE DISEASES.

VOMITING—gastro-intestinal allergy: See article ALLERGY.

VOMITING—germ invasion: See INFECTIOUS DISEASE, article THE PREVENTION AND TREATMENT OF INFECTIOUS DISEASE.

VOMITING—glanders: See article TRANSMISSIBLE DISEASES.

VOMITING—indigestion: See article DIGESTION AND DIGESTIVE DISEASES.

VOMITING—infantile paralysis: See

CHILDHOOD DISEASES, article INFECTIOUS DISEASES OF CHILDHOOD.

VOMITING—infants: See INFANCY, article CARE AND FEEDING OF THE CHILD.

VOMITING—infectious diseases: See INFECTIOUS DISEASE, article THE PREVENTION AND TREATMENT OF INFECTIOUS DISEASE.

VOMITING—intestinal obstruction: See article DIGESTION AND DIGESTIVE DISEASES.

VOMITING—kidney disease: See KIDNEY, article THE KIDNEY: ITS DISEASES AND DISTURBANCES.

VOMITING—pneumonia: See RESPIRATORY DISEASES, article THE RESPIRATORY DISEASES.

VOMITING—pregnancy: See BIRTH, article CARE OF MOTHERS BEFORE AND AFTER CHILDBIRTH.

VOMITING—radiation may cause: See article OCCUPATION AND HEALTH.

VOMITING—reaction to stress: See article STRESS AND DISEASE.

VOMITING—scarlet fever: See CHILDHOOD DISEASES, article INFECTIOUS DISEASES OF CHILDHOOD.

VOMITING—sick headache: See article FIRST AID.

VOMITING—stomach cancer: See article DIGESTION AND DIGESTIVE DISEASES.

VOMITING—ulcers: See article DIGESTION AND DIGESTIVE DISEASES.

VOMITING—uremia: See KIDNEY, article THE KIDNEY: ITS DISEASES AND DISTURBANCES.

VOMITING—ways to provoke: See article FIRST AID.

VOMITING—worms: See article DIGESTION AND DIGESTIVE DISEASES.

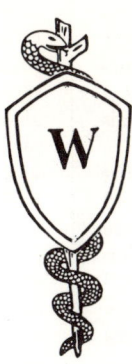

WARTS When warts are studied scientifically, they are found to be growths of the skin. Many doctors believe that they are infections. They appear to be slightly contagious. In fact inoculation of material from warts has been followed by the growth of new warts.

Warts seldom produce any symptoms except when they are on the soles of the feet, in which case, of course, they may become painful.

It has been found that picking of warts and spreading of the blood or material from the wart over the adjacent skin may result in multiplication of the warts in the same person by autoinoculation. It is better, therefore, not to attempt to treat them unscientifically.

When a specialist in diseases of the skin is called upon to treat warts, he applies any one of a number of treatments, including injections of bismuth directly into the wart, destruction of the warts by strong chemicals, freezing with carbon dioxide snow, electric desiccation of the wart, and surgical removal if the warts are large or multiple in any one spot.

Radium and X rays are also used for warts and in some instances seem to work most satisfactorily. This method is used especially when there are many warts around the fingernails. When the warts appear on the scalp, it is customary to treat them first by softening them with the application of various acids and then to make the final removal by freezing with carbon dioxide snow or by the electric needle. However, none of these materials or methods should ever be used except by those trained in the technic.

Warts on the soles of the feet are most resistant to treatment. Frequently they are best removed by surgery. After the horny material has been properly cut away, caustics are used on the base of the wart to prevent regrowth. In these cases also the X ray is frequently used to destroy the wart-bearing area and to prevent the growth of new warts.

Although warts disappear spontaneously in many cases, it does not seem to be desirable to wait too long for this to occur.

In addition to the common wart there are similar growths associated with venereal infections. These are called venereal warts. They develop around places where the mucous membranes join the skin. They are usually aggregate collections of overgrowths like warts. Because of irritation, friction, heat, moisture, and a large supply of blood they grow luxuriantly and spread rapidly. Such warts demand special treatment because of their nature. Most important, however, is the application of treatment as promptly as possible in order that the condition may be fully controlled before it has spread too widely.

Old people have a special form of wart known as senile wart. These also demand prompt attention because continued irritation may cause them to develop the malignant growth that is characteristic of cancer. It is best in such instances to have each wart removed as it develops and to have a careful study made of the tissues under the microscope to make certain that cancerous changes have not occurred. Such warts develop most often on the body rather than on the hands or the exposed skin. As far as is known, this type of wart never disappears spontaneously.

WARTS, PLANTAR—One of the most difficult situations that confronts the specialists who deal with the skin and also those who are concerned with the feet is the formation of warts on the soles of the feet. Various treatments have been suggested from time to time including surgical removal of the warts or their destruction by application of caustic material like glacial esthetic acid. A new treatment involves the use of a drug called euphorbium which is commonly known as the wart weed. A solution of 30% euphorbium in 95% alcohol was used on 60 patients by one physician who reported only two failures. First the surface of the wart was removed by a knife; then this solution was applied to the wart and the area was covered with adhesive tape. After 48 hours in which the dressing was left in place, the surface of the wart was again pared, the euphorbium was applied again and the surface again covered for 48 hours. Then the wart was readily removed.

The causes of warts on the soles of the feet are not definitely known. They seem to be associated with irritation but possibly also with infection by a virus which has not yet been isolated.

WARTS—See SKIN, article THE SKIN.
WARTS—cancer mistaken for: See SKIN, article THE SKIN.
WARTS—cancerous: See article CANCER.
WARTS—change may indicate cancer: See article CANCER.
WARTS—foot: See FOOT, article THE FOOT.

WASSERMANN TEST People with syphilis are usually submitted to an examination of the blood by a test called the Wassermann test which determines the presence or absence of the disease. Various modifications of this test have been discovered, most prominent of which is the so-called Kahn test, also the Eagle and the Hinton tests. Such tests are necessary at the earliest possible moment to determine whether or not the disease is present and at fairly frequent intervals throughout the course of the disease to determine the extent of improvement.

WASSERMANN TEST—See BLOOD, article THE BLOOD AND ITS DISEASES; article DIABETES; VENEREAL DISEASES, article THE VENEREAL DISEASES.

WASSERMANN TEST—in blood transfusions: See BLOOD, article THE BLOOD AND ITS DISEASES.

WASSERMANN TEST—not positive in first stage of syphilis: See SKIN, article THE SKIN.

WASSERMANN TEST—syphilis of the heart: See HEART, article DISEASES OF THE HEART AND CIRCULATION.

WEIGHT, FACTORS WHICH INFLUENCE Neither body build (physique, or body shape) nor body size (body surface area), taken by itself, is a good indication of the appropriateness of a person's weight. Individuals of many different shapes may be the same size, that is, have the same body surface area. The tall thin man and the short chubby woman may be peers in this respect; yet the weight of neither one may be desirable. Conversely, individuals of assorted sizes may resemble one another in body build, or shape. A six-sided solid block is a cube, whether it be one of a pair of dice or a cornerstone. During the growth period the healthy child shows a tendency to preserve the same physique, or shape, through the changes in size which occur at successive ages. However, among adults outside of fairy tales or circuses it is seldom that we see miniature or greatly enlarged replicas of various body types. It is only when we relate body build to body size that we can get a useful conception of the suitability of a person's weight with respect to health and good looks.

INFLUENCE OF FRAMEWORK ON HEIGHT AND BUILD—Body build is largely a matter of bony structure. We are as tall and as broad as our skeletons. The skeletal pattern is set by heredity and roughed in by the forces which bring the body to maturity. The dimensions of the long bones and the spinal column, which largely determine height, are little susceptible to fluctuations in dietary fortune (except in cases of marked calcium and vitamin-D deficiency) but are greatly susceptible to fluctuations during the growth period in the amounts of certain hormones secreted, particularly those of the anterior (front) portion of the pituitary gland. Upon reaching maturity the skeleton stops growing. Hence height and the contributions made to weight by the skeleton become stable features of the human body.

The trunk with its powerful bone structure and tightly packed visceral contents contributes more to weight than do the head and limbs. Hence a person with a long and roomy trunk, with broad shoulders, and wide pelvis would be classified as having a heavy frame irrespective of total height. And the individual with a medium or short trunk would be classified as medium or slight in build, depending upon the ruggedness or delicacy of his skeleton.

Unlike height, which is a stable feature of the mature body, weight is a variable feature. This is true because total weight, which is a measure of mass, is made up partly of the weight of soft tissues, and the substantial proportion of body weight contributed by these tissues can be added to or reduced according to our living habits and circumstances.

INFLUENCE OF MUSCULATURE ON WEIGHT—The type of skeletal build with which a person is endowed appears to be related in some measure to the amount of muscular tissue allotted for the operation and support of his bones. A person with a large bony framework requires large muscles for its operation, while a lighter framework requires smaller muscles. Also a big frame is well equipped structurally speaking to carry a relatively large amount of muscular tissue, whereas the slight frame is built for smaller loads.

In general, muscle tissue makes up about 40 per cent of body weight. In the adult, degree of activity probably has the biggest influence on muscular development. Given the raw materials (food elements) required, each tissue tends to produce more like itself when it is actively engaged in doing its proper work. Hence the extent to which a person uses his muscles in work and play will have a great deal to do with the comparative heaviness or lightness and the comparative strength or weakness of his musculature.

How much the bulkiness or flabbiness of one's muscles ought to be taken into consideration as a factor influencing desirable weight for health is a debatable question. Certainly we have all had the experience of hearing someone accused of being too fat come back with the retort, "But that's not fat—that's muscle. I'm hard as a rock—just feel!" To this it might be said, "But excessive poundage is overweight no matter what tissues are involved or how it was accumulated." Nevertheless, insurance studies have shown that the solidly built large-boned overweights do have better longevity records than the flabby overweights.

Exercise, while it enlarges and toughens muscles and improves nerve-muscle tone and posture, cannot make up for a lack of the food materials required for muscle building, nor can the increased energy output occasioned by exercise adequately counterbalance the excessive storage of fat resulting from overeating. For example, a man weighing 300 pounds who walked a mile on level ground would use up only about the amount of extra energy contained in a piece of chocolate fudge.

THE INFLUENCE OF BODY FAT ON WEIGHT—The least stable factor affecting body weight is fat. Hence it is by far the most controllable factor. So firmly entrenched in the popular mind is the idea that excess fat is chiefly to blame for overweight that the terms fatness, or obesity, and overweight are practically synonymous. And obesity is closely associated, even etymologically, with overeating; the word obese comes from the Latin *obesus* (the past participle of the verb *obedere*, to devour), which literally means "having eaten itself fat."

In the average well-nourished person fat makes up from 10 to 15 per cent of the body weight. It has a more or less passive but none the less important role. It is found in every cell, tissue, and organ of the body, but in certain regions great numbers of specific fat-containing cells are normally packed closely together to form the storehouses of fat, or fat depots, of the body. The largest internal fat depots are located in the abdominal cavity, around joints, and between muscles. Most of the fat under the skin (subcutaneous fat) is found in the abdominal wall, in the lower part of the back, and in the buttocks. However, fat is normally present with few exceptions in all other subcutaneous regions.

The relative fullness or emptiness of the fat depots is a matter of great concern in body economy. Fat is stored in them because the body does as Joseph advised Pharaoh to do; that is, it sets aside a store of fuel food to be used in time of famine so that it will not perish through the famine.

The contents of the fat depots may be compared to goods placed in dead storage. They consist of fat droplets produced from the fuel food (chiefly fats and carbohydrates) remaining over and above the amount required by the body for immediate use and for live storage in the liver and muscles.

The fat held in storage primarily to take care of possible shortages in the body's fuel supply serves many other useful purposes in the body. The internal fat depots form soft elastic shock absorbers between various organs, and the fat deposits beneath the skin help to regulate body temperature, cushion blows, and round out body contours. The delightful chubbiness of little children and the streamlined curves of youth owe their existence, in part at least, to the paddings of fat below the surface of the elastic skin. And the thinning out of these paddings is usually responsible for the baggy wrinkled skin seen in many old folks and in persons who have lost a great deal of fat quickly as a result of illness or of too drastic a get-thin-quick routine.

WEIGHT, NORMAL FOR HEALTH (See also, *Weight, Over and Under*) This question can be answered only for the individual and even then only when the answers to several other questions are known. For example: How tall are you? Is your framework small, medium, or large? How long is your trunk in relation to the length of your appendages? Has your weight pendulum tended to swing back and forth within rather narrow limits after attaining maturity? Or are you a great deal heavier—or lighter—than you were at twenty-five? For a person younger than twenty-five the question, "How old are you?" would also have to be answered, because physical growth obviously is accompanied by increase in size. Terminal stature is reached in the average girl at about age sixteen and in the average boy at about age seventeen, but there are many individual variations. To allow for these variations and also to give the structural pattern of the body time to settle, so to speak, twenty-five is the age generally accepted as marking the arrival of full-blown physical maturity.

HEIGHT-WEIGHT-AGE TABLES—In old-fashioned tables showing average weights for height of men and women cognizance is taken of the age factor. In constructing such tables the average, or mean, weight for height at various ages of very large numbers of individuals is computed, and the average weight for a particular height and age is then set up as the standard of comparison for any individual of that height and age.

It would be rare indeed for the weight of a single individual to be exactly the same as that arrived at by averaging the weights of thousands of individuals. All that can be expected is that his weight will fall within the weight range of a substantial fraction of the total number of persons of his age and height measured. Hence in using height-weight-age tables a person is considered to be overweight or underweight only if his weight is from 10 to 15 per cent above or below the mean reported for each height at different ages.

Tables for adults giving average weights for height and age show sizable increases with advancing years. Is this all right? Is it "normal" or healthy for the little woman to put on thirteen or fourteen pounds between the ages of thirty and fifty or for the big woman to get heftier by fifteen pounds or more? Is it necessary or desirable for the middle-sized men to pick up twelve extra pounds between the ages of twenty-five and fifty?

The tables indicate that men and women of various heights do make such gains. But after the anatomical dimensions of our fellow mortals have been tabulated and averaged we have simply a collection of mathematical averages of weights for height at various ages. Because a person is within the weight range of the majority of those who were measured to arrive at the averages does not mean that he is "normal" or that his weight is optimum. He is only average. He represents what *is,* not necessarily what ought to be. But who is to say what ought to be?

DESIRABLE WEIGHTS FOR MEN AND WOMEN OF AGES TWENTY-FIVE AND OVER—If there were such creatures as an "ideal" woman and an "ideal" man, physically speaking, to whom we could approximate real men and women, we might get an exact idea of what is normal, or ideal, weight for health. Some of us may remember when the dimensions of the Venus de Milo were held up as the ideal female measurements. But who knows whether the young woman who modeled for the sculptor of the Venus de Milo was healthy and how long she lived?

Instead of asking, "What is normal weight for health?" we may properly ask, "What do healthy people weigh?" If health also is an abstraction—that is, a conception practically impossible to define in concrete anatomical and physiological terms—we may select one easily determined factor associated with health—length of life.

Having escaped the hazards of infancy, childhood, youth, and early maturity represented by the infections which still are the most common causes of death by disease in these age periods and, barring accidents, the individual who has the best chance of coming closest to the limit of the human life span is the constitutionally toughest. Inborn constitutional traits are largely responsible for compelling strengths and weaknesses, and sometimes the health of the individual stands or falls by his constitution alone. In other words, he may be a "good egg" or a "bad egg" so far as his ability to resist the hazards and the usual wear and tear of life is concerned. However, inherited constitution has never been given a free hand, and perhaps never will, in determining health and length of life. We have ample evidence that environment, circumstance, and living habits can create marked ups and downs in individual resistance to disease and to the insults or injuries to various tissues which complicate the physiological process of aging.

Numerous medico-actuarial studies of hundreds of thousands of insured men and women show that body weight plays a leading part in creating such ups and downs. All in all, those who stay within the average weight range have the best longevity record, the frank overweights the worst. Also, it was found that, irrespective of age, but allowing for differences in body build, the most favorable weights for health and longevity for adults are those which come closest to the averages observed at ages twenty-five to thirty.

These findings make it possible to answer "no" to the question, "Is it all right—desirable—for men and women to make sizable gains in weight after attaining complete physical maturity at about twenty-five years of age? They have also made it possible to construct tables showing the range of desirable weights for men and women of various heights and body build, irrespective of age, after reaching or passing their twenty-fifth birthday. These tables are intended as a guide for judging correctness of weight rather than as a standard to which all individuals must conform— or else!

Although the classifications of slight, medium, and heavy body build are used in the tables, it must be remembered that there are many graduations in body build, or physique. The classification into which an individual falls will depend upon the characteristics that are predominant.

IDEAL WEIGHTS FOR MEN. AGES TWENTY-FIVE AND OVER

These tables are based on numerous medico-actuarial studies of hundreds of thousands of insured men and women. Weight in Pounds According to Frame (as ordinarily dressed)

Height (with shoes on)		Small Frame	Medium Frame	Large Frame
Feet	Inches			
5	2	116-125	124-133	131-142
5	3	119-128	127-136	133-144
5	4	122-132	130-140	137-149
5	5	126-136	134-144	141-153
5	6	129-139	137-147	145-157
5	7	133-143	141-151	149-162
5	8	136-147	145-156	153-166
5	9	140-151	149-160	157-170
5	10	144-155	153-164	161-175
5	11	148-159	157-168	165-180
6	0	152-164	161-173	169-185
6	1	157-169	166-178	174-190
6	2	163-175	171-184	179-196
6	3	168-180	176-189	184-202

Weights for men in the age group eighteen to twenty-five can be estimated by subtracting one pound for each year under twenty-five from the limits at each height. Examples:

Age	Height (with shoes)		Small Frame	Medium Frame	Large Frame
	Feet	Inches			
18	5	2	109-118	117-126	124-135
	5	10	137-148	146-157	154-168
19	5	2	110-119	118-127	125-136
	5	10	138-149	147-158	155-169

IDEAL WEIGHTS FOR WOMEN. AGES TWENTY-FIVE AND OVER

Height (with shoes on)		Small Frame	Medium Frame	Large Frame
Feet	Inches			
4	11	104-111	110-118	117-127
5	0	105-113	112-120	119-129
5	1	107-115	114-122	121-131
5	2	110-118	117-125	124-135
5	3	113-121	120-128	127-138
5	4	116-125	124-132	131-142
5	5	119-128	127-135	133-145
5	6	123-132	130-140	138-150
5	7	126-136	134-144	142-154
5	8	129-139	137-147	145-158
5	9	133-143	141-151	149-162
5	10	136-147	145-155	152-166
5	11	139-150	148-158	155-169

Weights for women in the age group eighteen to twenty-five can be estimated by subtracting one pound for each year under twenty-five from the limits at each height. Examples

Age	Height (with shoes) Feet	Inches	Small Frame	Medium Frame	Large Frame
18	4	11	97-104	103-111	110-120
	5	6	116-125	123-133	131-143
19	4	11	98-105	104-112	111-121
	5	6	117-126	124-134	132-144

WEIGHT, OVER- AND UNDER-

People get fat because they eat too much. After a good many years of study experts have come to the conclusion that the only source of fat for the human being is food. As pointed out by Dr. Edward H. Rynearson, there are many people who by the inherited structure of their body are more likely to be fat than other people. Exceedingly few people are fat because one of their glands of internal secretion fails to work.

A great many people are fat for psychologic reasons. For instance there are children who eat as a means of escape from personal distresses. There are people who eat as a habit to pass time just as there are others who smoke as a habit to pass time. However, none of these modifications of the situation in any way alters the statement that the only source of fat in the human body is the food taken into the body. Therefore the only successful way to cut down on the fat is to restrict the total amount of food taken into the body. This was called by Professor Lafayette B. Mendel "physiologic bookkeeping."

The proteins taken into the human body are necessary to repair the cells and to correct new tissue. Vitamins and minerals also act in the essential metabolism of the human body. The fat taken into the body need only be sufficient to carry the essential fatty acid and the fat-soluble vitamins and to make it unnecessary to eat too large a total amount of food. All the rest of the calories necessary for maintenance of weight and for the energy of the body can be taken in the form of carbohydrates or sugars. In fact the highly refined grains and sugars are the cheapest sources of calories. They need to be supplemented always, however, by the protective elements such as the essential amino acids, the vitamins, and the minerals.

People who are underweight have much less trouble than those who are overweight because they can be comforted by the fact that life insurance statistics indicate that they are likely to live long and have, in general, better health than the people who are overweight. However, people who are thin because of illness or who suffer from lack of appetite and inability to eat represent a problem for both the psychologist and the nutrition expert. Just as the person who is overweight can improve his condition by physiologic bookkeeping, so also can the one who is underweight produce a gain if he will decrease expenditure of energy and increase the intake of calories.

As to those people who prefer to put all the blame for overweight or underweight on the glands, Dr. Rynearson says, "The race horse and the draft horse are not 'endocrine problems.' They are the result of intentional breeding, feeding, and training. No one in his right mind would attempt to convert a draft horse into a race horse, but by diet alone he can convert a fat draft horse into one of normal size."

Diet—See Diet, article Advice on the Diet.

Diet—appetite as guide: See Diet, article Advice on the Diet.

Diet—beverages: See article Digestion and Digestive Diseases.

Diet—bland: See Diet, article Advice on the Diet.

Diet—calorie requirements: See Diet, article Advice on the Diet.

Diet—classification of foods: See Diet, article Advice on the Diet.

Diet—fads: See Diet, article Advice on the Diet.

Diet—importance in control of dietary diseases: See article Digestion and Digestive Diseases.

Diet—infants: See Infancy, article Care and Feeding of the Child.

Diet—meat: See Diet, article Advice on the Diet.

Diet—Mosaic laws of food: See Diet, article Advice on the Diet.

Diet—normal: See Diet, article Advice on the Diet.

Diet—preparation of food important: See Diet, article Advice on the Diet.

Diet—reducing: See Diet, article Advice on the Diet.

Diet—rice: See article Blood Pressure.

Diet—salt-free: See article Blood Pressure.

Diet—sample: See Diet, article Advice on the Diet.

Nutrition—skin: See Skin, article The Skin.

Overweight—adolescent girls: See Women, article Hygiene of Women.

Overweight—dangers: See article Diabetes.

Overweight—diabetes preceded by: See article Diabetes.

Overweight—hypertension treatment emphasizes correction: See article Blood Pressure.

Underweight—reduces life expectancy: See article Diabetes.

Weight—diabetes related to: See article Diabetes.

Weight—loss as result of fever: See Infectious Disease, article The Prevention and Treatment of Infectious Disease.

Weight—normal, at various ages: See Diet, article Advice on the Diet.

WEIGHT - REGULATING MACHINERY OF THE BODY—The body is equipped with a great many automatic checks and balances for preserving healthy conditions in its internal environment and for safeguarding its vital processes. Is there any self-regulating machinery for stopping the storage of fat when the depots are comfortably full? It would seem that regulation of the deposition of fat would be an important task, since both the reduction of fat reserves below the danger mark and the accumulation of fat to the extent of making the body "a bloated bondholder" are detrimental to health.

The regulation of body weight by automatic control over the amount of fat deposited in the fat depots would mean the application of a simple mathematical formula. Food intake (in terms of calories) must exactly equal energy output (in terms of calories) to maintain body weight at a constant level. To gain weight food intake must exceed energy output. To lose weight food intake must be less than energy output so that the body will use, or burn, its excess fat to make up the difference between food income and energy expenditure.

The assumption that the body does have an automatic weight-regulating mechanism is based on the fact that a great many people, especially those of slender and medium build, maintain practically the same weight throughout adult life. Although medico-actuarial tables show that the *average* man or woman has a tendency to gain weight year after year, it has been pointed out that these average increases were arrived at by measurements obtained from a mixed population including some individuals who do not change their weight at all and others who gain in weight at a faster rate than the average. Another bit of evidence is the fact that the frankly obese, who seem to put on weight at every turn and twist of life's journey, do reach a limit, that is, a point at which their weight remains static.

The nature of this weight-regulating mechanism is obscure. Both heredity and the nervous and endocrine systems undoubtedly influence its operation. It is a well-established fact that stoutness and leanness are hereditary variations of body build.

And endocrine or nervous-system disturbances, or both, whether inherited or acquired during life, have been found in many cases of generalized obesity and of grotesque distributions of body fat.

WEN The wen is scientifically known as a sebaceous cyst. It is due to the fact that the sebum or material excreted from these glands in the skin does not get out because of some obstruction; therefore, a black plug of sebum will be found choking the outlet to the gland.

The material is dammed back and sooner or later is reacted on by itself and by the material from the blood so that the semisolid mass becomes semifluid. The material is likely to have a rancid odor.

If the wen does not become infected, it can go on swelling as long as the release of the material is prevented. Such bumps have been known to grow as large as a golf ball or even larger before the person concerned consulted a doctor and had the material let out.

Because of the inflammation that may set in, the skin over the bump may become adherent to the wen. Moreover, the clothing rubbing against a bump of this kind will irritate it.

Should these cysts become infected, they are a much more serious matter. Frequently the bumps on the scalp will be multiple and if they are allowed to grow too large, it may be necessary to remove a considerable amount of skin to get all of the material out.

When the wen becomes infected, merely cutting the opening in order to cause the material inside to flow out will not cure the wen. The difficulty is in the structure of the tissues; the lining of the cyst continues to secrete the sebaceous material, which again hardens and begins to collect.

The permanent cure, therefore, involves a complete surgical dissection which will take away the lining walls of the cyst and thus prevent a repetition of the swelling.

WENS—See SKIN, article THE SKIN.

WHEAT SENSITIVITY (See also discussion under *Allergic Conditions, Allergy, Food Allergy*) A case has recently been reported of a woman who, two hours after eating any wheat products, developed a great swelling of the parotid glands on each side of the face below the ears. The condition resembled mumps. Actually however it was caused by a sensitivity to wheat. One of the manifestations of allergy may be the swelling of various portions of the body such as the area around the eyes, the area in front of the ears, the area inside the throat—in fact almost anywhere —due to accumulation of fluid in the area. When wheat was eliminated from the diet of this woman, she remained well. Some fifteen similar cases have been reported in medical writings.

WHOOPING COUGH Doctors call whooping cough pertussis. They prefer pertussis because not every patient with whooping cough whoops. The disease got its name because it is characterized by a series of repeated, spasmodic coughs which cause the patient to get out of breath. As a result he is forced to draw air into his lungs, and the sound of this forced inspiration is the whoop.

Whooping cough has been known to the medical profession for a great many years. The earliest reference to it appeared in medical literature as far back as 1540. In those early days the condition was called quintana.

Often vomiting follows the coughing spell, and this was noted as far back as 1578.

Many people consider whooping cough a trivial disease of childhood. It is, nevertheless, one of the most serious conditions that affect mankind, causing more deaths than measles. Most of the deaths from whooping cough are associated with secondary conditions like bronchopneumonia or infection of the intestinal tract, and thus they are not always reported as whooping cough.

The number of days lost from school by children with whooping cough is greater than that for any two other infectious diseases. Most of the cases of whooping cough occur in children under five years of age, but it may affect people of any age and is more serious in the very young and in the very old than in those of intermediate ages.

For years there has been an argument as to the cause of whooping cough, but now bacteriologists are convinced that the disease is caused by a germ to which the name *Hemophilus pertussis* is given. It is found almost invariably in the throat during the early stages of the disease. It is seldom found in people who have not been exposed to whooping cough. Inoculation of the germ into animals will produce infection. Conceivably the case of whooping cough is complicated early by the invasion of other germs. This happens to be the case also with the common cold, in which infection with a virus is associated with secondary infections.

The modern technic for establishing with certainty the existence of whooping cough is to have the child cough on a plate which contains a substance on which the germs grow easily. The plate test is now used to prove, first, that the child has the disease, and, second, that the child is free from the germs and recovered from the disease. This is particularly important because it prevents wider dissemination of the disease from healthy carriers.

The first stage of whooping cough is a period of about ten days, in which the symptoms are like those of a person catching cold. This is the incubation period. After five or six days, however, the cough usually gets worse instead of better. Then come the typical seizures of whooping. This introduces the second stage of whooping cough. If the coughing spells are severe, the face becomes deep red or purple; the veins of the face and scalp swell; and the eyes fill with tears. Very young children vomit immediately after a spell of coughing, particularly when the coughing follows the taking of food.

Since the cough is provoked by exposure to cold, tobacco, or overexercise, much can be accomplished by keeping the child quietly at rest during the severe period of the disease.

The doctor diagnoses whooping cough not only by the typical coughing spells but also by changes in the blood. The white blood cells increase in number, particularly one form known as the lymphocytes, which are cells with a single nucleus, or central body, when seen under the microscope. The cough is so characteristic in whooping cough that special studies are seldom necessary to establish with certainty the nature of the disease.

For the prevention of whooping cough children with this condition should never be allowed to attend school. Tiny babies particularly must be guarded against contact with those who have the disease. Since the child should be kept closely confined for periods of nearly six weeks or even two or three months, other children in the family for whom exposure would be dangerous may, when possible, be sent away from the house. If the child is permitted to play outdoors during the time of gradual recovery, arrangements should be made to guard carefully against contact with other children.

I have heard children with whooping cough contaminating the air of motion picture houses, trains, busses, streetcars, and even churches. Parents ought to be more careful about the danger the child with whooping cough presents to other children. In some communities it has been suggested that the child who is recovering from whooping cough ought to wear a red band with the words "Whooping Cough" prominently displayed.

For the prevention of whooping cough all sorts of methods have been tried, such as those that have proved efficient in other diseases. Children may be inoculated with the blood of people who have recently recovered from whooping cough. They may be injected with vaccines made from germs that have been isolated, permitted to grow, and then suitably killed. These vaccines are believed to be useful in shortening the attack of whooping cough and making it milder. They are used also now in the treatment of whooping cough. Their development has taken more than thirty years; they were first prepared in 1914.

Gradually they have been improved, tested in epidemics, and studied as to dosage and duration of efficiency. Furthermore, technics have been developed by which the efficiency of the vaccine can be tested. The vaccines now available have been proved to be useful and to provide considerable protection. They are given preferably after the child is six months of age. It is now accepted that they reduce the total number of cases of infection and greatly minimize the severity of the disease when infection does occur.

Parents can be of great help to the child with whooping cough. On the first appearance of the symptoms the child should be put to bed and isolated from members of the family who have not had the disease. In bad weather the child should be kept away from drafts and should be protected suitably with light but warm bed clothing. Since there may by considerable strain on the muscles of the abdomen during coughing, a binder such as is worn by babies may be wrapped around the abdomen to support the muscles.

Due to persistent vomiting, children with whooping cough may become undernourished and particularly short of fluids. The diet is watched closely. Preferably small amounts of food are given at frequent intervals. Food should be chosen by the doctor especially for its nutritious and easily digestible qualities. By all means make certain that the child gets and retains enough water in the body. Large amounts of food must be avoided because they cause irritation and more vomiting. The best time to give a small amount of food is ten or fifteen minutes after a coughing spell. Among the foods particularly recommended are small amounts of meat, carefully chopped or sieved, and vegetable soup properly prepared. Foods to be avoided in whooping cough include excess of bread, starchy foods, sweet pastries, and potatoes. Dry and crumbly foods like crackers and nuts should be avoided. Particularly helpful are drinks of fresh fruit juices.

The doctor can do a great deal toward diminishing the severity of coughing spells by the prescription of drugs which lessen the severity of the cough. These drugs are potent and cannot be given without a doctor's prescription. The doctor will prescribe those that are just up to the strength of the child concerned. For many years it has been known that inhalations of steam with various soothing oils may be useful in lessening the severity of coughing spasms.

An interesting observation is the fact that children sometimes imitate the coughing of others. Even a small baby will soon learn that a handsome demonstration during a spell of coughing brings presents, sympathy, and attention which otherwise he might not receive. The wrong mental attitude, therefore, may make a serious invalid out of what might otherwise be rather a mild attack of whooping cough. Children need to be encouraged to control coughing as much as possible.

Most dangerous of all the complications of whooping cough is secondary pneumonia. The child with a combination of whooping cough and pneumonia is probably best cared for in a hospital.

In 1940 whooping cough and tetanus immunizing agents were available, but combined preparations had not yet gained acceptance. Now the use of a combined triple antigen for infant immunization against diphtheria, tetanus, and whooping cough is well established.

A new technique for treating long-lasting cases of whooping cough involves placing a patient in a decompression chamber under low air pressure. Six or 8 patients are put into the chamber along with a trained attendant. At first they remain in the chamber 20 minutes; later the time is extended to 45 minutes. The method is apparently useful, but it is still being investigated.

During a period of $5\frac{1}{2}$ years, 903 patients were treated this way, and in 782 the results were evaluated. Of the 782, 28.2% showed rapid, significant improvement in 4 to 7 days; 34.1% had slower but significant improvement; the remainder were not affected. Of the patients who had been vomiting, 57.7% stopped within a few days, and 20% more were greatly relieved. The treatment was unsuccessful chiefly when given during the first $2\frac{1}{2}$ weeks of the cough. The method is not used when the patient has a fever, when he has had congestion in his chest, or when he is blue from lack of air. The treatment was first suggested in 1927, when a doctor in Strasbourg, France, took a number of children with whooping cough up in an airplane to an altitude of 10,000 feet. At that time any beneficial results were thought to be wholly psychological.

WHOOPING COUGH—See CHILDHOOD DISEASES, article INFECTIOUS DISEASES OF CHILDHOOD.

WHOOPING COUGH—cause determined: See INFECTIOUS DISEASE, article THE PREVENTION AND TREATMENT OF INFECTIOUS DISEASE.

WHOOPING COUGH—childhood disease: See CHILDHOOD DISEASES, article INFECTIOUS DISEASES OF CHILDHOOD.

WHOOPING COUGH—contagious disease: See INFECTIOUS DISEASE, article THE PREVENTION AND TREATMENT OF INFECTIOUS DISEASE.

WHOOPING COUGH—deaths annually: See CHILDHOOD DISEASES, article INFECTIOUS DISEASES OF CHILDHOOD.

WHOOPING COUGH—diet: See CHILDHOOD DISEASES, article INFECTIOUS DISEASES OF CHILDHOOD.

WHOOPING COUGH—incidence: See INFECTIOUS DISEASE, article THE PREvention and Treatment of Infectious Disease.

Whooping Cough—incubation period: See Childhood Diseases, article Infectious Diseases of Childhood.

Whooping Cough—measles frequently precedes: See Childhood Diseases, article Infectious Diseases of Childhood.

Whooping Cough—pneumonia frequently follows: See Childhood Diseases, article Infectious Diseases of Childhood.

Whooping Cough—prevention: See Childhood Diseases, article Infectious Diseases of Childhood.

Whooping Cough—quarantine: See Childhood Diseases, article Infectious Diseases of Childhood.

Whooping Cough—treatment: See Infectious Disease, article The Prevention and Treatment of Infectious Disease; Childhood Diseases, article Infectious Diseases of Childhood.

Whooping Cough—tuberculosis frequently follows: See Childhood Diseases, article Infectious Diseases of Childhood.

Whooping Cough—vaccine for pertussis: See article Allergy.

WOMB See *Uterus*.

Hygiene of Women

BY

MORRIS FISHBEIN, M.D.

Former Editor, *Journal American Medical Association,* Chicago; Editor, *Excerpta Medica, Bulletin World Medical Assn.; Post-graduate Medicine.*

T<small>HE BOY AND GIRL</small>, until the age of twelve, may be reared in much the same manner. Their health problems are approximately the same. Thereafter, however, the problems of the girl are distinctive. At this period in her life her organs begin to differentiate to prepare her for her functions as a mother. It is taken for granted that the mother will have prepared the daughter suitably for recognition of the changes that are to come. In the majority of girls these changes take place so gradually that they are not noticed.

The startling change which appears is the development of the menstrual flow. In far too many instances, notwithstanding the advance in health education that has been made in the last quarter century, girls still come to this phenomenon without any knowledge, and some of them sustain mental shocks which mark their lives thereafter. Until menstruation appears, the girl is not likely to bear children; with the coming of menstruation, the organs develop and the possibility exists.

Before that time, the body configuration of most girls has been much like that of the boy. After puberty, which is the time when the menstrual flow appears, the breasts, the pelvis and neck enlarge, hair develops in the armpits and over the sexual area, and the voice changes.

The onset of the menstrual flow is not always an abrupt and complete development. The first flow may be very brief; it may disappear and not appear again for weeks or months; it may, at first, be irregular and then later regular. Just as soon as the flow appears regularly at a definite interval for several months, the menstruation may be said to be established.

Associated with this physical change are also mental changes. Many of these changes are associated with interests in the male sex, in more mature occupations, in a different type of reading, and in many new interests. For this reason, parents should have surveillance over their daughters and use proper understanding of the nature of the change that is occurring.

Our views have greatly changed in the last quarter century. Girls used to be sick in every sense of the word during the menstrual period. Nowadays they are likely to go through without the slightest alteration in their habits. There are, of course, instances in which the function is accompanied with severe pain or with physical disturbance. When these occur, they should have the attention of a physician.

The adolescent girl is undergoing rapid development. For this reason her posture must be carefully watched. If she grows too rapidly and is somewhat tall, there may be an inclination to slump the shoulders forward, the abdomen out and the chest in. Such posture is bound to lead to a poor figure later in life. Exercises, described in the article on posture in this book, will help to develop a proper position when standing and when sitting. The chin and abdomen should be kept in and the chest forward. Many young girls worry about the development of the breasts and, not understanding the changes that occur, attempt to hide them. Poor posture may result from holding the shoulders in such a manner as to draw in the chest.

The girl, at this period of life, needs plenty of sleep; ten or eleven hours in twenty-four is not too much. Extra relaxation in the form of a nap in the middle of the day, such as is given to smaller children, may be exceedingly useful in maintaining her body tone. There need be no special attention to the diet other than the certainty that it contains the necessary proteins, carbohydrates and fats, mineral salts and vitamins that are necessary in any well-balanced diet.

Many girls passing from adolescence into adult age feel that it is necessary for them to adopt sophisticated habits. Whereas they have formerly avoided tea and coffee in favor of milk, they want to partake of these and even of alcoholic beverages as giving them somewhat more of an adult status in the family. Smoking cigarettes is not necessary, and again may be considered as a habit to be controlled until it can be indulged in at a later date with intelligence and restraint.

Some girls at this age put on so much weight that they are seriously disturbed. The weight may increase so rapidly that the skin of the abdomen stretches and red marks appear along the curves of the hips. These should not cause worry because they will fade when the weight of the body is more definitely adjusted. For the control of the tendency to overweight, a suitable diet with a lowered amount of carbohydrates is desirable. Nowadays most people have learned enough about calories and carbohydrates in relationship to overweight to exercise a certain amount of control over this danger.

Special attention should also be given at this period to the condition of the thyroid gland. In some children there is a tendency to overactivity of the gland, which is marked also by rapid heart, nervousness, perspiration, and similar symptoms. If any sign appears of overactivity of the thyroid gland, the basal metabolism should be determined by a competent doctor and the condition of the thyroid gland controlled in relationship to the results. If there is overweight or underweight, the basal metabolism test should also be made to determine whether or not the activity of the thyroid gland is related in any way to this unusual development.

In the Great Lakes area and in the Northwest, the water and the soil lack iodine, hence there is a tendency among young children to develop simple enlargement of the thyroid gland that is known as simple goiter. There is a special chapter on this condition elsewhere in this book. Any tendency of the thyroid gland toward enlargement should, of course, be studied by the family doctor. In most cases, however, intelligent parents nowadays give small doses of iodine regularly each week to supply the iodine deficiency and thus effectively prevent the appearance of simple goiter.

Disorders of Menstruation

As I have already said, menstruation may be occasionally irregular during the first year without causing any anxiety. Certainly, by the end of the first year it should be regular, in the majority of women, occurring every twenty-eight days. Menstruation occurring regularly anywhere from twenty-one days to five-week intervals may be considered within normal limits.

Sometimes, in connection with the first appearance of menstruation, the usual signs of adolescence appear, including pimples and blackheads on the face, back, and chest, soreness and swelling of the breasts, and headache. These may appear as the result of the changes in the glands that occur at this time.

Ordinarily menstruation should cause no more pain than any of the other functions of the body. When the pain occurs, it is usually associated with a disturbance of the circulation or of the glands. Sometimes failure of the bowels to act properly is a complication, which may be easily corrected by establishment of regular habits, sufficient rest, drinking of plenty of water, and the other measures suggested in the section on digestion.

Doctors now recognize a period of a few days before menstruation when symptoms of distress, irritability, anxiety, flushing, nausea and such, make what is called premenstrual tension. Control may involve study of the glandular condition and prescription of suitable drugs, vitamins and glandular substances.

EXERCISES

Various exercises have been described for use by growing girls at this time. Some of these simple exercises involve not only the usual bending and standing, which are good for posture, but also kneeling in the knee-chest position, walking on the hands and feet as the monkey or cat walks, and other postures which help to develop the ligaments which hold the organs of the pelvis in position. Since menstruation is a normal function of women and involves several different organs, its control must involve study of the organs concerned.

Emotional shocks and nerve shocks may tend to be associated with pain at this time. A change in the altitude, extraordinary changes in the diet, over- and under-exercise, and many similar factors may yield difficult symptoms. For this reason, the routine of the girl's life during the menstrual period should be disturbed as little as possible.

She may take her baths daily as always, preferably a warm bath; but if she is in the habit of taking cold baths, she may take these also. There is no good reason why most women should not take a bath during the menstrual period. If the flow of blood is profuse, strenuous swimming may make it excessive; also a very hot tub bath may increase the amount of blood lost. A very cold bath taken just before or at the beginning of menstruation may occasionally stop the bleeding. The danger of infection from the water is very slight.

Indulgence in competitive games during the menstrual period should, of course, be carefully controlled. Such games involve emotional stress and high tension. They place a considerable burden upon the heart. They bring about shocks and jolts to the internal organs for which these organs are not competent. It is particularly important that every girl indulging in athletic sports have a physical examination in relationship to her feminine constitution.

PAINFUL MENSTRUATION

A tremendous number of remedies have been suggested for painful menstruation. Sufficient rest and sleep, proper hygiene and treatment for anemia, if that is present, are especially important. Some patients get immediate help from rest in bed and the use of an enema for emptying the bowels. Others are relieved by placing a hot-water bag over the painful area. Aspirin and similar drugs which relieve pain are used by many girls and are not harmful, if taken in small doses and preferably under the direction of a physician.

Sometimes it is necessary for the doctor to make certain modifications of the glandular mechanism of the patient. The administration of suitable glandular substances which are known to have control over the menstrual functions sometimes yields successful results in eliminating pain.

In the process of menstruation several organs are involved: the pituitary gland, adrenals, ovaries, and the uterus. Regular bleeding from the uterus, called menstruation, is nearly always dependent on proper functioning of the ovaries. These, in turn, are controlled by a portion of the pituitary gland in the brain. The pituitary gland has been called the motor of the ovaries. When there are unusual symptoms during the menstrual period, such as flushing, numbness of the finger tips, fainting spells, and crying, the glands and their secretions are ordinarily responsible, related in turn to various mental influences.

Because of the tendency to bleed at this period, some women bruise more easily during the menstrual time; others suffer with nosebleeds. These symptoms usually disappear when the menstruation ends.

When menstruation is exceedingly scanty, the state of the blood should be studied as to whether or not there is anemia. There should also be an investigation of the basal metabolism and the general nutrition.

During menstruation the vast majority of women wear a simple cotton pad, such as is now commercially available in many different forms. Vaginal tampons are also used satisfactorily and safely. Where there are unusual odors of any kind, a careful investigation should be made by a competent doctor to determine the presence or absence of infection. In most cases, annoying odors are a sign of infection, and they cannot be corrected by application of deodorants or powders of any kind.

The medical profession has not settled definitely the question of the advisability of using douches before and after the menstrual period or at any other time. About an equal number of specialists in diseases of women are arrayed on each side of this question. Women who are not infected in any manner and who do not have excessive discharges of mucus and other material from the genital tract need not employ douches regularly. Ordinary bathing will suffice for the purpose. However, in cases in which there are excessive dis-

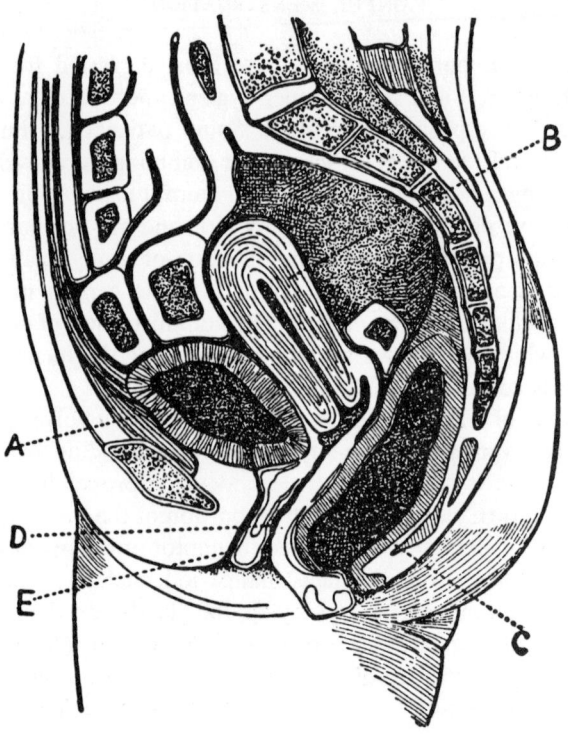

Lateral view of female pelvic organs. A. Bladder. B. Uterus or womb. C. Rectum. D. Vagina. E. Urethra.

charges, or in which, as has been mentioned, an odor is present, a physician should be consulted in order to determine the presence and nature of the infection. The infection should be treated by the means that the physician will recommend. This recommendation will in most instances involve the use of suitable cleansing and antiseptic agents used in the form of douches and in similar ways.

ABSENCE OF MENSTRUATION

Most people know that menstruation disappears when a woman becomes pregnant and is to have a child. It disappears also at a period known as the climacteric, which is also an important epoch in the life of women. This period is also called the menopause, as an indication of the fact that the menstruation disappears at this time.

There are, of course, other factors which occasionally produce a change in menstruation and in some instances even a temporary absence. A change of geographical location, which involves chiefly a change of climate and perhaps of altitude, not infrequently produces alterations in menstruation. Usually the flow may stop, but in some cases the amount of blood lost is excessive. Because the process of menstruation is controlled by glandular action, disorders of menstruation, including stopping for no apparent reason, are generally assumed to be due to some glandular difficulty.

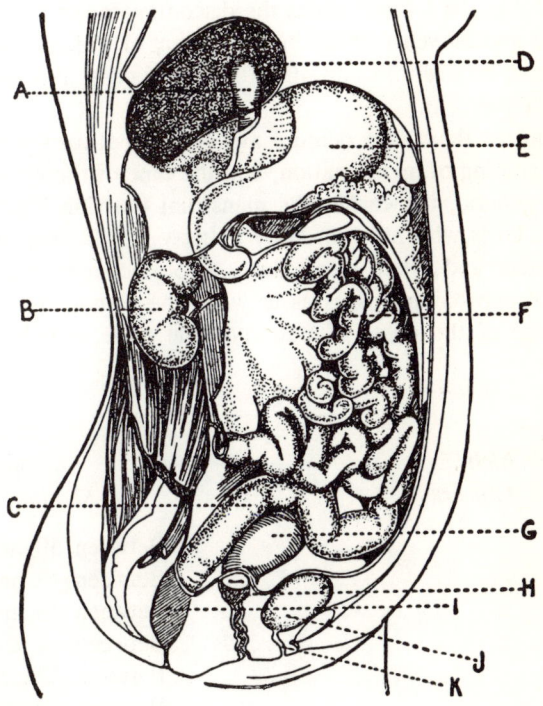

Abdominal female organs. A. Gall bladder. B. Kidney. C. Large intestine. D. Liver. E. Stomach. F. Small intestine. G. Uterus or womb. H. Vagina. I. Rectum. J. Bladder. K. Urethra.

Women who do not menstruate are not in any way inferior to those who do. They rarely show any abnormal symptoms, and their sex life is about the same. The whole difficulty lies in the minds of such women. They feel they are subnormal; they may become exceedingly disturbed mentally worrying over the condition. Frequently a physician can bring about menstruation in such patients by the experimental use of various glandular preparations.

The discontinuance of menstruation at the menopause is, of course, a different matter. The average duration of menstruation in women is from 30 to 32 years. The average age for the beginning of the climacteric or menopause in the temperate zone is about 47 years. However, there is an enormous variation in the ages at which the symptoms of climacteric may arise. Cases are known in which the change of life occurred as early as 27 years of age and as late as 59 years. Usually in the United States the discontinuance of menstruation occurs between 45 and 50 years of age in 50 per cent of women; between 40 and 45 in 25 per cent; between 35 and 40 in 12½ per cent, and between 50 and 55 years in 12½ per cent.

In most instances there is a definite association between the onset of puberty, or the beginning of menstruation, and the time of the appearance of the menopause. In general, the earlier the menstrual function begins, the longer it will continue. Girls who have an early puberty will have a long, potential, reproductive career and a late menopause. A physician named Gallant published a chart of approximate ages as to when the menopause would appear, based on the age of the onset of puberty. The table, which is for healthy women, follows

Year in Which Menstruation Appears	Menopause Should Occur
10	Between 50 and 52 years
11	Between 48 and 50 years
12	Between 46 and 48 years
13	Between 44 and 46 years
14	Between 42 and 44 years
15	Between 40 and 42 years
16	Between 38 and 40 years
17	Between 36 and 38 years
18	Between 34 and 36 years
19	Between 32 and 34 years
20	Between 30 and 32 years

Exactly as parts of the body change at the onset of puberty, so also do similar changes occur at the menopause. Usually the spleen and lymphatic glands decrease in size. There is an increased tendency to constipation, because of changes in the wall of the intestine. Most women have some physical discomfort and some mild mental or nervous changes, but some women cease menstruating with slight inconvenience. As a rule, the woman may miss one or two or more periods, then will have menstrual periods that seem almost normal; then she will miss other periods, and finally the periodic flow will cease altogether. This variability is due to the fact that the glandular changes which are occurring take place gradually.

There may be, during this period, slight inflammation and swelling of the sexual parts. These are, however, of little significance. The most difficult symptom which may develop at this time is excessive bleeding. Whenever excessive bleeding occurs, however, either at the menopause or at any other time, a physician should be consulted immediately so that he may make a study of the condition and determine its cause. It is well established that the appearance of blood is sometimes associated with the appearance of cancer. The only way to make certain is to have a direct examination of the tissue to guard against such a possibility.

Occasionally there is a good deal of itching, particularly after bathing. In such cases the use of an ointment, such as 12 per cent boric acid in an ointment of rose water, is helpful. If such mild treatment does not secure a good result, a physician should be consulted for the prescribing of something more powerful.

While it is true that states of mental depression and other abnormal mental states occur somewhat frequently at or about the age of menopause, it must be remembered that these are not really important abnormalities, and that they occur also in men around the age of fifty. Unless they are extreme, there is nothing to do in the way of treatment.

Since many different forms of mental disorder may occur at this period, it is always advisable to have a scientific diagnosis as to the character of the disturbance that occurs. In some women there seems to be increased sexual desire at this period. In such cases also the treatment is good hygiene, including also the avoidance of any unnecessary stimulants. The avoidance of coffee, and a good deal of outdoor exercise, may be helpful. In other cases there is a gradual loss of sexual desire. This also may be quite temporary. Many women continue to be sexually active for considerable periods after the menopause. Not infrequently there is a mild degree of overactivity of the thyroid gland, and, associated with this, increased excitability. There may also be a slight elevation of the blood pressure.

All of these symptoms, however, are associated with the gradual change in the glandular mechanism and, unless severe, need not be considered seriously. New substitutes for missing glandular substances may be prescribed by the doctor to overcome symptoms.

The changes associated with this period demand slight modification of the general hygiene of the body. Usually older people will want less food. Because of the difficulties of digestion, foods rich in carbohydrates, including sugars, cake, candy, preserves, and jelly, should be taken with moderation, as also foods that are known to cause indigestion in many cases; for example, foods fried in a good deal of grease, hot breads, pastry, cheese, and similar substances.

Since there is a considerable amount of congestion in the abdomen, the care of the bowels should be a special problem. A daily, free evacuation of the bowels is essential to health. The use of mild laxatives may bring a good deal of relief. The kidneys must be especially watched for the onset of any degenerative changes.

It is necessary to keep the skin in good condition by bathing—sometimes alternate hot and cold baths. Massage is helpful in toning up the nervous system and the circulation. Exercise daily in the open air is helpful in steadying the nerves and stimulating the body generally.

From the point of view of the mind, it is particularly necessary at this time of life that some pleasant occupation be followed. Usually by this time children will have passed the age when they need constant supervision, and the mother must take relaxation from her home cares. Many women at this time of life become expert bridge players or golfers, although previously they may have taken but little interest in such diversions. Any mental occupation that will take the woman into a new interest is the best possible safeguard against the slight mental difficulty which develops in some women at this period.

The estrogenic hormones including the natural and the synthetic, stilbestrol, will aid in overcoming headache, hot flashes, and melancholia, which are so distressing at this time. These substances should never be taken except when prescribed by the doctor. Physicians also prescribe some androgen or male sex hormone particularly when there is depression or fear of loss of sex-life.

The Rhythm of Menstruation

A definite relationship exists between the time a woman menstruates and the time when an egg cell or ovum passes from the ovary into the uterus. If a woman menstruates regularly every twenty-eight days, it is usually impossible for her to conceive between the first and tenth day of her menstrual cycle, the first day being the one on which the menstrual flow begins. She can conceive on the eleventh day and up to and including the seventeenth day, but she will not be able to conceive from the seventeenth day on. Therefore, the days on which conception is most likely are the days from the fourteenth to the sixteenth day after the first day of menstruation. This is the period in which the mother cell or egg cell is produced by the ovary. In a woman who menstruates every twenty-eight days, the egg cell comes from the ovary on the fourteenth day.

The period of nine days, referred to as the period when conception is most likely, includes three days for the production and discharge of the egg cell, one day allowed for variability, and two to three days for the survival of the fertilizing power of the male cell. It has been definitely shown that the male cell will not survive much over three days, unless it meets the egg cell of the female and brings about conception. The extra three days added to these seven are in the interests of safety against any irregularities.

Records have now been kept of many thousands of cases in which women have observed this safe period, and failures, when absolute observance prevailed, are exceedingly few. Of course, the matter is complicated when the menstrual cycle in the woman is more or less than twenty-eight days. For the majority of women, therefore, it will be necessary to determine the exact dates and variations of the menstrual cycle. This is done by keeping an accurate record for several months of the exact dates on which menstruation begins, how many days it continues, and the number of days from the first day of menstruation to the first day of the next menstruation. All sorts of calendars and devices have now been developed for keeping records of this kind.

It is known that a good many women have occasional variations in their menstrual cycle. Thus one authority said, "The only regular thing about menstruation is its own irregularity." Just as soon as the cycle is definitely established, it becomes possible for the woman to calculate the periods when she is likely to conceive, or the fertile period, and the period when she is not likely to conceive, or the sterile period.

The Temperature Control Method

Many people think there is a chance for conception whenever the male sperm cell is deposited in the woman's genital tract. Actually, the sperm cannot fertilize an egg cell or ovum unless the ovum is there when the sperm reaches the Fallopian tube. Only one ovum, smaller than a pin point in size, is released by the ovary during the woman's periodic cycle. This takes place about 14 days before the beginning of the next cycle. If pregnancy is to occur, intercourse must take place within 24 hours of ovulation, since the life of the ovum is not more than 24 hours, and the sperm cells have fertilizing power for only 24 to 36 hours. Hence, if a woman can determine the exact time of ovulation, she can increase her chances of conception by having intercourse then.

The most practical method of achieving this is to keep a careful record of body temperature on arising each morning. Whereas a man's temperature follows a regular pattern day after day, the temperature of a woman is altered by the normal functioning of the ovaries. For several years thousands of women have kept daily temperature records, which physicians have studied and interpreted. We now know that the release of the ovum raises the level of a woman's temperature during the latter half of the menstrual cycle.

Your doctor can help you get charts especially designed for **daily temperature records** and show you how to use them.

Take your temperature immediately after waking up in the morning. Do not get up to go to the bathroom first, or drink water or smoke a cigarette. Just reach over, get the thermometer, put it under your tongue, lie back and remain quiet for five minutes. Then record the temperature on your chart. If it differs from those recorded before, and particularly if it is lower, shake the thermometer down, put it back under your tongue and hold it for another five minutes to verify the reading.

Temperature drops 24 to 36 hours before the onset of the menstrual flow, reaching a low point during the first day or two after the flow begins. This low level continues until the middle of the interval between two menstruations. This is the time when ovulation usually occurs in the woman who has a 27- to 31-day cycle. A sharp drop often takes place just before the rise that indicates the ovulation is occurring. During the next 24 to 36 hours, the temperature goes up abruptly. It stays at the higher level until one to two days before the beginning of the next flow. Start a new chart when the next period begins. You should have records of two consecutive cycles to establish your personal cycle. Then you can be reasonably sure when the next shift in temperature, and ovulation, will occur.

After childbirth or a miscarriage, about three months are required for the cycle to return to normal.

At least four out of five women find that the temperature record is an accurate guide to the time of ovulation if it is recorded and evaluated intelligently. Emotional upheavals, infections, dissipation, overeating and colds can cause an irregularity in temperature; barring such disturbances, the record pursues a remarkably constant course.

A couple wanting a child should have intercourse at the time the temperature falls, just before the rise that precedes ovulation. Intercouse should be continued daily during the rise of the temperature and when it has reached its peak after ovulation; however, too frequent intercourse causes a decrease in the number of sperm cells and lessens a man's fertility.

A carefully kept temperature record will also indicate the beginning of pregnancy. If the elevated temperature that develops after ovulation does not drop in its customary fashion, the woman is pregnant. Failure of the temperature to drop during the first week of the missed menstrual period is reliable evidence.

This natural method of child-planning is within the normal range of human functions, and it does not require procedures that might cause objections for religious or esthetic reasons.

A successful marriage depends on the presence of children. Methods for the prevention of conception should be used only when they are definitely indicated, and most marriages are far more likely to be permanent and happy if children come soon to complete the marriage bond.

WOOD ALCOHOL OR METHANOL POISONING

(See also *Poisoning*) Poisoning with this industrial solvent may lead to blindness and death. Since it has been used as an antifreeze many deaths of drunkards have resulted from drinking antifreeze solution. The symptoms of wood alcohol poisoning are like those of ordinary drunkenness except for the symptoms that include blurring of vision or blindness. In treating wood alcohol poisoning the stomach is washed out by having the person drink copious amounts of salt solution which is then vomited back. Afterward a saline cathartic is taken to wash out the bowel. Thiamin and nicotinamide and Vitamin K are given to protect the nervous system. The pain, restlessness, or delirium should have prompt medical attention. The doctor may provide oxygen for breathing and necessary stimulation.

WORMS

A recent survey showed in certain Southern areas that from 50 to 60 per cent of the children had intestinal worms at one time or another. A survey made of children in Washington, D.C., revealed pinworms in from 35 to 65 per cent in various groups of children.

Apparently the worms may often be present in the bowels without causing much in the way of serious symptoms. In other instances they produce all sorts of disturbances.

By far the most common and most widely distributed of all of the worms that live on man is the pinworm, which is also called the seat worm or the threadworm. This worm is exclusively a human parasite. It is a small white worm about ⅛ to ½ inch long. When the eggs are taken into the human body, they hatch in the small intestine, where the worms mature and mate. The males are then passed out of the body, while the females move on to the large bowel and develop the eggs. As the worms are passed out of the bowel, the eggs are discharged. The entire life cycle is a matter of about two months.

The eggs of the pinworm may lodge in the area around the opening of the bowel, may get onto the sleeping garments or bedclothes. By scratching they get under the fingernails of the infected child and again contaminate his food, so that reinfection and dissemination go on constantly.

The most disturbing symptom from pinworm infestation is the itching which is associated with the presence of the female worms and their eggs at the lower end of the bowel. Scratching sometimes leads to secondary infection. Occasionally in girls the worms migrate to the genital area. Occasionally the trouble with the worms may be sufficient to interfere with eating, so there is loss of weight and some anemia.

In the control of pinworms the utmost care is required in maintaining cleanliness of the parts affected. There must be daily bathing. All infected members of the family should be treated at the same time. The doctor can prescribe suitable antiseptic ointments for application to the area involved.

All of the drugs that are taken for the control of this infection are of such character that they should be used only when prescribed by the doctor and in the amounts prescribed in each case. The dosage necessary for a child is quite different from that for an adult. In the treatment of the condition enemas of suitable amounts of hexylresorcinol are used. Reports are also made of the use internally of a dye substance called gentian violet. Here again the exact amount and the manner in which the drug is to be taken must be left to the doctor.

ROUNDWORMS—The roundworm is known as the *Ascaris lumbricoides*. This is exceeded in its frequency of infection in the human being only by the pinworm. In the Appalachian Mountain area investigators found over 40 per cent of infection with the roundworm among preschool and early school age children in rural and mining camp districts. Similar rates have been reported from the Gulf and Atlantic coasts. Infestation with this type of worm is much less common in the Northern states; a small survey made near Detroit showed only 2 per cent of children infected.

The roundworm is a large white worm which lives normally in the small bowel of the human being. The female is 10 to 15 inches long and is about as thick as a lead pencil. The male is 6 to 8 inches long and is more slender. They hold themselves in the bowel by a sort of springlike pressure with the two ends of the worm held against the intestinal wall. Throughout life the female worm discharges about 200,000 eggs each day. These develop to an infective stage on the surface of the soil in from two weeks to a month. They may survive for many months in a moist, shaded soil.

Infection is acquired only when the eggs are taken into the body of the human being. They hatch in the small intestine. The larvae then penetrate the intestinal wall and are carried to the liver and from the liver to the lungs. In the lungs they are coughed up and swallowed again and then develop to maturity in the intestine. The development of this worm in the body of human beings requires a month to six weeks, and it may live for six months thereafter.

This worm does not cause much in the way of serious symptoms in the human being except that sensitivities have been noted which produce some of the symptoms of allergy. Under various conditions like fever or when people are being treated with drugs the worms may wander from where they are and have sometimes shown up in the nose and mouth or even in the tube that passes from behind the nose to the ears. When the worms wander into a tube like the one that carries the bile or into the appendix, they can obstruct the passage of fluid and do serious harm. Obviously, therefore, anybody who has these worms ought to get rid of them. Fortunately such drugs as hexylresorcinol have been found especially effective against this worm. It is given to a patient after a minimum of twelve hours' starvation. It should be taken only when prescribed by the doctor and in the manner which the doctor prescribes. After the drug has been given, the person must abstain completely from food of any kind for at least five hours. Less disturbance follows if semifluid foods only are taken for the next five hours. Twenty-four hours after the drug has been given, a saline cathartic is taken so as to wash all of the material out of the bowel. Usually one treatment with the drug, properly given, will rid the patient of worms.

HOOKWORMS—The parasite that causes hookworm disease in the United States is known as *Necator americanus*.

The story of the way in which the hookworm infects the human being is one of the fascinating stories in medicine. A female hookworm can lay from 6000 to 15,000 eggs a day. When the skin of man is exposed to infected soil in which the hookworm eggs have been deposited, the larva of the hookworm penetrates the skin, enters a blood vessel, and is carried to the lungs, where it breaks out into one of the open spaces in the lungs. The worm then makes its way up the bronchial tubes into the throat, where it is swallowed. Next it passes to the small intestines, where it develops into an adult worm. It takes about six weeks for this program from the time when the larva penetrates the skin until the eggs appear in the human excretions.

A human hookworm is something less

than ½ inch long, and the females are a little larger than the males. The worm has teeth by which it attaches itself to the wall of the bowels, and the worms secrete a toxic fluid which causes dilatation and rupture of the small blood vessels and prevents coagulation of the blood. The worms feed mainly on blood.

From this description of the hookworm it is easy to understand the harm it does. First, when it penetrates the skin, it produces conditions that are called "ground itch." Second, when it passes through the lungs, it may produce an inflammation. Third, when it gets into the intestines, it causes anemia through loss of blood, weakness of the muscles, and a distaste for work. As a result of the long-continued, mild anemia a person with hookworm disease has a face that is dull, hair that is dry and lusterless, and usually an inordinate appetite. If the condition is not corrected, the anemia may become so severe as to cause permanent invalidism or death.

A doctor can easily establish a diagnosis of hookworm by examining the material excreted from the bowel. The eggs of the worm will be found through such studies. Fortunately we know today many different ways to eliminate hookworms from the bowel, including a variety of remedies like hexylresorcinol, oil of chenopodium, and tetrachlorethylene. All these remedies are poisonous and should be given only by the doctor according to the prescribed method. There are, however, several things that the average person can do when he lives in an area where hookworm is prevalent. First, he should wear shoes and, second, he should provide for sanitary disposal of material excreted from the bowel. Since the larva of the hookworm cannot climb up a vertical surface to any height, the use of places of disposal that are sufficiently deep in the ground will control the dissemination of the hookworm from infected excretions.

Notwithstanding all that has been learned, hookworm is still an important public health problem in many parts of the world and in certain portions of the southern United States.

TAPEWORMS—Among the worms that live in the human intestine the tapeworms are among the most frequent and perhaps also among the most interesting. The quacks who used to go about in buggies carried with them huge glass jars displaying tapeworms and peddled their worm medicine on the basis that one look at the worm in the jar would bring the customers around.

Although there are thirty or forty different species of tapeworms that can get into the human intestine, six of them, known as the beef tapeworm, pork tapeworm, fish tapeworm, dwarf tapeworm, rat tapeworm, and dog tapeworm are the most common.

A complete beef tapeworm will measure 1 to 15 feet long and contain as many as 2000 parts. Cattle pick up the eggs when grazing on moist pasture land that has been contaminated with human sewage. The meat of the cattle is infected, and when man consumes this infected meat, inadequately cooked, he can acquire the infection. This is especially frequent when people eat raw beef.

The pork tapeworm seldom reaches 10 feet long and has about 1000 parts. Hogs that feed on human sewage become infected, and then human beings become infected from eating insufficiently cooked pork.

The fish tapeworm occurs wherever human excrement is discharged into bodies of fresh water. The swimming embryos are eaten by water fleas; the fresh-water fish eat the fleas; the human beings eat the infected raw fish. Occasionally the water fleas are eaten by little fish, which are eaten by bigger fish, which in turn are eaten by human beings. This condition was formerly frequent chiefly in Europe, but immigration from the Scandinavian areas and Poland has brought the infection to the United States.

The dwarf tapeworm is less than 1 inch long and is correspondingly small in its other dimensions. Infection with this worm is more frequent in children than in adults. Usually this infection is passed from one person to another through the eating of food contaminated by human excrement.

The rat and dog tapeworm are relatively uncommon in the human being, although cases are known.

The damage done by a tapeworm to a human being depends on the size of the worm, the kind of worm, and similar factors. Often the existence of the tapeworm is marked by toxic diarrhea and false hunger pains, frequently by the appearance of secondary anemia, loss of appetite, and loss of weight. The diagnosis is made certain by examining the excrement and finding the parts of the tapeworm or eggs in it.

Many different substances have been used to get rid of these worms. The doctor will starve the patient for a while and then give him a large dose of salts. The next day the patient takes medicine as prescribed by the doctor, and after waiting another day, during which the patient takes nothing but water, he gets another dose of salts. This succeeds in destroying the worms and getting them out of the body. Several different medicines are known which doctors can use and which are effective against the tapeworm.

Infection with pinworms is common in the United States. During a two-year period, 1,768 children with this condition were seen in one Buffalo hospital. Three groups of children, approximately 50 children to a group, were treated for pinworms; one group was treated with piperazine hexahydrate, the second group with Terramycin, the third group with dehydrated garlic powder. A syrup of piperazine hexahydrate cured 85 per cent of the cases in the first group. Only 38 per cent of the children treated with Terramycin were cured. Although 7 per cent of the children treated with garlic were cured, this may have resulted from a change in habits.

Worms—See article Digestion and Digestive Diseases.

Worms—nose: See Ear, article The Ear, Tongue, Nose, and Throat.

WORRY (See also, *Mental Depression, Mental Disease, Mental Hygiene*) Worry is a protracted or recurrent act of the mind, which always fails to result in a constructive solution of the question and usually ends in confusion, fatigue, and emotional instability. You can concern yourself about an important problem, if this means merely a careful consideration in an orderly manner leading eventually to an acceptable conclusion. Even when the conclusion happens to be contrary to your wishes, it may be accepted as a conclusion and thus worry can be avoided. Such an effort is constructive, whereas worry is always destructive.

The ordinary dictionaries describe worry as feeling or expressing a great deal of care and anxiety; manifesting unrest or pain; fretting, chafing, being anxious or fearful. Since all of these reactions are undesirable from the point of view of their effects on the body, worry is a most undesirable characteristic.

Many people insist that they never worry. These are the people who have learned to reason themselves out of anxiety over situations in which they find themselves. The process is known as rationalizing. Other people develop mental tranquility or peace of mind by accepting a belief which eliminates from consideration anything displeasing to them. Such a process is not rationalizing but may achieve the same effect, if the person can shut out completely any problem that disturbs him.

Most people find peace of mind necessary if they are to accomplish their responsibilities in the business world or in the home. If one does not have such peace of mind there is a constant feeling of insecurity, a constant fear of a threat to life itself or to the life situation of the person concerned. As a result energy is squandered and the reserve of the nervous system is exhausted, so that the person becomes tired, worn, distressed and may eventually have what is commonly called a nervous breakdown.

When worry appears to this extent the effects manifest themselves on different portions of the body. If the worry is related to the heart the person feels palpitations, extra and light beats of the heart, and similar manifestations; such a person may focus attention unduly on the pulse or the blood pressure or some other factor related to the circulation. If the nervous condition brings the focus of attention on the stomach and bowels there may be constipation, diarrhea, or other manifestations even more serious.

Many a person endeavors to escape from worry by fleeing into an addiction to drink, to drugs, to sedatives, to gambling, or to other practices that are known to be against the best interests of humanity. The escape is only temporary, and the trouble returns just as soon as the liquor or the drugs have worn off. There is no doubt that a restful night's sleep, a vacation, indulgence in outdoor sports, or even the theater or the movies may be utilized to better advantage as means of escape from the reality of worry.

WOUNDS A wound is any injury that breaks the skin or the underlying tissues. Wounds are classified according to the way in which they occur and according to the type of the wound. Wounds may be made by a razor blade, a knife, a bullet, a pin, or a burn. The wound may be clean-cut, lacerated, punctured, or due to a breaking force.

The chief danger arising from a wound is the danger of secondary infection. Hemorrhage or bleeding may be dangerous if large in amount or persistent. Hence the treatment given to wounds is designed first to control the bleeding; second to prevent infection. The control of bleeding is usually accomplished by putting a gauze compress over the wound. It should be made of sterile gauze. Under circumstances in which a first-aid pack is not available and bleeding is serious, a recently laundered handkerchief may be used. It is especially advisable, however, for people who are hunting, fishing, or touring in motorcars or in areas far removed from access to medical care to carry a first-aid cabinet with proper amounts of sterilized bandages.

The antiseptics commonly applied to wounds include iodine, boric acid, hydrogen peroxide, mercurochrome, tinctures of metaphen and merthiolate, and many others. Soap and water also act to destroy germs. Since many of the antiseptic substances are poisonous, it is a good rule never to put anything on or in a wound unless you have used it before and know exactly what you are doing. If you are not positive, it is much better to cover the wound with a clean dressing and wait for the doctor. In the case of a small wound, thorough washing with soap and boiled water is helpful.

Following any injury, the injured place may heal slowly or may become reddened, hot, and painful. Large red streaks may appear running up the arm or leg or away from the wound. There may be swelling, pain, chills, and fever. This means that infection has occurred and that a physician should be called immediately to take care of the condition; otherwise death may ensue.

Whenever a wound is seriously contaminated with clothing, soil, or similar materials, the doctor must also take into consideration the possibility of tetanus, or lockjaw, and advise the use of the anti-tetanus serum.

WOUNDS—cauterization: See article TRANSMISSIBLE DISEASES.

WOUNDS—defined: See article FIRST AID.

WOUNDS—first aid: See article FIRST AID.

WOUNDS—open, paths of germ invasion: See INFECTIOUS DISEASE, article THE PREVENTION AND TREATMENT OF INFECTIOUS DISEASE.

WOUNDS—tetanus: See article TRANSMISSIBLE DISEASES.

WRY NECK   See *Torticollis*.

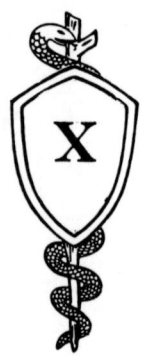

XANTHOMA Certain tumors develop a yellow color. The word "xanthoma" means yellow tumor. Quite often flat plaques of a yellow color appear on the skin due to deposit of fatty substances. These are called xanthomas. It is quite possible for these benign tumors to become mixed with malignant tumors, giving rise to such conditions as xanthosarcoma and xanthocarcinoma.

XANTHOMA—See SKIN, article THE SKIN.

XERODERMA This is a skin disease in which there is marked roughness or drying of the skin and in which there may be discoloration. The term merely means dry skin. The prefix "xero-" refers to dryness.

X RAY The discovery of the X ray was first announced in December 1895. Since that time the X ray has become one of the greatest aids of the medical profession.

One of the chief uses of the X ray continues to be for the diagnosis of broken bones. Nowadays pictures are made from different angles so that the exact relationship of the broken bones to the tissues may be determined.

An X ray of the skull shows the presence of disease of the bone, sometimes the presence of a tumor or changes in the blood vessels in the brain.

Once an X ray could be used only to show tissues like the bones. Nowadays, by the use of accessory materials, it is possible to visualize various organs and tissues. These materials include various dye substances which may be taken into the body and which localize in certain

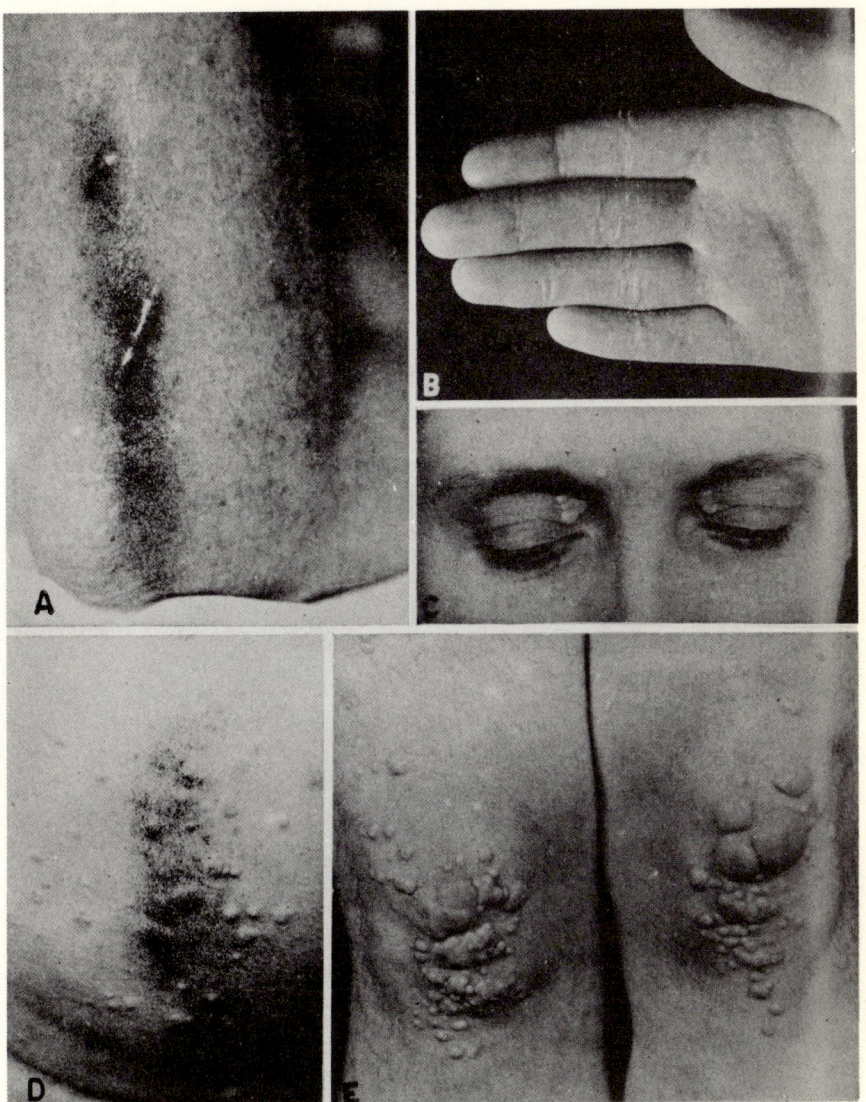

Five photographs showing different areas of the body where yellow patches or nodules of xanthoma may appear. The skin disease is found anywhere on the body's surface, but most often it occurs on the eyelids. Yellow, slightly raised plates in the skin form on the inner portion of the upper eyelid. Lesions on the hands develop in the creases of the palm.

Postgraduate Medicine

organs and tissues. Then by the use of the X ray these tissues and organs are made visible. One dye substance is used in taking X rays of the gall bladder; others are used for the kidney and the urinary bladder; still others for the female genital system or the spinal column. A substance called lipiodol may be injected into the lungs or sinuses and thus make them visible.

By the use of the X ray the exact size of the heart may be determined. The ability of the bowels to carry food forward may be studied and the outlines visualized.

The X ray is used also in the treatment of disease, particularly in the treatment of tumors, conditions affecting the skin, inflammations of various kinds such as bursitis, and, in fact, for a wide variety of purposes.

Since the X ray was described by Wilhelm Konrad von Roentgen, innumerable improvements have been made. Portable apparatus is now available that can be taken directly to the patient's bedside. In our armed forces there is portable X-ray equipment together with portable darkrooms for developing the plates, so that complete X-ray equip-

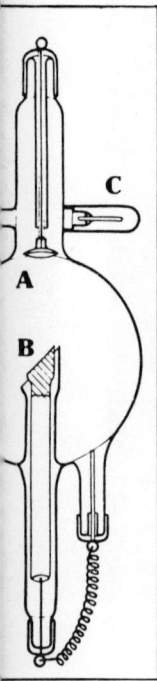
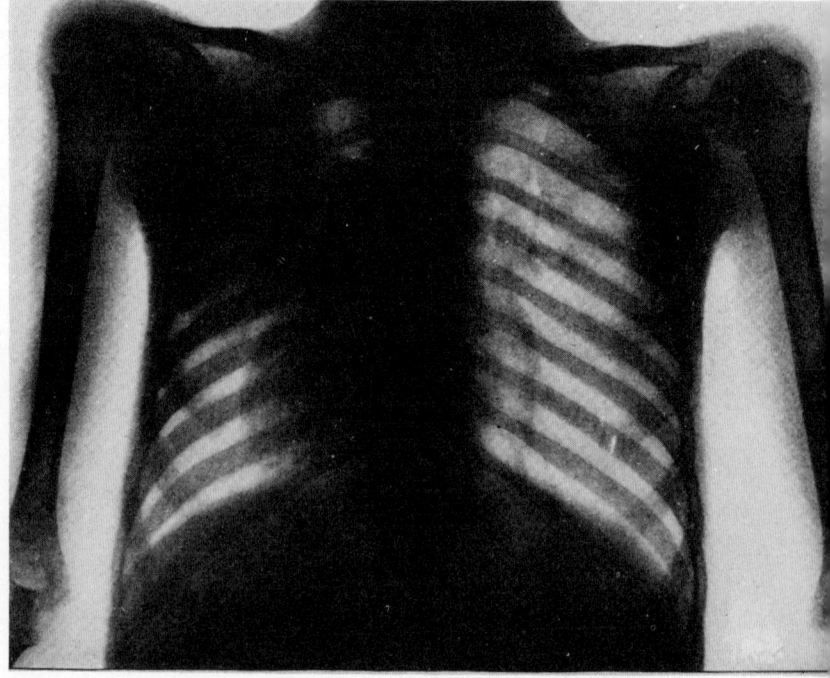

Diagram of an X-ray tube. A is the cathode; B, the anode; and C, the vacuum regulator.

Chest X-ray of a nine-year-old child, showing pathology in the left lung.

X RAY

ment is set up close to the front within twelve minutes after the arrival of the trucks that carry the boxes.

One of the most important developments in the use of the X ray has been the taking of a 4×5 chest film of every man in the armed forces as a means of ruling out the presence of tuberculosis.

X RAY OF HEART—Nowadays it is possible to get most accurate measurements of the size of the heart by the use of a seven foot film called a teleoroentgeno-

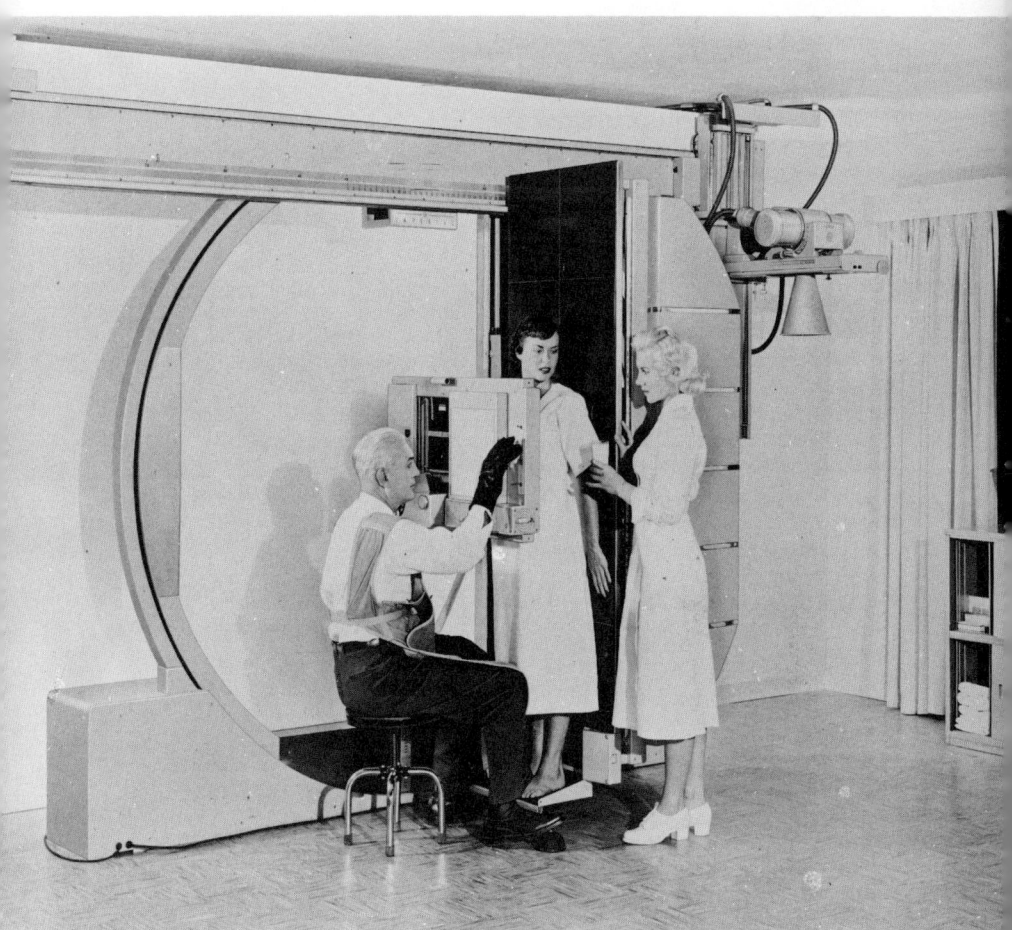

Modern X-ray apparatus has attained a high degree of technical perfection, as evidenced by this major X-ray unit. Here the patient is about to have her stomach examined. The physician, seated before the fluoroscopy screen, observes the action of her stomach as she drinks a special preparation.   General Electric gram or to have even a greater picture which is called an orthodiagram. For prolonged study of a patient with heart disease such X-ray pictures are made about once every year or two.

New methods have been developed during recent years for the use of the roentgen ray in studying the heart. These are extraordinary because of the accurate information that they convey regarding the functions of this vital organ.

Contrast fluids containing substances

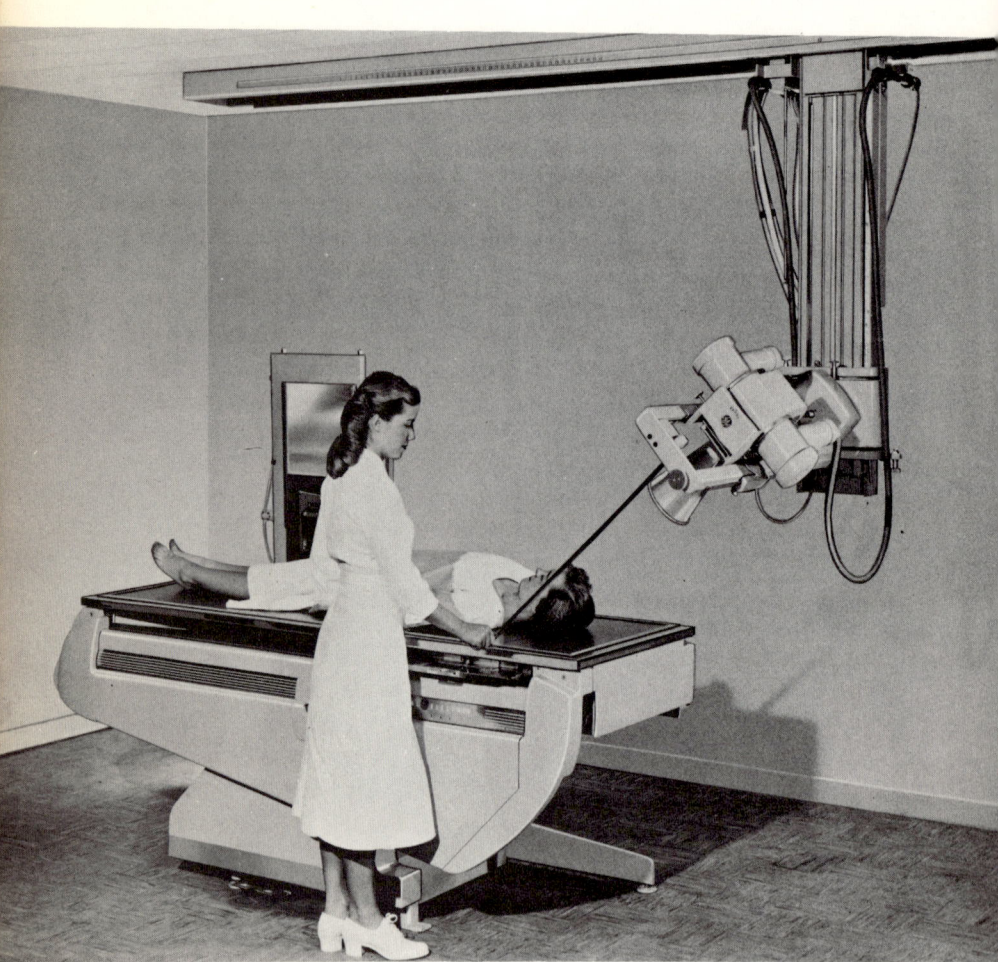

X-ray units serve your doctor by permitting observation of body functions in action (fluoroscopy), or taking X-ray pictures on film (radiography). In this view, the technician is aligning the patient, X-ray tube, and examination table prior to skull radiography.

General Electric

that are opaque to the X ray may be injected into the blood vessels or even into the heart itself. Then when an X ray picture is taken these structures are clearly outlined. The method is not a routine method but in difficult cases has been most helpful in making a diagnosis. The technique which is called angiocardiography has been found to be especially valuable in determining the nature of congenital abnormalities of the heart.

Another method called electrokymography translates the pulsation of the heart into graphic records through the use of a photoelectric cell which is placed over any desired portion of the heart or a border of a blood vessel and is then connected with a galvanometer. This method will show the presence of any portion of the heart wall which is not receiving blood supply from the coronary blood vessels and that remains inactive when the rest of the heart beats, or which will produce a change in the pulsation at the time when the heart contracts. The X ray film has been so greatly improved in its quality that it will now frequently show enlargement of the various chambers of the heart or calcification of the sacs surrounding the heart or of the valves or the healing of old areas which have formerly subjected to coronary thrombosis and this even without the injection of any contrast material.

Not long since scientists hailed the announcement that it had been possible to pass a small tube through a large blood vessel directly into the heart and thus to learn much more about its functions than could have been found out formerly. With the X ray the position of this rubber tube is easily observed. The method is especially valuable in permitting the withdrawal of blood from various portions of the blood vessel system or determination of the amount of oxygen that is being carried by the blood. The method serves also to show the changes in the blood pressure in various portions of the circulation.

X Ray—See Physician, article The Choice of a Physician; article Occupation and Health.

X Ray—acne: See Skin, article The Skin.

X Ray—after fall: See article First Aid.

X Ray—ankle, sprained: See Foot, article The Foot.

X Ray—aplastic anemia caused by: See Blood, article The Blood and Its Diseases.

X Ray—arterial calcification: See article Diabetes.

X Ray—birthmarks: See Skin, article The Skin.

X Ray—boils: See Skin, article The Skin.

X Ray—bowel cancer: See article Digestion and Digestive Diseases.

X Ray—brittle bones: See article Endocrinology.

X Ray—cancer caused by overexposure: See article Cancer.

X Ray—cancer diagnosis: See articles Digestion and Digestive Diseases; Cancer.

X Ray—cancer treatment: See article Cancer.

X Ray—difficulty in swallowing: See article Digestion and Digestive Diseases.

X Ray—discovery: See article Occupation and Health.

X Ray—eczema: See Skin, article The Skin.

X Ray—erysipelas: See article Transmissible Diseases.

X Ray—gastroptosis: See article Digestion and Digestive Diseases.

X Ray—herpes simplex: See Skin, article The Skin.

X Ray—horseshoe kidney recognized by: See Kidney, article The Kidney: Its Diseases and Disturbances.

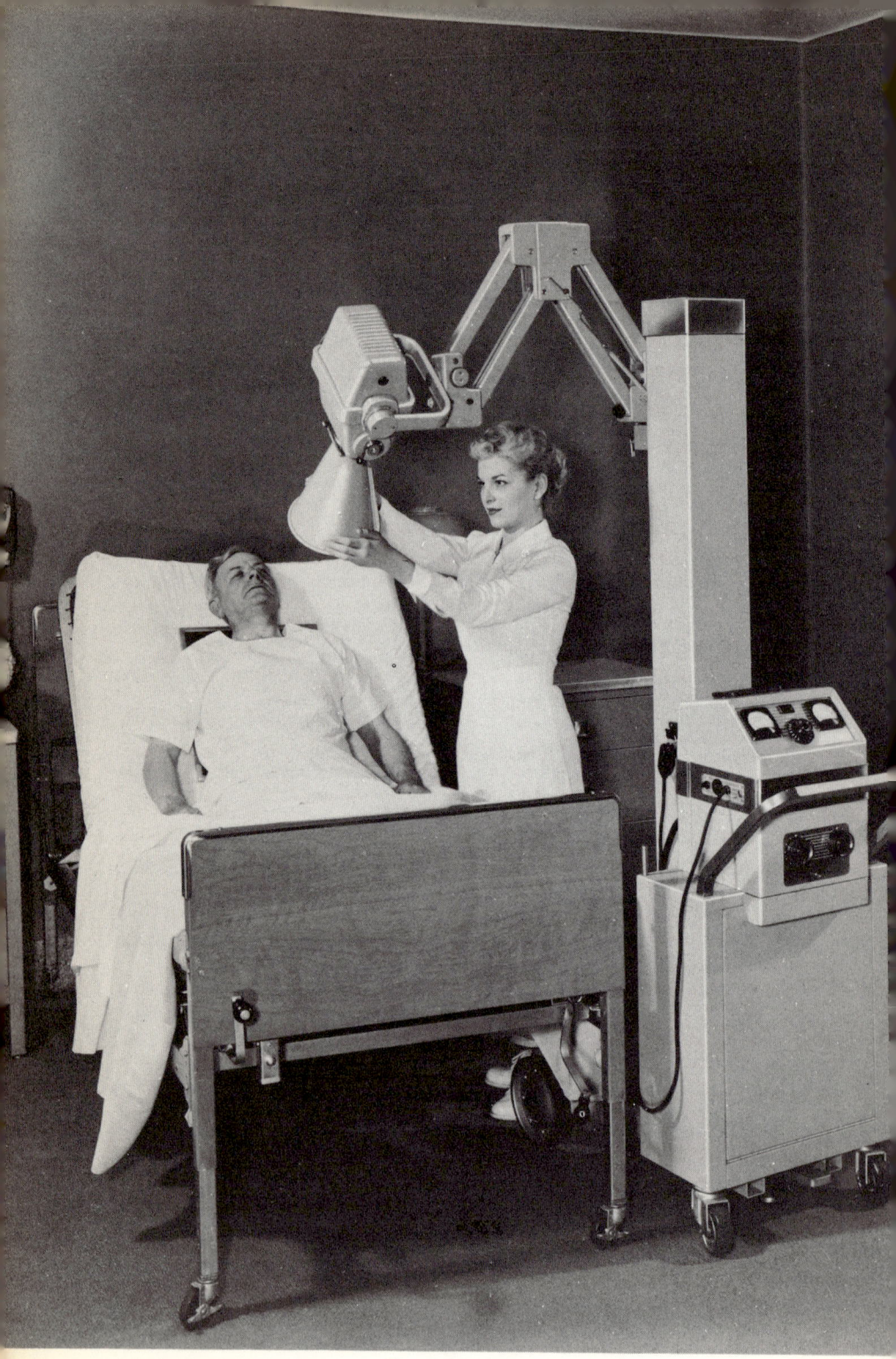

X Ray—keloids: See Skin, article The Skin.

X Ray—kidneys: See Kidney, article The Kidney: Its Diseases and Disturbances.

X Ray—kidney stones: See Kidney, article The Kidney: Its Diseases and Disturbances.

X Ray—leukemia: See Blood, article The Blood and Its Diseases; article Cancer.

X Ray—lung cancer: See article Cancer.

X Ray—lymphomas: See Blood, article The Blood and Its Diseases.

X Ray—occupational diseases: See article Occupation and Health.

X Ray—periodic examination for cancer: See article Cancer.

X Ray—pituitary tumors: See article Endocrinology.

X Ray—pneumonia: See Respiratory Diseases, article The Respiratory Diseases.

X Ray—polycythemia: See Blood, article The Blood and Its Diseases.

X Ray—rickets: See Infancy, article Care and Feeding of the Child; article Deficiency Diseases.

X Ray—ringworm of the scalp: See Hair, article The Hair.

X Ray—scurvy: See article Deficiency Diseases.

X Ray—sinuses: See article First Aid; Ear, article The Ear, Tongue, Nose, and Throat.

X Ray—skin unprotected from overexposure: See Skin, article The Skin.

X Ray—sprained ankle: See Foot, article The Foot.

X Ray—spurs: See Foot, article The Foot.

X Ray—stomach: See article Digestion and Digestive Diseases.

X Ray—stomach cancer: See article Digestion and Digestive Diseases.

X Ray—syphilis of the heart: See Heart, article Diseases of the Heart and Circulation.

X Ray—teeth: See Teeth, article The Care of the Teeth.

X Ray—treatment for certain types of rheumatism: See article Arthritis, Rheumatism, and Gout.

X Ray—tuberculosis: See Respiratory Diseases, article The Respiratory Diseases.

X Ray—ulcers: See article Digestion and Digestive Diseases.

X Ray—ureter: See Kidney, article The Kidney: Its Diseases and Disturbances.

X Ray—warts: See Skin, article The Skin; Foot, article The Foot.

In the daily routine of modern hospitals, it is often necessary to X-ray patients who cannot be moved from their beds. Mobile X-ray units such as this provide X-ray apparatus on wheels that can be moved right to the patient's bedside. The film is positioned behind the patient's chest and the technician is aligning the X-ray tube prior to making an exposure.

General Electric

YAWS Tropical disease which is contagious and in which there are raspberrylike growths on the face, the hands, the feet, and the genital organs is called yaws. It is also called frambesia. Occasionally it has been called leishmaniasis. While the condition is not seen frequently in the United States, it is likely to be seen more frequently when great numbers of soldiers have returned from tropical areas.

YELLOW FEVER In 1918 the eminent Japanese investigator Noguchi found what he believed to be the causative organism of yellow fever. The disease had previously been shown to be definitely related to a mosquito of a particular type. As a result of this investigation yellow fever has been eliminated from the United States; Havana, Rio de Janeiro, and Panama have been made safe places in which to live.

However, there seems to be plenty of evidence to show that yellow fever is capable of infecting the monkey, and that it can be found among monkeys in the jungles of South America. For that very reason cases occasionally break out in various parts of Brazil and even in Rio de Janeiro.

While studies were going on in Brazil, it was found that the organism discovered by Noguchi was not the organism of yellow fever, but rather the organism which causes infectious jaundice. Noguchi himself died of yellow fever in Africa, but even before his death he had become convinced that the cause of yellow fever was not the spirochete which he discovered but a virus—a toxic agent so small that it can pass through a clay filter.

In 1930 investigators at Harvard University developed a serum that would act against the yellow fever virus; still later, workers in the Rockefeller Foundation were able to prepare a vaccine against this condition. In the making of the vaccine against yellow fever they plant the virus on chicken embryos —the same type of procedure that is used for the making of vaccine against influenza. Today vaccination against yellow fever is a well-recognized public health measure. Almost 2,000,000 people have been vaccinated against this disease in Brazil.

It does not seem possible that the disease can be eradicated as long as there are jungles in which animals may be infected and in which mosquitoes may propagate, to infect human beings.

It takes six days for yellow fever to develop after a person is bitten by an infected mosquito. As part of the procedure which is used to keep yellow fever out of the United States airplanes are regularly inspected when they come from South America or other infected parts of the world. Fumigation is used to kill any mosquitoes that are present; passengers are examined and questioned as to whether or not they have been in contact with possible sources of yellow fever. The crews which fly the airplanes to South America and Africa have been vaccinated against yellow fever. With these precautions this menacing disease has been kept out of our own borders.

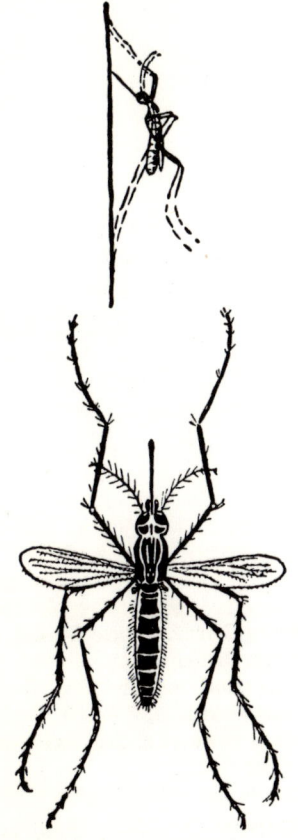

Female yellow fever mosquito (enlarged). These mosquitoes transmit the yellow fever virus from infected persons to uninfected persons. Vaccinations against yellow fever have helped to control the disease. Postgraduate Medicine

YELLOW FEVER—febrile nephroses may result: See KIDNEY, article THE KIDNEY: ITS DISEASES AND DISTURBANCES.

YELLOW FEVER—incidence: See INFECTIOUS DISEASE, article THE PREVENTION AND TREATMENT OF INFECTIOUS DISEASE.

YELLOW FEVER—mosquito: See INFECTIOUS DISEASE, article THE PREVENTION AND TREATMENT OF INFECTIOUS DISEASE.

YELLOW FEVER—mosquito (fig.): See article TRANSMISSIBLE DISEASES.

YELLOW FEVER—undulant fever less serious: See article TRANSMISSIBLE DISEASES.

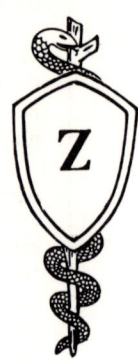

ZINC The uses of zinc in medicine are chiefly as a component of zinc chloride and zinc oxide and similar combinations used in the treatment of conditions affecting the skin. These drugs are combined with ointments and dusting powders.

Zinc—added to insulin: See article Diabetes.
Zinc—industrial poison: See article Occupation and Health.
Zinc—nephrosis: See Kidney, article The Kidney: Its Diseases and Disturbances.
Zinc Oxide—herpes simplex: See Skin, article The Skin.
Zinc Oxide—medicine chest: See Medicine Chest, article The Family Medicine Chest.
Zinc Oxide—rosacea: See Skin, article The Skin.
Zinc Stearate—See Skin, article The Skin.

ZYGOMA A portion of the temple bone in the head is called the zygoma. It is occasionally involved in fractures of the skull.

ZYME Zyme is a short word taken from the Greek which means ferment. Enzymes are ferments which develop inside the body. Many different forms of ferments are used in medicine.

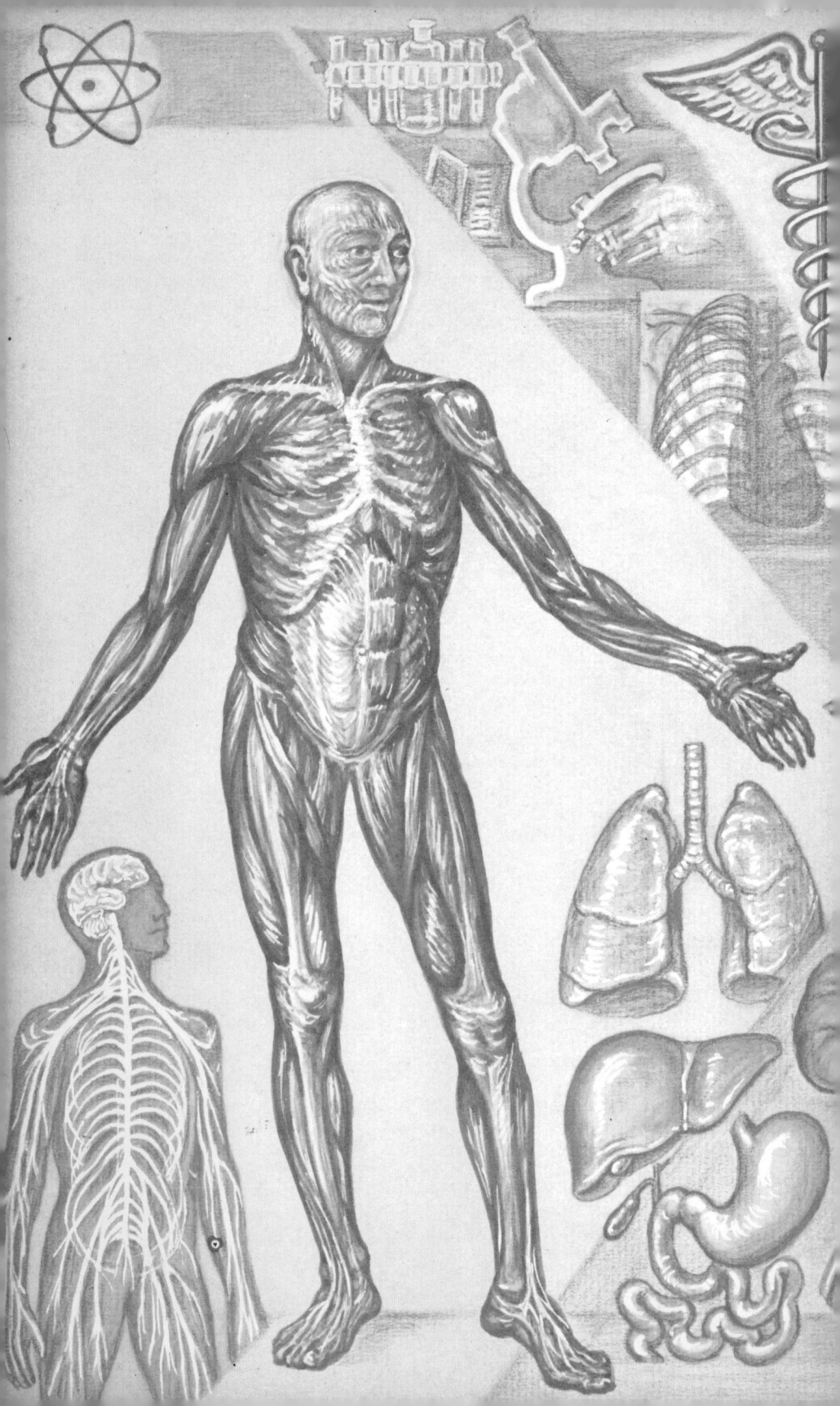